To Gilbert
with our best wishes
for a speedy recovery
Jan. 23d 1961

Hertha and Justin,

centaur

ESSAYS ON THE HISTORY OF MEDICAL IDEAS

centaur

ESSAYS ON THE HISTORY OF MEDICAL IDEAS

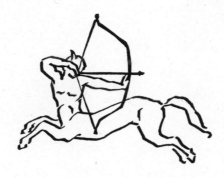

félix martí-ibáñez / m.d.

Professor and Director of the Department of the History of Medicine,
New York Medical College,
Flower and Fifth Avenue Hospitals, New York, N. Y.

Editor-in-Chief of MD Medical Newsmagazine

MD PUBLICATIONS / INC.

NEW YORK

First Printing, 1958

Second Printing, 1960

Grateful acknowledgment for permission to reprint is made to the following: Town & Country *for "The Lives of Leonardo";* Gentry *for "Psychiatry Looks at Modigliani";* Art & Architecture *for "The Strange Universe of Georges Braque";* Anatol Sivas, Inc., *for "On the Psychology of Symbolism in Oriental Rugs" and "Symbols and Life";* Journal of the History of Medicine and Allied Sciences *for "Sigerist and Spain."*

Library of Congress Catalog Card Number 58-59696

*This book is dedicated with
admiration and friendship
to my three dynamic colleagues,
Doctors Arthur, Mortimer, and Raymond Sackler,
who with their psychiatric research
have helped to write today
the psychiatric history of tomorrow.*

CONTENTS

Introduction: A Man and His Thoughts: A Confidence . .   xi

I. MEDICAL HUMANITIES

Books in the Physician's Life   3
Minerva and Aesculapius: The Physician as Writer . . .   29

II. THE TAPESTRY OF HISTORY

The Artist as Physician   59
The Physician as Alchemist   81
The Physician as Traveler   111
Padua and London: A Harveian Tale of Two Cities . . .   119
The Medico-pharmaceutical Arts of *La Celestina:* A Study of
   a Fifteenth Century Spanish Sorceress and "Dealer in Love"   149
Medicine in the Spain of Don Quixote   167
Fortunes of Cervantes and the Endeavor of Don Quixote . .   209
The History of Endocrinology as Seen Through the Evolution
   of Our Knowledge of the Adrenal Gland   213
The Mind and the World of Paul Ehrlich   257
As I Remember Him: Santiago Ramón y Cajal   271
Three Enigmas in the History of Curare Before Sir Walter
   Raleigh   277
Toward a History of Medical Thought   291
Sigerist and Spain   329
Medical Geography and History   335

The Spirit of American Medicine 349
On the History of Public Health 357
On the History of Neurology 361
On the History of Ophthalmology 367

III. THE PHILOSOPHY OF MEDICINE

The Biophilosophic Significance of Artificial Hibernation . . 373
Philosophic Perspectives of Motion Sickness 381
The Search for the Nature of Disease 389
A Footnote to Medical History 393
New Perspectives of Health and Travel 399

IV. ON MEDICAL COMMUNICATION

On a New Concept of Medical Journalism 405
Words and Research 409

V. THE MIRROR OF PSYCHIATRY

The Historical and Philosophic Background of Psychobiology 421
The Philosophy of Organicism in Psychiatry 433
The Great Physiodynamic Therapies in Psychiatry . . . 447
The Quest for Freud 455
The Challenge of Bio- and Chemotherapy in Psychiatry . . 467

VI. THROUGH THE PSYCHOLOGICAL GLASS

On Christmas and Neuroses 475
On the Psychology of Symbolism in Oriental Rugs 483
Symbols and Life 497
On the Psychology of Chess 501

VII. THE ARTIST'S WORLD

The Psychological Impact of Atomic Science on Modern Art . 511
The Lives of Leonardo (A Short Story) 541
Psychiatry Looks at Modigliani 555
The Strange Universe of Georges Braque 561
The Brush and the Bottle: Maurice Utrillo 573
The Theatre in Our Age of Anxiety 595

VIII. EDITORIAL MESSAGES

The Fabric of a Dream 611
The MD Concept 614

Children of Apollo 616
The Strings of the Lyre 618
Aesculapius in the Kitchen 620
To Walk and to See 624
The Endeavor of William Harvey 627
A Place in the Sun 630
The Angelic Conjunction 632
The Neuron Jungle 635
Per Ardua ad Astra 639
Half Woman and Half Dream 642
The Holiday and the Holy Day 645
The Physiology of an Endeavor 648
To Navigate—The Essential Thing 650
De L'Amour 652
The Sun Queen 654
Give Me of Your Dreams 657
The Joy of Leisure 660
Bright Twilight 662
Fashion as Dimension and Symptom 664
Disease as Biography 667
Lady with the Lamp 669
A Light in the Window 671

Bibliography 673
Subject Index 689
Name Index 705

A MAN AND HIS THOUGHTS: A CONFIDENCE

Every man in his progress through the years and distances leaves behind fragments of his thought, which are a mirror of his preoccupations, his longings, and his dreams. Sometimes such fragments crystalize into an artistic work or a scientific discovery, and sometimes they are translated into written words. Taken separately each of these fragments is like a piece of a jigsaw puzzle, revealing only a fraction of a man's spirit, but even combined they rarely ever fit together perfectly like the pieces of a puzzle. Instead, like a row of concave mirrors, they often reflect the same image but from different angles and even in different colors, thus reflecting the time and place, when and where, they were conceived. In any event, they do mirror the image, sometimes dull and blurred, sometimes bright and colorful, of what he thought, felt, and did regarding his dreams and his problems and those of his times.

In my life, literature, psychiatry, and medical history have been the burning lights that lured my roving spirit, which, born on the blue shores of the Mediterranean, has never since ceased to feel that same restlessness that launched Ulysses on his Mediterranean wanderings.

Fragments of my thoughts during a life that has participated in war and revolution and toiled in three continents, creating a new life on strange soil, are two novels, a number of short stories, about two thousand cultural and journalistic articles, more than a thousand lectures, several medical journals, and a handful of works in progress, including an historical novel about Vesalius. All this is no more than the modest result of the efforts of a man for whom, as for the ancient

Greek seafarers, "the essential thing is not to live; the essential thing is to navigate"—to navigate with pen and paper as oars and galley across the shoreless waters of thoughts and dreams.

From all this mass of words scattered through time and space in domestic and foreign magazines, I have selected for this volume a few of the articles that have appeared since 1950 in American medical journals, several others on art, and one short story with an historical interest, as well as one or two cultural lectures and some unpublished works. All these works have as a common denominator their historico-medical background and the fact that they were inspired by my love for, not just history, but *living* history, and by the desire to impress upon the physician that every one of his professional endeavors and thoughts is ineradicably clothed in the fabric of such history.

I have been moved to publish these essays in book form by the repeated requests of colleagues and friends. This volume is accompanied by *Men, Molds, and History,* and will be followed by three others: *An Outline of Medical History, The Fabric of Medicine,* and a semipopular book tentatively called *A Prelude to Medical History.* Then, freed from the burden of this task, I hope to set out on other literary paths, which I have had to bypass in order to devote myself to more pressing endeavors.

Reviewing the items contained here, reproduced exactly as they appeared originally, with all their imperfections, several questions come to my mind, which I willingly anticipate to simplify the reader's task.

First of all, these articles are only *essays,* a type of literature all but forgotten today but which in the past half century was a vital nourishment to all intellectuals. The essay, particularly on historical problems, never attempts to take the place of the scientific treatise. It is light, it is unfinished, a fragment of a sculpture, a stanza of a poem, a preliminary sketch of a picture, a bar from a symphony, an orator's gesture rounding out the phrase not completed by his lips, the silent farewell of a fluttering handkerchief that speaks louder than words. That is the misery of the essay.

But the essay also has its greatness. This lies, if we put our ear to its heart, in the vast swarm of suggestions throbbing within it, which scarcely stirred by the reader's hand darts out humming around his brow like a nectar-laden cloud of bees. For if the essay is like an unfinished sculpture, there is also inherent in it something of what occurs to a sculpture abandoned at the mercy of the elements on a beach. Over a period of years the angles and edges are smoothed down, leaving only a soft elusive form in which is imprisoned the very essence of the original sculpture. And so it happens with the essay: after repeated waves of meditation over the years by an author, a multi-edged geometry of ideas becomes an essay of elusive lines and soft profiles.

The value of an essay lies in the fact that instead of exhausting a theme, the essay simply draws the curtain on it and spotlights it. Like the magician who suddenly conjures a handful of sparkling coins and then quickly juggles them out of sight, leaving us filled with curiosity, the essay presents a theme in short vivid flashes that incite the desire to know more about it, to seek out more erudite treatises on the subject. The essay can be fascinating because it is alive and exciting, in contrast to the rigid crystallization of the exhaustive treatise.

The articles in this book are but leaves torn from the notebook of a restless man, who has moved through the world of the history of medicine in much the same way he moves through the world itself and through life: gazing with wonder-filled, loving eyes at men, facts, and things, jotting down his notes about them with more enthusiasm than meticulousness, leaving others more expert to complete the task.

There is also some repetition of ideas which I beg the reader to forgive. But is learning possible without repetition? Repetition is indispensable in education, and, whether authors admit it or not, every written work, however humble or commonplace, seeks in some degree to educate, though in the worst of cases it may find no other pupil than the author himself. For this reason, and also because each article was written as a unit and to mutilate them for the sake of avoiding editorial repetitions would only defeat their original purpose and might disappoint the reader who wishes to know them in their original form, I finally decided to overlook the repetition of concepts in some of the articles. Besides, like tunes in a music box, certain themes repeat themselves regularly in every writer's mind.

The third point in this self-criticism is that in several instances I have expressed personal opinions and conclusions not in accordance with those of much higher authorities than myself, thus giving rise to points that may be labeled, perhaps correctly, inaccurate. But, as Sigerist said in speaking of himself and of the history of medicine, "Like every artistic creation, a book of history has a strong personal note. It is *my* experience that I am passing on, *my* interpretation of history, what *I* as a result of my labors have come to consider the truth. This is why so much depends on the personality of the historian. The work of a historian of genius will have tremendous persuasive power, while the work of a mere craftsman will pass away without any repercussions."

Rereading these articles has also made me acutely aware of my immeasurable indebtedness to those philosophers and historians whose thoughts, and sometimes even their words, are faithfully reflected in many of the concepts expressed. It often occurs that an author buries his gratitude to other authors in the eight-point-type graveyard of a bibliography. But for me this would not even begin to clear the vast debt that I owe some of them. Hence, I wish to single them out here and express with warmth and emotion my ineradicable debt to them, second only to that which I owe my parents—my beloved father, the late Professor Félix Martí-Alpera, humanist, encyclopedist, and educator, and my brave and noble mother, Josefa Ibáñez de Martí-Alpera, still living in Spain—for the idealism and intellectual aspirations with which they nourished me.

First of all, José Ortega y Gasset, perhaps the most lucid and fertile philosophical brain of the twentieth century and the greatest Spanish stylist of our day, whose pupil I was and continue to be, and whose thinking and words taught me, as had been previously taught me by my own father, that one's duty in life is to think high, feel deeply, and speak plainly. I then wish to acknowledge the profound influence of another of my teachers, Dr. Gregorio Marañón, for though ideologically a gulf exists between us, I feel closely identified with him because of his devotion to medicine, to history, and to a noble prose, which in his case is also deep, fresh, and limpid like a Castilian mountain stream. And there is another Spaniard, the great historian and philosopher, Pedro Laín Entralgo, who, barring also the political distance between us, commands my greatest admiration for his unique learning, and whose philosophy and literature permeate many of the pages of this book.

Other than Spaniards, I wish to mention a great friend and admired medical historian, the dynamic Scotsman, Dr. Douglas Guthrie, whose work has been for me a source of inspiration. I specially wish to cite the beloved master, Henry Sigerist, who gave me so much through his friendship, his conversation, his writings, and, above all, his Quixotic ideals that carried him to voluntary isolation in Switzerland so that he might devote himself exclusively to the vast empire of culture and liberty to which he sacrificed everything else. Sigerist's writings, like those of Ortega, are reflected throughout this book, which, inspired by his concepts and quoting many of his words, is therefore a spiritual monument to his memory.

Ortega y Gasset said that true life is doing one's authentic work and not just anything. One must find one's authentic path in life and then follow it faithfully to the end. Only then do we really find ourselves, and life instead of nature becomes history. The following pages follow the path that I traced for myself many years ago as a student: to do everything possible to conciliate in my work art and medicine, humanism and technology, science and conscience, the physician's realistic view of the world with the poet's romantic view.

When the historic situation of my own life was destroyed by historical events in my native country, and I found myself in another land with my life thrust back into my hands, I realized that articles and lectures were not enough to evolve the message of universality that I had dreamt of as a student and that I started to develop during the heroic days of the Spanish Civil War. This message became crystallized, with the help of my American colleagues, in the pages of the medical newsmagazine *MD* and I hope in some of my writings.

As a student in my hometown on the shores of the Mediterranean, in the still hours of the siesta I enjoyed strolling on the beach and conjuring atop the aquamarine sparkle of the legendary waters the vine-wreathed hirsute head of Chiron, the divine Centaur of Greek mythology who taught Aesculapius art and medicine. This fantasy of an impressionable adolescent has crossed my memory in other lands, when in the evening the last gold of the sun or the silver of the moon sparkles the waters, recalling the noble head of the Centaur who knew all and taught all in the green woods of Attica. Alas, never in my life have I seen Chiron; but I have heard the rushing gallop of his cloven hooves upon the marble floors of universities and medical schools, in the long silent halls and pain-filled rooms of clinics and hospitals, in the still, white mystery of laboratories, on the solitary roads traveled by the country doctor, on the battlefield once the cannons have been silenced, and in the hushed peace of libraries where the gilded spines on ancient volumes embroider the walls with a tapestry of centuries and dreams. May these pages go forth across the golden fields of this hospitable land of hope, to which I owe so much, under the sign of the divine Centaur, who, besides medicine, taught Aesculapius the love of man for man.

Félix Martí-Ibáñez, M.D.

NEW YORK

xv

ACKNOWLEDGMENTS

I warmly express my everlasting gratitude to the persons without whose help this book would not have been possible:

To Josephine Martí Ibáñez for her devoted, tireless, and skillful editing of the articles in this book; Charles Stern and Martin Nozick for their excellent and accurate translations; Verna Sabelle for her talented editing and her dedicated work in organizing the articles in book form; Betty Hamilton, Elaine Grohman, and Glen Gould for their loyal and efficient editorial assistance and help in the research that went into some of the articles; Dr. Michael Fry for his expert editorial advice on some of these articles; Ted Bergman for his exquisite design of the book and the jacket. Through these persons I am also thanking others who helped in various capacities. I am especially indebted to Doctors Arthur, Marietta, Mortimer, and Raymond Sackler for their continued scientific encouragement in my historical endeavors and for their collaboration on some of the psychiatric articles included in this book.

centaur

ESSAYS ON THE HISTORY OF MEDICAL IDEAS

l. medical humanities

BOOKS IN THE PHYSICIAN'S LIFE

This essay is dedicated to W. Somerset Maugham, my admired friend, the greatest living example of the physician as homme de lettres.

Give me the power to speak beautiful words: keep the rest. Walt Whitman

BOOKS AND MEDICINE

Books and patients are the two poles of the axis about which revolves the professional life of a physician. Without patients, Medicine would not be an art; without books, it could not be a science. Medicine is based on experience, and the only way of recording and perpetuating that experience is the written word. "In the beginning was the Word," says the Gospel. Without words there would be no transmission of thought; without thought there would be no humanity, no science. All the professional experience of the best physicians in the world would mean little unless verified by what books say about those same clinical phenomena. The book is the silent record of medical thought, just as the patient is the living record of human pain.

As long as Medicine was only an *ars medendi,* the desire to cure the sick, it was transmitted orally from teacher to pupil. It was an art of the public square, the gymnasium, and the forum, passing from the pale dry lips of the master to the eager ears of the pupil. But as soon as Medicine had at its disposal a graphic record—Assyrian cuneiform tablets, Egyptian papyri, Aztec stones, or medieval parchments—the era of Medicine as Science began.

The book was to medical science what the spoken word was to the art of healing. Whereas the teacher of Medicine taught a group of contemporary students, the medical author, from Hippocrates

From *International Record of Medicine 168:650,* 1955.

on, taught posterity. Hippocrates himself needed no books because he was his own library; but when his *Corpus* was compiled, he bequeathed reading matter to countless generations of physicians.

Books have always been the best index of the cultural progress of the physician in history. The only book the primitive witch doctor had was the patient himself, but the physician's library has always been a window open to the lights and shadows of his intellect.

From Hippocrates' day on, the physician has accumulated in his library books dealing with Medicine, the humanities, and the fine arts. At first, those books were an integral part of the threads depicting the immense polychrome tapestry of human knowledge. But from the middle of the seventeenth century to the beginning of our own century, the physician was interested almost exclusively in medical books, and there was great need for the counsel of wise men—such as the Spanish physician-philosopher Letamendi who said that "the physician who knows only Medicine, does not know even Medicine" —to *ritornare al segno,* return to the concept that to know a little about medicine the physician must know a lot about other things.

There was a time—so remote that it seems mythological—when the physician could boast that he had read everything or almost everything of any importance written on Medicine. In Galen's time, medical literature had scarcely begun, and the Hippocratic *Corpus* was practically the only basis of scientific medical knowledge. By medieval times, however, the physician, who was often a monk, already had at his disposal a great number of medical manuscripts pouring in from Greece and Rome, which multiplied to a fantastic number during the Renaissance, when the famous schools of medical translators were established in cities like Toledo.

When the printing press was invented, facilitating the transmission of knowledge, it became difficult for the physician to assimilate everything printed concerning medicine. Yet the task of acquiring a medical culture was still comparatively simple, because for centuries medical knowledge tended to crystallize into heavy texts, unchallenged by the present-day avalanche of medical journals.

Only at the beginning of the nineteenth century, when the ocean of medical knowledge, already overflowing the dikes of cardboard and cloth built by book covers, fanned out into journals and other types of publications, did the professional life of the physician become truly difficult.

The idea then emerged, and still prevails, that medical books are the crystallization of classical knowledge only and therefore are condemned eventually to pass out of fashion, and that anything of value can only come out of medical journals. Thus the physician has become a galley slave in perpetual servitude to thousands of medical journals published today throughout the world, which relay anything old that medical writers can recollect or anything new they can think of.

Half a century ago the physician learned Medicine from textbooks. Today he learns Medicine from the medical journals and uses textbooks only as "reference works" whose formidable appearance and weight make them elephants to be put away and taken out for a slow tedious walk only once in a while. The general trend now is to run, even if it leaves one breathless, with the impatient noisy hounds of current medical journals.

There was a time when the physician enriched his knowledge by the simple expedient of observing his patients and occasionally heeding the advice of an old colleague or listening to a lecture by one of the wise old mentors of Medicine. He acquired medical wisdom through the windows of the senses. The ear was especially important, for it absorbed the words of the teacher, while the other senses served in the attainment of as perfect a knowledge as possible of the person of the patient.

The introduction of the medical textbook radically changed the teaching of medicine. From a discipline acquired by listening, it became a lesson to be read. Medical knowledge was no longer transmitted orally from master to pupil, usually at the patient's bedside; it became instead a rather lonely learning process, carried out sometimes at the patient's bedside, but more often in the office, library, or workroom alone, with a book containing the sediment of medical knowledge deposited by several generations.

Today Medicine is taught with emphasis on the visual elements through books, journals, and other forms of printed matter, supplemented by medical films and that other great vehicle which may hold the key to medical teaching in the future: television.

If we limit ourselves to printed matter, we may say that nowadays the physician learns Medicine from books (textbooks, medical books, monographs, or encyclopedias), medical journals, and, I would add, the copious flow of medical literature issued by pharmaceutical companies, which for the most part is today so accurately and tastefully done that it has bestowed a new dignity on that much discussed and often misunderstood and undervalued art, medical advertising.

Bombarded from all sides with popular and scientific medical literature, the physician cannot help being completely submerged in it. Medical literature is perhaps the most dynamic of all literatures, because it embraces both the science and the art of saving human lives. Medicine is action and, as Stendhal said, *"La joie de l'âme est dans l'action"* (The soul finds its delight in action).

What does, what should the physician read?

Let us remember that even more important than being a physician is being a man and that the physician's professional value is closely linked with his status as a human being. One cannot become a great physician without being, to a degree, "great" in one's personal daily life. Spiritual *savoir faire* and dignity in private life very often underlie competence and skill in the art of healing. A great physician also usually bears the mark of a great man.

Reading and studying act as catalytic agents on human greatness. One does not become a great man simply by reading great books, but such books may act as shafts of light to illuminate the treasures of greatness that lie dormant in the deep, dark mines of the human spirit. It is therefore even more important to the physician to determine what he *likes* to read as a man than what he *must* read as a physician; lastly, he should consider what he aspires to read as a member of society.

We are therefore confronted with three concentric circles of intellectual activity, each embracing its own horizon of reading: the physician as a man, the physician as a professional, the physician as a member of society and maker of history.

The first of these categories crystallizes the physician's most intimate desires and human needs; the second takes care of his need for information as a professional; the third satisfies his confessed or unconfessed social mission in space—in his country—and in time—in his own period and in history. Let us examine, then, what these three types of reading matter are and what they should be: recreational for the physician as a man; informative and educational for the physician as a professional; and progressive for the physician as a member of society and of a culture.

THE MAGIC DOOR

What is reading?

Quevedo (1580–1645), the Spanish poet and satirist, defined it in an immortal quatrain as "listening with the eyes to the dead":

> "Retirado en la paz de estos desiertos
> con pocos, pero doctos, libros juntos,
> vivo en conversación con los difuntos,
> y *escucho con los ojos a los muertos.*" [1]

> (Withdrawn into the peace of this desert
> With few but the wisest books,
> I live in converse with the dead
> And *with my eyes I listen to their speech.*)

For Descartes, reading was *"une conversation avec les plus honnêtes gens des siècles passés"* (a conversation with the wisest men of bygone days). And Arthur Conan Doyle defined reading as opening a "magic door" to the world of the great.*

We may then broadly classify the physician's reading as reading for *pleasure,* reading for *work,* and reading *out of duty.* With the first he learns to develop as a man and to fly on the wings of the spirit; with the second he learns to master his profession, navigating with the sails of his knowledge; and with the third he learns how to become worthy of his country and of his period, thus leaving behind him a cultural mark on the face of humanity.

RECREATIONAL READING

Reading for pleasure is not the same as reading for escape. Art is escape, flight from reality, for the artist; but the enjoyment of art— and art includes reading—should not become that *vice impuni* mentioned by Valéry Larbaud. The pleasure of those who read voraciously and indiscriminately, preferring a sloppy concoction of beans to a delicate dish of intellectual caviar, is nothing but an unpunished vice. So great is the pleasure of this type of reader that they read anything, anywhere, at any time, in a deliberate attempt to

---

* Arthur Conan Doyle, physician and writer, spoke thus of the "magic door" of his library: "I care not how humble your bookshelf may be, nor how lowly the room which it adorns. Close the door of that room behind you, shut off with it all the cares of the outer world, plunge back into the soothing company of the great dead, and then you are through the magic portal into that fair land whither worry and vexation can follow you no more. You have left all that is vulgar and all that is sordid behind you. There stand your noble, silent comrades, waiting in their ranks. Pass your eye down their files. Choose your man. And then you have but to hold up your hand to him and away you go together into dreamland. . . .

"No matter what mood a man may be in, when once he has passed through the magic door he can summon the world's greatest to sympathize with him in it. If he be thoughtful, here are the kings of thought. If he be dreamy, here are the masters of fancy. Or is it amusement that he lacks? He can signal to any one of the world's great story-tellers, and out comes the dead man and holds him enthralled by the hour. The dead are such good company that one may come to think too little of the living. . . . But best of all when the dead man's wisdom and the dead man's example give us guidance and strength in the living of our own strenuous days.

"Come through the magic door with me, and sit here on the green settee, where you can see the old oak case with its untidy lines of volumes. Smoking is not forbidden. Would you care to hear me talk of them? Well, I ask nothing better, for there is no volume there which is not a dear, personal friend, and what can a man talk of more pleasantly than that? The other books are over yonder, but these are my own favourites—the ones I care to re-read and to have near my elbow. There is not a tattered cover which does not bring its mellow memories to me." 2

escape from a world of reality into a world of fantasy. Such reading is an opiate, or a refuge that masks the reader's world and hides from him his own soul.

True recreational reading satisfies the spiritual needs of the physician as a man.

What is the main value of such reading? I would say it is the same as it was at the beginning of history: entertainment. Early man loved to sit around the fire, under the blinking stars, and listen to tales of adventure and mystery. When those stories were perpetuated in written form, man continued listening to them with the inner ear of the intellect.

Today, man is more than ever interested in tales that divert him for a while from his pressing daily tasks and bear him over land and sea on the Pegasus of his mind to remote places where adventure fills the air. He still loves to listen, ". . . in the eerie hour between dog and wolf . . . when the last day departed and we settled ourselves in the smoking room for a sleepy evening of talk and tobacco," [3] to stories of bold men who, like John Buchan's heroes, dared to seek out "unpathed waters, undreamed shores."

The physician does not exist who, after a few hours of such diverting reading, does not return to his task with a spirit lightened by the conflicts of the heroes he has just met, by their fate-tossed lives, for, as the *Aeneid* says, *Quisque suos patimur manes,* each one must suffer his own destiny.

The physician should enjoy even more than others this type of purely recreational reading, whether it be detective novels, books of travel and adventure, or, more recently, scientific fantasies, for it pours a balsam on his soul battered by the constant spectacle of human suffering. By means of the spiritual ennoblement of reading, the physician may escape becoming an automaton incapable of displaying emotion or a cynic wearing the mask of professional skepticism.

Why should the physician read literary works? Primarily, as we said before, for entertainment, since this is, after all, the greatest mission of literature. "Literature," said G. K. Chesterton, "is a luxury; fiction is a necessity. The simple need for some kind of ideal world in which fictitious persons play an unhampered part is infinitely deeper and older than the rules of good art, and much more important."

After an hour or two of recreational reading, the physician may return to his daily task—that exacting, often harrowing, emotion-laden task—refreshed in spirit by the vision of horsemen galloping at breakneck speed over frost-covered highways under a faint silvery moon; of mysterious travelers in dusty capes rapping their whips on the closed shutters of a deserted inn; of snowy paths in a silent forest, crimson under the setting sun; of taverns with frozen black windows framing an interior of candlelit tables, jugs of wine, and men embarked on a night of drinking, gambling, and singing by a blazing fire.

The love of story and fable belongs to all times and all places. Physicians once gathered around storytellers in ancient Mesopotamia; today they go to their St. James Street or Fifth Avenue clubs to read stories. The mission of recreational literature is not to educate but to entertain. In quest of such diversion, the physician has recourse to reading during those hours that the Romans called *otium,* the hours of rest from the pressures of life, in contrast with *nec-otium,* the negation of rest and leisure which is business or duty.*

There are physicians who entertain a sense of guilt over their fondness for recreational reading and try to justify it by calling it a pastime or a *hobby,* a somewhat derogatory word often used by people who do not understand that a pastime frequently represents the truest, most authentic aspect of living, especially when that pastime is reading instead of bridge or television.

This matter is especially important because nothing reveals the true silhouette of a person's soul better than his favorite pastime. The active repertory of any given person is amazing in its limitations and boring in its uniformity. We may be physicians or carpenters, painters or farmers, clerks or cab drivers, lawyers or dancers, yet our daily tasks are extraordinarily alike, as alike as eating, loving, sleeping, and dreaming. What distinguishes one person from another is not his occupation but the activities he chooses in his leisure time. From that angle, there are no two people alike. There are no two physicians who spend their free time in exactly the same way, even though we may all have the common denominator of our love for reading.

Sometimes recreational reading may be valuable in supplementing

---

* Robert Louis Stevenson pointed out most eloquently the importance of the novel: "The most influential books, and the truest in their influence, are works of fiction. They do not pin the reader to a dogma, which he must afterwards discover to be inexact; they do not teach him a lesson, which he must afterwards unlearn. They repeat, they rearrange, they clarify the lessons of life; they disengage us from ourselves, they constrain us to the acquaintance of others; and they show us the web of experience, not as we can see it for ourselves, but with a singular change—that monstrous, consuming *ego* of our being, for the nonce, struck out. To be so, they must be reasonably true to the human comedy; and any work that is so serves the turn of instruction. But the course of our education is answered best by those poems and romances where we breathe a magnanimous atmosphere of thought and meet generous and pious characters." [4]

our professional education. Let us recall Thomas Sydenham's immortal answer when the physician and poet Blackmore asked him what he should read to learn Medicine.[5] "Read *Don Quixote;* it is a very instructive work." Although that puzzling remark has been interpreted as expressing Sydenham's contempt for the "official" medical textbooks of his time, the fact remains that when we read *Don Quixote*[6] we learn about the Medicine, not only of Philip III's time but of all time. That book teaches us an impressive lesson in traumatology—comparable only to that of the *Iliad*—another in physiognomy, and several lessons in Galenic pharmacy, besides providing us with a wonderful psychiatric and endocrinologic typology. Above all, we learn about the human being, in sickness and in health, from a psychologic viewpoint that is universal because it is so human.

Many literary works could teach the physician to recognize the medical processes affecting their characters, for instance, Don Quixote's madness, Camille's tuberculosis, the epilepsy of Smerdyakov in *The Brothers Karamazov,* the endocrine obesity of the fat boy in *The Pickwick Papers,* and he could then apply his knowledge to real life. They can also teach us to describe disease with that literary flair —so lacking today—that can change a cold, dry clinical history or scientific paper into a beautiful warm piece of writing.

History, like science, is continually created by scholars and artists, as Sigerist has so brilliantly demonstrated.[7, 8] Disease is a supreme aesthetic experience, and the artist, the most sensitive of men, cannot help being affected by it. The literary works of a given age afford us a much more vivid medical picture of the times than any technical work. Casanova's *Memoirs,*[9] besides being a monument of artistic story-telling, depict a dazzling panorama of Medicine—sometimes as vertiginous as a saraband, sometimes as graceful as a ballet, but always as merry as a tarantella—involving quacks, doctors, and patients in the Venice and Europe of the 1700's, as well as in the Russia of Catherine the Great.

Literature has indeed made a generous contribution to Medicine— in Erasmus' *Praise of Folly,* in James Joyce's *Ulysses,* in Thomas Mann's *Magic Mountain,* in the novels of Stendhal and Dostoevski.

Writers have always enjoyed creating literary figures inspired by living physicians.[10] In his *Symposium,* Plato gives us Eryximachus, the physician who advised Aristophanes to sneeze in order to cure his hiccoughs. In the *Canterbury Tales,* Chaucer describes the medieval physician who claimed to have cured his patient through "natural magic" and was modeled after John of Gaddesden, the author of the *Rosa Anglica.* Rabelais, a physician of Lyons and a graduate of Montpellier, generously sprinkled his immortal works with physicians. Shakespeare, with his knowledge of Medicine and with characters like Dr. Caius in *The Merry Wives of Windsor,* modeled after the great John Caius,[11] illuminated for us that sterile period in medical history stretching from Vesalius' death to Harvey's discovery of the circulation of the blood. Browning glorified Thomas Linacre, one of the greatest humanist-physicians in history, in his *A Grammarian's Funeral.* And in his *Anatomy of Melancholy,* a consecration of the melancholy that was the author's constant companion, Robert Burton parades before our eyes an impressive cavalcade of physicians and their patients.*

In Louis XIV's time, Molière satirized physicians in his *Le Malade Imaginaire,* and Le Sage, in his *Gil Blas de Santillana,* created in the figure of Dr. Sangrado a frightening example of the blood-letter of the "vampire age" in Medicine, a man as drunk on vein openings as Guy Patin, who bled his family, his friends, and himself into anemia.

In the eighteenth century, Daniel Defoe wrote his *Journal of the Plague Year,* a fictional but faithful account of the same events witnessed and related by Samuel Pepys. Sterne created the querulous Dr. Slop in his *Tristram Shandy,* and Tobias Smollett satirized Dr. Mark Akenside in *The Adventures of Peregrine Pickle.* Jenner penned a tribute to the birds he adored in his *Address to a Robin,* and Keats, physician and poet, dreamed during his anatomy classes of those diamantine phrases that later made him the greatest jeweler in words of the English language. In his vast work, Charles Dickens satirized fifteen doctors and seven surgeons, some of whom, like Dr. Bob Sawyer of the incomparable carousals, are unforgettable. Thackeray and Trollope followed in Dickens' footsteps. Robert Louis Stevenson created, among other physicians, the schizophrenic Dr. Jekyll and in *Treasure Island* the brave surgeon, Dr. Livesey.

THE PHYSICIAN AS MAN OF LETTERS

The medical profession has produced more writers than any other, more than law, engineering, and the other liberal professions. The only exception is the clergy, which, because of perennial meditations on man and God, has in the past produced as many great writers as Medicine.

Since we cannot mention the entire roster, we shall limit ourselves to pointing out that in England the literary tradition of Keats, Thomas Dover (who in real life discovered Alexander Selkirk, the original model for Robinson Crusoe, on the island of Juan Fernández), Oliver

---

* "Browsing in the *Anatomy of Melancholy,*" H. S. Carter said, "is like spending a sunlit afternoon in a dusty old library, for Burton's book is a bookman's book, an endless mosaic of many-colored patches." [12]

Goldsmith, Tobias Smollett, and others who were not physicians but nevertheless wrote medical books (like Robert Burton, a contemporary of Rembrandt, Velázquez, and Shakespeare, who wrote "the greatest medical treatise ever written by a layman") has been continued by physicians like Arthur Conan Doyle, Ronald Ross, A. J. Cronin, and, above all, the prince of contemporary English novelists, my admired friend, W. Somerset Maugham.

With his habitual elegance, Maugham has explained why a physician may very well become a great writer: "I do not know a better training for a writer than to spend some years in the medical profession. I suppose that you can learn a good deal about human nature in a solicitor's office; but there on the whole you have to deal with men in full control of themselves. They lie perhaps as much as they lie to the doctor, but they lie more consistently, and it may be that for the solicitor it is not so necessary to know the truth. The interests he deals with, besides, are usually material. He sees human nature from a specialized standpoint. But the doctor, especially the hospital doctor, sees it bare. Reticences can generally be undermined; very often there are none. Fear for the most part will shatter every defense; even vanity is unnerved by it. Most people have a furious itch to talk about themselves and are restrained only by the disinclination of others to listen. Reserve is an artificial quality that is developed in most of us but as the result of innumerable rebuffs. The doctor is discreet. It is his business to listen and no details are too intimate for his ears." [13]

The best contemporary Spanish novelist is a physician, Pío Baroja, and years ago Spanish writers like Pedro Mata, Vital Aza, and Armando Palacio Valdés were also physicians.[14] In France the tradition of physician-novelist started by Rabelais has been continued by Georges Duhamel. In Germany and in Switzerland the glory of Schiller, surgeon and playwright, was reborn in contemporary medical figures such as Albert Schweitzer. In Austria we can point to the novelist and poet Arthur Schnitzler. In Russia, alongside Dostoevski, a physician's son brought up in the medical tradition, we have Anton Chekhov, physician, storyteller and playwright. In the United States, there are S. Weir Mitchell [15] and Oliver Wendell Holmes, William Carlos Williams, and Frank Slaughter.[16] From Sweden came one of the greatest physician-writers of our age, Axel Munthe, whose immortal book, *The Story of San Michele*,[17] has drawn pilgrims from the world over to his villa in Capri, there to lean —as I have done—on the stone balustrade, guarded by pink marble sphinxes, that overhangs his beloved *mare nostrum* of Homeric legends, and gaze out over the scintillating silver-blue waters.

There is no pleasure so rewarding as having for lifelong friends a few selected writers, whose inspired ideas, crystal-like prose, idealism, and lyrical essence enliven with enchanting colors the gray monotony of our daily lives.* As Hazlitt said: "There are only three pleasures in life pure and lasting, and all derived from inanimate things—books, pictures, and the face of nature."

In literature, the physician looks for a screen on which to project the images of his own fancy. For, as Sir Thomas Browne said in his *Religio Medici*, "We carry within us all the wonders we seek without us. There is all Africa and her prodigies in us." [18]

PROFESSIONAL AND SCIENTIFIC READING

It is the physician's duty to read and study textbooks and reference works, medical journals, and other publications that will refresh his basic knowledge and keep him abreast of the latest happenings in Medicine. Ever since man developed the written word, medical information has been transmitted down the generations in incalculable amounts; certainly no one would even dream of reading all this exhaustive material.

We shall mention only a few of the most famous medical books—the list compiled by Ralph Major[19] plus a few more—and even this short list will resound like clarions, like a roll call of warships ready to enter an epoch-making battle in history.

The Egyptian *Ebers Papyrus* (c. 1500 B.C.), which described contraceptives and conditions like angina pectoris; the *Corpus Hipocraticum* (460–375 B.C.), basis of modern naturalist medicine; the works of Galen (138–201), landmark of experimental medicine; The *Canon* of Avicenna (c. 1028), the Bible of Medicine for more than a thousand years; *De Humani Corporis Fabrica* of Vesalius (1543), prelude to modern science; *De Motu Cordis* (1628) by William Harvey, herald of modern physiology; *De Sedibus* by Morgagni (1761), basic pillar of pathological anatomy; *An Inquiry into the Causes and Effects of the Variolae Vaccinae* (1798) by Edward

---

* I myself have four constant companions among British authors alone: Stevenson, Chesterton, A. Conan Doyle, and John Buchan. I do not refer, of course, to the Stevenson of *Treasure Island,* but to the Stevenson of *The Master of Ballantrae, The Weir of Hermiston* and other less known masterpieces; nor do I mean the Chesterton of the Father Brown series, for I prefer his poems, biographies, and literary criticisms; I do not admire the A. Conan Doyle of Sherlock Holmes as much as I do the author of the historical novels *Micah Clarke* and *The Refugee;* and I love the John Buchan of *The Man from the Norlands* and *The Moor Endureth* more than I do the author of *The 39 Steps.*

Jenner, foundation of immunology; *De l'Auscultation Médiate* by Laënnec (1819), which introduced one of the most valuable diagnostic methods in clinical practice; *Die Cellularpathologie* by Virchow (1858), which revolutionized pathology; just as the *Principles and Practice of Medicine* of William Osler (1892) revolutionized the teaching of Medicine, and Cajal's *Histología* the teaching of modern histology.

These are but a few of the immortal medical books which, like the runners of the classical marathon, have passed the blazing torch of medical science from hand to hand through the generations.

IN PRAISE OF BASIC TEXTBOOKS

Of course, the physician needs to read and study basic texts of Medicine, the so-called *reference books,* which furnish essential information on any specific medical question.

What qualities should we look for in the books we consult?

First of all, *accuracy.* A reference book should include no opinions of the author except those that help clarify or define the subject under study. Anything hypothetical or experimental should first be published in the form of articles in some journal and in a textbook only when research or clinical application and confirmation by other scientists have proved it to be valid.

Clarity of exposition generally goes hand in hand with beauty. I have never believed that a book must be obscure in order to be scientific. The best teachers of Medicine all over the world were good writers in the sense that they were clear. Frequently, they were also given to beauty of literary style, but even then the art of writing well was simply the crystallization of clear thinking. The works of Oliver Wendell Holmes, Osler, Cajal, Claude Bernard, Harvey, Cushing, and Sherrington are as limpid as they are beautiful. Their concepts stand out on every page like polished pebbles in the crystal-clear waters of their prose. The "light" that Goethe frantically begged for on his deathbed has always been the guide of good medical writers.

Many of the obstacles that stand in the way of the progress of modern psychiatry derive from its grotesque terminology, a vast multiform jargon unnecessarily confusing, and from the compulsion felt by many psychiatrists to express themselves technically so that, since only a few will understand them, they will be subject to a minimum amount of criticism. "Not only don't I understand the mysterious dialect of psychiatrists," said Marañón, "but when I hear them speak, I comprehend but half of what they say." This is the more deplorable since the "verbal" style of Freud himself—and before him Charcot's dialectic and Kraepelin's didactic styles—set one of the finest examples of clarity and harmony. Their prose was beautiful because of its pellucid *simplicity*.

Accuracy, clarity, simplicity—these should be the attributes of a good medical reference book if it is to become a constant and pleasant source of information for the physician.

The reference library of a practicing physician should contain, above all, the basic texts he used in his student days,*† for their contents form a part of his professional subconscious. These should be supplemented by other more recent basic works in those disciplines in which the greatest progress has been made. A modern anatomy textbook differs little from the Testut's anatomy from which we studied, and the basic chapters of a histology like Cajal's or a physiology like Gley's or Sherrington's have changed little except for sections such as endocrinology, which in Falta's day had an anatomic, morphologic, and constitutional range, and today is a laboratory science. From the study of glands, endocrinology evolved into the study of hormones and then into the study of the latter's biochemical principles.

Pharmacology has changed only in the sense that new substances

---

* "When a young physician asks me what books he should read," Marañón has said, "I always tell him the same thing: For the present, I say, read again the little abstract from which you studied for your examinations; keep it at your bedside and every night, before you fall asleep, go over a few pages. Later on, choose any modern book, but study it thoroughly; and use whatever time you have left over from such work to read the journals, only *try to get those journals that carry a selection of abstracts, and which, fortunately, are so much in fashion. One of these abstract journals is as valuable as ten other journals read at first-hand.* Only when you wish to do research into a given area of Medicine is it logical and necessary for you to go conscientiously through those piles of journals which some people think are indispensable to fulfill the mad ambition of 'keeping up to date.' " [20]

† "Present-day science suffers from an excess of 'scientism,' from an immoderate avidity for everything that springs up under the name of science but which is really detrimental to true science. For true science is signalized by submission to the strict quarantine of the present. 'Scientism' can be recognized in the fetish-worship of the latest information. Strict science, however, demands that last-minute discoveries have time to settle before they acquire definite status. True science always takes such precautions, and is, by definition, built from material acquired the day before yesterday.

"True science therefore does not take the form of the book right off the press, but of the treatise, the well-thought-out manual, and, even more important, the epitome, that small volume the student carries around in his pocket and leaves at his bedside at night. And not only the student, for the epitome should also be the inseparable friend of the teacher. There is nothing more valid than the advice that everyone should go back to his school-books every thirty years. Despite the disconcerting torrential progress of learning today, there are certain invariable starting-points without which all the latest erudition is a flower that lasts but a day." [21]

have been added to the pharmaceutic arsenal, often with unnecessary haste, as happened with some antimalarials and chemotherapeutics, which, because of their toxicity, turned out to be as ephemeral as the smoke from a straw fire. But the basic pharmacology of the main drugs has changed little.

Bacteriology has enriched its panoply with so many new microbes that it requires new supplementary works.

Some disciplines, like psychiatry, which twenty years ago were eminently philosophic, have become biochemical and physiodynamic and have extended their influence to disciplines formerly far removed from them, such as dermatology, physiology, and gynecology.

The basic texts from which we studied pointed out the broad paths along which medical thought in the different specialties runs, and we should not replace them by other texts until these have definitely proved their value by the influence they exercise on contemporary medical thought.

But the medical book, the forgotten and even despised medical book, has (with the exception of disciplines such as anatomy, physiology, and pharmacology, which still defend themselves behind the solid walls of huge thick volumes) fought and lost a battle against that elegant and nervous aerodynamic publishing expression of our day—the medical monograph. The monograph is not a book but the x-ray of a book; it is not a matron but a girl; not a symphony but its constituent chords condensed into an intellectual shorthand to satisfy the haste of an impatient generation.

Just the same, the medical book is still, as it was in Vesalius' time, the cornerstone of the monumental fortress of medical knowledge in our atomic age. Medicine is a science whose progress is announced in medical journals but is consolidated only in books. For the young physician the medical book is a guarantee of the classic solidity of his know-how, just as for the aging practitioner it is a companion whose wisdom has grown alongside his own through the years.

Faced with the frightening number of medical books incessantly published all over the world, the physician must learn to discriminate in his reading. He must *select*. Life is short and complex and no man can visit *all* countries, as Marco Polo did, nor can he work in *all* professions, as Leonardo da Vinci did; he cannot love *all* women as could Casanova, nor read *all* the books as did Thomas Linacre. There was a writer, Thomas Wolfe, whose zest for life "and more life" made him want to do all things himself. The result was confusion—bewitching perhaps in literature but pathetic in life—in all his works and even in his life, as evidenced by his leaning on the age-old stone embankments of the romantic Seine only to dream of the dank smells at the Brooklyn Bridge.

The physician's library can be selective and still range from the austere simplicity of Thomas Sydenham and John Radcliffe* to the splendid humanism of Guy Patin and William Osler.

MEDICAL JOURNALS AND THEIR MISSION

Medical journals constitute the principal source of medical information today. Every year about three thousand medical books are published, nine hundred of them in the United States, and from four thousand to five thousand medical journals, nearly fifteen hundred of these in the United States. These journals are classified into three groups: monthly (thirty-three per cent), bimonthly and quarterly (thirty-three per cent), and the remainder weekly, annually, or sporadically. The volume of medical journals today is so great that there are special journals devoted to abstracts *of* abstracts appearing in other journals.

It has been calculated (Nathan Flaxman)[23] that five thousand of the medical journals published in a single year represent about eleven million pages of text which, if lined up, would stretch from Chicago to Seattle, Washington.† No one, therefore, can possibly even scratch the surface of such a huge mass of literature; but it *is* possible to pick out the highlights of medical information. Above all, we must decide what it is that we *must* read, what we *should* read, and what we *want* to read. These should be our three criteria in the selection of reading material.

We should read everything of immediate practical significance to

---

* "The business he [John Radcliffe] was intent upon was no less than the Preservation of Mankind, and this he did not endeavor to make himself Master of, by an useless Application to the Rubbish of Antiquity, in old musty Volumes, that requir'd Ages to be thoroughly perus'd in, but by a careful Examination of the most valuable Treatises that saw the Light from modern. His Books, while he was a Student of Physick, for so we must term him, 'till he becomes a Practitioner, were very few, but well chosen: So few indeed, as to make Dr. Bathurst, the Head of Trinity College, who, notwithstanding his Seniority in the University, kept him Company for his Conversation, stand in a Surprize, and ask, Where was his Study? Upon which, pointing to a few Vials, a Skelleton, and a Herbal, he receiv'd for Answer, Sir, this is Radcliffe's Library." [23]

† The subjects of articles appearing in journals fluctuate with medical fashion. In 1945 there were published fifty articles on cortisone; in 1952 there were eleven hundred articles. There are topics, such as peptic ulcer, which are "old friends who never die" and thus manifest their professional importance. In the United States, in one year alone there appeared one hundred and seventy-five articles on surgical treatment for peptic ulcer and one hundred and twenty on medical therapy for the same disease, also two hundred articles on arteriosclerosis and as many more on child sex hygiene.

our daily clinical tasks, scientific research, or professional teaching. In selecting such material, the practicing physician can be guided by his own daily clinical practice, which requires him to keep informed of new diagnostic methods or new therapeutic weapons that may help him save a patient's life.

The research worker is in a different position. Not only must he know almost everything other research workers are doing—in case he can use any of it in his own research and thus save himself years of work—but he must also keep up-to-date on the most trivial developments in his own field of research, even though such data may not be of immediate practical importance, because in research anything may become important at any time.

The professor of medicine must know everything that improves or changes the subject matter he teaches, everything that expands the area of medical learning; he must enrich his basic material with the newest contributions, e.g., antibiotic medicine, which has changed the teaching of the natural history of infections. In addition, he must be informed about everything that may widen the cultural horizon of teaching and, finally, everything that contributes to the progress of Medicine.

Thus we see that the practicing physician must be guided by his daily *needs,* the research man by his *duty* to expand his research, and the teacher by his *desire* to enrich and improve his teaching. But to a certain degree all three—the practitioner, the research worker, and the medical teacher—should engage in all three categories of reading, devoting the greatest part of their time to what they *must* read, what time they have left over to what they *ought* to read, and any time they can steal to what they *want* to read.

Frequently, what one *must* read can be found in the basic medical texts and reference works; what one *ought* to read, in the most important medical journals; and what one *wants* to read, in the classic books we discussed earlier.

But reading medical journals is in itself a problem, however much we may limit our selection. There are three ways of acquiring the medical articles we want to read: by subscribing to the journals that publish them, by visiting medical libraries, or by writing to the authors for reprints. First, however, we should find out *what* is being published, so that we may select what to include in our daily curriculum of reading.

THE VALUE OF MEDICAL ABSTRACTS

The answer to this problem lies in the journals of medical abstracts, which, if well done, enable us to pick out quickly the best grain from the fertile crop of recent findings.

There are two types of journals of medical abstracts. One carries practically everything published in a given specialty. The other is selective rather than exhaustive; it gives the practitioner only what is of immediate practical importance, particularly in such specialties as internal medicine, obstetrics, and gynecology. Other specialties, such as endocrinology and psychiatry, require that the physician know, if only for reference, all that is happening in these fields in order to exercise his profession with skill.

Medical abstracts, unfortunately, are not always well done, as a physician is hardly the fittest person for this task. Perhaps the solution would be a standard form for abstracts, of a predetermined length and structure, calling only for the fundamental data of the work. Medical editors would then polish and round out such abstracts into an acceptable final form. This certainly would simplify the reader's task. At present, however, the reader must be content with what is available.

Actually, an abstract should be a complete "short short" story, with a beginning, a middle, and an end. A medical abstract should follow, figuratively, the same procedure used by the Indians of Ecuador when they shrink a human head to the size of an orange without spoiling the harmony of its proportions.

Of course, physicians must be careful not to fall victims to what Marañón called "scientism." To have absolute faith in everything labeled science, or to convert into dogma anything published by well-known journals, is to emulate the physicians who for hundreds of years believed blindly in the books of Galen and Paracelsus.

The danger of dogmatism in Medicine lies not in whether the dogmas are good or bad, but in their being dogmas. There is danger in replacing experience and research by authority and in attributing infallibility to the least infallible of all sciences, Medicine.

Many physicians, bewitched by scientific dogma, sacrifice the simplicity of basic information, which can be as placid as a little water cupped in the palm of the hand, to the turbidity of a torrent of scientific erudition, muddled even further by the mass of bibliography with which some authors burden their work, perhaps to cover up their sterility of thought.

We often forget that the immortal works bequeathed to us by the greatest teachers of Medicine are built on a solid framework of classic data, with personal ideas and experiences woven around it and a pertinent quotation only here and there.*

* In this respect, Marañón said: "Our information should be, in a whole, made up of some exact truths, those which emerge from the sea of notions to be revised. In other words, to know is not only to know, but to know and to doubt, and therefore not to know everything."

The third important source of scientific information for the doctor today, a source worthy of a place alongside textbooks and medical journals, is the scientific literature prepared and sent to doctors by pharmaceutical companies.

Only a few years ago such literature was considered—rightfully so—mere advertising propaganda in the worst sense of the term. Today the medical literature issued by pharmaceutical companies, and often prepared by medical advertising agencies, has become an important source of study, consultation, reference, and medical education. Specifically in the fields of antibiotics, vitamins, biologic products, and hormones, it can be said that pharmaceutical literature is not only abundant but also precise, effective, ethical, and educational.

To a certain degree, the evolution of pharmaceutical advertising has followed a course that I would compare to the evolution of painting. Classic painters represented especially the physical bulk of objects and persons; the impressionists relegated photographic representation of physical bulk to a subordinate level and represented lights and shadows; modern surrealists represent the idea of things, the very soul of an object. For Velázquez, a human being was the specular image of his physical make-up; for Seurat, the human being was a conglomerate of tiny polychrome dots of light; for Picasso, he is a geometric abstraction. Summing up, classical art represented *things;* impressionism, the *light* of things; modern art, the *idea* of things. Classical art is photographic and visual; impressionism appeals to the sensory and emotional image; modern art is attractive to the intelligence as it presents the *concept* of things.

Pharmaceutical advertising began by presenting a photograph of the *products* followed by a verbal description and a cumbersome iconography. All past pharmaceutical literature is cluttered up with pictures of bottles, pills, ampules, and salve tubes. The revolution began when such advertising represented the *properties* and *uses* of the products involved. Modern pharmaceutical literature presents the *idea* behind a given product, the philosophic concept that motivates and justifies it. A recent advertising campaign on the combined use of antibiotics and vitamins for treating the etiologic agent of an infection and the stress caused by it was based successfully on the introduction of such a concept into medical thought and later on the introduction of the product incarnating the idea.

In my opinion, the medical literature of the future—including medical advertising—will shed its present form and become *educational literature*. When a drug is universally accepted and has become a part of the basic therapeutic arsenal of the physician, it no longer needs any advertising: it is enough to inform, guide, and educate us as to how to use it. A vaccine, a hormone, an antibiotic already tried and proved does not need advertising; all we need is technical information on how to use it. As I see it, medicopharmaceutical advertising in the future will be limited to announcing new products, while its primary mission will be educational—to complete the work of preventive medicine, which is the Medicine of the Future.

Meanwhile, for the physician who can winnow the bad from the good in the praises heaped on a drug, who has an eye for picking the nuggets out of the cluttered mine of information, for him pharmaceutical literature is a precious source of medical knowledge and an educational vehicle of unique value. This is especially true of physicians who practice in isolated regions where it takes months for a book or a journal to arrive. This "country doctor" keeps abreast of the progress of medicine through advertising pamphlets and leaflets, as colorful as a peacock's plumes but which also contain information as scientific and precise as the calculations done by a Princeton mathematician.

READING FOR IMPROVEMENT

Now we come to the reading done by the physician as a member of society, as an individual participating in the life of a nation, a period, a culture, a civilization.

As a human being, a physician may enjoy recreational reading: novels, short stories, poetry, travel books, or humorous literature. As a professional, he must read informative literature: scientific books, medical journals, and other technical publications. But as an individual functioning in society, who must contribute to his country's growth as a nation and to its universal function, he must read works that help him to improve himself and thus enable him to improve his environment through the influence of his thoughts, his • words, his pen, and his actions.

Such reading for improvement may be classified as scientific (on the progress being made in the biologic, natural, and physical sciences), philosophic, historical, sociologic, or reading in the miscellaneous arts.

Yet how can one ask the overburdened practitioner to devote time to reading that is not directly related to his profession? If he can hardly keep abreast of the latest developments in his own speciality, how will he find time for abstract or theoretical reading?   \

To such objections, I would say that one does not *have* time: one *makes* it. We must be time's ragpicker, following the example of those great teachers who snatched up the snippets of "the gold dust of time," those minutes, quarters of an hour, or half hours wasted during the day in unnecessary chatter, the overlong telephone calls, the newspaper or popular magazine that fell into our hands and that we read out of mere curiosity, the time-stealing visit from some stranger, and those long evenings spent with eyes glued to the television screen. Elimination of such unproductive activities would yield the hour or two for the reading we so badly need.

HOW TO FIND TIME TO READ

If we intend to devote an hour or two every day to reading, we must organize our time with the greatest caution. Perhaps it would be wise to follow the advice a teacher once gave me to imagine at all times that we are about to embark on an extended journey. The day before we leave we do the work of several days, take care of any number of details rapidly and efficiently, give each minute its just due, and leave everything in order. If we could manage to consider each day as the day before the beginning of a long trip, we might work harder and fill our lives with effective activity and success.

There are four sources of time where we can find those precious moments so necessary for rounding out our cultural lives. The first and most important source we have just described: gathering up the gold dust of time and making each minute yield its maximum value.

WAR ON THE "CHRONOPHAGES"

There is a second source in Goethe's advice, so wisely summarized by André Maurois: Let us eliminate from our lives all time-devourers, the cannibals who feed on our minutes and hours, Molière's *fâcheux* whom Montherlant called *chronophages* (time-eaters).

"*Chronophages*," Maurois said,[24] "have no mercy. If you allow it, they will steal your very last moment, never realizing that if they had left you alone you might have accomplished something worthwhile. *Chronophages* have no scruples. On the very day war is declared, a callous time-eater will break in on the Chief of Staff to discuss his janitor's conscription. *Chronophages* operate by means of visits, telephone calls, and letters. If you show them any patience or kindness, you commit a grave sin. You must treat them without any consideration, for to allow them into your presence is sheer suicide."

Goethe once said that "if one wishes to do something for the world, one must not allow the world to take hold of one." This is legitimate advice, for if we do not succeed, the world reproaches us for being too easygoing. "You should not go anywhere," the *chronophage* will say, "for you would be neglecting your work." And with his very next breath he adds, "Come to dinner tomorrow." And you must refuse, for he who allows himself to be swallowed up by such people will never see his work completed.

The third source of time lies in cutting to the bone the time we allow daily to reading too many newspapers or news magazines. As citizens of a nation and participants in a historical epoch, we should aspire to be well informed about everything happening in the world. But to exaggerate such an ambition leads us to devote too many hours a week to reading the same news in different newspapers and articles on the same subject in different magazines, to listening to the same news over the radio at different hours, and—*vade retro, Satanas!*—to watching television programs that we would have shunned on the motion-picture screen. Thus the time we could devote to useful things is sacrificed to a false sense of accomplishment.

In general, it is sufficient to read one newspaper a day. Nor do we need to read it from beginning to end. We should learn to read "vertically" by catching the essence of what every article or report says. As for news magazines, one a week is enough to supplement what we have learned from our daily newspaper. Everything else makes us spread ourselves thin, throwing away our time on superficial commentaries or anodyne tales, thereby misspending the most precious of treasures and the most difficult to keep: time.

The next source of time is our spare time. What should we do with it? Should we read, study, indulge in some sport, some distraction, or what is called a "hobby"? I confess that I am a mortal enemy of hobbies. Man's life should be divided into three parts as harmoniously balanced as possible: work, rest, and recreation. When our work is also our recreation, we can take away a part of that recreation and give it over to lighter, different, or more agreeable tasks, such as reading. An obsessive hobby that becomes the Moloch of all of one's free time is a fatal error. If a hobby—collecting stamps, assembling toy trains, breeding canaries—is really so interesting, we should devote our lives to it: it should become our profession. Let us drink from all the cups of entertainment without getting drunk on any one. A hobby carried to extremes may be the reason why a physician has no time for any reading aside from professional texts and news magazines. Many of us love chess, the movies, and the theater, and there is no need to give up such pastimes altogether; but we must decide what is more important in the scale of life's values: to be an "expert" in one or several hobbies, or to be a good physician and a valuable member of the society in which we live. The choice should not be open to any doubt.

To summarize this subjective evaluation of what a physician should do to make time for reading and studying: we must not allow details to consume our lives; we must delegate to others everything they can do for us; we must live *deeply* rather than fast, doing the important things first and the unimportant ones never.

What should the physician read in history, philosophy, the arts, and the sciences? Let each person choose his own road to humanism.[25] The roads leading toward that goal are as infinite as the roads toward the sea, but each man's or woman's road is as individual as the road to Damascus was for Saul of Tarsus.

It is a good idea to select a *basic* text in each one of the fields mentioned, using it as a compass on our voyages over the seas of culture. It should be a clear, complete, and not too lengthy text that can be mastered without undue effort and supplemented with monographs, short books, and magazine articles on the topics of greatest interest to us.

Along with this general cycle of basic reading, on which we graft epicycles of complementary reading, we should include the classics in science, philosophy, history, literature, and the arts, for their voices not only bring back the past, but allow us to commune with the great historical figures whose thoughts are always an inspiration and whose lives may yet teach us something about our own. Allenby's campaigns in Arabia and Schliemann's discovery of the jewels of Helen of Troy derived from the fact that they had read the *Iliad*. When General Lyautey was unjustly relieved of his post in Morocco, he consoled himself by reading Shakespeare's *Coriolanus*.[25] Poincaré found enlightenment in Tacitus and Marcus Aurelius, two writers who have always provided guidance for statesmen, just as Kipling and Cervantes have inspired men of action, and Romain Rolland, Aurobindo Ghose, and Ramakrishna have pointed the way to humanists and thinkers.

Naturally, reading for improvement demands respect and concentration. While a medical journal, a monograph, or a recent article can be read between visits to patients, on the subway or in a plane, in one's office or in a hospital corridor, the great classic texts in medicine or other sciences, in philosophy or history, require the proper place, time, and state of mind. That is the minimum respect we can show to their authors. The reader should become worthy of those great books, for, as Miguel de Unamuno said of *Don Quixote,* the important thing is "not what the author meant, but what each reader sees or even creates."

To obtain the most out of the great books, we must approach them as travelers approached the old Spanish inns in Don Quixote's time. Since generally no food was to be had at those inns, the abundance and savor of a traveler's repast depended on how well his knapsack was stocked. When we read Gibbon or Oliver Wendell Holmes, Taine or Osler, Voltaire or Cajal, what we derive from them is in direct ratio to the devotion and respect we give them. From books, as from love, we receive as much as we give.

IN PRAISE OF READING IN THE HISTORY OF MEDICINE

The physician must include in his program of reading for improvement books of medical history and the great works of the classical physicians. The rebirth of the history of Medicine has impelled many physicians—at first out of intellectual curiosity and later because of a spiritual need—to peer into the well of medical classics, and to recognize with astonishment that many elementary basic truths, long forgotten, can be learned from them. From Cajal or Claude Bernard we may not learn to diagnose the rickettsiae; but these masters can help us to develop medical and clinical acumen and to apply it competently and with assurance in diagnosis and therapy. Such classical books are like the ancient, worn-out but indispensable tools bequeathed by a watchmaker to his son and by the latter to his own son, tools which often are of greater value than the most modern instruments, for old tools were fashioned on the basic requirements of the trade as instinctively foreseen by the born artisan. I personally read the classics often—although not as often as I would like—and I reread *Don Quixote* every night at bedtime, opening the book at random, for I know that, like a healthy tree that yields only good fruit, any page will provide food for thought.

There are physicians who rebel at mixing required reading with the reading of medical classics, which they in any case consider a boring and even dangerous pastime. Perhaps they are, at bottom, afraid that the classics may disagree with the ideas and methods they often accept uncritically, like the caliph who caused the library at Alexandria to be burned because "if all these books are in agreement with the Koran, we do not need them, and if they disagree, they lie."

There is another type of physician who is somewhat afraid of too much reading, unconsciously subscribing to the proverb, "The librarian who reads is gone!" He therefore refuses to read anything not directly related to the practical needs of the moment. Sir Thomas Browne, for instance, limited his pocket library to three books: "a Greek testament, some of the aphorisms of Hippocrates and a text by Horace."

But fortunately there are many physicians who love good books, and for them reading—and dreaming about what they read—is one of the most pleasant occupations of their lives. With Edgar Allan Poe, they can say "to dream is the work of my life." At the head of that legion stands the Goethe of modern medicine, Sir William Osler, who adopted Thomas Linacre as his model because he was "an example of a life of devotion to learning, to medicine and to the interest of humanity." It was Osler who said: "For the general practitioner a well-used library is one of the correctives of the premature senility which is so apt to overtake him. . . . It is astonishing with how little reading a doctor can practice medicine, but it is astonishing how badly he may do it." [26]

But we should never hasten to buy a book unless we are first certain that we wish to "live" with it and not just to pass the time away.* We should buy only those books worthy of being read, reread, and kept, which incidentally would discourage bad writers who waste the time of unsuspecting readers. And in selecting such books, let us not be guided only by the critics—often biased and wrong—for they are only human, many times too human in their judgments.

C. G. Osgood [27] adopted Bacon's habit of differentiating between books "to be chewed, swallowed and digested" and "books to be relished." He recommended that we read first the index, the preface, and one or several basic chapters, then in both directions, forward and backward, until we have a perspective of the entire book, as the test of whether we want to buy it or not. That was also the practice of the great Spanish historian Menendez y Pelayo, who possessed the amazing gift of grasping in less than half an hour the essence of a four hundred-page book, the "something good" which Don Quixote said that even the worst book contains.

I confess that I am guilty of reading too rapidly. Yet, although my *tempo* is rather fast and although I have developed a method of keeping seven or more books—excluding medical readings—"moving" each week, thus averaging about a book a day over the period of a year, I have noticed that time is making me more selective in my reading, for I humbly recognize the enormous difficulty of acquiring in our limited lifespan even a small part of human knowledge.

HOW TO SELECT READING MATERIAL

In selecting basic reading for improvement, we should be on guard against books of passing interest that appear and disappear as quickly as certain species of butterflies, leaving no trace other than the dust into which they are crushed by the critic's unmerciful fist.

In general, we should follow Emerson's dictum "never to read a

---

* Arthur Conan Doyle thought differently: "Reading is made too easy nowadays, with cheap paper editions and free libraries. A man does not appreciate at its full worth the thing that comes to him without effort. Who now ever gets the thrill which Carlyle felt when he hurried home with the six volumes of Gibbon's "History" under his arm, his mind just starving for want of food, to devour them at the rate of one a day? A book should be your very own before you can really get the taste of it, and unless you have worked for it, you will never have the true inward pride of possession." [2]

book less than a year old." Perhaps it is wise not to read books that are too recent. A reasonable amount of time should elapse after their publication to give us the opportunity of comparing them with other books and authors.

Some books have survived through the ages because they are veritable monuments of learning, such as Sir Thomas Browne's *Religio Medici* or Hippocrates' *Aphorisms*. These books are like museum halls filled with wonders that we can visit whenever we have the time and the inclination; but in no circumstances should they replace books of permanent relevance, the true classics that are classics not only because of their literary value but also because of their philosophic depth.

The physician should learn to discriminate in his reading for improvement. He should learn that it is better to know a few classic authors and universal themes thoroughly than all authors and themes superficially. I admit I am inclined to worship encyclopedic knowledge, but only a *cultural* encyclopedism, the kind that affords one a panoramic view of human learning through time and space. On the other hand, I believe that the physician should, above all, know his specialty thoroughly before wandering into other professional fields.

Just a few friends from among the giants of classical Medicine are enough to enrich the life of a physician. If a physician knows thoroughly only the works of Claude Bernard, Ramón y Cajal, William Osler, Charles Sherrington, Sigmund Freud, and Ivan Pavlov, supplemented by recent works on Medicine, he is a cultured man, a humanist, and a true scientist.

The value of the history of Medicine increases enormously when we allow the great medical philosophers to be our guides, as the classical Vergil guided Dante, through the caverns of Hell which are the complexities of life today.*

Sydenham's healthy Hippocratic criteria, Oliver Wendell Holmes' humorous philosophy, Claude Bernard's skillful experimental eye, Cajal's noble precepts are more important to the physician's professional education than the flock of hastily written little books flooding the publishing market, which try with a torrent of bibliographic ma-

---

* A physician should make a list of the great philosophic, historical, and scientific works he should know, for unless one is acquainted with those monumental works one loses some of one's human value. Whether it is read chapter by chapter religiously every day, or on vacation, or during a siege of illness, I believe that *Don Quixote* should be read in its entirety alongside *The Decline and Fall of the Roman Empire,* Plutarch's *Lives,* Balzac's *Comédie Humaine,* the works of Dostoevski, Tolstoi, Dickens, Marcel Proust, Burton's *Anatomy of Melancholy,* the works of Shakespeare, Osler, Kant, and Spinoza. And when some of these have been read, our moral weight is increased and life takes on a new dignity.

terial to make up for their lack of those clear fundamental concepts within which the physician's learning should be framed.

There is one infallible criterion in choosing the authors who are to be constant spiritual companions of our lives, and that is to select those who are consecrated by history. A person or even a whole generation may be mistaken in their judgment of a contemporaneous work, but Humanity is never mistaken when it consecrates the works of great men.

L'ENVOI

To read—and to read is to dream—is as important in the physician's life as clinical experience. At the Mayo Brothers House there is a multicolored stained-glass window representing the evolution of Medicine and bearing the following words by Dr. W. J. Mayo: "Take of my experience but give me of your dreams."

To conclude, let us listen, before we close the "Magic Door," to the fitting words of the Scottish physician and storyteller, Arthur Conan Doyle: "And now, my very patient friend, the time has come for us to part, and I hope my little sermons have not bored you over-much. If I have put you on the track of anything which you did not know before, then verify it and pass it on. If I have not, there is no harm done, save that my breath and your time have been wasted. There may be a score of mistakes in what I have said—is it not the privilege of the conversationalist to misquote? My judgments may differ very far from yours, and my likings may be your abhorrence; but the mere thinking and talking of books is in itself good, be the upshot what it may. For the time the magic door is still shut. You are still in the land of faerie. But, alas, though you shut that door, you cannot seal it. Still come the ring of bell, the call of telephone, the summons back to the sordid world of work and men and daily strife. Well, that's the real life after all—this only the imitation. And yet, now that the portal is wide open and we stride out together, do we not face our fate with a braver heart for all the rest and quiet and comradeship that we found behind the Magic Door?" [2]

MINERVA AND AESCULAPIUS:
THE PHYSICIAN AS WRITER

LITERATURE AND MEDICINE

*t*his Atomic Age of ours has witnessed the downfall of many traditions. Only a few weeks ago I stood once again entranced by the palaces in fabulous Venice and their reflections, wan and faded, on the dead, green waters of the canals. Within their walls the tragedy immortalized long ago by Alfred de Musset is still unfolding: suits of armor are rusting away piece by piece; tapestries are fading away blossom by blossom, while the cressets stand empty of candles, and, for lack of powder, the wigs of the lackeys hang limp. There they stand, these ancient palaces, as though waiting to be closed forever or at best converted into prosaic flights of offices. In a like manner modern medical culture has been denying its proud classical heritage and has been contracting its once vast encyclopedic and humanistic domains into an aggregate of ever more and more specialized techniques.

Since, as time goes on, the physician exercises less and less his imagination and literary ability, scientific expression is slowly being stifled. As Sir James Barrie, the magnificent creator of *Peter Pan,* once said, "The man of science appears to be the only person who has something to say just now and the only man who does not know how to say it."

And yet, paradoxically enough, the physician, more so than other professional persons, has truly artistic strains hidden within his being, though he seldom allows them to burst from their shell for the edification of his fellow men. The physician, for reasons we shall shortly

From *International Record of Medicine 169:*723, 1956.

see, experiences, as few others can, the desire to relate what he knows or thinks, what he sees or dreams. The proof is that no other profession has provided so many famous writers as medicine. In the course of the world's history, physicians have outshone all other professionals in the writing of romance and philosophy.

Let us then look into medicine's contribution to literature and literature's reciprocal assistance to medicine and find out what are the psychologic reasons that determine the physician's urge to write and the connections between art and science, so that in the end we may descry what the art and the science of the future may expect from the development of a more "literary" type of physician and a more scientific type of writer.

THE COMMON ORIGIN OF THE PHYSICIAN AND THE ARTIST

"And I'd leave the hurry, the noise, and the fray for a house full of books and a garden full of flowers," once said the Scottish poet, Andrew Lang.

Throughout history the physician has always felt attracted to flowers and books. In the classical Greece of the blossoming groves, as in the old Spain of the Moorish gardens, in the Rome of the splendorous palaces, as in the France of the great chateaux, the physician always sought refuge from the hazards and sufferings of his work in those book-filled, flower-begirded houses sung by the poet.

Let us not forget that the primitive doctor was an artist and that art and medicine are but two sides of that cyclopean quarry which is the civilization of a country or of an epoch. The blocks carved from that quarry, whatever their shape or size and whoever their quarrier was, are all of the same stone, for all originated from the same mountain.

From the beginnings of the history of medicine, the physician has felt the urge to relate what came before his eyes in the practice of his profession, thus weaving with the raw hemp of human suffering the fine gold cloth of story and legend.

The physician and the artist have common roots in history. In primitive societies the physician was both priest and witch doctor. His triple mission was to cure mild ailments with drugs and potions, to appease the gods with prayers, and to master the demons through conjurations and magic. Later, he was a priest in Babylon, where, clad in a scarlet tunic and bearing a raven on one hand and a falcon on the other, he appealed to the kindness of the gods; a scribe in ancient Egypt; a naturalist in the Greece of Pericles; often a slave in Rome; a monk and "library doctor" in the Middle Ages. At all times art and medicine have remained united in the person of the physician, perhaps because, like art, medicine, which professionally was and is a service, must always be creation if it is to yield fruitful results.

The tradition of the physician as artist and philosopher is then as ancient as it is distinguished. In Plato's *Symposium,* among the men of action and the philosophers gathered in the quiet shade of the silvery olive trees sat Eryximacus, a physician whose voice rang with science and conscience.

Since Plato, the physician has felt, as few other professional people have, a burning desire not only to impart his knowledge by means of the spoken and the written word, but also to wander whenever possible off the arid road of science into the green meadows of art and literature. On a previous occasion,* I discussed the physician's contribution to that monument compounded of the masterworks of medical literature accumulated through the ages. Here I will speak of what physicians have done as writers in the course of history. And in order to appreciate this achievement better, let us first examine medicine's contribution to literature.

MEDICINE IN LITERATURE

The writer's mind, like a weathercock, turns in whatever direction the social wind of his times blows. Medicine has perhaps been the strongest of all the winds bearing upon this weathercock of the mind, probably because sickness, pain, and death, being the greatest antithesis to health, joy, and life, are the most dramatic and the most universal subjects about which man can write.

There is room indeed for a literary history of medicine embracing an analysis of the greatest medical problems of mankind as seen through the eyes of men of letters in each period. For throughout history writers have frequently used as background to their stories the most pressing medical problems of their age. For instance, Homer, faithful chronicler of ancient Greece, left us in the *Iliad* a vast mural of traumatology depicting arrow, sword, spear, and stone wounds, contusions, and traumas of every type. In those times man lived by his fist and the main national worry was about the lesions resulting from such a violent way of life.

In the Middle Ages, an era of collectivism, as pointed out by Sigerist, "collective" illnesses, such as the plague, leprosy, and St. Vitus' dance, held fearful sway, to say nothing of contagious "fevers" propagated by the extremely low standards of hygiene prevailing in medieval cities. Thus it came about that there flourished at that time poems and legends depicting the cruel tragedy of leprosy, the

---

* In "Books in the Physician's Life," page 3.

foulest horror next to the plague to scourge the whole of Europe throughout that period.

The plague, the fearsome "Black Death" that in a few short years killed off a quarter of the population of the globe and half the inhabitants of London, could not but exert a powerful impact upon literary minds. On the macabre canvas of a plague, Boccaccio laid the scene of his roguish *Decameron* and Daniel Defoe wrote (1722) his *Journal of the Plague Year*.

During the Renaissance, an age of intense individualism in living as in art, there was an abundance of "individual" diseases, for example, syphilis, which inspired Fracastoro to write in 1530 his famous poem to which this disease owes its name.

Later on came diseases caused by nutritional deficiencies and poverty, such as typhus and ergotism, as well as others derived from overindulgence, like gout and dropsy, the scourge of the *bon vivants* in seventeenth and eighteenth century Europe.

Syphilis continued to lurk like a serpent in ambush behind the deceptive flowers in the Renaissance gardens of love. Both syphilis and gonorrhea rear their ugly heads in the pages of Boswell's *Memoirs,* for that faithful chronicler of the great Dr. Johnson caught these venereal diseases as an unexpected souvenir for his pains in pursuing the wanton ladies of his passions. Sir John Davenant, reputed son of Shakespeare, lost the whole of his nose, eaten away by syphilis, as the result of an unfortunate embrace with "a handsome wench in Axe Yard."

Syphilis continued for a long time to be the favorite theme of writers, who were its principal victims in France, where after having first driven some of them mad, it killed off writers like Baudelaire, Goncourt, de Maupassant, and Daudet.

Molière, obsessed against physicians and patients alike, assailed the profession in many of his works and has left us an ironical picture of iatrogenic diseases and of the harm involuntarily done by the physician who does not police his language and whose careless words may plant the seed of dismay in the ears of his patients. This new way of killing—by means of worry that ends in terror—echoes through the whole of Molière's satirical works like the anguished cry of a child smothered in the sumptuous folds of his prose.*

---

* Physicians have been the favorite target of satirists throughout the ages. In 1638 Francis Quarles said: "Physicians of all men are the most happy: Whatever good success soever they have the world proclaimeth, and what faults they commit, the earth covereth." It was Voltaire who said: "Doctors are men who prescribe medicine of which they know little to cure diseases of which they know less in human beings of which they know nothing." And Franklin said: "God heals and the physician takes the fee."

Shakespeare's knowledge of medicine is proverbial and has great historicomedical value, since it helps to fill in the period between Vesalius and Harvey. It may be that the great dramatist had some influence on the work of the brilliant physiologist, since the whole of Shakespeare's writings is imbued with preoccupation regarding the motion of the blood and the beating of the heart. No other poet's work is so abundant in the use of these words. In one scene in "Hamlet," Shakespeare describes the course of the poison administered to Hamlet's father as it makes its way through all "the passages" of his body. It is quite possible indeed that the noble verses of the Bard of Avon, heard by Harvey in an age when the baroque was reaching its peak and art was all vibration and movement, sharpened his anxiety to perfect his *anatomia animata* or physiology, which was to culminate in his discovery of the circulation of the blood.

The romantic period awakened an unwonted predilection for laudanum among the poets, who took it as carelessly as we take aspirin nowadays. Thomas de Quincey, Coleridge, and Shelley frequently wrote under the influence of the poppy, whose tincture was freely available to the public at any apothecary's. The romantic French poets, as we have commented elsewhere,* who used hashish to spur the Pegasus of their fancy, were the forerunners of the recent scientific experiments with mescalin, LSD, and other hallucinogenic agents now used in the experimental study of psychoses.

THE ROMANTIC MALADY: THE MYTH OF CHLOROSIS

A favorite subject of the authors of the romantic period was the "romantic malady" par excellence, a form of consumption accompanied by pallor, swooning, and sighs, which afflicted all the great literary heroines in Europe for practically a whole century. This malady attacked mostly young maidens with a greenish or cameo-like paleness, a nervous disposition, and anemia. In 1620 Varandeus of Montpellier gave this illness the name of chlorosis. Frequently, the process ended in fatal tuberculosis, as occurred to the Lady of the Camellias in Dumas *fils'* famous novel and, in actual life, to Julia Charles, the inamorata of Lamartine.

Nowadays we know that chlorosis, as Marañón has so brilliantly explained, was nothing but a literary myth, an ailment created by poets to whom pallor was synonymous with purity and love. In world literature pallor has always been a symbol of sexual passion. Pallor

---

* In the paper "Contemporary Physiodynamic Therapeutic Trends in Psychiatry" by Arthur M. Sackler, M.D., Raymond R. Sackler, M.D., Félix Martí-Ibáñez, M.D., and Mortimer D. Sackler, M.D., in *The Great Physiodynamic Therapies in Psychiatry,* published by Paul B. Hoeber, Inc., New York, 1956.

in woman, already noted by Ovid in his *Ars amandi,* became the classic *febris amantium.*

The romantic movement, which gave new values to the scene of drama and to the sickness and sin that were enacted thereon, played an important psychogenic part in making chlorosis the romantic malady of its period, reaching its apogee in 1830. Chlorosis was supposed to have affected Mimi in *La Bohème,* who in fact suffered from tuberculosis. Chlorosis, which was nothing more than puberal and postpuberal symptomatic anemia, was an imaginative psychologic entity contributed by the poets to medical literature only to disappear when customs became more liberal and the love life and daily habits of young women more normal.

THE INFLUENCE OF CLAUDE BERNARD AND SIGMUND FREUD ON LITERATURE

When with Claude Bernard the evolution of medicine changed into a revolution, Bernard's experimental and naturalistic method exerted a powerful influence upon the French writers of his period and their successors.

Verlaine versified on hospitals; Saint-Beuve was an *externe des hôpitaux* in Paris; Balzac, in the words of Taine, was a "doctor" who "dissected" his characters instead of depicting them. His pet physician among the many appearing in *La Comédie Humaine* was Bianchon, to whom Balzac on his deathbed appealed as the only one capable of curing him. Balzac was inspired by a humble health officer from l'Île Adam, Jacques Boisson by name, to create that other model physician, full of wisdom and kindliness, called Doctor Benassis.

Under the inspiration of Claude Bernard, Renan adopted the rationalist, experimental method in history, Taine in art, and Émile Zola—who dealt with medical subjects ranging from abortion to drunkenness—in literature. In imparting to the novel Claude Bernard's impersonality, Zola placed it at the service of science, thus being true to his own words: "I do not want like Balzac to make decisions on the affairs of mankind, or to be a philosopher or a moralist; I shall be satisfied with being a savant."

Flaubert, son and brother of physicians, was born in a hospital (just like Verlaine, who lived in hospitals "under the wing of my mother, *l'Assistance Publique*"), and was chained to the galley of medicine by his epilepsy. In *Madame Bovary* he proved his medical knowledge in his descriptions of Hippolyte's club foot, the purulent sores of the blind beggar, and the poisoning of Emma.

Claude Bernard with his new approach to physiology initiated the transition from the determinism of the ameba in biology to that of man's free will in literature, which was parallel to the transition from Hegel's philosophic fatalism to Virchow's physiologic fatalism.

When many years later Freud revolutionized psychopathology, his influence was felt in every novel written at the end of the nineteenth century and in the twentieth century, neurosis becoming from that time on the favorite theme of novelists, just as leprosy and the plague had been favored by medieval writers. From then on, deep psychology after the Freudian manner was contrived by such writers as Paul Bourget, who coined the medical terms "pathomimy" and "mythomany" and maintained that in every French novelist from the middle of the preceding century on there was a "physiologist . . . who yearned to bring to art the same freedom that the hospital and the operating theater granted the physician"; the Goncourts; Paul Valéry, whose "visceral obsession" has already been commented upon; Marcel Proust, whose works could not have been produced without the groundwork provided by Freud; and later still by a flood of writers who either were physicians themselves or wrote about medical themes, such as, in Norway, Henrik Ibsen in whose psychiatric dramas syphilis and alcoholism played such an important part; in France, Roger Martin du Gard with his monumental work on the Thibaults, Jules Romain and Georges Duhamel; in England, Virginia Woolf, George Bernard Shaw, and James Joyce; in the United States, Eugene O'Neill.

Medicine has been, therefore, a perennial fount of inspiration for literature, and has provided the keynote for many of the greatest masterpieces in the world by drawing the attention of writers to the great dramas of history in every period.

Let us now consider the impact that physicians as writers have had upon the history of literature.

THE PHYSICIAN AS WRITER: RABELAIS, HALLER, GOLDSMITH,
KEATS, OLIVER WENDELL HOLMES, S. WEIR MITCHELL,
CHEKHOV, ARTHUR CONAN DOYLE, W. SOMERSET MAUGHAM

If men of letters have found in medicine and its eternal themes of pain and death an inexhaustible source of inspiration, physicians, too, have at one time or another felt the desire to peer more deeply into the life rushing like a swollen river beyond their office windows.

What have been the distinguishing features of the literary work done by physicians? We can do no better than apply to the medical writer the same clinical procedure followed in the study of various cases of the same disease. Let us first examine each case separately, though with the brevity obligatory in an essay, so that we may then try to find the common denominator connecting all these physicians.

To some of them writing was as important in their life as medicine, others forsook altogether their profession in order to plunge into the sea of literature. Of the former class we might say, to parody Chekhov, that they took medicine for a legal spouse and literature for a mistress; and I would add that they had an overwhelming desire to divorce their wife and wed their mistress and thus legalize their "scandalous" passion for literature.

Of the physician-authors whom we shall review briefly, and of many others whom we cannot mention for lack of space, such as Arthur Schnitzler and Albert Schweitzer, one outstanding feature is the wide variety in their literary themes and styles, settings and techniques, which are almost as diversified as the medical specialties themselves. One can, however, discern a common thread running through all of them, which we shall analyze further on when dealing with the key to the psychology of the physician-author and of the physician who, like Molière's famous character, is an author *"malgré lui,"* despite himself.

What did the classical physicians write about? At first, the physician wrote mostly philosophy. This is understandable if we remember that classical medicine was born within the shadows of the temples, and the temple has always been a favorite resort for meditation. The priestly physicians of antiquity were at the same time philosophers and thinkers. The doctor of classical times devoted his leisure to philosophy.

This was what Aristotle did. He studied medicine, although he did not practice it, and along with his biologic learning, which was accepted right up to the Renaissance, he accumulated the polished nuggets of his work on politics, ethics, and philosophy; so did Celsus, the most sophisticated Roman of his day, who clothed his *De re medicina* with the elegant trappings of his Latin.

However, in order to come to the really lettered physician, we must traverse the days of the collapse of the Roman Empire beneath the double assault of clouds of anopheles and hordes of barbarians. Classical learning had survived only in the papyri that, next to the spices and myrrh, were transported on the backs of Arabian dromedaries along the great caravan routes and, later, by Moorish steeds, finally to be translated in Italian convents and in the palaces of Toledo. There monks and translators, working in the light of the medieval sun that embroidered their floors with the brilliant colors of the stained-glass windows, transferred the Hellenic wisdom from the Syriac vessels into the classical amphoras of the Latin language. Thereafter, from the height of the Middle Ages on, the physician commenced his incursions into the literary field. And with the medieval poet-physicians the road was opened that would lead to Schiller, Keats, and Schnitzler.

All the roads of literary medicine and medical literature lead to **Rabelais** (1490–1553)—that great peer of Cervantes, Shakespeare, and Dante, according to Coleridge—with whom the great tradition of the physician-littérateur really commenced. Rabelais had the supreme ability of reconciling his religious education, imparted to him by Benedictines and Franciscans, with his scientific education at the University of Montpellier, harmoniously combining his work as a physician in the 200-bed hospital, the Hôtel-Dieu of Lyons (where he dissected a few corpses yearly and designed certain surgical instruments for the reduction of ruptures and fractures of the femur), with his taste for literature.

Every physician ought to read *Gargantua and Pantagruel,* Rabelais' great satiric epic, not merely because he poured into it so much of the medical learning of his age, but because it also contains the satiric spirit of an epoch in history made great by Thomas Linacre, Paracelsus, Vesalius, and Leonardo da Vinci. *Gargantua and Pantagruel* is a gleesome guffaw from the medieval world, a joyous shout of rebellion as mighty in its impact on literature as was the impact of Paracelsus on the world of medicine. In this story Rabelais created that captivating character, Panurge, a swashbuckling scoundrel, based on François Villon, who with his carousals and jesting is perhaps the happiest figure to adorn the colorful pages of this work.

Besides the figure of Rabelais the Rebel, there stands out in contrast that of the conservative **Albrecht von Haller** (1708–1777). This prodigious physician from Bern was one of the marvels of the Age of Enlightenment, which comprised the latter half of the eighteenth century and which was the third great turning point of modern history after the Renaissance and the Baroque. At the age of nine, Haller had already compiled two dictionaries, Greek and Latin, and over two thousand biographies. After this stupendous start, he followed a medical career, at the end of which he left behind more than two thousand papers published in his medical review, *Göttinger Gelehrten Anzeigen,* fourteen thousand letters, the records of his clinical practice, a chair in botanical research, a multitude of books on medicine, and a whole galaxy of poetic, philosophic, and religious works. Although he maintained a friendly correspondence with libertines like Casanova and atheists like Voltaire, Haller in his poems sang above all the praise of God, as in his famous poem on the Alps. Haller sought to combine faith with logic, creating a poetry imbued with Christian revelation and love of nature. His verses reveal that he looked on mankind with the same tenderness with which he classified in his herbarium the plants and flowers of the Rhone Valley, since to him, as to St. Francis of Assisi, flower and man were brothers in the great communion of Nature before God.

If Haller's poetry causes us to reflect on the greatness of Nature, the work of that physician of Irish ancestry, **Oliver Goldsmith** (1728–1774), brings us in touch with the human being on the sentimental stage of his stories. Goldsmith was a fugitive from medicine. He studied at Edinburgh, Leyden, and probably Padua, receiving his diploma to practice medicine in London. Prior to trying his fortunes unsuccessfully in the field of medicine, he tramped through the whole of Europe with only a guinea in his pocket, playing the flute and teaching English for a year in a lonesome vagabondage that put to the test all his wits and fortitude. It may be that the society of such artistic geniuses as Dr. Johnson, Boswell, the painter Reynolds, and the novelist Samuel Richardson, set him off on the road to writing. He composed a series of poems that we can still read with delight, and a novel that Goethe considered the best in the eighteenth century and that Dickens himself took to bed every night. Reading the *Vicar of Wakefield* we can understand why Dr. Johnson said, "Goldsmith writes like an angel." I myself have read this novel many times, always with increasing pleasure. It is full of warm humanity with a bucolic strain of shabby-genteel sentimentality, rich in humor and tenderness. The prose is quiet, soothing, and translucent like the crystal-clear waters of a brook through which one can glimpse the pebbles on its bed. There is no better way, perhaps, to learn to write with clarity than to study carefully the Cervantesque "difficult simplicity" of this novel.

Goldsmith's limpid prose was still an influence in literature when another English physician, **John Keats** (1795–1821), graduated in 1816 at the Apothecaries' Hall in London after his studies at St. Thomas' and St. Guy's hospitals, was filling his poems with a visionary world stirred by chimerical breezes and warmed by the sun of youth. Keats died a tragic death at the age of 26, his hazel eyes glazed, his face waxen beneath the red mop of hair, his lungs eaten away by tuberculosis as he lay in bed facing the white stone steps of the Piazza di Spagna in Rome. But his poems, conceived during his anatomy classes, still lull the ears of the romantics all over the world.

The greatest contribution of the New World to the realm of physician-authors has been **Oliver Wendell Holmes** (1809–1894), of whom Osler said he was "the most successful combination the world has ever seen of the physician and the man of letters." Holmes was one of those rare cases of a genial child born to a genial father. (The year he was born also saw the birth of Darwin, Lincoln, Gladstone, Chopin, Mendelssohn, Tennyson, Edgar Allan Poe,

Gogol, and Edward FitzGerald!) Oliver Wendell Holmes won his place in the hall of honor of the history of medicine with his work *The Contagiousness of Puerperal Fever* (which preceded that of Semmelweis), which he wrote after doing only theoretical book research, with almost no clinical experience, relying solely on his extraordinary intuition, thus proving what the scientifically trained mind can do in the realm of theory.

Holmes was also the author of the poem, "Old Ironsides," which saved the frigate "Constitution" from the scrap pile. He wrote other poems and "psychiatric" novels, but the best known is his delightful *Autocrat of the Breakfast Table,* in which a philosopher, thinker, humanist, and humorist teaches us what many men of science have forgotten: that it is possible to reconcile science and conscience, learning and wit, without losing prestige as a scientist while gaining it as a human being.

Though I have great admiration for **S. Weir Mitchell** (1829–1914) as a writer, I have still more for him as a physician (he received his doctorate in medicine at the Jefferson Medical College in Philadelphia and studied under Claude Bernard in Paris), since it was his work that gave the status of a science to the study of neurology, which had started scientifically in 1820 with Bell and Magendie and clinically, later, with Duchenne of Boulogne, Broca, Charcot, Erb-Westphal, Jackson, and Gowers. Mitchell published a series of admirable "psychiatric" novels and of these, his *Constance Trescott* is a must for the present-day physician, since it consists of fictionalized clinical histories in which the author anticipated many of Freud's theories.

It is symbolic that Mitchell, a gentleman from old Virginia, should recommend as professor of medicine a Canadian by the name of **William Osler** (1849–1919), whose manners he tested at a gala dinner by having him served cherries with their pits to see if he could eat them as elegantly as he himself did. Osler not only survived the test, but, in addition, became the supreme example of the harmonious combination of physician and man of letters. Though Osler wrote no "pure" literature, his philosophic and medicohistorical works suffice to assure him a place of honor in the Hall of Fame of modern medicine. Osler was the Goethe of medicine. His genius for teaching and writing, so far excelled by no one, was partly transmitted to his pupil, Harvey Cushing, another fine example of the modern medical humanist.

One of the greatest examples of the physician who sought to combine the art of writing with that of medicine was **Anton Chekhov** (1860–1904).

Russian literature, like all Russian arts and sciences, had a late start in history. In 1837, while the poems of Pushkin were still echoing around Europe, Gogol published his novel, *Dead Souls*. With this and, two years later, the first novel by Dostoevski, a doctor's son bound to medicine by the tragic ties of his epilepsy, a new and powerful literature of universal appeal raised its head above the ermine-covered Siberian steppes. Half a century later, following Dostoevski, Tolstoi, Turgenev, and Goncharov, came that brilliant author-physician, Anton Chekhov.

Son of a liberated serf, Chekhov graduated in medicine at Moscow, led the struggling existence of a country doctor, and died at the age of 44 from tuberculosis and exhaustion, far from home, in the shade of the pines of Germany's Black Forest. In addition to his journeys through Siberia, his struggle against cholera epidemics, his studies on the bad conditions in the penal colonies on Saghalien Island, and his sojourns on the French Riviera to combat his tuberculosis, Chekhov also wrote stories, dramas, and novels of a heroic pessimism, over which, however, there hovered a fleeting shadow of humor.

Chekhov was raised above his colleagues by those three hours daily and part of the night which, throughout his life, he devoted to the "secondary" task of writing. Writing was the mistress with whom he spent the night when weary of his legitimate spouse, the practice of medicine.

Chekhov's portrayal of the Russian people is remarkable. His use of the scientific, experimental method in studying them in no way diminished his affection for them. His work sometimes lacks shape, perhaps because he preferred to take a cross section of Russian humanity and reveal it in its stark, naked reality. The reading of his works is to be recommended not only for the esthetic pleasure it affords (his short story, "The Siren," for instance, is a marvel of wit and humor), but also as a lesson in the art of telling a story with simplicity and realism, though always with elegance and artistry, which are equally desirable in the writing of novels and of clinical case histories.

A contemporary of Chekhov was the Scottish physician, **Arthur Conan Doyle** (1859–1930), whose professional life lasted barely ten years. First he served as a ship's physician on whalers in the Arctic and on the West African coast; then he waited eight years for patients who never came, first in his consulting room in Portsmouth and, later, in the neighborhood of Harley Street, only around the corner from the fame that years later would come to him through the literary road. His professional failure, however, was well redeemed by his success in literature, which transmuted into gold the lead of his existence as a doctor. His teacher, surgeon Joseph Bell, who by mere observation could diagnose the disease as well as the profession and life history of his patients, excited Arthur Conan Doyle to create his famous sleuth, whom he surnamed "Holmes" in honor of his much admired friend, Oliver Wendell Holmes.

Sherlock Holmes brought Arthur Conan Doyle fame and fortune —and a psychologic conflict. For above all, Arthur Conan Doyle wanted to be recognized as a historical novelist. His eight historical novels (my favorites, which I have read and reread time and again, are *The White Company* and *The Refugees*) are great models of the novel of action, admirably in line with Arthur Conan Doyle's personality as soldier, sportsman, traveler, crusader, poet, and historian. These really are his best works, although one is equally fascinated by his detective stories embroidered on the backcloth of Victorian London. Here, by the light of the gas lamps, through streets shrouded in fog and mist, the clip-clop of a horse drawing a carriage heralds the arrival of a mysterious damsel in rustling silks and another adventure for Holmes and the reader alike.

The best of Arthur Conan Doyle in my opinion is his historical work. All of it is tinged with a spirit of romance and chivalry. It gives a picture of the Crusades and of medieval France far superior to anything we can read in the often trashy "best sellers" of today. Arthur Conan Doyle's work bears the clinical, experimental stamp of the naturalistic physician, yet it lacks none of the humanistic and loving spirit that inspired his crusading life. In Sherlock Holmes are combined an analytic, scientific mind with understanding, kindliness, and a sense of humor, attributes of both a great detective and a great physician.

Another lover of detective novels, such as those of Arthur Conan Doyle, is my admired friend, **William Somerset Maugham** (b. 1874), with whom we end our list. Maugham's masters in writing technique were de Maupassant and Chekhov and in style Swift and Hazlitt. Graduating from St. Thomas' Hospital at the age of 24, he assisted at 63 child deliveries, working in the Borough of Lambeth (London) which he has immortalized in one of his novels. Though he retired early from the practice of medicine, preferring to struggle as a dramatist and writer, he was of the opinion that every writer ought to have a good knowledge of physiology and psychology "for he must know how the basic elements of literature are related to the minds and bodies of men."

Somerset Maugham, who I trust will soon be awarded the Nobel Prize for Literature which he ought to have received years ago, has applied the naturalistic, experimental method to his work as no other writer-physician has. His writings afford us some remarkable clinical and psychiatric sketches and, particularly, a picture of deep psychologic searching into the human mind. Although his novels, unlike those of Cronin, Slaughter, Sinclair Lewis, Georges Duhamel, and Lloyd Douglas, are not of a medical nature, they nevertheless bear the stamp of his medico-psychologic education. With him as the best example of the physician turned man of letters we end this chapter, remembering that the ingredients that Maugham recommends for the writing of good literature are also vital to the writing of good medicine—namely, *lucidity, simplicity,* and *euphony.*

If we now reflect for an instant on the examples here introduced of physicians who brought their clinical education to the art of writing, we perceive that in all of them there is present one common denominator—the application to the technique of writing of their training in the scientific, naturalistic, and observational methods of medicine. All of them, from Rabelais to W. Somerset Maugham, wrote realistic literature. Even those who, like Keats, were romantic poets never lost the sense of external reality and of man's humanity that they had gained through contact with pain and death in the course of their professional work. A medical career is, therefore, a good ground for literary training, since it provides that practical sense of reality so essential to a good writer. If the feelings do not become atrophied by daily clinical practice, it also provides that kindliness toward and respect for one's neighbor which have always inspired the truly great literature of all nations.

THE PHYSICIAN AS MAN OF ACTION

There is one interesting aspect in the life of all these physician-writers—common also to all nonmedical writers and even to other artists—that is evidenced in their own life stories. This is the lack of action in their lives. As a rule, the more prolific an artist's output is, the less active is his life.

The cases of writers who were men of action, such as Cervantes, Lope de Vega, Dumas, and Joseph Conrad, are the exception that proves the rule. As a general rule, however, great painters like Velázquez, great writers like Dante, great poets like Shakespeare, great thinkers like Kant, great historians like Renan, or great novelists like Tolstoy have been confined most of their lives to one place and have known few adventures or even excitement of any kind. This is explained not only by the fact that the task of creation demands that the artist withdraw from all active occupation, that he break away from the hustle-bustle of active life, but also by the marked psychologic difference that exists between the intellectual and the man of action.

The physician is basically a man of action. Perhaps this is why it is such a labor for him to practice reflection and contemplation once he has decided to substitute creation for action. This is not difficult to understand.

There are two basic types of man: the *occupied* and the *preoccupied*.

The *preoccupied* man is the intellectual, the artist, the creator who feels no need for action and shies clear of it for fear that it might stifle his creative impulse. The intellectual lives within himself, engulfed in his own inner wealth of thought. This is at once his glory and his misery. The intellectual needs nothing, he needs no one, he is a microcosm. The mind of an intellectual is a perpetual festival of thought, a treasure chest filled with wonders, a music box forever playing intimate sonatas which he alone can hear.

In contrast to this preoccupied intellectual man we have the *occupied* man, the man of action. The physician belongs to this group. *Preoccupation* precedes occupation. It is the act of thinking first *before* taking action; it interposes ideas between the desire and its execution. *Occupation* is actual action; it is the jump from desire to execution; it means living in a state of reflexes, on an instinctive conative plane instead of on the intellectual plane. The intellectual is a little apraxic; the man of action, on the other hand, vibrates with reflexes.

The man of action, the real adventurer, like Marco Polo, Casanova, or Pizarro, lacks an inner life. He lives extraversively, ever looking outward, and for him words are merely tools and so are the ideas they contain. The intellectual lives an inner life, always looking inward, heedful of his ideas and emotions. The man of action does not exist for himself, and the hubbub of the outer world to which he is always tuned does not allow him to hear his inner voice. He is dominated by impulse, not by imagination, which he lacks completely. And imagination is the key to the vocation of the intellectual.

The physician's psychologic conflict is that medicine in all its fields, even in research, is eminently a profession of men of action. This is particularly true of the surgeon, that swordsman of medicine, who thinks with his fingertips and writes with his scalpel, who lives in a perpetual race against the clock, and on whose ability for quick decisions as he works the lives of his patients depend. Even the general practitioner is ever more the man of action as he tries to outrace disease or, at least, to keep up with the present swift pace of science.

The physician was a contemplative man in the times when medicine was mainly theoretical and patients were diagnosed by looking not at their faces and bodies, but at the treatises of Galen and Avicenna. Today the physician is a man of action, living in a perpetual whirl of activity, like the country doctor, or immersed in an endless series of short, broken episodes enacted by the long stream of patients at his office or at the hospital.

The physician therefore may very well decide as the days whirl by that he cannot allow himself the luxury of writing, for it would mean, he feels, turning his back on impulse and action only to favor imagination and art. And yet cultivation of the imagination would make of him the ideal physician anticipated by Osler: the physician who can alternate hours of intense action with hours of meditation and reflection that might result in a great medical treatise, just as the hours of action might result in a scientific discovery or a new clinical method.

The physician should realize that writing is another form of action, indeed one of the most dynamic, and that the use of words to communicate his ideas can also make him a man of action, not only in space, by being able to reach physicians the world over, but also in time, by leaving behind him written thoughts to assist his successors from generation to generation. It is the duty of the physician, who is one of the makers of modern history, to believe in himself not only as a man of action in space, but also as a creator in time. The only way of doing something worth while in time is to use the written word, our only means of reaching the future, just as reading is our only means of communicating with the past.

THE PSYCHOLOGIC MOTIVES OF THE PHYSICIAN-WRITER

(a) *The Premature Choice of a Profession.* Why does a physician write literature? We are not referring only to those physicians who have become famous as writers, but also to those others who, apart from their professional work, translate their literary leanings into poems, short stories, novels, or philosophic and historical essays.

The first answer that comes to mind is that many physicians choose a medical career because, their minds not being as yet mature, the profession appears to them romantic, sentimental, and humanitarian. Medicine to them is the *camino real* to the fulfillment of their dreams. This was what happened to Maeterlinck, a frustrated physician who thought of medicine as a golden key to the most secret recesses of the soul.

Years later, many physicians discover that they are interested in life not so much as a general philosophic problem, as in the case of the "pure" scientific researcher, nor as an individual practical problem, as with the practicing physician, but as a psychologic problem.

This impels them belatedly to write as a means of expressing their most secret yearnings.

It is a curious paradox that during the romantic movement, a period of intense individualism, life mattered more as a general and abstract problem, while today, at the very height of a collectivist period, life matters more as an individual and psychologic problem.

(b) *Escape from Professional Life.* The physician, whether he has literary leanings or not, is attracted to literature more than other professionals, perhaps as a reaction against the painful, many times hopeless, surroundings of his work. The hospital, the laboratory, the medical institution would probably end by exhausting him and drying him up spiritually were it not for the vital sap that he can derive from a mere glimpse into the world of letters. Literature, more than painting or sculpture, can provide the door through which the physician may escape temporarily from the shadow-world of disease into the light-world of fancy. Just as Goethe, by "killing" Werther, sublimated through artistic creation his sorrow at losing his own Carlotta, so does the physician sublimate through literature his anguish in the face of pain.

(c) *The Secret Vocation.* The human being generally is not born a physician, a lawyer, a mason, or a carpenter. He often harbors within himself an ideal program of achievements in life which more often than not the need for survival compels him to forego. We all harbor in our minds a whole world of success dreams, and our success in life is measured by the extent to which the realization of such dreams fills out our social profile. There are some professional people whose life seemingly has a wide, well-filled social profile; but let one peer intently into it and one discovers within the elaborate frame of success a pitifully wasted creature, languishing under the defeat of his youthful illusions. In the eyes of many a successful physician there lurks the figure of a melancholy child who never saw his dreams fulfilled.

Literature opens the gate to those possibilities that every one of us entertains in his mind, to those "unlived lives" that we all conceal in our hearts, and to the complex vocations that form a constellation around our "official" calling. There are times, however, when, after timidly allowing it leash, one of these secondary vocations swells to gigantic stature, sweeping us off our feet and compelling us, like a triumphant and all-powerful demon, into a path quite different from that which we had been following. For this secondary vocation, not the "official" one, this secret and private vocation, not the public and social one, was indeed our true vocation. This is what happened to those physician-fugitives from medicine who became successful writers.

(d) *A "Reserve" Preoccupation.* Literature, moreover, can compensate for that monotony inevitable in the medical and any other profession. A physician who is only a physician and nothing more can grow very bored with life; so can an engineer or a lawyer. Contact with our professional environment to the exclusion of everything else has a mechanizing effect; it turns us into automata. We can be saved only by a "secondary" existence with a certain amount of that disorder, that negation of regularity, that is intrinsic to artistic invention.* There is a sort of creative chaos that can save us from the boredom of the mechanized profession (the artist himself sometimes gets fed up with the world of inspiration and seeks relief in some manual labor), and by offering us a "reserve" preoccupation, it can preserve us from deadly tedium, just as our organic reserves of fat and sugar, as Marañón has pointed out, protect us from the dangers of fasting.

Now, it so happens that many times literature, which the physician adopted as a secondary activity, ends by getting the upper hand as a revenge against his false vocation and to the triumph of his true vocation. The physician then ceases to be an actor in life and becomes what the artist is—an observer of life. Even the most famous men of science do not escape this inexorable need to combine science with art in their life, whether it be writing short stories, as Cajal did in the cafés of Madrid, or composing sonatas and philosophic essays, as Albert Schweitzer has done in the heart of the African jungle.

Moreover, the physician has more things to tell than the ordinary writer, for he accumulates a rich store of human subjects in the course of his professional duties. The specific medical range of subjects, however, is extremely limited, since conflicts with pain, as with sin, are limited in themselves. A physician or a sinner who relates exclusively the sufferings of pain or the pleasures of sin would soon prove himself unbearably monotonous and boresome unless he embellishes his tales with the trappings of literature. This Axel Munthe did with medicine and Casanova with sin. They wrote literature because they painted their stories with the magic brush of their art.

(e) *The Craving for Immortality.* Another reason the physician has for "making" literature is that he is aware that a medical document not only is comparatively anonymous, but has a relatively short life. Medical writing and medical discovery outside the

---

* "While medicine is your vocation, or calling, see to it that you have also an avocation—some intellectual pastime which may serve to keep you in touch with the world of art, of science, or of letters. Begin at once the cultivation of some interest other than the purely professional. The difficulty is in a selection and the choice will be different according to your tastes and training."—Osler, *Aequanimitas and Other Addresses.*

professional sphere receive very limited or no recognition. (How many "men in the street," for instance, know today who was the discoverer of the antidiphtheria serum, or of chloramphenicol, or of the microscope?) The name of the medical discoverer or writer is all too soon forgotten. On the other hand, artistic creation lasts forever. The same "men in the street" who do not know the name of the inventor of the thermometer they so often use, or of the discoverer of streptomycin to which they may owe their lives, can probably tell you who did the "Moses" or "The Night Watch." Scientific discovery lasts through the ages, but it is never identified with the name of its discoverer. The work of Aristotle, Einstein, Descartes, and Vesalius, though everlasting, is not associated with the personalities of their authors. But artistic work not only is itself immortal, but also gives immortality to its creator. This is what subconsciously impels the physician and the scientist to turn to literature; it is a means of gaining the immortality that is forbidden to them as physicians.

People are rather suspicious when dealing with physicians who are also writers. A plumber in the building in which I live recently asked me to recommend a physician, "but not one of those who write books." These people are right to mistrust the physician who devotes more interest to his writing than to his patients; but they ought to know also that the physician who knows only medicine and nothing else does not even know medicine, and that creative activity makes a much better physician by making him a better man.

THE DUTY OF WRITING

For a considerable time now I have been preaching (no doubt in the desert, which is where all preaching, inevitably, begins and ends) the duty of the modern physician to write, a duty that is forgotten and neglected more and more.

Today many people write when they want to dazzle others with their knowledge, or when they hanker to see their name on a book. But very little is written communicating each one's spiritual experiences. It is vital that the physician write more. For this purpose, he must learn to meditate; he must withdraw from the madding crowd and concentrate on the search for that inner light almost extinguished under the glitter of city lights.

Once, when planning one of his major works, El Greco shut himself in his darkened studio while, outside, the imperial city of Toledo glittered like a fine-cut gem under the golden Spanish sun and doves fluttered in the clear blue sky like white kerchiefs waving good-by. "Come out into the sunshine," his disciples cried out to him, and El Greco answered, "My light is in myself."

Cultivation of belles-lettres in any of its forms would also be of great value to the physician in improving his professional writing. By helping him to be more articulate, it would improve his technique, which, in turn, would induce him to write more. "A bad book is as much a labor to write as a good book," Aldous Huxley has said.

CLARITY IS IMPERATIVE

"Speak clearly, gently, truly, properly."

(The Oath of the Hindu Physician, c. 300 B.C.)

It is vital to cultivate the habit of writing with clarity, simplicity, and euphony. Everything must be sacrificed to clarity. Even truth itself ceases to be truth when it becomes entangled in the coils of a verbose prose. There have been orators in history who, before addressing their audience, have read over several pages of a dictionary or of the Bible in order to impart simplicity and conciseness to their speech. Reading the great masters of prose is a means to this same end. It all helps to acquire the great classical frame of learning compounded of serenity, tradition, and judgment.*

Writing has to be a labor of love for the physician. His books must be the result of well-planned meditation. In *Don Quixote,* Cervantes had this to say about historical literature:

> History is a sacred kind of writing, because truth is essential to it . . . notwithstanding which there are those who compose books and toss them out into the world like fritters. . . .
>
> There are few books so bad, said the bachelor, but there is something good in them.
>
> There is no doubt of that, replied Don Quixote, but it often happens that they, who have deservedly acquired a good share of reputation by their writings, lessen or lose it entirely by committing them to the press.
>
> The reason of that, said Sampson, is that printed works being examined at leisure, the faults thereof are the more easily discovered; and the greater the fame of the author is, the more strict and severe is the scrutiny. . . . And therefore I say that whoever prints a book runs a very great risk, it being of all impossibilities the most impossible to write such an one, as shall satisfy all kinds of readers. . . .
>
> Does the Author aim at money and profit?—said Sancho Panza. It will be a wonder then if he succeeds, since he will only stitch it away in great haste

---

* An artistic pastime helps the physician to acquire greater culture, replacing his erudition by humanism, his specialization by encyclopedic knowledge, since the best specialist is he who has a more universal mind, not he who is symbolized in the sarcastic definition made by a nasty joker: "A specialist is a man who knows much about little, and who successively knows more and more about less and less, until finally he knows practically all about nothing. An encyclopedist is a man who knows very little about much, and who successively knows less and less about more until finally he knows practically nothing about everything."

like a tailor on Easter-eve; for works that are done hastily are never finished with that perfection they require.*

A knowledge of literature helps to develop clarity in scientific expression. "In science," as Marañón has said, "the form in which truth is clothed is part of truth itself, and truth being clear by nature, the art of clarity is a scientific factor of the first importance." Writers would have much to gain if they were to read, as the Cubist painter, Juan Gris, did in his leisure hours, scientific works to temper down their rhetoric, just as scientists would also gain beauty of style by practicing a literary discipline.

Scientific prose can be clear without sacrificing beauty, as shown by Cajal's works, and beautiful literature can also be scientifically accurate, as shown by Vergil's exquisite versified description of swine fever. The elegance of medical writing lies in clarity. When it is nonexistent, as in present-day psychoanalytic texts, it impedes the progress of science, as has happened in psychiatry.

In order to communicate effectively, the physician must learn the technique of gracefully alternating short and long periods. He must use adjectives sparingly and substantives lavishly. The Spanish philosopher, Miguel de Unamuno, once remarked, "We must speak in substantives!" The physician-writer must not fear the repetition of concepts, since without repetition it is difficult to impart knowledge.

I have elsewhere said that I do not believe in the so-called "rules for good medical writing" laid down, in many cases, by nonmedical writers who, with no other encouragement than the patience of their readers, have presumed to arbitrate on such matters. I believe in clarity. I also believe in beauty of style, in the metaphor, in the lengthy phrase when it suits the case, in the unusual word when it is exact in definition and rich in meaning—in short, I believe in quite a lot that is now being banished from medical writing by those who evidently do not know that these very qualities made the prose of Osler and Cajal great and imperishable.

I also advocate something else that American medical literature has almost completely eliminated—the literary quotation and poetic, philosophic, and classical allusions. In this respect, I salute the *British Medical Journal* and *Lancet,* which, like *La Presse Médicale* in France and the medical journals of Spain and Italy, have preserved a humanistic tradition in medicine. I believe that it is now time to reinstate this noble tradition in this country.

WORDS AND IDEAS

To write is to communicate ideas by means of words, which, ac-

* From the World's Classics edition of *Don Quixote,* translated by Charles Jervas, Oxford University Press, London, 1928, Book II, Chapter iii, pp. 31–32.

cording to Aldous Huxley,* are man's foremost and greatest invention.

The social need for writing was born in the dawn of civilization. After the grunt, the shout, and the spoken word came the transmission of thought by means of graphic and plastic signs. At first, writing, being more ideographic than phonetic since it represented ideas rather than sounds and words, consisted in drawing objects and things, after which followed hieroglyphic or symbolic writing, and finally artistic or plastic writing.

"Writing," in the words of Abraham Lincoln, "the art of communicating thoughts to the mind through the eyes, is the greatest invention of the world—great in enabling us to converse with the dead, the absent and the unborn; and great not only in its direct benefits, but greatest help to all the inventions."

Now writing is done by means of words, and these should be "invisible" while clearly revealing the ideas they embody, just as a fine glass brings out the rich color of a red wine while it itself remains imperceptible. Language should fit ideas in the same way that tights fit the acrobat, accentuating the contours they cover, instead of deforming or concealing them as crinoline skirts once did to women's figures.

Nowhere is clarity so important as in the description of scientific methods and apparatus. This type of writing puts the writer to the supreme test of clarity. The monk Benito Feijóo, in his *Theatre* and

---

* "That is the test for the literary mind, the feeling of magic, the sense that words have power. The technical, verbal part of literature is simply a development of magic. Words are man's first and most grandiose invention. With language he created a whole new universe; what wonder if he loved words and attributed power to them? With fitted, harmonious words the magicians summoned rabbits out of empty hats and spirits from the elements. Their descendants, the literary men, still go on with the process, mortising their verbal formulas together and, before the power of the finished spell, trembling with delight and awe. Rabbits out of empty hats? No, their spells are more subtly powerful for they evoke emotions out of empty minds." (Chapter XX.)
"The pleasures of human contacts are much exaggerated. . . . It seems to me doubtful whether they are equal to the pleasures of private reading and contemplation. Human contacts have been so highly valued in the past only because reading was not a common accomplishment and because books were scarce and difficult to reproduce. *The world, you must remember, is only just becoming literate.* As reading becomes more and more habitual and widespread, an ever-increasing number of people will discover that books will give them all the pleasures of social life and none of its intolerable tedium. At present people in search of pleasure tend to congregate in large herds and to make a noise; *in the future their natural tendency will be to seek for solitude and quiet.* The proper study of mankind is books." (Chapter XXVIII.)— Aldous Huxley, *Crome Yellow.*

Cartas, created scientific Spanish, as borne out by his descriptions of the "magic lantern" (*Teatro,* III, 11, 12 and 13) or of the air-pump (*Teatro,* V, IX, final note). Cajal left descriptions of laboratory techniques that are unsurpassable models of clarity and conciseness. Such manner of writing is not to be learned in correspondence courses, but by extensive reading of good literature.

WRITING IS A SOLITARY ART

This kind of writing demands solitude, something rarely granted to the physician unless he sacrifices his hours of rest or pleasure. Writing is the most solitary of all occupations. It is also the most sublime of the arts. While other arts always require certain special and sometimes costly tools—canvases, paints, brushes, chisels, marble, a grand piano, models—writing requires only the most humble of tools—a pencil stub and a few sheets of paper—yet it is possible with these to create a masterpiece that may embody the melody of a symphony, the rhythm of a ballet, the coloring of a fresco, and the cadences of a poem, transcending all barriers of time and space. Literature indeed is the embodiment of all the arts.

Writing is, we repeat, the most solitary of the arts. The best place for writing is inside the writer's head, as Hemingway has said. And Vicente Blasco Ibáñez recommended as the writer's best equipment "a good set of kidneys" and the fortitude to remain seated eight or ten hours a day. Writing being then a lonesome task, most famous writers led a quiet, uneventful life. When they indulged in some action, they did little or no writing. To write their best, they had to withdraw from the world and even from love and happiness and be a slave to their pen. When a man of action such as Casanova turns writer, he has to cease being the man of action and become a spectator of his own life. The writer (so I heard the philosopher, Ortega y Gasset, in Madrid, describe him) is a man who does not live, but contemplates how others live.

GOOD WRITING STARTS WITH THE CLINICAL CASE HISTORY

From what has been said herein, it can be deduced that I advise the physician to "make" literature even when he is writing on medicine. Even if he has but little creative talent, he should assiduously encourage it, counterbalancing his hours of research and clinical practice with the cultivation of good writing, using for material the thousand facets of life that file daily before his eyes. Let him begin by exercising his imagination when writing his next case history.

Elsewhere I have pointed out the historicomedical importance of the case history as a record of the medical learning at any particular period in history. A good case history can be of more importance (may laboratory workers forgive me this heresy) than an extensive examination complete with analyses, for a good case history reveals not only the patient's past and present life, his morphology and the biographico-pathologic course of his existence, but also the repercussions of his organic, humoral picture on his soma and psyche.

A good clinical case history makes it possible today to diagnose the disease of a slave of the Egyptian Pharaohs or of Imperial Rome, of a warrior from the times of the Incas, or an Emperor of the Ming dynasty, or a Doge from Venice, or a King of the Austrian dynasty in Spain. A clinical case history was of yore a precious document, fashioned with love and respect by the physician. Today, it is indifferently committed to the hands of a subaltern. In this manner we are losing the habit of careful anamnesis, without which there can be no truly scientific medicine.

The clinical case history is the basic medicoliterary document of medicine. A good clinical case history, like a well-written short story, should have a "beginning," the patient's personal and family antecedents, a "middle," the patient's present problem, and an "end." This "end," of course, is foreshadowed projectively by the prognosis.

To demand clinical case histories based on observation by the physician of the patient as a human being is to compel the physician to write better and to write more. To write a good clinical case history is to be a clinical novelist. It is to know how to observe shrewdly and how to describe vividly. It is to make the reader subconsciously identify himself with the patient, just as the good novelist makes his reader identify himself with the hero.

There is one other essential quality: to know how to apply one's imagination in interpreting a chart or in reading a laboratory tabulation. A table containing a patient's diastolic and systolic pressures, blood viscosity, pulse, temperatures, etc., to the untrained person is no more than a mass of figures. But to the clinician, unless he has grown insensitive and callous, such a table is the drama of a human being fighting for life.

To train his mind in literature will help the physician to see, to interpret, and to describe better—all attributes of the great artist and the great physician. Medicine is the most dramatic of all the professions. Why are we bent on mechanizing it? Why not follow the example of the great classical masters? They never allowed science to destroy their sense of the tragic or their compassion for mankind.

Today's clinical case histories are arid documents without any dramatic worth, except perhaps for psychiatric cases. These, unfortunately, are crammed with such psychoanalytic jargon that they are unintelligible even to the psychiatrists. Hippocrates' clinical histories, the medieval *consilia,* Sydenham's and Freud's case histories—reading these one feels once more that sense of greatness in clinical narration which has been lost in the ruling craze for "technical" expression.

A true portrait in words, a vivid verbal image of the patient's past and present, and a preview of his future—this is what a clinical case history should be. And this would be not only good writing but, above all, good medicine.

THE NECESSITY OF KNOWING HOW TO "FIND" TIME

Of course, the busy physician will contend that it is extremely difficult to write when one has no time to spare, and besides not everybody possesses the natural talent to become a writer.

Granted that not everyone can be a mine of productivity like Lope de Vega,* who was more prolific than anyone else in the history of literature, and that not everyone can produce a complete novel in one day like Georges Simenon, the Belgian novelist. On the other hand, nothing, not even illness, can stop a man if he really craves to write. The Italian writer, Giovanni Papini, though completely paralyzed, went on writing until the time of his death. He had cards made bearing the letters of the alphabet and, by winking his eyes, he would indicate to his niece the cards that would form the words he wanted. It would take him a whole week to write a very short piece. The contemporary Austrian poet, Hieronymus Lorn, lost his sight and hearing at the age of eight; but right up to his death in his seventy-second year, he composed verses and other pieces by pressing his fingers on the hand of a relative.

The secret of prolificness in writing is simple: first, to be methodical and persevering; and, second, to employ fruitfully those precious minutes and seconds, that "golden dust of time," wasted in unnecessary telephone conversations, in reading rehashed news, in watching

---

* No writer in history wrote so much and so fast as the Spaniard Félix Lope de Vega. He averaged more than twenty sheets a day all his life and wrote more than 400 plays in less than twenty-four hours each. He wrote books in prose and poems by the hundreds, ranging from religious sonnets to light odes. But, above all, he wrote plays—*more than 2200!* They include 1800 plays and more than 400 *autos sacramentales* or religious plays. For over half a century Lope de Vega, *"el mónstruo de la naturaleza"* (nature's "monster"), satisfied world audiences from Mexico to the Sultan's seraglio at Constantinople. He alone created an entire literature like the force of nature he was.

worthless television programs, and, particularly, in abating those de-
vourers of time, "chronophages" as Molière called them, who having
nothing to do themselves will allow no one to do anything either.*

THE THEMES OF THE "NEW" LITERATURE

The physician interested in writing literature has one thing in his
favor: the fondness of former times for stories of distant lands entailing long sea journeys has disappeared. We still remember the
France of Balzac, the Italy of Mazzini, the Russia of Tolstoy, the
Spain of Cervantes; but the vehicles that brought them to us, those
long volumes of yesteryear, have all but vanished, except maybe for
some historical novels which provide modern man's escape on the
plane of time just as the aforementioned long tales provided escape
from the limitations of space.

Formerly reading was the only road to dreamland. Nowadays there
is the cinema and television. Then there are the complexities of modern life which leave no time for lengthy stories nor the peace of mind
for following the comings and goings of a vast number of characters.
The present trend toward the short novel was anticipated a long time
ago by Chekhov when he stated, "The art of good writing is the art
of abbreviation."

Today people crave to explore the landscape of the mind, the jungle of the instincts, the wildwoods of all the passions. No one is better
prepared than the physician to satisfy this craving. Man today anx-
iously searches for man. Beyond anything else, he is interested in
dissecting, fiber by fiber, the human soul on the smooth marble slab
of succinct, lucid writing. The mature man of today prefers to read
about real human beings rather than about fictitious characters, as in
former days. This psychologic preoccupation in today's art is not
merely a token of the impact of Freud; it is also a proof of the "in-
trahumanization" of art. The literature of today is studded with
hearts throbbing with the same immortal stimuli—love, jealousy,
power—that throbbed behind the tightlaced stays of the women portrayed by the Impressionists.

No one indeed is so apt as the physician for writing the naturalistic, experimental, psychologic literature craved by people today,
which shrouds the mystery that lies behind our present age.

The most successful novels still rely on a few worthy literary
themes—the vagabond, the return of Ulysses to Penelope, the damnation of Faust, the quest of Don Quixote, the conflict of Hamlet,
the journey to eternity in the Divine Comedy. These themes recur

* See page 22.

time and again, for they are archetypes with a universal appeal and a firm hold on the human mind. Nor is there anybody better equipped than the physician to know and explore these archetypes in literature.*

MINERVA AND AESCULAPIUS

Our age is still witnessing the antagonism between Truth and Beauty, Minerva and Venus, incarnate in the antinomic conflict (so brilliantly outlined by my teacher the psychiatrist Emilio Mira) between artists interested in form and the incommensurable, whose tool is passion and whose goal is beauty, and scientists interested only in the measurable and the substantial, whose tool is logic and whose goal is that truth as they see it shall be made incontrovertible. Each of them from his lofty ivory tower is hampering the progress of science and art.

Pure art has become dehumanized and abstract or industrialized and strictly utilitarian. The artisan is replacing the artist. A similar occurrence in science is responsible for today's "pure" scientist and the scientific technician. Nevertheless, in pure science, research does reach a point where intuition is of more avail than reason and where there is a need for that passion which Pavlov recommended as an essential quality in the man of science.

Science and art can and must help each other, as has indeed already happened in the field of the cinema, in functional architecture, and in applied psychology. It is imperative to bind and bind again the scientist and the artist. Let us not forget that the inner meaning of the word "religion" (from the Latin *religare*) is to bind the human mind to that which is essential for its spiritual life.

Minerva and Aesculapius must come together again, as they were originally in the brain of Jupiter. From the union of Minerva and Aesculapius, from a Medicine accepting the principles and ideals of art, and from an Art accepting the experimental method and the humanism of Medicine, there shall arise the physician who will recon-

---

* "It helps a man immensely to be a bit of a hero worshipper, and the stories of the lives of the masters of medicine do much to stimulate our ambition and rouse our sympathies. If the life and work of such men as Bichat and Laënnec will not stir the blood of a young man and make him feel proud of France and of Frenchmen, he must be a dull and muddy-mettled rascal. In reading the life of Hunter, of Jenner, who thinks of the nationality which is merged and lost in our interest in the man and in his work! In the halcyon days of the Renaissance there was no nationalism in medicine, but a fine catholic spirit made great leaders like Vesalius, Eustachius, Stenson and others at home in every country in Europe."—Osler, *Aequanimitas and Other Essays.*

cile learning with kindness, reason with passion, and truth with beauty. In the words of Hermann Boerhaave (*Institutiones Medicae,* 1708):

> "Imagine a man applying himself to study the first principles of medicine. . . . He learns by precept and example how to distinguish clearly the evident from the obscure, the false from the true. . . . He builds for himself a clear idea of the human frame. To this he adds a knowledge of the vital fluids; and tests it in the living person and his excretions by the aid of anatomy, chemistry, hydrostatics and even of the microscope. . . . Now he opens and explores the bodies of those whose maladies he has noted; now he studies the disease he induces upon animals; again he groups together all the results of diseases and of remedies he has tried; again he learns the same things from the best authors; finally, arranging and pondering, he adjusts all things to one another, and, by the means which Theory has shown, he obtains at length a certain grasp of the history and cure in each disease. See then before you the finished picture of the perfect doctor!"

If the physician will add writing to his other tasks, and if he will read and write outside the limits of his particular professional field, he will find himself looking with newly opened eyes upon the wonderful world around us. He will gain a dramatic sense of existence which he will apply to his professional life, just as he will bring to his literary work the sound experimental, naturalistic judgment he has gained from medical training. The physician of today, if he is to help the physician of tomorrow, must learn to speak to them through written words—more and better words. The physician of today can make it possible for Minerva and Aesculapius together to guide him in the performance of his professional duties and in the assertion of his creative rights. Together they can point to him the path at the end of which proudly stands the physician-artist of the future.

II. the tapestry of history

THE ARTIST AS PHYSICIAN

If we had to decide what figures incarnated the greatest medical knowledge available at each period in the history of medicine, we should choose the seer for Mesopotamia, the priest and the philosopher for ancient Greece, the physician-soldier for imperial Rome, the erudite monk and the alchemist for the Arabian and European Middle Ages, and for the Italian Renaissance—the artist and the humanist. Each one of these figures was the leader who provided new impetus for the medicine of his period.

Medicine in the Renaissance made three fundamental advances that paved the way for modern science: it undermined the authority of the old dogmatic medicine, which crumbled like an ancient castle under the weight of the centuries; it laid the scientific foundation for modern anatomy; it took a decisive step forward in pharmaceutical chemistry.

Of these revolutionary advances—personified in the iconoclastic genius of Paracelsus and the naturalistic thought of Vesalius—the most important was the contribution Vesalius made to anatomy with his book, *De Humani Corporis Fabrica*, keystone of modern science. Vesalius' famous anatomic illustrations crystallized all that Renaissance artists had evolved before him.

The psychologic and historical analysis of Renaissance art and culture will help us ferret out the secret of that amazing outburst of anatomic illustration underlying the Renaissance progress in medical sciences.

A lecture delivered at the Fourteenth International Congress of the History of Medicine, Rome, Italy, September 13-20, 1954; published in *International Record of Medicine 167*:221, 1954.

Most histories of medicine record medical ideas as emerging one from the other in logical and inevitable sequence. Human intelligence, however, does not function in this self-contained manner but is directed by the imperative needs in our life. Thought is a reaction to pre-intellectual human needs. Any given intellectual occupation is preceded by an emotional *pre*-occupation. Man does not concern himself with knowing simply because he is endowed with a mind. Underneath that generic knowledge called science, there is a vital function that inspires it: belief. And when man wavers between two beliefs without choosing one or the other, he is living through a historical crisis. That is what occurred in the Renaissance.

In the thirteenth century—apex of the fabulous period starting with Albertus Magnus and ending with Saint Thomas Aquinas—man pitched his tent in a world where he was guided by one single idea to which all the needles of the medieval compass pointed: the Divinity.

From the Crusades, the most extravagant adventures ever undertaken by human beings, Western man returned a military failure but facing a glorious future. For in his travels he established contact with an Arabic civilization impregnated with Greek culture, and when he returned home he brought, strapped on the back of his horse, the rich booty of Arabico-Hellenic wisdom.

And so there fell upon warring Christian Europe—which was hardly intellectual and not one bit scientific—a shower of new knowledge fed by ancient Greek science and based therefore on pure reason. Instead of resisting Aristotelian science, Christianity accepted it and tried to assimilate the fruits of lucid Greek thinking. Albertus Magnus and Saint Thomas Aquinas, the two great medieval philosophers, polished the facets of the Christian diamond in the manner dictated by Greek ideology.

This was the second attempt, after Saint Augustine, to Hellenize Christian thought. The Christian *theos* united with the Greek *logos;* the result was a reform of medieval *theo-logy.* The Gothic-evangelic inspiration of the Middle Ages was buried beneath the avalanche of Aristotelian *Corpus.* For the Greeks, courage and ingenuity were the keys to existence, just as for the Romans they were a militarized state and a regimented bureaucracy. The Asians, on the other hand, were content simply to live, guided by the hand of God.

During the Renaissance, the relation of man to God changed radically. In primitive societies, man was concerned with seeking a relationship with God; in the Renaissance, with nature; whereas in our era man attempts to find his relationship with man.

When Constantinople and Byzantium fell into Turkish hands, Hellenic knowledge was transposed to the West in the form of Greek manuscripts hidden in the travel pouches of Byzantine scholars. Thus, the vast impetus of Hellenic humanism was set in motion. The word *humanist* became international and was synonymous with that cultural viewpoint that saw in man the measure of all things (the *uomo mensura* of Protagoras). Humanism stimulated scholars to become reacquainted with true Latinity.

Renaissance man joyfully proved that the hoary classical clock of his Greek forebears could still mark the right time. The *humanities* began to challenge the *divinities,* although humanism also embraced religion and established—through Erasmus and Vives—a balance between God and man. In order to compensate for these ideologic and scientific complications, Renaissance man attempted to simplify existence by turning to classicism.

Paradoxically enough, the Renaissance began as man took a step backward and then took the great jump forward. Man was determined to return to a simple culture and even to the stage preceding culture: he wished to return to bare nature. And as man threw off the heavy raiments of medieval philosophy, in that process of simplification which always characterizes despair, he was also ready to unclothe himself artistically.

Science became a wall between man and the symbolic medieval universe. Nature became a screen separating God from man. As man began to predict the future course of cosmic and biologic events, he recovered his lost self-confidence and followed a new humanism, with his very own self as the starting point. From the fifth century, history had traced a Christian path along which man, pushed by despair toward religion and the next world, ascended steadily until the thirteenth century, and then in the Renaissance plummeted back to the earth he had wished to leave behind. In the *quattrocento,* the exhausted medieval skyrockets sputtered down to earth while new ones soared above the horizon.

Renaissance man followed a dramatic pattern of life and required vital tasks to occupy his attention. Although his faith was far less fervent than it had been, he still believed in a medieval God but felt a new confidence in himself and in his world. Having faith, however, is quite different from having concrete knowledge. A historically demonstrable objective truth persists even without men of faith. In the Renaissance, *cognition,* or unlimited knowledge, and *sentire et scire,* or natural perception, replaced faith and medieval scholasticism as basic elements of predominant thought patterns.

Enthusiasm about nature, then, provided the impulse for the study of nature. At first it was only a vague interest in natural things—partially resembling earlier mysticism—which encouraged demonology, astrology, magic, dream interpretation, and alchemy; but then came the desire for the methodical investigation of nature that characterized neo-Platonism. Aristotelianism survived only as a speculative concept of nature.

In the Middle Ages theology led science in the same manner that a totally blind man might lead a half-blind man. It is true that the thirteenth century was a flash of lightning in the dark. But if we recall that the fourteenth century brought a relapse into the darkness of earlier centuries, we see, with Osler, that the thirteenth century was not the dawn that slowly turns into daylight, but an *aurora borealis* that flared up and then went down in the arctic night of medievalism.

THE TIME-AXIS AND THE "VISCERAL" COUNTRIES

In every period of history certain areas of the planet acquire a sudden staggering importance. Karl Jaspers pointed this out when he referred to that *time-axis* when China, India, and Greece became, circa 500 B.C., the spiritual axis of mankind. In every period of history there are certain countries that act as the vital organs of the world, while others remain on the periphery and are mere adipose tissue. In the fifteenth century, three nations stood out as focal organs whose rhythm provided the answer to the problems of that era: Italy, the Low Countries, and Spain.

At the beginning of the fifteenth century, Italy was the heart of Europe, being the most advanced country intellectually and emotionally and almost completely free of the mystical, ideologic circle of the Middle Ages; the Low Countries represented the greatest religious advancement; while Spain made the greatest strides politically. In the Renaissance, the Low Countries planted the seeds of modern religion and Spain founded the modern State; but to Italy belongs the glory of creating the *nuova scienza*.

The historical phenomenon of the Italian Renaissance is essentially Mediterranean. This sudden rebirth of classical ideas, this almost springlike resurrection, recurs periodically in Mediterranean history. Minoan culture was reborn in Periclean Athens. Hellenism reappeared in Alexandria and then again in the Renaissance. This historical rebirth always occurs around the Mediterranean for biologic reasons, among them a propensity to emotionalism and a mental alertness created by paradisiacal climates and by the intermingling of a great number of civilizations. If the history of medieval Europe is contained in the history of Spain, the heart beat of Italy synthesizes the history of the Renaissance.*

---

* The center of gravity was then displaced. If ancient life was cosmocentric and medieval life theocentric, in the Renaissance modern life suddenly became anthropocentric. Though at the beginning of the Renaissance the Gothic still predominated, medieval thought had already become independent of God.

The Renaissance represented a crisis. It was a rebirth. And to be reborn is more important than to be born, for rebirth comes about with full awareness of the fact that one is going to live again. Resurrection has always moved men more deeply than birth itself.

Between the uncertainties of the Middle Ages and the all-embracing intellectualism of the seventeenth century, the Renaissance emerged in deep crisis. As man realized that his world was disintegrating, he fell victim to an uneasiness that lasted from 1400 to 1600. At the dawn of the seventeenth century, he finally found his place in a new world. Galileo and Descartes were his patron saints in the tremendous spiritual exodus.

Man, then, began to live between the sword and the wall. Behind him he left a formulistic Christianity; before him rose a world that looked unalterable. The horizon was closed off on the side of the future. His only alternative was to return to the past philosophically and to enjoy the present physically. Since a disintegrating tradition failed him and he foresaw only a confused, dark future, man had to turn inward, upon himself, upon his body, and to nature as his last resources.

Many different factors were involved in this formidable growth of individualism and relaxation of authority: rationalism, freedom of thought and opinion, the circumnavigation of the globe by Spaniards and Portuguese and later by the English and Dutch, the discovery of the printing press which aided in the diffusion of culture (among the incunabula were works on popular medicine as well as the Bible), the discovery of gunpowder which destroyed feudalism, and the discovery of heliocentric astronomy by a Polish physician called Copernicus.

In Italy, the Renaissance began in the fourteenth century with two poets: Dante, critic, historian, and political rebel, and Petrarch, who heralded a return to nature and the classics. Italy, still recovering from pestilence and war, felt the need for new intellectual triumphs— a triumph over the constellations in the heavens, over the countries beyond the seas, over the secrets of the human body. Man replaced God Himself as the center of interest.

It was a portentous era. Great names rose on the horizon like new dawns. It was the era of Lorenzo the Magnificent and the House of Medici, of Ludovico il Moro and the House of Sforza, of Popes Julius II and Leo X, the Borgias—Rodrigo, Cesare, Lucrezia— Machiavelli, Michelangelo, Savonarola, Castiglione, Cellini, Gutenberg, Titian, Holbein, Erasmus, Dürer, Bramante, Pico della Mirandola, François Villon, Botticelli, Isabel and Ferdinand, Columbus,

Torricelli, Pinturicchio, Calcar, Charles V, and Luther. It was the era of Raphael, El Greco, Giotto, Fra Angelico, Cortés, Balboa, Pizarro, Magellan, Rabelais, Servetus, Cervantes, Lope de Vega, Chaucer, Shakespeare, Calvin, Saint Theresa, Saint Ignatius of Loyola, Tycho Brahe, Galileo, Kepler, Cesalpino, Paré, Bacon and Copernicus, Leonardo, and Vesalius.

It was an era of sumptuous palaces, fabulous jewels, gorgeous velvets and silks, exquisite gold and silver work, magnificent weapons, proud statues, and gigantic cathedrals. It was the era of the Inquisition, of struggles among barons, popes, feudal lords, and *condottieri*. The class struggle had begun with the Magna Carta, but the struggle of faiths reached its height with the Reformation. It was a period that marked the foundation of universities run like democracies at Freiburg, Basel, Thuringia, Toledo, and Valencia. Granada was conquered and the Moors were expelled from Spain. And the Americas were discovered.

PURPOSES AND ORIENTATION OF RENAISSANCE MEDICINE

During this glorious rebirth of culture, the *leaders* of medicine were the artists, who made the greatest contributions to anatomy.

The renaissance of medicine developed parallel with the *re*birth of the arts and literature. The new ideal of human and political individuality brought in its wake the study of the forms and functions of man. Illness ceased to be a divine punishment and became a derangement in the harmony of nature.

Medicine sprang originally from primitive terror of the unknown. It allied itself with magic and later with philosophy and religion; but in the Renaissance, medicine joined forces with art. The rigid, hieratical figures became more human, and anatomic drawings began to reveal the human body. The artist became an anatomist and the physician an artist, as in the cases of Berengarius and Fracastoro. For the new *uomo universalis,* who replaced the *uomo sanctus* and *uomo doctus* of former days, anatomy became the basis for the teaching of medicine.

A passion for exploration and the worship of antiquity were antagonistic forces in the Renaissance. But the *nuova scienza* won the battle. In 1543 and 1546, three books, which were to become decisive in the history of scientific thought, appeared: *De Humani Corporis Fabrica* by Vesalius, *De Revolutionibus Orbium Coelestium* by Nicolaus Copernicus, and the *De Contagione et Contagiosis Morbis* by Girolamo Fracastoro. These three men had studied medicine at the University of Padua and were the standard-bearers in the struggle against the entrenched principles of Galen and Ptolemy. Before them, medical texts had been mere philosophic tracts, and teaching had been syllogistic and theoretical dialectic. But from Vesalius on, editions of the old Hippocratic *Summa* and Galenic *Corpus* with commentaries sprang up everywhere.

The Middle Ages, especially the thirteenth century, were in a sense a period of splendor. Men built magnificent cathedrals with huge stained-glass windows through which the sun dressed the faithful kneeling in prayer in glittering colors. Dante, too, marked a high point in the history of the world. But if in theology the thirteenth century produced an incomparable trio—Abelard, Albertus Magnus, and Thomas Aquinas,—in the field of medicine it produced nothing, and man remained enslaved to Greek and Arabic theories. The flame of medical knowledge kindled by the Arabs with Greek lamps, which had shone without interruption from the eighth to the thirteenth centuries, was a flame that yielded no creative warmth.

In the Renaissance, interest in the classical world was revived when humanists like Linacre, Fracastoro, Gesner, and Caius, who were naturalists and botanists as well as physicians, rediscovered Greek philosophicoscientific thought and, "with the New Testament in one hand and Aristotle in the other, resuscitated Greece." (Osler)

In addition, there was an awakening of interest in the anatomic structures of the human body, a movement spurred on by artists with a physician's mind, like Leonardo, and by physicians with the soul of an artist, like Vesalius. The printing press made the diffusion of classic texts possible and anatomic illustrations replaced symbolic drawings.

If Renaissance architecture and painting were national, medicine, science, and the universities assumed an international character. In sixteenth century Europe, the University of Padua, wisely governed by the Republic of Venice, protected freedom of thought, which was constantly persecuted in other universities. In Padua, astronomers, mathematicians, and physicians opened new vistas on the future. Copernicus prepared the way for Galileo, Vesalius for Harvey, Fracastoro for modern pathology. That century saw a revolution against the dogmatism of the medical classics—especially against the authority of Galen and Avicenna—which had kept physicians intellectually enslaved for over two thousand years. It was a real revolution, with Paracelsus as leader. And in the seventeenth century, men gave meaning and function to the anatomic structures of the human body discovered in the Renaissance.[A]

ART AND MEDICINE

In order to comprehend the role played by Renaissance art in the development of medicine, we should remember that medical science and art have been closely related for long periods in history. In ancient civilizations, medicine, art, and religion formed an indissoluble trinity. The priest of primitive cultures was also the medicine man, and, besides acting as an intermediary between the gods and the people, he used his influence with the deities to cure the sick. He was also the first patron of the arts, since he had to present the deities to his people in the most artistic form, which forced him to seek artists who could fashion the best images of the gods. The priest, therefore, was not only a healer but also a Maecenas.

In the Middle Ages, the trinity disintegrated and the medicine man and the artist became specialized figures, although art continued subserving religion. But in the Renaissance, art and medicine were again united. The need for representing the parts of the body with exactness forced the artist and the physician to become one and the same. But until dissections were authorized, the artist was forced to use diagrams of animals or to make imaginary drawings of the human body.

Because disease is a dynamic process it can be fully described in words or, as it is done today, shown on a screen. Plastically, however, only one phase at a time in the course of the disease can be portrayed. This the Renaissance artist did when he painted the portrait of an important person who happened to be sick. He did realize, however, that anatomic structures could be better depicted with a brush or a mallet than with words. The human body, a *terra incognita* that, like the new continents that were then being discovered, had to be explored, began to yield its secrets to the artist, who had the advantage over the physician of having a keen eye—*sapere vedere,* as Leonardo said.

The history of anatomy changed the day that an Italian artist, in order to carve a wooden crucifix for a church in Florence, obtained permission from the prior to remove the skin from a corpse and study its muscular anatomy.

ART IN THE RENAISSANCE

The historical period that stretched from the birth of Leonardo da Vinci to the death of Michelangelo was characterized by a return to nature and the study of the human physical form. Florentine painting and sculpture, the essential arts of the Renaissance, reveal a mystical softness and sad vigor which reflect their medieval roots and the religious fanaticism of Savonarola and the popes. They also reveal a pagan humanism that is a faithful image of the licentious court of the Medicis.

Renaissance art is turbulent and restless. It is the expression of a society continuously torn by religious and civil strife and by somber visions of the hereafter, which are still an integral part of the Florentine school. Enthusiasm about nature, and about man as nature's noblest manifestation, encouraged a methodical investigation of nature through neo-Platonic philosophy. Moral life was reinvigorated, and the human mind turned back to the models of ancient art. In the social order, manners were elegant but corrupt and violent. *Virtu,* that compound of despotism and cunning which Machiavelli advised the Prince to cultivate as an indispensable quality; *onore,* described by Baldassare Castiglione in his *Il Cortegiano;* religious fanaticism; and excessive violence encouraged by the silence of public opinion— these were the determining factors in the shaping of Renaissance art.

Reflecting this restless atmosphere, Florentine art leaned to melancholy and languid grace as easily as to happiness or tormented painful realism. The major reason for this was Christianity which, primarily through the voice of St. Francis of Assisi, defied pain, anathematized the flesh, and adopted an attitude of mystic tenderness. Exuberant vitality and admirable anatomic precision were evident everywhere. Sculpture had a delicate firmness of line with a high level of tactile values; it represented a careful study of the morphology of man in repose or in action. Every line and color in painting throbbed with life.

The contribution that Renaissance artists made to medicine was more than mere inconographic documentation or a series of static and dynamic morphologic observations; it was an awakening of interest in biologic man, a bending of studious minds to the observation of the form and functions of the human organism.

Disregarding symbolism and the mystical subtleties of medieval disquisitions, the artist aroused popular attention through his simple representation of nature and of man in his complex and beautiful nudity. Thus, the mind was directed toward science along the royal road of beauty.

Before the Renaissance, the artist created only stylized, almost imaginary, figures. But the Renaissance artist believed that the greatest beauty lay in a faithful copy of reality. In order to become acquainted with the human original, the artist studied details of external morphology as well as internal structure. Man became an object of physical study. A knowledge of man could be obtained, the artist realized, not by drawing away from him, as in the Middle Ages, not by depending on occult philosophies and astrology, but by closely observing the human being. Landscape became a backdrop. Michelangelo, dictator of this school, declared that the true object of art was man. With the decline of great art, landscape would be painted again, but it would still be only "a setting for pastorals and pomp" (Taine), a noble, measured accompaniment of "mythological gallantries and lordly outings."

This artistic interest in man had strong repercussions in medicine. The physicians of the time were influenced by the artistic trend and, instead of studying man and his pathology through symbols and vague analogies, they proceeded by deduction and the linking of facts substantiated by data gathered directly from man himself.

Italian painting in the Renaissance ceased to be mystical and theological, as it had been from Giotto to Fra Angelico, and became sensual and pagan. Paintings no longer depicted the dreamy Magdalenes, pensive Virgins, and tragic martyrs of the old school of Bologna. The primary objective of painting was "to paint well a nude man or a nude woman," as Benvenuto Cellini stated. Artists used sculpture as their starting point, for they could palpate the muscles, curves, and bones. They wished to create a healthy, dynamic human body. Theirs was the Greek ideal of man: athletic, caught in a fine plastic posture, as if to tell God what He could have done with man if He had so desired.

Renaissance man experienced a strange dualism: to the dreams of the fanatic he joined the keen insight of the intellectual. Like the former, he thought in images, and like the latter, he arranged them. Perfect physical forms were born and stylized in pictures.

THE PSYCHOLOGIC MEANING OF RENAISSANCE ANATOMIC ART

What underlay the interest that the Renaissance artist took in the human body, in vigorous dynamic figures?

The answer is based on a psychologic fact. Art is escape. Art is flight from reality. The painter entrusts his most intimate feelings, desires, and anxieties to canvas. The "outer" art of a given period mirrors only the external appearance of that period, its *mise-en-scène*, its pretexts. But true painting reflects what did *not* happen at the time, the "unlived lives" of the artist—everything the reality of his times denied him.

The main trend in Greek art was to banish from statuary and painting all sensation of effort; but in doing so, they also eliminated inner life. The anatomic perfection of Greek statues hides an inexorable emptiness. Those polished marbles representing athletes with their muscles fully flexed cover up *man in a state of mental repose*. Medieval art shows *man frightened* by the idea of life beyond death; it is an art of terrorized men who pooled their individual fears in a gigantic collective panic. To the Renaissance belongs *man on the defensive*, a mixture of saint, bourgeois, and adventurer endowed with intense inner vitality.

In order to understand the Renaissance artist's interest in the human body, an interest that ushered in a tremendous rebirth of anatomic studies and that, through Vesalius' efforts, was to open the doors to modern science, we must recall the historicosocial conditions of the period. It was an aggressive and cruel era, without peace or justice, during which exquisite manners covered up violent instincts. Machiavelli justified murder in his writings. Benvenuto Cellini, protected by Pope Paul III, boasted of his innumerable crimes in his *Life,* perhaps the best mirror of the times, and bragged about the blood his sensual indulgences had caused to flow in the streets of Rome. The Borgia Popes, members of a sensual, cruel Valentian family (Borja) that had settled in Rome, used terror as their principal weapon. The fear of death at the hands of tyrants or professional assassins tempered the Renaissance man and tautened his nerves. Such conditions could not but forge a biologic example of man on the defensive, fiery and restless, of ebullient intellect, impetuous in behavior, with an imagination seething with sensual or religious images.

A way of life that commands to kill or be killed naturally awakens a passionate interest in the human body. Every muscle, every movement of the body, acquires suddenly a vital importance, for they can deal life or death. Men therefore were trained à la Cesare Borgia through all sorts of physical exercise, for they were aware of the importance of a quick limb and a mighty muscle in times when ambushes and skirmishes were everyday occurrences.

The lack of justice and the omnipresence of danger engendered great passions in Renaissance man, making him capable of equally enjoying paintings and statues depicting strength and grandeur or innocence and simplicity. People derived the same pleasure from the sight of nude Madonnas as of vigorous warriors. Out of involuntary sympathy, Renaissance man equally enjoyed the bulging muscles of Michelangelo's figures, the health and softness of Raphael's Madonnas, the bold vitality of Donatello's bronzes, the strange beauty of da Vinci's creations, the animal sensuality and athletic power of Titian's or Tintoretto's figures.

Benvenuto Cellini wrote enthusiastically of the "admirable bones of the head, the shoulder-blades which, when the arm is raised, produce magnificent effects, and the five floating ribs which, when the torso is bent back or forward, form marvelous projections about the navel." He also said, "You will draw the bone that is located between the hips; it is very beautiful and is called the coccyx or sacrum. . . . You will draw the vertebrae because they are magnificent." When Luca Signorelli lost his beloved son, he removed all the clothing from the dead body and drew its muscles with great care. Pollaiuolo and Verocchio flayed corpses and committed to memory bones, muscles, and tendons, which they later reproduced in bronze or on canvas. Thus they were able to convey to the spectator the notion that beneath the skin there was depth and living flesh and bones. This effect is evident in the six executioners of Pollaiuolo's "Saint Sebastian"; their anatomies are displayed to the most minute detail. Another impressive study of muscles in action is the "Battle of the Ten Nude Men," by the same painter.

Artists filled the homes of Florentine nobles with muscular nudes in which not a single muscle was overlooked. To do so was to mutilate the human being.[B]

At the end of the fifteenth century, the study of corpses marked a return to nature. The human figure represented on canvas ceased to be stiff and acquired life and dynamism. Broadsides on anatomy for students appeared one century later in Bologna, Paris, Nuremberg, and Venice. Among them were the "Six Tables of Venice" printed by Bernardino Vitali and signed by a physician named Andreas Vesalius.

ANATOMY AMONG THE RENAISSANCE MASTERS. THE SCHOOLS OF FLORENCE, VENICE, UMBRIA: VEROCCHIO, BOTTICELLI, SIGNORELLI, DONATELLO, RAPHAEL, MICHELANGELO

Verocchio was one of the first Renaissance artists to revive anatomic exactness in paintings. Ten years before his birth, John and Hubert Van Eyck had attempted the exact reproduction of figures on canvas. Masaccio, too, in his "Adam and Eve" depicted a middle class Florentine couple with all the imperfections of flabby nude flesh. But Verocchio represented a tremendous advance over his predecessors. In his "Virgin and Child with Two Angels," the Virgin is a simple woman with a serene countenance, long, slim fingers and well-delineated anatomy; the child is a healthy, chubby infant so well reproduced that his big toe shows the so-called Babinski neurologic sign, normal in children of his age.

Somewhat younger than Verocchio was Sandro Botticelli, a disciple of Pollaiuolo and of the Fra Filippo Lippi who painted buxom virgins and fat little angels. Botticelli was one of the most original of the Renaissance painters. Restless and unhappy, he translated his feelings into such exaggeratedly expressive lines that he induces a nervous vibration in the spectator. His paintings immortalized the tall, thin woman. The virgins of his "Primavera" are the quintessence of Florentine distinction, and their heavy abdomens reveal the painter's knowledge of the asthenic habit, the leitmotif of Botticelli's work.

Signorelli was the Dante of fifteenth century painting. Impersonal and cold, he created stiff figures, tormented but stoic. However, the fierce emotions hidden beneath the stoic countenances can be sensed even in his virgins.

Florentine sculpture boasts of a Donatello, whose statues of saints are characterized by a sharp naturalism and whose children ("David" or the "Angel with Timbrel") possess an exquisite grace. In his bronzes, Donatello has left us examples of robust anatomies, like his "Saint John" and "Anatomy of a Miser's Heart," and heads of sweet, sad virgins.

The second half of the fifteenth century witnessed the development of the Venetian school, deriving from the school of Padua and synthesizing Florentine elegance. It reflected the social life of the city, its people, their pastimes and their rich attire, in a setting of luminous landscapes under skies of silvery clouds. The Virgins of this school are beautiful young girls with golden hair, and the saints are happy youths attired in precious stuffs. Light, color, well-being, cheer are the characteristics of this art, characteristics that cannot be accounted for by the mild climate, but rather by that sort of moral and physical health usually associated with the opulent Flanders that Rubens painted. The red or golden hair and pink flesh stressed by the Venetian school derived most likely from the fact that these painters were especially sensitive to the chromatic impressions of red and yellow, colors usually associated with "primitive" men in full possession of their virile instincts. This school immortalized the type that Landouzy would later translate into medical language by the term "Venetian habit": pink skin with blue veins, golden or red hair, and somatic frailty usually associated with tuberculosis. As verification, we need only recall the softly rounded virgins of Cima da Conegliano, the thin, nervous virgins of Crivelli, the dwarfs of Paolo Veronese, and the vital silver tones of Titian and Tintoretto.

The Umbrian school, characterized by poetic freshness, childlike grace, and translucent coloring, had its most brilliant exponent in Raphael Sanzio of Urbino, who died at the age of thirty-seven from overwork, tuberculosis, and his amorous excesses with the lustful dancer la Fornarina.

Raphael was influenced by Timoteo Vitti and the French school; hence his fondness for round, opulent figures. For four years he was inspired by Perugino and Pinturicchio. He then went to Florence and there for another four years painted his immortal Virgins, in imitation of Leonardo and Michelangelo. He became the favorite painter of Julius II and Leo X and decorated the loggias of the Vatican with half-mystical, half-pagan Virgins. In his unfinished "The Transfiguration," he made some magnificent contributions to anatomy, such as the relief of the muscles, the lumbar slope, and the flexed back of a young woman kneeling.

Raphael's anatomic exactness may be ascribed to the years he spent in Perugino's studio studying the forms of mystical figures or of sweet Madonnas. With these impressions and his earlier memories, he forged an ideal of strength, youth, and cheer. Raphael succeeded in thinking in terms of form and translated all his aspirations into contours and postures. It is no wonder that at the age of twenty-five he was the outstanding painter of his time.

Raphael made some admirable medical observations in his "Saint Peter and the Lame Man" and in "Tommaso Inghinami" in which he depicted divergent strabismus. His portrayal of the timid virgin in the "Madonna di Foligno" is a psychologic study and reveals great mastery of anatomy, particularly in the child, whose soft thigh shows an inguinal fold that was doubtlessly significant to the artist. Raphael loved the contour of a vigorous naked thigh and the vitality of a muscular back. His "Descent from the Cross" is a hymn of praise to the adolescent body; his "Graces" are heavy, fleshy girls, and the cupids of his "Psyche" have the pink, thick-textured flesh of well-nourished children.

But plasticity, strength, and dynamism of the living body reached their apogee with the Florentine, Michelangelo Buonarroti. Michelangelo was a poet, architect (he built the Basilica of Saint Peter), painter, and, above all, sculptor. "I, Michelangelo, sculptor," was the signature on his letters.

From early youth, Michelangelo worshiped beauty of form. Dante Alighieri's immortal poem and Savonarola's fiery sermons forged the temperament of that Michelangelo whose greatest urge was to impose his genius on marble and canvas. Only man interested him. And the men he created were giants, their gestures eloquent, their sharp postures tormented, their muscles tense almost beyond possibility. His Virgins are fiercely naked; his captives arch their backs with formidable strength. Michelangelo played on the human body as on a musical instrument from which he extracted overpowering, menacing, awesomely beautiful sounds. He created a school of gigantism which became artificial and mannered in the hands of his successors.

In order to attain realism, Michelangelo used live models. With the permission of the prior of the Monastery of Santo Spirito, who assigned him a cell for the purpose, he dissected corpses which he secured from the gravediggers of Florence in exchange for statuettes he had made. In his improvised bare studio, he would insert a candle in the navel of the corpse and minutely study the muscles, tendons, and ligaments, the same muscles, tendons and ligaments that stand out so fiercely under the polished marble of his "Solitude" and his "Moses."

Thus Michelangelo became acquainted with the mechanism of human dynamics and the structure of bones and muscles. He familiarized himself with all the postures of the human body and learned how to make them portray the hidden torments of the soul. His

"David" is a masterpiece of anatomy; in his "Virgin and Child" one can almost see the trembling of the Madonna's fingers; and his "Florentine Soldiers Bathing in the Arno and Surprised by Pisans" is an anatomic wonder.

Michelangelo lived alone. He was a chaste giant, without any love other than that he felt for Vittoria Colonna, the wife of Pescara. And his figures bear the impress of his lonely, tormented soul. They are somber creatures, with a world of their own, showing (such was Michelangelo's mastery of musculature) anger or fear even in an inguinal fold or in the relief of a shoulder blade.

Before decorating the ceiling of the Sistine Chapel for Paul III, a work that occupied him for four years, Michelangelo sought inspiration by reading Dante among mausoleums. The Sistine Chapel displays tremendous figures, radiant with the strength of flexed muscles, beings who belong to a superhuman race. His "Moses" (the statue in the Church of San Pietro da Vincoli in Rome which Freud psychoanalyzed) overflows with "repressed emotion," passion, and anger. There is even greater strength in his four statues lying on sarcophagi, with their exuberant and exasperated musculature. But all the possibilities of motion are exhausted in his fresco "The Final Judgment," painted at the command of Paul III on the back wall of the Sistine Chapel, which took him seven years to complete. In this work he created a sinister world of angry, nude giants with prodigious musculature. The herculean Jesus gives the impression of a feverish Titan on the verge of insanity. This work alone, "an apotheosis of nudity," symbolizes the Renaissance.

AND—LEONARDO

Leonardo da Vinci personified all of Renaissance culture, all dreams of progress and glory, all love of beauty and science.

I have already written the story of Leonardo's life and the romantic legend that grew about him.[c] Although Leonardo's wanderings were limited to only three places—Florence, Milan, and Amboise-sur-Loire—his intellectual range was universal. Leonardo the scientist was an encyclopedia of things to come. But here we are interested only in Leonardo the anatomist.

Leonardo underwent his artistic apprenticeship in Verocchio's studio, where he spent innumerable hours dissecting dead bodies, developing a passion for anatomy as a vehicle for beauty. Later he performed dissections at the Hospital of Santa Maria la Nuova. In his own studio he worked on clay figures which he later painted, imitating relief with his brush, thus introducing into painting the sensation of solidity. Even his first work, "The Adoration of the Magi," is a miracle of anatomy.

Leonardo's personality has not yet received the thorough study it deserves. Unfortunately, the artist has eclipsed the scientist, and interest in the picturesque artistic atmosphere in which he moved has withdrawn attention from his scientific accomplishments. The five hundredth anniversary of his birth brought to light new facets of his genius and confirmed him as perhaps the most extraordinary being that ever existed. Others, like Goethe, may have possessed as vast a knowledge and may even have surpassed him in their ability to integrate harmoniously all the facets of their life; but no one has ever matched the radiant flame of genius that burned in him.

In the six thousand or so closely written pages of his diary, studded with brilliant illustrations, we find the seed of modern science. Recently, English and American medical journals published a series of studies on Leonardo's work in the various fields of anatomy, physiology, and medicine. The outstanding anatomists, physiologists, cardiologists, geriatricians, and ophthalmologists of today were amazed to discover that Leonardo knew the basic principles of their specialties, and in many cases they find his views to be identical with those held today. The anatomic studies that he started in 1472 were not published until modern investigators uncovered them. Had they been made public in Leonardo's time, the circulation of the blood might conceivably have been discovered in the sixteenth century instead of in the seventeenth. The loss the scientific world suffered at the disappearance for several centuries of Leonardo's amazing scientific work can be matched only by the loss to the artistic world of his equally amazing anatomic illustrations. One of these illustrations, lent by Elizabeth II to the centenary exhibit, shows a fetus in the womb with an incredibly expressive face. The child's face seems illuminated by a prophetic vision of imminent life and its drama. It is perhaps the most beautiful anatomic figure ever created.

Leonardo's achievements in anatomy are only a small part of his prodigious work, which included engineering, mechanics, and science in general. He completed nothing that he started, spread himself too thin, changed his direction too often, and his work was almost completely unknown until the last century. His methods were still being discussed by painters when, thirteen years after Leonardo's death, Vesalius came to Italy and found his compatriot van Calcar still under Leonardo's influence. Between them, they reconstructed a part of Leonardo's spirit in the field of scientific anatomy.

Leonardo, who accepted Galenism but advanced the notion of the circulation of the blood which Harvey would later discover, adequately described the position of the liver, spleen, and kidneys. In his drawings he anticipated by a century the discovery of Highmore's maxillary sinus. His studies of the influence of age on the organs, deriving from his dissection of corpses of old men, are the forerunners of contemporary geriatric research; his studies of the human eye are likewise notable.

Refuting Galenic ideas that had been accepted for twelve hundred years, Leonardo demonstrated that the heart was a muscle and described two new cavities—the auricles—which he added to the two ventricles Galen had described.

Leonardo's *Diary* contains one hundred ninety pages devoted to anatomy, of which fifty are about the heart alone. His approach to anatomy was that of an artist who, although guided by Galenic ideas, formulated mechanical laws to replace supernatural principles and the ancient analogy between the macrocosm and the microcosm. For example, while watching the farmers in Tuscany slaughter their pigs by driving a *spilla* or long pin into the heart, he observed the contraction and dilatation marked by the pin and thus discovered the cardiac systole and diastole.

Leonardo dissected more than thirty corpses and planned to write a one-hundred-twenty-volume treatise on anatomy.[D] His drawings superseded Galen and restored the anatomic dignity of man. He studied the fetal membranes and denied that the fetus can cry in the uterus. He described bone textures and muscular functions and placed bones in wire boxes to study their dynamics. Fascinated by mechanical laws, he studied muscular antagonisms and correctly ascertained the points of insertion and outlet of a muscle. He injected the cerebral ventricles with liquid wax and also described the pleura and lungs, but did not emphasize the circulation of the blood, since to have done so would have been heresy. With such work, he created the experimental method.[E]

As a painter, Leonardo represents the culmination of the realistic trend started by Andrea da Castagno. His theory of painting is summarized in the advice he gave his disciple Giovanni Beltraffio: "The painter's soul should be like a mirror: it should reflect movement and color while it itself remains motionless, limpid and pure."

Leonardo believed that a scientific knowledge of artistic anatomy, quite different from the intuitive knowledge of the static or dynamic nude figures that the Greek sculptors created, could be acquired only on the dissecting table. Many were the times his cold blue eyes explored the dead human body, his delicate, almost feminine, hands felt anatomic structures, measured longitudes with goniometers, figured out proportions, and reduced parts of the organism to mathematical formulas.

He studied people and their expressions in various states of excitement, making sure that they did not perceive what he was doing so that they should not become self-conscious. "Study the expressive movements of deafmutes," he counseled. He was obsessed by the desire to translate states of mind somatically on canvas. "Diversity of movement is as infinite as diversity of feeling," he said. "The loftiest aim of the artist is to express the passions of the soul on faces and in movements." Painting was his religion: *"Chi biassima la pittura biassima la Natura."* His painting is a blend of perfect figuration and precise chiaroscuro. His anatomically impeccable figures combine a singular gelatinous softness, personified in Mona Lisa's molluscan smile, and a disturbing lack of consistency. He used both qualities to translate a state of mind.

His "Last Supper," painted in oil on the wall of the refectory of the Monastery of Santa Maria delle Grazie, is a miracle of psychologic observation. Today it is smoke-blackened and mutilated at the bottom, where the Renaissance monks cut a door into the kitchen so that their food would not reach them cold. His painting of Mona Lisa, the Gioconda, third wife of the Florentine Francesco del Giocondo, took him four years. To make the lady smile he surrounded her with all sorts of pleasant objects and even provided music.[F]

Leonardo's chalk drawings laid the foundations for artistic anatomic iconography. Buried in oblivion for two hundred years, these drawings, copies of which may be found in the works of Dürer and in the Uffizi skeletons in Florence, are surrounded by marginal notes of great exactness, written from right to left—which Leonardo found easy to do since he was left-handed—perhaps for fear of plagiarism or of the Holy Office.

In all, Leonardo made more than seven hundred fifty drawings of muscles, the heart, the lungs, the cervical, thoracic, abdominal and femoral blood vessels, bones and nerves after performing minute visceral dissections and sagittal and frontal cuts of the brain.

Among his curious physiologic observations are those he made of facial muscles in laughter and tears. His desire for exactness led him to study dispassionately the facial anguish of men condemned to death, engraving on his brain their slightest gestures during execution for future use. To be able to recall these faces later, he thought of a method, which anticipated the Bertillon system now used in forensic medicine, based on a division of noses into straight and curved, the straight into short and long with round or pointed extremities, and the curved into three groups according to the curvature. These divisions and subdivisions were given numbers. He did the same with the mouth and the eyes. All he had to do, therefore, to be able to recall a face later on was to jot down the corresponding numbers. He also worked out a gradation of the colors of the rainbow. His collection contains many drawings of monsters and abnormal beings, dropsy victims and goiterous old men of the Bergamasc Mountains, strange animals, porcupines, cats, fish, flies, and birds.[G]

Leonardo's accomplishments in medicine were prompted by his desire to achieve the greatest possible knowledge of anatomy to help him in his art and by his desire to know per se, which inspired his frenetic search for scientific truth.

His medical studies established an anatomic canon based on a "natural" ideal, in opposition to the canon based on a "divine" or unattainable ideal. Leonardo called himself *"il pittore anatomico,"* but never allowed anatomy to impinge on his art. He urged painters not to show the entire play of the muscles in their nudes.

Leonardo was the first to approach science as an artist and to use the scientific study of nature as a vehicle that would lead him to the supreme mastery of the artistic sketch. It was not enough for him to reduce natural laws to mathematical formulas; he had to go further: he had to dramatize them in drawings. In this sense, his work was a crusade against the esoterism that had enveloped science before his time. His great desire was to show man's knowledge encyclopedically. It is possible that had Leonardo not exhausted himself in so many directions and had he systematized his work, it might have embraced the following fields: mathematics and optics as the basis of all observation; mechanics as the science of all physical—organic and inorganic—forces; biology as the science of life and growth in organic nature; and cosmology as the study of inorganic forms.

To the religious fanatics of his time Leonardo was a skeptic. It has been said that during a fiery sermon delivered by Savonarola to a horde of people cringing at his feet, Leonardo, his corpulent figure erect under a black and red tunic, stood nearby, listening impassively to the preacher's apocalyptic prophecies. And as he listened he scornfully drew a caricature of the tormented priest.[H]

Leonardo da Vinci, poet, man of letters, musician, sculptor, physicist, painter, architect, engineer, geologist, anatomist, psychologist, alchemist, naturalist, anthropologist, philosopher, and constructor of flying machines and tanks, was the most amazing personality of the Renaissance. His was the spirit of the Renaissance, ever eager to soar to new horizons. His contribution to modern medical science began to take shape when, thirteen years after his death, there arrived in Italy a Belgian anatomist with a restless mind and a firm hand. This man was Vesalius. With Vesalius, the physician was to become an artist *and* a scientist.

NOTES

A. Before the Renaissance, anatomy had had to struggle against obstacles put in its way by religion. The history of the development of anatomy is the history of the popular attitude toward dissection. Even in 1750 the prisoners in Newgate trembled at the possibility of their being used after death for anatomic research. In 1820 when a felon who was hanged at Carlisle was dissected, his friends attacked the physicians who performed the dissection.

It is true that Talmudic literature contains references to the dissection of dead slaves or of those condemned to death by the Egyptian monarchs. Herophilus, the father of anatomy, practiced vivisection in Alexandria, where Galen did his studies in osteology and myology. But then followed hundreds of years of paralysis in these fields. The two principal reasons for this historical fact were, first, Christianity, which neglected the body in favor of the soul, preferring to wait until the Day of Judgment to know about the body; and, second, the idea that the human body was a miniature universe and therefore could be studied astrologically by looking at the heavens instead of at the body. That is why when anatomic studies began to make headway astrology declined.

B. The principles governing anatomic illustrations before the Renaissance were: (1) servile adherence to tradition and (2) observation of reality. The first made for diagrammatic anatomy which attempted to deduce nature from a structure of the function assigned to it by the Creator. The second made for artistic and morphologic anatomy, true living anatomy, the precursor of modern physiology.

In the fifteenth century, Florentine painters were already buying their pigments from the apothecary and thus had the opportunity of fraternizing with physicians. Artists like Masaccio joined the *League of Physicians and Apothecaries*. For two and a half centuries science and art constantly drew closer. Masolino, Roselli, Lucas Cranach, all apothecaries' apprentices, became great painters. Giotto had friendly relations with the physicians Dino del Garbo and Torrigiani; Luca della Robbia and Benivieni were friends, and so were Leonardo and Marco Antonio della Torre. Giotto wished to break with the flat dimension (in the fashion of the Byzantine mosaic) of his master Cimabue; he sought a tridimensional depth and solidity in the field of painting. The paintings of Stefano, his assistant, were studied by barber-surgeons before they opened the veins of their patients.

C. "Leonardo da Vinci," Universidad de Madrid (Spain), 1934; and "The Lives of Leonardo," *Town & Country, 106*:55, December, 1952.

D. In October, 1517, Cardinal Luis of Aragon and his secretary paid a visit to Leonardo da Vinci at his home in Amboise. The secretary wrote: "This gentleman has written on anatomy with great detail, showing by illustration the limbs, muscles, nerves, veins, ligaments, intestines, and whatsoever else there is to discuss in the bodies of men and women, in such a way as had never yet been done by anyone else. All this we have seen with our own eyes; and he said that he had dissected more than thirty bodies both of men and women of all ages. He has also written of the nature of water, of diverse machines and of other matters which he has set down in an infinite number of volumes all in the vulgar tongue, which should they be published will be profitable and very enjoyable."

E. Thus spoke Leonardo: "And you who say that it is better to look at an anatomical demonstration than to see these drawings, you would be right if it were possible to observe all the details shown in these drawings in a single figure, in which with all your ability you will not see, nor acquire a knowledge of more than a few veins. While in order to obtain an exact and complete knowledge of these I have dissected more than ten human bodies, destroying all the various members, and removing even the smallest particles of flesh which surround these veins. . . . And as one body did not suffice for so long a time, it was necessary to proceed by stages with so many bodies as would render my knowledge complete; and this I repeated twice over in order to discover the differences.

"Though possessed of an interest in the subject you may perhaps be deterred by natural repugnance . . . or fear of passing the night hours in the company of these corpses quartered and flayed and horrible to behold."

F. The "Mona Lisa" may be the image of his mother, since it is possible that Leonardo was a timid type because of superdifferentiation of instinct. He sought an inaccessible ideal and fled from women because he needed absolute calm and liberty to work. It is said that he loved only once in his life and even then it was a scientific experiment. All his life, however, he evinced aversion for the sexual act. "He who does not control his sensuality lowers himself to the level of the beast," he said. "The carnal act and the organs it involves are so coarse that were it not for the beauty of the faces and the adornments of human beings, and the unbridled impetus that carries them away, mankind would be lost." "Mona Lisa" may be the portrait of the artist's most cherished ideals, for her smile is perpetuated in all of Leonardo's works, especially in "Saint Anne" and "Leda." Leonardo and "Mona Lisa" are two mirrors reflecting the same image. The outer aspect of "Mona Lisa" conceals a portrait of Leonardo himself, for when he looked upon his model, La Gioconda, he felt that the entire physical being of that woman lay hidden in himself.

G. Leonardo invented a many-stringed lute of silver in the form of a horse's head which Ludovico il Moro greatly admired. Leonardo took advantage of this opportunity to offer his services to Ludovico as inventor of instruments of war, builder of collapsible bridges and tanks, engineer, an expert in artillery and the art of sieges, sapper, astronomer, sculptor, and painter. It was at Ludovico's court that Leonardo showed himself to be a polemicist in paleontology and geology by outlining the scientific bases of prehistory. He worked seventeen years on an equestrian statue of Ludovico's father, Francesco Sforza, and in his polyfacetism he showed himself to be the refined inventor of all modern ideas and the precursor of all modern advances. After carefully observing the flight of birds, he constructed a batlike flying machine heavier than air. He did not, however, succeed in his ambition of enabling man to fly, and he put his machine away in a corner of his studio along with his dissected crocodiles and embryos in alcohol. He was also a chemist, geologist, and a researcher in camera obscura.

H. Leonardo was neither an atheist nor a devotee of black magic. His was a universal religion, for he worshiped the divinity in flowers, insects, and the stars. He would not eat meat because he believed that animals had souls and should not be slaughtered. "The carnivorous man, in his cruelty," he said, "is *re delle bestie*." His enthusiasm for nature led him to scorn physicians, whom he called "liars and destroyers of life." He had the opportunity of dramatizing this scorn for doctors upon the death of Dux Jean Galeas and during the illness of his pupil Andrea Galaino, when he tossed the pills prescribed by their doctors out of the window.

His imagination was so vivid that he could see figures in the stains made by dampness on the walls and could hear voices in the ringing of far-away bells. Everything stirred him to psychologic observation, which he recorded in mirror writing with his left hand (he was naturally left-handed).

THE PHYSICIAN AS ALCHEMIST

TAWADDUD, THE FABULOUS SLAVE GIRL

It happened in medieval Baghdad. "When it was the 436th night, Scheherazade resumed her story, saying, 'And among my tales is that of Abu al-Husn and his slave-girl Tawaddud.'" A Abu al-Husn was the prodigal son of a rich merchant of Baghdad. After his father's death, Abu al-Husn soon squandered his inheritance by listening too long and too often to the "giggle of the daughter of the vine as she gurgled from the flagon," and the jingle of the silver anklets worn by the slave girls as they danced to the rhythm of the lutes. Only one slave girl called Tawaddud remained with him, a girl with "eyes like gazelles' eyne, with strait arched brows twain, as they were the crescent moon of Sh'aban, and nose like the edge of scimitar fine, cheeks like anemones of blood-red shine, mouth like Solomon's seal and sign, and teeth like necklaces of pearls in line." In addition to these divine gifts, Tawaddud boasted of a navel "holding an ounce of oil of benzoin," and "hind parts heavier than two hills of sand."

This fabulous creature one day suggested to her impoverished master that he sell her to the Caliph Harun-al-Rashid for ten thousand dinars, which money would rescue him from his financial plight.

Once in the presence of the Caliph, amid silks, tambourines, fountains, divans, lutes, geraniums, pillows, and mosaics, Tawaddud offered to answer all questions put to her on "syntax, poetry, juris-

From *International Record of Medicine 168:399*, 1955.

prudence, exegesis, philosophy, the Divine ordinances, arithmetic, geodesy, geometry, ancient fables, the Koran, the exact sciences, medicine, logic, rhetoric and composition, the lute, dancing, and fashions."

The questioning of Tawaddud by a solemn jury made up of the sensual Caliph and the most learned men in his empire occupies twenty-seven nights (436th to 462nd) of *The Thousand and One Nights*. Tawaddud provided wise and correct answers on all the aforementioned subjects. Her answers to the questions on medicine, anatomy, and physiology give us a faithful picture of medical knowledge during the Golden Age of Arabic medicine.

Tawaddud explained that man, according to the Koran, had two hundred forty-nine bones, two hundred sixty veins, and "three souls or spirits—animal, rational, and natural," and that "Allah made him a heart and spleen and lungs and six intestines and a liver and two kidneys and buttocks and brain and bones and skin and five senses," and that "the heart He set on the left side of the breast and made the stomach the guide and governor thereof. He appointed the lungs for a fan to the heart and established the liver on the right side, opposite thereto. He made, besides this, the diaphragm and the viscera, and set up the bones of the breast and latticed them with the ribs."

In the slave girl's subsequent answers we get snatches of Talmudic anatomy, Galenic physiology, Hebraic clinical experience, and Mesopotamian astrology, all of which had been incorporated into Arabic science.

Then Tawaddud explained the principles of diagnosis based on the "patient's actions, what is evacuated from his body, the nature of the pain and the site thereof, swelling and the effluvia given off his person," adding that "a physician who is a man of understanding is guided by the feel of the hands, according as they are firm or flabby, hot or cool, moist or dry," as well as by the patient's eyes. She described the symptoms of illnesses caused by variations in the bile, and advised bread sopped in broth and mutton meat as the most profitable to man, but she condemned fermented liquors. She explained when and how cupping should be applied and vegetable medicines administered. "He who would live long," she advised, "let him be early with the morning meal and not late with the evening meal; let him be chary of such depletory measures as cupping and bloodletting; let him make of his belly three parts, one for food, one for drink, and the third for air." She recommended walking gently, for "it will be better for the body and more in accordance with the saying of the Almighty: 'Walk not proudly on the earth.'" She also extolled the virtues of copulation, explaining that moderate indulgence "lighteneth a body full of black bile, dilateth the heart, calmeth wrath and banisheth trouble, and is good for ulcers," but she warned that copulation with old women was "deadly."

The silvery tongue of the lovely Tawaddud affords us an outline of the medical knowledge of the fourteenth century. If a slave girl, however intelligent, could accumulate such a treasure of medical science, we can safely surmise the extraordinary amount of knowledge that an Arab physician of that period must have possessed. By restoring the colors, faded by the passing of centuries, of the luxuriant tapestry of Arabic medicine, we shall be better able to understand the history of medieval Europe and the magnitude of the legacy inherited by modern medicine from the Arabic world.

ARABIA BEFORE MOHAMMED

The geography of Arabia has changed little since the times when the rocket of Mohammedan civilization burst over the horizon of the ancient world.

At the beginning of the seventh century, Arabia was a vast wasteland surrounded by flourishing cultures: the Chaldean, the Assyrian, the Egyptian, and the Mediterranean. Through the center of the Arabian peninsula stretched an immense desert of burning sands whipped by terrible storms, but bordering this barren country, strips of pasture lands and bits of productive soil formed a belt of fertile promise extending from Yemen all the way to the south.

Before the seventh century Arabia was made up of nomad Bedouin tribes and of sedentary farmers huddling near wells and springs. Self-protection had spurred these farmers to construct walled cities, like Medina and Mecca, with clumps of palm trees, wells with bitter tasting water, and populations of fifteen to twenty thousand inhabitants. Medina, inhabited by Yemenites, was more exposed to the influence of Judaism, Christianity, and Zoroastrism. Mecca was inhabited by Bedouins, and its walls protected men with a thirst for knowledge that manifested itself in poetry and singing contests.

The nomad tribes, on the other hand, preferred to wander incessantly across oceans of sands, alternating days of warring adventures with nights of story-telling, huddled around the fire under the cold lofty stars while camels and scimitars rested nearby. Each tribe chose its own chief and even its own god. One of these gods was a meteorite that had fallen on the sacred city of Mecca and around which a Kaaba was built like a casket. To this crude black basalt temple the faithful flocked from all over at least once a year.

Before the appearance of Mohammed, the neighboring lands, viz., Egypt, the Mediterranean coast, and Mesopotamia or the Land Between the Two Rivers, had been overrun by Semitic invaders who mixed with Sumerians, Babylonians, Assyrians, Phoenicians, Egyptians, and Canaanites. Arabia's strategic geographic situation—it lay like a wedge between Egypt, Palestine, and Mesopotamia—made of it a stopping-point much coveted by the hierarchs of the ancient Oriental empires. On numerous occasions, these neighboring empires had attempted to subjugate Arabia, and in name at least incorporated it to their imperial possessions. They even introduced the Saracens—as the Romans and Persians called the nomad Arabs—in their folklore.

THE ADVENT OF THE PROPHET

As has happened so many times in history, the trigger that set off the tremendous Arab explosion was released by the word of one man.

At the beginning of the seventh century there suddenly appeared in Arabia an unknown merchant who, emulating Buddha who retreated to the hills and Christ who retired to the desert, withdrew to his tent and even covered his head completely with his burnoose to intensify his introversion. And the anonymous merchant who entered the tent emerged as Mohammed, a prophet illuminated by a message.

This happened at a time when the Byzantine empire was being ravaged by a plague (probably bubonic plague) that had originated in lower Egypt and, in the space of a few years, had caused ten thousand deaths in Constantinople. The corpses were piled up in the wall-towers which once filled were sealed to protect the survivors.

In this decadent and disintegrating empire of lovely mosaics and exquisite stained-glass windows, Mohammed, the prophet of Allah, started to preach, impelled by the dream of uniting all the nomad tribes of Arabia within the iron bonds of a single religion. Some tribes remained faithful to the gods of Mecca, but others readily accepted Mohammed's message, for he promised them a paradise with innumerable couches for every warrior, where sinuous houris, their eyes as black as the night, awaited them wrapped in the somnolence of a heavenly seraglio.

Mohammed was born in Mecca. In his youth he worked as camel driver for a rich widow called Kadija whom he later married. He led the life of a prosperous merchant until, at the age of forty, he was seized by the urge to go forth and speak of a religion that would replace the pagan gods of Mecca with a single god.

Faced by a growing hostility in Mecca, Mohammed sought the support of Medina, whose inhabitants had already felt the influence of other religions. At the age of fifty-one, Mohammed had to flee Mecca (a flight known to history as the Hegira), and after many a mishap crossing the desert he took refuge in Medina. From this city for several years he waged constant battle against his enemies—

Bedouins, Jews, and nomad tribes—until he finally subjugated all Arabia.

Mohammed died at the age of seventy-two. This lusty, fanatic man had one redeeming feature: his passion for books, the result of his own illiteracy which made him long for culture as for some forbidden fruit. The Arabs, fervent lovers of books, later came to divide people into "those who owned books and those who did not," possibly in memory of the time when Mohammed, wishing to extol his god to the highest degree, said that it was Allah who "taught man to move the pen."

IN THE WAKE OF MOHAMMED

The Arabic conquest of the ancient world (it began in 622 A.D., the first year of the Mohammedan calendar) was an explosion of sheer will, a collective manifestation of fanatic ambition for power. Mohammed was dead, but the trail he blazed with his preaching remained. Under the leadership of Abu Bekr and Omar I, the Arabian empire expanded by giant leaps until it stretched from Medina to Finisterre.

At first, Arabia sent emissaries to neighboring countries inviting voluntary submission. When this failed, the Arabic swords glittered under the sun of history. One after another the neighboring countries succumbed, even powerful Persia whose emperors used war-trained elephants: in the glow of a scarlet twilight, both pursuer and pursued stared at the huge beasts, fatally wounded, staggering through their lines.

The Arabian warriors, not satisfied with trailing their hooded garments over the hot sands of Arabia, spurred their horses and, with the winds of the new Mohammedan gospel howling behind them, reached India, swallowed up Persia and the Caucasus, invaded Sicily, and finally cut a wide crescent into Spain when Tarik leaped from Africa to Gebel-Tarik, or the mountain of Tarik, later called Gibraltar, and created the Western Caliphate in Cordova.

This vast empire, which began with the Caliphate of Baghdad in the eighth century, came to an end with the sack of Baghdad by the Tartars in the thirteenth century, the expulsion of the Arabs from Spain, and their defeat in the East by the Turks.

THE ARABIC CIVILIZATION, MOSAIC OF RACES

The Arabic civilization, therefore, comprised a conglomerate of peoples—united only by the same language—of which but a few were born in Arabia and the rest were Syrians, Persians, Spaniards, Mohammedans, Christians, and Jews. For the Mohammedans were as tolerant as the primitive Christians were intolerant. Perhaps that is

The Physician as Alchemist

why Christianity survived. A materialistic, indolent, sensual, skeptical people, the Arabs accepted their religion as a self-imposed moral law, but they never attempted to impose it on the peoples they conquered. They never forced anyone to accept their religion; they required only that the Koran be recognized as the vehicle of the divine word, and since the sacred book was written in Arabic, the conquered peoples had to learn the tongue of the victorious invaders. Thus the vast Moslem Empire came to be united by one single language. Before the acceptance of Arabic as the "official" language among learned men, Greek was the preferred language, later replaced by Syrian in west Asia; but from the ninth century on, both the humble rug vendor in the public market and the haughty physician at the caliphs' courts spoke in Arabic.

The only other term imposed by the Arabs upon the conquered peoples was the surrender of Greek manuscripts. At the end of the eighth century, all of Arabic knowledge consisted of a translation of a Greek medical book and a handful of books on alchemy; but before the end of the ninth century the Arabs were already acquainted with all the Greek sciences. The glory of Greece vanished and the might of Rome destroyed, there remained the work of the Byzantine copyists and the Arab translators as the only bridge of light spanning a thousand years of darkness until the outburst of light in the Renaissance.

During this historical transition from classical Greece to the Arabian caliphates, a vital role was played by the Syrian translators. Except for medieval Spain, never in history have translators played such an important part as they did at the beginning of Islamic expansion. Thanks to their work, the Arabs could add the dazzling treasure of the philosophic and medical knowledge of Periclean Greece to their war booty.

THE NESTORIANS AND THE PERSIAN ORIGINS OF ARABIC MEDICINE

Medicine was one of the most important facets of Arabic culture during the halcyon days of Mohammedan civilization. Arabic medicine joined Byzantine and monastic medicine to provide the three channels along which medieval medical thought flowed.

In order to understand Arabic medicine it is necessary to cast a glance back at its Persian origins. Two centuries before the birth of Mohammed there lived in Constantinople one Nestorius, an Aramaic priest of eloquent tongue and subtle metaphysical mind, who was named patriarch of the city in the year 428. At a time when Christianity still glowed with the light kindled by Paul of Tarsus, Nestorius dared found a religious school that challenged Christian dogma by attributing two personalities and two natures to Jesus Christ and by proclaiming that the Virgin Mary was not the Mother of

God, but the mother of Christ. Because of this slight semantic difference, Nestorius was denounced by the Council of Ephesus (431 A.D.) and banished from his native land.[B]

Nestorius and his followers fled to Edessa (today Orfa) in upper Mesopotamia and later moved on to Djondisapur in southwestern Persia, where they founded a school of medicine that lasted until the tenth century and was the cradle of Arabic medicine. For the Nestorians, forced to abandon theology for lack of dialectic opponents with whom to argue out theologic subtleties, turned to medicine. Since their aspirations to heal man's soul had cost them so dearly, they decided to heal man's body.

Disappointed with their own times, the Nestorians turned their eyes back to classical Greece, drinking deeply of the medicophilosophic waters of the Greco-Roman school. Later, generous with their newly acquired knowledge, they poured the ancient Hellenic nectars into Syriac vessels, translating Greek medical works into Syriac, in the hope of continuing the brilliant Hippocratic tradition, and establishing medical schools in Edessa and other Persian towns.

When the Arabs conquered Persia, therefore, they suddenly found their shepherds' pouches filled with the medicophilosophic treasures of the Greeks recorded on old Nestorian parchments.

THE WORK OF SYRIAN TRANSLATORS

Arabic medicine therefore was of Persian and, indirectly, Hellenic origin. It represented not a uniform canvas but a multicolored mosaic of races and nations held together by the sword and prestige of the Saracen crescent.[C]

In the year 700, when the Omayyad caliphs were reigning in Damascus, learned men—mostly Nestorian Christians—migrated to the Islamic capital. The Nestorian physicians and the graduates of the school of Djondisapur took care of the first caliphs. Their medical emissaries often traveled to Salerno where the first European medical school was located, thus establishing the first "official" medical link between Asia and the western world, later continued by the schools of Bologna and Padua during the Renaissance.

The rise of the Abbasid caliphs (750), with Baghdad as their capital, inaugurated the Golden Age of Arabic civilization. Medical literature had not yet made an appearance in Arabic dress. The second Abbasid caliph, Abu-Ja'far al-Mansur, recognized the need for translating Greek works into Arabic. Once when he was sick he sent for the chief physician of the hospital of Djondisapur, the Nestorian Jurjis ibn Bukht-Isho, the first of a dynasty of no less than seven generations of eminent physicians and translators. Impressed by the physician's knowledge, the Caliph extended Greek medical science all over his empire. To the Bukht-Isho family belonged Jibrail, physician to the fifth Abbasid caliph, Harun-al-Rashid, who made a fortune of three million dollars and was one of the wealthiest physicians in history; and Hunain ibn Ishaq, who translated into Arabic almost the whole immense corpus of Galenic writings and other works and received in payment the weight in gold of all the manuscripts, among them *Ten Treatises on the Eyes,* the most famous Arabic text on ophthalmology.

The production of books at this time was facilitated by the introduction of paper, invented in China and imported by Arabia to replace papyrus and parchment.[D]

In the ninth century, Syrian translations from the Greek were made for Christians and Arabic translations for Mohammedans. The Abbasid caliph al-Ma'mum (reigned 813–833) instituted a regular translation school in Baghdad equipped with a library, and encouraged Arabic translations of Greek works by offering generous fees and by sending learned men to Alexandria in search of Greek manuscripts.

And so the Arabs, then masters of half the world, attempted to acquire the knowledge that was the only pearl missing in their crown.

The heroes, therefore, at this stage in Mohammedan medicine were the translators. To the two most famous families of translators, the Bukht-Isho and the Messuas, should be added the "prince of translators," the Syrian Christian Honein, or Johannitius (809–873), who translated almost all the works of Hippocrates, Galen, and Aristotle.

Prominent at the court of Caliph Moawiyha I was the brilliant physician Maser Djawah Ebu Djeldjal of Basra, who translated into Arabic the *Pandects* of Haroun, the Alexandrian physician. Under the auspices of Harun-al-Rashid, the Rabbi of Seleucia, Joshua Ben Nun, converted Baghdad into an international intellectual oasis.[E]

Those were happy times when even beneath the warrior's mail beat a heart avid for culture. When Michael III of Constantinople was defeated in battle, the penalty imposed upon him was that he send a caravan of camels laden with ancient manuscripts to Baghdad. On one occasion, an Arab sheik offered a powerful friend of his not a precious jewel, but a manuscript of Dioscorides. The book was mightier than the sword! Other schools began to flourish in Samarkand, Isfahan, Alexandria, Sicily, and later in the Spanish cities of Cordova, Seville, Toledo, Granada, and Saragossa.

During the ninth century, medical practice was in the hands of Christians in Baghdad. If a physician bore a foreign instead of a Mohammedan name, spoke Syrian or Persian instead of Arabic, and wore black silk instead of white cotton, he could be assured of a great many more patients than a Mohammedan physician. This predilection in every country for foreign physicians is an interesting phenomenon of medical sociology still observable in our own times.

The first great book written at that time was concerned with pharmacology; it was the *Great Book of Medicine* of the Christian Sabur ibn Sahl, the first director of the hospital of Djondisapur and physician (850–869) to al-Mutawakkil, Caliph of Baghdad. For three centuries this book was a basic text at the hospitals and pharmacies of Baghdad and Persia. The Persian al-Tabari, converted to Islam as an adult, wrote *Paradise of Wisdom,* which covered the entire therapeutic armamentarium of the Arabs. In its pages there are references to tamarind, melon seeds, sugar candy, sandal, nux vomica, senna, indigo, manna, gum arabic, resins, sugar cane, cocoa, betel nut, areca nut, and bamboo, as well as recipes of incense and essences. Although Indian medicine did not influence Arabic medicine, Indian drugs enriched the Arabic pharmacopoeia.

Pharmacology more than any other branch of medicine seems to have fascinated the Arabs. Century after century there was not a single medical writer who did not devote some of his writings to this science, thus incessantly increasing the list of medicaments which already swelled Arabic pharmacy. Arabic pharmacology spread throughout Persia in the tenth century in the form of works written in Neo-Persian. In one of these books, written by Abu Mansur Muwaffaq, five hundred and forty-nine medicaments and their effects are mentioned, and in the *Hami* (thirteenth century) fourteen hundred drugs are studied.

RHAZES, THE EXPERIMENTER

The first of the four great medical figures—Rhazes, al Tabari,[F] Haly Abbas,[G] and Avicenna, all Arabs or Persians—of the Eastern Caliphate was Abu-Bakr Muhammad ibn-Zakariya al Razi (c.860–c.932), called Rhazes because he was born in Rai (Tabaristan, northern Persia) near present-day Teheran. Because of his Hippocratic spirit, Rhazes won for himself the noble name of "the Experimenter." Rhazes, who in his youth was more interested in music than in medicine, did not begin his medical studies until the age of forty, on the occasion of a visit to Baghdad. It is not unusual in the history of medicine to find men whose interest in this science was aroused late in life and yet achieved great fame, as if all their earlier years had been a sort of prelude to their consecration to science.

Rhazes became chief physician of the great Baghdad hospital where he had been educated, an honor vouchsafed to few doctors. Because of his important post, his services were much sought by the nobility of several Persian courts. He practiced in Rai and Baghdad. It is said that once, anxious to choose the very best site on which to build a hospital, Rhazes hung out pieces of meat and buried others at several points in the city, and then had the hospital built where the meat took longest to rot. This experiment in medical ecology shows great perspicacity and wisdom.

Rhazes was an eminent historian and philosopher and a clinician of the stature of Hippocrates, Aretæus, and Sydenham.[H] Contrasting with the polypharmacy of his time, he recommended a sparse therapy and a sober treatment; he preferred a few simple remedies to the copious pharmaceutic bill-of-fare served at the banquet of Arabic chemistry.

Rhazes compiled more than two hundred volumes on philosophy, religion, mathematics, and medicine. His *opus magnum* is *Kitab al-Hawi Li'l-tibb,* or *Liber Continens.* Of almost equal importance is his little book *Mansurio* or *Liber Medicinalis ad Almansorem,* dedicated to Almanzor the Victorious, and still consulted in Elizabethan London at the time of the plague. The *Liber Continens* is a gigantic compilation of all Arabic medical knowledge at the beginning of the tenth century and is considered one of the greatest books in the history of medicine. The first edition weighed more than twenty-two pounds and is one of the heaviest incunabula extant. The ninth book of the *Liber Continens,* translated by Vesalius, was the principal source of therapeutic knowledge until after the Renaissance.

Andalusian, Arabic, Persian, Berber, Egyptian, and Hebrew students came to listen to Rhazes the physician speak the magic words "according to my own experience."

Unfortunately, Rhazes quarreled with the hierarch of Bokhara, who ordered that he be beaten over the head with his own book until one or the other broke. Rhazes' head broke first. The lesions caused by this "intellectual" beating brought on blindness in Rhazes' later years. A true philosopher, he refused to be operated on because "he had already seen enough misery in this world."

AVICENNA, THE PRINCE OF ARABIC MEDICINE

The greatest medical figure of the Eastern Caliphate and one of the greatest physicians in history, a man whose encyclopedic knowledge has earned him comparison with Aristotle, Leonardo, and Goethe, was the Persian Abu 'Ali al Husayn ibn'Abdullah ibn-Sina (980–1037), generally known by the Latinized name of Avicenna.

The so-called "prince" of Arabic physicians and author of the most famous book ever written in the history of medicine was born in Kharmesan, near present-day Bokhara. A child prodigy, at the age of ten he knew the Koran by heart, a feat difficult even for a wise man of mature years, and had also mastered the *Isagoge* of

Porphyrius, the *Geometry* of Euclid, the *Almagest* of Ptolemy, and Aristotle's *Metaphysics,* which he reread more than forty times. In his early teens he studied Indian philosophy, numerology, logic, and jurisprudence.

At the age of eighteen Avicenna cured the king of an illness, whereupon he was appointed royal physician and granted, as a special reward, access to the royal library. To one as hungry for knowledge as Avicenna, it was like opening the doors to paradise. Legend has it that when he had learned by heart everything of any value in the vast library of the Samanids, he set fire to it to hide the source of his knowledge.

When the Samanid dynasty came to an end, Avicenna fled to Khiva and Rai, where he wrote a great many books, and then on to Kazwin. In Hamadan he cured the Emir Shams Addayla of colic and in reward was appointed prime minister. When the Kurds rebelled against such an unqualified political appointment, Avicenna hid in the house of a friendly sheik, a refuge he left when the Emir fell ill again with the colic. Avicenna cured the ruler once again and was appointed vizier.

Avicenna was a peerless scholiast in Arabic, Latinity, and dialectic, and the definitive codifier of Greco-Latin medicine. His life was an extraordinarily active one. During the day he practiced medicine and performed the duties of the statesman. At night he studied, dictated his works, and gave lectures. When the stars were already pale in the heavens, Avicenna would interrupt his meditations to engage in more material entertainment; it was then he gave himself over to old wine and young maidens. When he laid away the pen that wrote of mathematics, astronomy, physics, chemistry, geology, philosophy and theology, poetry, music, and medicine, the lute played, wine flowed, and girls danced.

It was a strange adventurous life he led, punctuated by flights, disguises, voyages, and political honors. When a problem was especially difficult he would withdraw to a mosque to pray until he felt illuminated by his inner light, or he would retire to sleep and let his subconscious solve the problem in his dreams. Some historians have believed him to be the author of the *Rubáiyát,* but although Avicenna's personal philosophy is comparable to that of Omar Khayyám's poem, attribution of authorship is nothing but poetic license.

Avicenna's philosophy is worthy of Plato. His writings are at times frankly Platonic in their allegories, as when he compares men to caged birds that are liberated from their prison only by the Angel of Death. He admitted the influence upon the physical world of souls dwelling in celestial regions, and believed in the omnipotence of spiritual forces to crystallize in action and matter. Thought could make a camel in the desert move; victory over a rooster could make a hen so proud that she could grow spurs.

The vizier's baton of authority, the cutlass in the *razzias,* the lute, wine, and women, along with excessive work, proved to be too much even for Avicenna. At the age of fifty-eight he felt that death was near. He accepted his approaching end philosophically, distributed his wealth, read the Koran from beginning to end several times in periods of three days, and died during the holy month of Ramadan. His tomb in the ancient romantic Ecbatana of the Oriental poets is still a shrine.

Avicenna's *magnum opus* was his *al-Q'anun fi'al-Tibb* or the *Canon Medicinae,* which runs to a million words and made of Avicenna the dictator of world medicine during the long period from the coming of the *almorávides* to Spain to the advent of Vesalius. It was the medical bible for several Asiatic and European civilizations for more than six centuries and was considered an infallible oracle. If Galen dominated the medicine of the ancient world, Avicenna ruled medical thought during the Middle Ages.

In the thirteenth century the *Canon* was translated into Latin in Spain, and in the fifteenth and sixteenth centuries it was reprinted almost thirty times in Latin. It is a book as monumental in facts as it is in errors. Each page is a garden where weeds grow next to the rosebush. For example, Avicenna attempted to deduce the pharmacologic properties of drugs from their taste, color, and odor, and advised such treatments as the insertion of a louse into the meatus of patients suffering from urine retention.

The *Canon,* epitome and summary of Greco-Latin medicine, achieved for the Arabs what Galen's works achieved for the Romans: complete and absolute authority. To criticize it was considered sacrilege. In 1650 the *Canon* was still used as a text at the universities of Montpellier and Louvain, and today it is still applied in the East.[1]

Avicenna, the greatest physician of the Eastern Caliphate, died in 1037, but almost a thousand years later his system continues to heal the sick of Persia.

MOSLEM SPAIN

The history of Arabic Spain is the history of medieval Europe and its medicine.

The conquest of Spain by several thousand Arabs and Berbers lasted five years. The reconquest of Arabic Spain by Catholic Spain lasted eight hundred years. This difference in time provides the key to the secret of Arabic Spain.

Musa, governor of North Africa, and his lieutenant, Tarik, conquered Spain with twelve thousand Arabs and Berbers who had come to the Iberian peninsula without their families, married Spanish women, and created Celto-Iberian, Visigothic, and Afro-Semitic mixtures in Andalusia. It was the scions of such Andalusian stock who set sail from Cadiz and Seville for the New World.

"I do not understand," Ortega y Gasset has said, "how something that lasted eight centuries can be called 'Reconquista.' " One should remember that the Moslems of the Iberian peninsula were true Spaniards in temperament and spirit. The Arab Abd-ur-Rahman III, King of Spain, was as much a Spaniard as the Spaniard Trajan, Emperor of Rome; Arabic Averroës, who was born in Cordova where he lived and prospered all his life, was as Spanish as the Spanish-descended Seneca, who was also born in Cordova but lived and worked in Italy.

During the Moslem domination of Spain, the Iberian peninsula was shaken by continuous wars, yet in the intervals between these wars, Christians, Mohammedans, and Jews learned to live together in relative harmony. The Berbers and the *almorávides* and their enemies the *almohades* (the unitarian Moors of Morocco), as well as other natives of north Africa converted to Islam, were the most fanatical, as has always been the case with religious converts. But to the Arabs themselves Islamism and unitarianism were only tools with which to achieve their conquests and an ultimate goal: pleasure. It is true that the Arabs were given to pillage, but as soon as they attained their goal, religious tolerance became the rule. The *mozárabes,* or Christians acclimated to Islam, and the *mudéjares,* or Mohammedans who accepted Christianity, received better treatment at the hands of Islam than the *marranos,* or converted Jews, and the *moriscos,* or converted Mohammedans, later received at the hands of the Christians. Christians and Mohammedans observed the same religious festivals and often worshiped in two separate wings of the same temple. The Jews, who had been persecuted by the Visigoths, went over to the Arabs and became prominent figures in the intellectual renaissance of Cordova and Toledo.

The Western Caliphate, which succeeded the Caliphate of Baghdad in importance, endowed Spain with a progressive cultural organization. Literature flourished together with art, science, and philosophy; libraries were constructed along with schools and hospitals; medical societies were established, and agriculture and industry developed. Except in mathematics and literature, the Mohammedans were assimilators and transmitters rather than creators. Their architecture, rich in domes and profusely ornamented planes which can still be seen in North Africa, derived from the Byzantine; the inside cloistered *patios* of their houses in medieval Spain derived from Rome; their medicine derived from Greece through Syria and Persia—all of which seems to indicate rather uninventive minds. But if we descend from the lofty disciplines of the mind to more earthy matters, we observe that the Arabs were responsible for notable progress in everything having to do with bodily comfort. The Arabs subordinated the soul to sensual delights. That is why even their religious paradise is endowed with all physical comforts and pleasures, including numerous houris. Their cities attested to the fertility of their gift for material comfort and pleasures, for they boasted of glass windows, street lights, spices, drugs and perfumes, gardens, and stringed instruments.

THE WESTERN CALIPHATE: MEDICINE IN CORDOVA

Once the Arabs were definitely established in Spain, the Western Caliphate of Cordova (755–1236) began to achieve great prosperity under the Spanish dynasty of the Omayyads. Their greatest medical writers were the surgeon Albucasis, the philosopher Averroës, and the Jewish physicians Avenzoar and Maimonides, all of whom were born in or near Cordova. It is difficult to understand why Spanish historians even today, guided by a false patriotism, do not consider these four men, who wrought a glorious page in medieval Spanish history, as Spaniards.

The capital of Moslem Spain was then Cordova, a city of one million inhabitants, three hundred mosques all housing schools, fifty hospitals, a municipal library of more than two hundred and twenty-five thousand volumes, seventeen universities, and as many public libraries.[J]

This frenzied adoption of ancient teachings, which the Arab clothed in the opulent apparel of his own fantasy, lasted well into the ninth century. The caliphs became Maecenases to a retinue of studious investigators. At their courts the twanging of the *guzlas* alternated with solemn discussions on medicine. Side by side in every palace were to be found the blue-shadowed seraglio, perfumed with the sensual flesh of the women, and the dim library filled with ancient, musty-smelling, yellowed parchments. During the rule of the Omayyad caliphs, whose vast empire stretched from Spain to Samarkand, the sumptuousness of the Arab courts provided a setting worthy of the remarkable work of its intellectuals.

Notable analogies exist between the awakening of medicine in the Golden Age of Arabic civilization and that of Renaissance Italy. Arab physicians, like Renaissance physicians, were also philosophers, so much so that the title of *Hakim* applied to both physicians and philosophers. The medical humanists of the Renaissance had their precursors in Arab physicians. If Renaissance Italy boasted of a *uomo universale* like Leonardo da Vinci, who was physician, architect, poet, musician, sculptor, painter, and geologist, or like Paracelsus, who was

philosopher, physician, physicist, astronomer, and geologist, Arabic
Spain could point to Abu-Bekr-Zakarias, favorite Koran expounder
of the Omayyad caliphs of Cordova, astronomer, naturalist, physician,
historian, and outstanding publicist in the *aljamiada* language; and to
Geber and Maimonides, whose many-sided achievements are related
elsewhere in these pages.

There is even a similar dramatic flavor in the lives of representative
men of both epochs. If Leonardo da Vinci led a life of silent loves
and of struggle against religious fanaticism; so did Maimonides, who
could distill philosophies as vaporous as the flower of sulfur he dis-
solved in his crucibles; and if Benvenuto Cellini, that brilliant goldsmith and charlatan, bespattered the walls of Rome with the blood
of his enemies, filled the Roman streets with his drunken songs,
and figured in audacious love-escapades, Avenzoar led a wild existence among the gypsies of Albaicin, and Avicenna only too often put
his lips to the silver jug filled with warm red wine and roamed the
streets plucking the strings of a guitar and singing love songs.

These men of Arabic Spain, fascinated by the marvels of life, tried
to discover the secrets of the universe through astrology and alchemy.
Their experiments fathered Arabic polypharmacy, that conglomeration of mixtures and unguents, and while their dark hands were busy
compounding gilded pills, their minds tried to crack the mystery of
space in search of the secret correlations between the position of the
stars and the destiny of men.

The Spanish Arabs were not mere compilers of Greco-Latin knowledge. They did more than pour the waters of Greek wisdom into their
own receptacles; they added to this water the essence of their intuition, the warmth of their humanism, and the fragrance of their imagination. Bearing witness to their work was the library of Al-Hakim
II containing four hundred thousand volumes, which spelled out
Arabic wisdom in a rich, vibrant, supple, virile style as perfectly
suited for the poetization of medicine as Virgilian Latin was for singing the glories of agriculture.

The Caliphate of Cordova (755–1031) by itself could be considered the Golden Age of Arabic civilization just as Cordova may be
called the Baghdad of the West. The coming of the Arabs marked
an upsurge in Spain's economic wealth. Arab vessels brought food
plants from Asia and Africa, while the Arabs raised domestic animals, constructed roads, gardens, and canals, and stimulated the
manufacture of silk, embroidery, ceramics, hides, and majolica. In
Andalusia and Valencia attendance at school was compulsory for
children from the age of six. The closing years of the Western Caliphate saw the creation of the *medressen* or centers of theologic,
legal, philosophic, and grammar studies; these were joined to the

mosques and had libraries and lecture rooms with professional lecturers.

The Caliphate of Cordova reached its peak with Abd-ur-Rahman III, who received embassies from the Emperor of Byzantium and Otto I of Germany and patronized scientific and medical meetings. Hakem II invited the outstanding scholars of Baghdad to visit Cordova.

Cordova would fall into Christian hands in 1236; Baghdad would be sacked by the Mongols in 1258; and Granada would succumb in 1492. But during the golden centuries of Arabic Spain, medicine flourished while in the rest of Europe it was buried in the prevailing semibarbarism.

Arabic Spain abounded in families, like that of Avenzoar, that produced physicians for several consecutive generations, in some cases as many as seven. Statues were erected to physicians, a tribute never again paid to the profession until our day. There even were women physicians despite Islamic restrictions. Latin medical compilations dating from before the twelfth century, still to be found in the Spanish libraries of those days, looked like poor relatives next to the sumptuous works of the Moslems.

Even during the reign of Philip II, Moorish tradition continued. When King Ferdinand of Aragon was sick, he requested the courts of Valencia to send him a healing woman known as the "dancing Moor of Mislata." Pinderete, a Valencian Moor converted to Christianity, treated Philip II's son, Don Carlos, with an ointment he had invented, notwithstanding the fact that physicians like Vesalius were living at the royal court. The Moorish physician Alonso del Castillo was summoned by Philip II to classify Arabic manuscripts at the Escorial.

The first concern of any Arabic city was the organization of a hospital, which in Andalusia served also as an asylum for the insane and destitute. These hospitals attested to the Moslem love of water, for they were embellished with lions spurting water from their mouths. One of these, built by King Nazari Mohammed V, can still be seen opposite the *Torre de las Damas* in the Alhambra at Granada. Since washing and cleansing were as necessary to the Arab as prayers, they constructed nine hundred baths in Cordova alone. Mohammedan civilization, born in hot countries, made a fetish of bathing and continued the practice even in the cold climate of Toledo. Christians thought such baths sinful and weakening, and Alfonso VI had them destroyed after the battle of Uccles.

Strange contrast! The Christian Crusades brought nothing but destruction and death to the East; the Arabs were lavish with the treasures of their wisdom and brought progress and prosperity to the West.

Medicine was taught privately. Only after acquiring the necessary general education at the *medressen* and only after learning the art of the mortar and the spatula from some pharmacist did the student enter the service of an experienced physician, in whose library he could study medical works bound in fine Cordovan leather embossed with golden or polychrome reliefs.

Cordova became a charming cosmopolitan city. Its streets bustled with the traffic of caravans from distant lands. A belt of tents marked the perimeter of the city and there were displayed lovely woven stuffs, rugs and carpets, delicately wrought metals, jewels, glassware, pottery, and dried sweetmeats. In the lazy shade of the awnings, merchants sipped their bubbly drinks fragrant with the essence of lemon and roses. The Arab, who only a few centuries earlier had not even dreamed of leaving Arabia, learned to live like a Sybarite far from his native soil. In the gardens of the Alcazar of Seville, the Alhambra of Granada, the Alpujarras, and the Albaicin, the indolent Moslems lazily followed the flight of the bees to and fro, from the flowers to the hive in the hollow trunk of a pine tree, the tiny dots of pollen on their legs glistening in the sunshine like drops of dew, while carnations, myrtles, sweet basil, passion flowers, lilies, and roses swooned in the sultry air, and the multicolored tile fountains spurted water as warm as blood. At sunset music was heard everywhere. It was here that the *cante jondo*[K] was born.

Astrology and magic were important areas of study for the Arab physician. Arab medicine was the mother of alchemy, which combined with magic. In ancient Chaldean pantheism, the doctrine of an *anima mundi* or a spirit animating all things was applied to any substance that could be extracted from fire. Hence the spirits of wine, niter, and other essences. The seven planets corresponded to the days of the week and to the seven known metals, which were thought to have been engendered in the entrails of the earth.[L] There also prevailed the notion of an elixir of life in the form of potable gold that could cure all ailments and confer eternal youth. Investigation of this *aurum potabile* led to the discovery of *aqua regia* and strong acids, just as the idea of an elixir of life led to the foundation of pharmaceutic chemistry.

ALBUCASIS, THE SURGEON

The first great physician of the Cordovan scientific quadrumvirate was Albucasis (Abu-al-Qasim Khalaf ibn 'Abbas al-Zahrawi) (912–1013), a native of Cordova and the greatest surgeon in Arabic medicine. It was Albucasis who recognized the deplorable state into which surgery had fallen and dedicated himself to writing a monumental medical and surgical compilation called *al-Tasrif*, with illustrations of instruments and certain operations common among the Arabs.[M] Oriental revulsion at touching the human body with the hands was responsible for the fact that Arab physicians seldom reproduced ancient surgical drawings. Albucasis' book was the beacon of European surgery until the advent of Ambroise Paré.

The part of Albucasis' book dealing with surgery was based on the work done by Paul of Aegina and was the basic surgical text (it was translated many times into Latin, once by Guy de Chauliac) of the Middle Ages until after Salicetus. The section devoted to medicine was copied from Rhazes, for among Arab physicians it was not considered dishonest to copy from one another.

Albucasis' book contains descriptions of cautery, lithotomy, amputations in cases of gangrene, fractures, and obstetric positions; it praises iron cautery which Albucasis used on more than fifty patients. Albucasis classified operations into "those that do the patient good and those that generally kill him."

Albucasis might be called the Arabic Vesalius, for he dared defy the Koran itself. "Never operate," he told his pupils, "without knowing the exact site of the veins, nerves, and tendons." Like Vesalius, he himself illustrated his text although his religion prevented him from drawing nude bodies, especially of women. He used bandages hardened with earth, and for the treatment of ulcers he devised bandages with windows. On the other hand, he neglected obstetrics and gynecology, which never made any progress among the Arabs, again because the Koran prohibited women from appearing in the nude even before a physician.

At the age of one hundred, Albucasis, still active as private physician to Abd-ur-Rahman III, composed his *Liber Servitoris,* a manual for pharmacists, and even engaged in the extraction of dead fetuses with serrated forceps in the Caliph's seraglio. His works, translated by Constantine the African, penetrated as far as Salerno.

AVENZOAR, THE CLINICIAN

If Albucasis was the greatest Arab surgeon, Avenzoar was the greatest clinician and physician of the Western Caliphate and one of the few courageous enough to rebel against Galen.[N]

The scion of a Sevillian family which for five generations produced teachers of the Koran, Avenzoar in the daytime would tread the plush carpets in the gilded Alcazar and at night would consort with beggars and galley slaves in the gypsy quarter of the Albaicin. One minute he would be feeling the pulse of the sick, and the next minute he would be plucking Apollo's lyre. Avenzoar rejected Avicenna's *Canon* and was the most Hippocratic of the Arab physicians. His list of antidotes was the bible for toxicologists, while his *Liber Orna-mentis,* a book on cosmetics, was "the beloved guide that every Mohammedan woman kept in her sandalwood box."

AVERROËS, THE PHILOSOPHER

Averroës (Abu-al-Walid Muhammad ibn-Ahmad ibn-Rushd) (1126–1198), a disciple of Avenzoar and an Aristotelian philosopher, lived in Cordova and, like Avenzoar, died in Morocco. He studied law, mathematics, philosophy, and medicine, and was physician to Caliph Abu-Ya'qub Yusif in Marrakesh. His master work was the *Colliget,* a treatise containing a complete system of medicine based on Aristotelian philosophy and expounding the pantheistic doctrine that the soul or the nature of man is absorbed upon death into the universal nature. His denial of man's immortality made him a lifelong victim of persecution; together with some of his disciples he was anathematized throughout the Middle Ages.

Averroës' works were burned, and the Infidels spat on him for his heresy, while Christian hands nailed his image beside the anti-Christ in the Orcagna fresco in the cemetery at Pisa. But Averroës' greatest claim to glory is that even his most virulent enemies, Raimund Lull and St. Thomas Aquinas, were deeply influenced by his theories.

MAIMONIDES, THE HUMANIST

Maimonides (Musa ibn Maimun, Rabbi Moses ben Maimon) was born of a prominent Hebrew family, March 30, 1135, in the city of Cordova.

The boy, who loved to play in the narrow sun-baked streets and stared spellbound at the water flowing from bronze and silver statues into marble troughs, was educated by his father in the Talmud and the Bible, law and science, astronomy and literature. When the intolerant *almohades* occupied Cordova, Maimonides had to flee to Fez where, together with his father, brother, and sister, he pretended to embrace Islam. Later, Maimonides went with his father and his brother to Jerusalem and from there to Cairo where, after his father's death, he became a dealer in jewelry, although he devoted most of his time to literature into which Abdul-Arab ibn-Muisha had initiated him in Fez. When his brother was drowned in the Indian Ocean, Maimonides found himself laden with debts and with a sister to support. It was then that he took time from his literary work and began to practice medicine. In Egypt he married the sister of a royal secretary who, in turn, married Maimonides' sister.

Maimonides became personal physician to the Sultan Saladin, the first Ayyubite sultan of Egypt (1138–1193), a living symbol of Mohammedan unity. The caliphs of Baghdad had then only nominal power; the viziers were the real rulers. One day there arrived in Acre a powerful-looking Englishman wearing a glittering coat of mail and an enormous sword. It was Richard I of England, the Lion-Hearted, who tried unsuccessfully to acquire Maimonides' services for his own court. But Maimonides had the Egyptian sun to remind him of his beloved Cordova and he refused to exchange it for the mysterious fogs of England.

Maimonides would work until the afternoon in the royal palace; then, tired and hungry, he would return home, have some dates, figs, grapes, and fowl, drink the watered wine from his silver cup, and go back to his consultations with Moorish and Hebrew patients. Only Saturdays did he set aside for studying and writing. Sometimes his pen would remain suspended in mid-air while he went into a trance, dreaming of the olive, orange, and lemon groves that perfumed the Cordovan hills under a brilliant blue sky.

Maimonides lived this sort of life to the very end. He preferred to regard medicine as an art, not as a science; he studied the sick, not sickness; and his actions and thoughts were guided by that teleologic criterion which today governs modern medicine. At the age of fifty, when he thought he would soon die, there was born to him a son. Both the son and a grandson became physicians in Cairo. Maimonides' aphorisms were seeds which took roots in the souls of his descendants.

Meanwhile, while the victorious banner of the Christian conquest advanced across Spain, Maimonides wrote books in Arabic that were later translated into Hebrew and Latin and that, along with the works of Averroës, would be decisive factors in the formation of a medico-philosophic school in western Europe.⁰

In all his writings Maimonides rejected astrology and even portions of the rabbinical tradition, and reconciled reason and faith. In his *Guide for the Perplexed* (1190) he analyzed Aristotle, establishing himself as an outstanding philosopher. When he died at the age of seventy (1204), he had already been recognized as a great teacher. But the greatest merit of this scholar lies in the fact that he was always frank about what he did not know. On one occasion he was moved to say (anticipating an idea later expressed by Roger Bacon): "Teach thy tongue to say 'I do not know,' and thou shalt progress."

Maimonides' principles of diet.

The Sultan Al-Malik-Al-Afdal, son of the Sultan of Egypt, was a neurotic young man forever worrying about his health. The sweet sounds of the silver *guzla* plucked by expert players, the shimmering bodies of girls dancing in the scarlet light of torches, songs and red wine—none of these amused him. Obsessed by his health, he consulted Maimonides, the court physician. The letters the latter wrote almost eight hundred years ago to his royal master, giving him advice concerning what to eat, have become immortal. Despite their naive simplicity, they are of such practical value that any modern physician might recommend them as a popular code of dietetic hygiene.

"Man," said Maimonides in these letters, "should lead a life pleasing to God, should do nothing to harm his health, and should eat and drink only when it is necessary. He should always eat a little less than he requires to surfeit himself; he should drink very little water during his meals and during the period of digestion, and the little he does drink should, if possible, be mixed with wine." On this point Maimonides agreed with some nutrition experts who have established the daily quantity of wine to be taken at fifty grams. He continued: "If possible, before eating, the body should be rested, warmed by a bath and evacuated; one should not eat in a sitting position, never walking or riding; nor should one do exercise or hard work in the first four hours after a meal."

Maimonides fully appreciated the value of the very same fruits that modern hygiene considers most nutritional. "Good fruits—grapes, almonds, figs, melon—are good laxatives," he said, "and should be eaten by themselves just before the meal; they should not be eaten from the tree or when they are dry or green, and never become too dependent upon them." Maimonides was warning against a diet too rich in sugar, a caveat of modern medicine.

"Eat," advised the good Maimonides, "what is easily digested, fowl rather than ox meat and beef rather than bull meat. In the summer or in warm climates, eat cold meats, acid foods and no spices. In winter and cold climates, eat very hot food, rich in mustard and spices." (Thus was laid the basis of calorie diets.) "These are harmful foods which should be avoided," he continued: "large salted fish, old cheese [danger of fermentation!], pungent foods, young wine and food that is bitter or too fragrant. Nor would I recommend milk more than a day old, meat from an old ox, peas, unleavened bread, onions and radishes. Of all the foregoing," advised Maimonides, "eat little and only in the winter. Never eat dried beans or lentils; have honey and wine in moderation and only in the winter, and never give them to children." It is almost as if we were listening to Montaigne or Luis Vives.

Then Maimonides discussed regulation of the intestines, a prosaic but necessary preoccupation and one of great importance among the Arabs. "Always try," he said, "to combat constipation; with this view in mind, young people should eat foods with a great deal of salt and oil, and vegetable soups; and old people should take honey with hot water in the morning. Above all," he insisted, "be temperate. Solomon said that he who stands guard over his mouth and tongue avoids many ills."

He advised against the excessive use of venesection, which was then very much in fashion. He also gave advice about bathing. "Take a hot bath at least once a week. Never bathe in cold water, except if you make it colder gradually; do not bathe while digesting your food, nor when hungry; cover your head to avoid drafts; during your bath drink watered wine or water with honey instead of plain water, rub your body with oil, and rest." What more could a contemporary hygienist in a hydrotherapy clinic recommend?

Finally Maimonides advised against sleeping during the day. Only at night should one sleep and for eight hours, waking at dawn; one should sleep first on the left side and then on the right. "He who follows these rules," his letters to Saladin concluded, "will live long without infirmities; but if he is ill he should consult a physician. If he does so, he will die from old age without needing one."

THE ARABS IN HISTORY

The Arabs made their appearance in world history with the Islamic explosion, an explosion that was not only religious, but also political and emotional. When the Arabs set out to conquer the world, they were an uncouth people, cruel and primitive in their ways, a horde of men with horses and camels, tents and scimitars, subsisting on goat's milk and palm dates. But they were also a people with a craving for culture and an innate respect for the written word.

Scarcely forty years after the death of Mohammed, the Atlantic shores were stained scarlet by the Arab onslaught. Before the century was out, the banners of Islam waved from the Pyrenees and the Pillars of Hercules in Gibraltar to the Heavenly Hills in China. During the course of this astounding cavalcade, the Arabs, who until then had been but lords of the winds and the sands and knights of the sun and the stars, were suddenly confronted with medieval castles and draw-bridges, Roman aqueducts and war machines, medical potions that worked better than any prayer, and mysterious manuscripts soaked in age-old wisdom. And avidly they added to their own scanty knowledge the mysteries of Persia, the Egyptian cabalas, Oriental magic, and Greco-Latin culture. They were wise enough not to enslave the peoples they conquered, as the Romans did, and they even encouraged their search for knowledge. They turned Damascus, Baghdad and other cities into modern, sophisticated, flourishing metropolises contrasting with the dirty, drab cities of medieval Europe. It was the fame of these eastern cities—marvels of culture and opulence—that provided one of the principal incentives for the Crusades.

Stimulated by their discoveries in the West, the Arabs made their own contributions to the general welfare. They perfected fireworks—the multihued explosion of their own colorful souls—put panes in windows, until then covered only by boards; installed lights in the streets; created a numerical system that is the basis of our own numerology; established the scientific bases of geology, algebra, and especially chemistry; and distinguished themselves for their work in gold, silver, bronze, steel, textiles, glass and ceramics, dyes and paper, sugar cane, viniculture, horticulture and botany.

The Arabs were not allowed by their religion to perform dissections and therefore accepted without question Galen's monkey anatomy and physiology; but they made three fundamental contributions to medicine: medicinal chemistry in the form of alchemy and botany; the organization of pharmacy; and the founding of hospitals.

ARABIC CONTRIBUTIONS TO MEDICINE

Medicinal chemistry.

The development of Arabic medicinal chemistry is the work of Geber's genius. It was he who distilled vinegar, sublimated sulfur, and crystallized mercury, and put all known compounds into his furnaces, sublimating pots, and retorts. Geber was the champion of therapeutic sobriety in contrast with the extravagant practices of the apothecaries in his day.

Following the path of alchemy, the Arabs discovered a whole fascinating world of drugs, including alcohol, sulfuric and nitric acids, silver nitrate, mercury bichloride, naphtha, benzoin, camphor, saffron, myrrh, laudanum, and potassium. While the rest of Europe was busy with prayer, the Arabs were introducing alchemistic techniques of crystallization, distillation, and sublimation, and were using anesthetics and practicing clinical medicine.

The organization of pharmacy.

The Arabs organized pharmacy, establishing two types of pharmacists: those who sold herbs, sirups, and simple medicines, and those who filled medical prescriptions. Arab pharmacies were supervised by an inspector who threatened the pharmacists with bodily punishment if they adulterated their drugs. Pharmacies were clearing houses for over five hundred drugs, not including their combinations. They also sold civet to Moorish women, and distilled water of orange blossoms, myrtle, roses, and carnations for physicians to wash their hands. And they sold honey, then the most fashionable medical panacea, in the form of sirups which are still used today.

The pharmacies were also centers of information, conversation and culture, dispensers of news, gossip, and rumors, and popular academies where people were informed of medical progress. Many Arabic words, which were later incorporated into our language, viz., alcohol, drug, alkali, sirup, sugar, spinach, alfalfa, admiral, arsenal, pillow, cipher, star, algebra, zero, zenith, and julep, were created during the interminable conversations held between the pharmacist and his customers while they gazed at the spurting waters in the blue tile fountains.

The pharmacist could immediately judge the importance of a physician calling on him by the height of his turban and the richness and length of the sleeves of his robe. Some physicians charged as much as one hundred and twenty-five thousand *duros* for a consultation and made as much as ten million *duros* in medical practice.

Paradoxically, physicians tended to rely on the vegetable medicaments provided by nature, while pharmacists alternated the preparation of drugs with horoscope readings, allowing the stars and alchemistic philosophy to rule their chemical manipulations. For the benefit of their credulous patients, pharmacies prominently exhibited bottles containing fetuses, frogs, scorpions, owls, dissected crocodiles, as well as flasks with mysterious liquids. Even physicians frequently combined science with the necromancer's tricks.

Arab physicians and pharmacists were pioneers in chemistry and pharmacology, for, driven by a consuming ambition to find the philosopher's stone that would transmute lead into gold or silver, they did extensive experimentation which led to the development of the basic methods in chemistry, viz., distillation, sublimation, calcination, and filtration. They also experimented with their drugs on animals. Rhazes, for instance, tried mercury on monkeys.

The Arabs also invented the art of filling prescriptions, an art inherited with few changes by our modern pharmacists. They introduced sirups, juleps, oils, poultices, court plasters, pills, powders, alcoholates, and aromatic waters. They discovered a form of surgical anesthesia consisting of a sponge soaked in narcotic and aromatic substances which the patient sucked or inhaled before an operation. *The Thousand and One Nights* abounds in stories involving hypnotic drugs that probably had been inherited from Chinese pharmacology.

To the Arabs then belongs the glory of having created medicinal chemistry, for the Greek attempt at chemistry was limited to casting metals.

Another contribution made by Arabic pharmacy was the manufacture of drug jars and bottles that were veritable works of art. The ancient Egyptian alabaster vases for ointments, the square Roman glass boxes for poultices, the Persian vessels embellished with figures of animals and fruits—all were outdone by Arabic ceramics, the result of a flourishing pharmacy. These Arabic ceramic jars were richly colored and ornamented with fruits and leaves, the same motifs used on jars for preserves and marmalades, and on tiles and majolica. They had such artistic value that later they were copied by Italian craftsmen. When Caliph Harun-al-Rashid wished to present Emperor Charlemagne with a gift, he chose the finest Arabic majolica jars and had them filled with ointments.

The founding of hospitals.

The Arabs further contributed to medicine by founding magnificent hospitals in Djondisapur, Baghdad, Damascus, Cordova, and Cairo.

The Mansur Hospital in Cairo had separate wards for men and women, wards for general diseases, and wards for eye diseases. For patients with fevers, it boasted of wards decorated with fountains so that the patients might be soothed by the chanting water.

This hospital was an immense quadrilateral construction with four courtyards, and had such features as lecture halls, a library with six librarians, chapels, and an asylum for the poor along with a dispensary and a kitchen, all attended by qualified male and female nurses. Day and night, fifty reciters intoned the Koran aloud. At nightfall, musicians played soft melodies to induce drowsiness in the patients. Professional storytellers entertained the sick with their tales. When the patient left the hospital he was given enough money so that he would not have to resume work immediately. The hospital was completed in 1384 by carpenters who had come from Egypt, but even passers-by were forced to help in its construction, thus making a compulsory contribution to a good cause.

In the year 1160 Baghdad had more than sixty hospitals, according to an old Jew who traveled there at that time. The same year saw the foundation of the famous hospital of Damascus, which for three centuries cared for the sick gratis. In 1427 it was destroyed by fire. Baghdad also had several insane asylums, where patients were treated with a gentleness and kindness never known before. All hospitals were also centers of medical teaching where new techniques were tried out, such as the use of cautery instead of the scalpel, which became the basis of Arabic surgery.

There were also many special hospitals for eye diseases. The Arabs were particularly interested in the eye, not only because of its religious symbolism ("the eye of Providence"), but because of the preponderance of blindness due to "Egyptian ophthalmy," or trachoma, and other eye diseases caused by perennial sand storms. This explains why ophthalmology made greater progress than other facets of anatomy or physiology, and it provides a good example of how a sociologic need forces the progress of a given branch of medicine. The Arabs, however, dared not go so far in their meticulous study of the eye as to violate the religious ban on dissection.[P]

In the eleventh century the Arabs published the *Book of Alhazen*, the most important treatise on optics in the fifteen centuries between the Alexandrian period of Euclid and Ptolemy and the initiation by Kepler and Newton of modern physics. All this progress in ophthalmology was made empirically, for when the Arabs operated on cataracts, for example, they were not even aware that they were removing a darkened lens.

Thus, through the great medical figures in the Eastern Caliphate, the Arabs bequeathed to the West a rich legacy in botany, pharmacology, pharmacognosy, and chemistry, together with the organization of hospitals and alchemical techniques. And in the Western Caliphate of Moslem Spain, Arabic medicine, propelled by the genius of a few Arabico-Spanish physicians, achieved new scientific and cultural heights.

COLOPHON

Such, then, is the imprint made on history by the Arabs during the centuries that witnessed the birth, the growth, and the decline and extinction of their mighty empire. The plain Mohammedan farmer and the warring nomad Bedouin, who led a primitive existence with but the barest necessities of life, after they reached strange lands, developed into a highly civilized people who knew how to adapt themselves to their new surroundings, how to create comfort and luxury, and how to nurture the seeds of an art and a science that had classical roots but gave forth genuine Mohammedan blossoms.

Deep within themselves, however, the Arabs remained a primitive people who preferred the barren desert to the verdant oasis, for they knew that it is in the desert, bereft of everything but sky and sand, that man may truly face himself and his Creator. This nostalgia of the western Arab for the life of the nomad was reflected in the *casidas* of eleventh century Andalusia, the melodies that influenced the poets of Dante's times and inspired the lyrical poetry of Shakespeare's predecessors.

We have seen in the foregoing pages the rich medical legacy left by the Arabs. Perhaps this legacy was not as indelible as that of other

Oriental nations; nevertheless, to the Arabs, besides the medieval monks, we owe all the medical progress made during the many years of darkness in medieval Europe. More than creators, the Arabs were "transmitters and transmuters" of classical science. But then, in those periods in history when there are no creators, the work of the transmitter acquires the importance of the only path for civilization and science to continue their journey.

At the end of the journey of Arabic civilization there was a night as Scheherazade could have never dreamed about. It was the night *one thousand and two,* on which medicine was suddenly illuminated by the dawn of the Renaissance.

NOTES

A. This and subsequent quotations are from *The Thousand and One Nights,* Sir Richard F. Burton's translation, New York, Heritage Press, 1934.

B. Ultimately, Nestorius retired to an oasis in Libya where he died.

C. Actually Arabic medicine is a misnomer since Persians, Syrians, Spaniards, Jews, and Copts contributed to it; it should rather be called Moslem or Islamic medicine, for it was not racial characteristics but the religious banner and the Arabic tongue that provided the unifying forces.

D. In the year 794 a paper factory was established in Baghdad.

E. The Jews exercised considerable influence on Arabic medicine, for they figured prominently at the courts of the caliphs. A common belief in an inner monotheism created strong ties of sympathy between Mohammedans and Hebrews. Another point of contact was that Hebrew and Mohammedan physicians, with their gift for analysis, intensive thinking, and appreciation of values, soon developed a materialistic way of looking at concrete things. Whereas Christian physicians were preoccupied with spells, amulets, saints' relics, and superstitions, most Jewish and Mohammedan physicians had no regard for such things.

During the Middle Ages and for a long time thereafter Hebrew physicians suffered varied fates. When the Persian King Chosroes established the school of Djondisapur in Arabistan, Jews as well as Christians were invited to teach; by the time the Islamic Empire had spread from Mecca to Finisterre, the Jews had gained ascendancy at the court of the Caliph Moawiya I. In the tenth and eleventh centuries they were a sort of forbidden luxury, much sought after by princes and bishops because of their superior abilities but often harshly treated for religious reasons. The Jews also distinguished themselves as translators of Greek works, and greatly contributed to the foundation of the School of Salerno, where Ben Salim translated Rhazes. In 1267 the Council of Vienna prohibited them from practicing among Christians. Under the Western Caliphate they were highly respected in Spain. When they were exiled from Spain in 1402, the School of Salerno engaged them as teachers but only until it was able to proceed on its own without outside help. The same thing occurred in Montpellier, which closed its doors to Jews in 1301.

F. Ali al-Tabari was a contemporary of Hunain, son of Isaac, the Persian-Jewish scholar. He wrote on cupping and amulets, and composed a manual called *Paradise of Wisdom* in which he discussed pathology from head to toes. He compared his book to a garden that should be viewed not from the gate but by strolling along its walks.

The Physician as Alchemist 107

G. Haly Abbas, a Persian magician, was born of a Zoroastrian family. His *Liber Regius* is a four million word compendium of the entire medical knowledge of the Arabs in the tenth century.

H. Rhazes was the first to describe and differentiate between smallpox and measles. He treated more than a thousand patients for sciatica, studied hiccough and the origins of jaundice, wrote the first treatise on pediatry, introduced several drugs, studied gonorrhea thoroughly, described seton application and pupilar reflex to light, wrote monographs on poliomyelitic endemiology, tuberculous fistular osteitis, and eruptive fevers, and even studied the allegoric dreams of his patients.

I. Avicenna's clinical observations are worthy even of our times, especially his comments on the physiology of dreams, the purification of water, medical ecology, dietetics, urethral medication, the use of vaginal plugs, oral anesthetics, the treatment of insanity by artificially induced malaria, tic douloureux, tetanus, pleuritis, the contagious nature of tuberculosis, anthrax, and diabetes mellitus.

Like other Arab physicians, Avicenna did not practice dissection of the human body because of religious reasons, and his anatomy therefore is Galenic. He used surgery only in extreme cases, preferring cautery to the scalpel. The application of cautery lasted until Ambroise Paré rejected it, lessening thereby the suffering of the wounded but increasing the number of infections. Which proves that progress in medicine is not always made in a straight line but often by detours.

J. To the north of the Caliphate of Cordova—which from 756 to 1031 embraced the major part of the Iberian peninsula—were the Visigothic kingdoms of Asturias, Leon, Castile, Navarre, and Catalonia, which were focuses of continuous rebellion during Moslem domination. The frontier lay to the south of the Duero River, and Aragon was in enemy territory. In 1150 this frontier had shifted down to the Tagus River, and in 1276 all that remained of Moslem Spain was the small kingdom of Granada.

Toledo swarmed with Arab manuscripts and became a great center for translators, eventually eclipsing Cordova in medicine, philosophy, and theology. Archbishop Raimundo of Toledo (?–1150) formed a society of Hebrew translators under the direction of Archdeacon Dominicus Gundisalvi, which later was converted into an institute for Saracen studies under Christian tutelage.

K. The *cante jondo,* a style of singing associated with the Spanish gypsy, is a symbol of the Spanish soul. Semitic winds carried plaintive melodies from Oriental shores to the Mediterranean coast of Andalusia. On the soft, dark Andalusian soil, while guitars strummed in the shade of proud cypresses and kind olive trees, Moorish and Christian tresses tangled with Jewish tresses, forming a braid that cracked like a whip into the popular soul. Thus was the *cante jondo* born.

L. The legend of a medicine that could cure one out of every six lepers would later be considered (by Boerhaave) as an allegory of the philosopher's stone that could transform the six basic metals of the world into gold.

M. Albucasis extracted arrows from the bodies of wounded men and ligated arteries to stop hemorrhages. He was the first to describe the position for lithotomy on women and to treat fractures with bandages. He performed transversal tracheotomies and differentiated between thyroid cancer and ordinary goiter.

N. In his book *Theizir,* Avenzoar describes the acarus that causes scabies; he therefore could be considered the first parasitologist. He also described serous pericarditis and pharyngeal paralysis. He practiced tracheotomy on sheep, used artificial feeding through a catheter introduced in the esophagus, and treated hernia with baked bread, boiled sparrows, two months' rest "without even praying except in the heart," milk baths to feed the patient through the pores, and food enemas. He claimed that "the interpreter of the soul of the brain is the tongue, and the most noble of the senses is the eye."

O. Among Maimonides' most famous works are his translations into Hebrew of the *Canon* of Avicenna, his medical aphorisms, his treatise on poisons and their antidotes, a treatise on asthma, and particularly his treatises on dietetics, which he wrote in the form of letters to al-Malik al-Afdal, son of the Sultan Saladin of Egypt.

P. The most ancient diagram in existence of the human eye is to be found in a manuscript of the Arab Hunain ibn Ishak.

THE PHYSICIAN AS TRAVELER

It is both a pleasure and an honor to greet the distinguished guests and audience of this First International Conference on Health and Travel. We have brought together here a brilliant array of internists, pediatricians, specialists in aeronautical, naval, and space medicine, medical geography, and physiology to discuss what happens to *Homo sapiens* today when he is transported out of his customary environment by plane, train, boat, automobile, or submarine to new lands, new seas, and new skies. We shall also study what happens to man under such circumstances at different times in his life, and in health and sickness.

Man is the most restless of all living beings. From the very beginning of his existence man has incessantly roamed the earth, at first on foot and later on horseback. One day man invented motor-propelled vehicles that helped him to conquer the earth and the seas. Finally he soared into the air in his supreme longing to conquer space.

Living is traveling *par excellence*. Life itself is a stormy voyage from the shores of light marking our birth to the shadowed threshold of death leading into the land of mystery. The Greek Argonauts symbolized this concept of life as incessant travel when they said: "The essential thing is not to live; the essential thing is to travel."

When man is confined to one point in space because of a lean pocket or for other reasons, he travels vertically on the wings of his inspiration, like the mystics and poets; or in an armchair, like Jules

An address delivered at the First International Symposium on Health and Travel, New York, June 23, 1955; published in *International Record of Medicine 168*:480, 1955.

Verne and his readers; or through time on the Pegasus of his art, like the artists of all ages.

But here we shall study travel as a physical displacement through time and space because traveling is the characteristic *modus vivendi* of modern man. In prehistoric times, man traveled only when impelled by fear or hunger. Primitive man traveled when threatened by the icy avalanches of invading glaciers or the frightful droughts that turned the earth into sterile ground, by the invasion of fearful monsters or floods, the approach of enemy tribes or geologic cataclysms. Later, in the ancient world, traveling became the living expression of the learned man's longing to learn more. Ancient Greece differentiated between sedentary and traveling physicians, or *periodeutes,* as the latter were called.

The medieval world witnessed great waves of migration resulting from war or invasion, contrasting the restless life of the knight errant and the crusader with the sedentary life of the scholar, the monk, or the scribe in the monasteries, those stone coffers closed to everything from the outside world but the sun that poured cascades of sparkling colors through the stained-glass windows.

The Renaissance marked the beginning of the great explorations, among them the travels of Marco Polo in quest of the riches of Kublai Khan, perhaps the most important historical gesture and an unequivocal expression of Renaissance man's yearning to discover what lay beyond the confines of his land, to venture beyond the edge of darkness of the world when it was considered a flat, saucer-like disk. It was not until the seventeenth century, however, that man dedicated himself to a methodical fulfillment of his yearning to explore every room and corridor of the planet of which he knew but a tiny parlor.

By the nineteenth century, the great land and sea expeditions had covered almost the entire earth so that little was left to explore in our century. Hence, twentieth century man was overcome, as Lawrence of Arabia prophesied, by a passionate longing to explore his planet vertically, as if to compensate for twenty centuries of horizontal explorations. He descended to the endless depths of the ocean with Picard and he soared into the limitless stratosphere.

Meanwhile, thinkers, mathematicians, and poets have continued to make the greatest voyage of all, through space as well as through time—astride a poem, a philosophy, a scientific theory. Even the ordinary individual keeps pace with the great explorations. Travel today is a necessity for some, an integral part of the work of many, and the ambition of almost everyone. As Chesterton foresaw, the modern world expanded under the microscope, but it has contracted with the airplane. Thanks to the plane—some countries have made a direct transition from the mule to the airplane—travel has become so rapid and countries are brought so close that today what happens in one place resounds throughout the world.

The best part of traveling, or *dépaysement,* as the French say, is not the rest from work that it affords, for all travel involves certain tasks more or less burdensome—the best part is that it tears us away from our responsibilities. The traveler lives for himself, not for his family or his habitual milieu. A new country is a play in which we cease to be participants and become onlookers. A trip is not only a physical displacement in space but also a leap into freedom, guaranteed—except for politicians or screen stars—by blessed anonymity.

As the most distinguished physician-writer of our time, Somerset Maugham, said in his travel book, *The Gentleman in the Parlour,* nobody has expressed the joy of travel better than Hazlitt in his essay *On Going a Journey:* "Oh! It is great to shake off the trammels of the world and of public opinion; to lose our importunate, tormenting, everlasting personal identity in the elements of nature, and become the creature of the moment, clear of all ties; to hold to the universe only by a dish of sweetbreads and to owe nothing but the score of the evening, and no longer seek for applause and, meeting with contempt, to be known by no other title than the 'gentleman in the parlour.' "

The physician could not resist this lure of travel, which has today become an accessible pleasure and even a necessity. Tied down to his patients or his hospital like a galley slave to his oar, the physician has suffered perhaps more than others from the impact of *Wanderlust.* The pages of history bear the names of many physicians turned explorers, travelers, and adventurers who carried their science and their dreams to the four corners of the earth.

We can appreciate what travel has meant to the physician and what the physician has meant to travel simply by mentioning two books, one medical, the other a masterpiece of literature. One is the first treatise on public health compiled for the *periodeutes,* or wandering physicians, from the lectures of Hippocrates (c. 460–355 B.C.) under the title *Air, Water and Places.* It contains all kinds of advice on changes of air, water, and environment that might affect the human being. The second book is Jonathan Swift's *Travels Into Several Remote Nations of the World* (1726), a satire for grownups that also fascinates children. Lemuel Gulliver tells us that he was a surgeon's apprentice in London and that he had gone to study in Leyden, then one of the most enlightened centers of European medicine. "There," Gulliver says, "I studied physic two years and seven months, knowing it would be useful in long voyages."

Actually, the honor of being the first physician-traveler and explorer belongs to Democedes of Croton (sixth century B.C.), who, according to Herodotus, traveled throughout Asia. Physician to Polycrates, Democedes treated Darius, King of Persia, for a twisted ankle and established a medical link between the learned classical world of democratic Greece and the turbulent world of Asia.

Two basic motives have linked the physician with travel: first, his own desire to move about and acquaint himself with the world in which he lives; second, the innumerable medical problems raised by travel in its evolution from something accidental or adventurous into something essential to modern life, problems that stem from the ecologic changes affecting the traveler, who is subject to incessant variations in diet, climate, atmospheric pressure, and other environmental factors.

Paradoxically, in former times, travel involved fewer mental and other health risks than it does today. It was slow, on foot or on horseback, as in the case of the Mongol explorers, or by ship, as in the case of the Greek Argonauts, and the traveler had ample time to become acclimatized physically and mentally to new environments.

The plane, even more than the train or ship, has revolutionized all that. A century ago, traveling by stagecoach, the voyager mentally arrived at his destination days, even weeks, before his poor broken body. Today, the body that leaves New York and in less than twenty hours is in Paris, Brazil, Hawaii, Cairo, or Greenland arrives at its destination long before the mind has time to adapt itself to the new situation. This anomaly has given rise to several new psychosomatic problems.

Furthermore, advances in locomotion have created new dangers, for nowadays not only man travels—so do disease carriers. A mosquito traveling by plane from Africa to Brazil brought in its wake a malaria epidemic that might have become catastrophic. A bus traveling from Mexico to New York brought, lodged in the body of a sick passenger, the smallpox virus that caused a near epidemic in Manhattan. Cattle ticks, plants, rodents, rats, flies, insects, birds, mammals of all species, traveling by auto, rail, ship, and plane, can today spread disease all over the world with the speed of the vehicle carrying them. That is why the World Health Organization tries to cope with problems of disease and to watch over human health on a worldwide scale. Travel may improve or restore a person's physical or mental health, but it may also cause disease and even death. "Where the body goes, there goes death," says an ancient Spanish proverb.

In medieval times, frightful epidemics—bubonic plague, cholera, smallpox—followed the great caravan routes. Death galloped on the heels of the interminable processions of pilgrims, crusaders, and nomads who, on foot or on horseback, slowly crossed the burning sands of Asia and Africa. Today combustion motors have contracted the world, shortened our trips, and even freed us from dependence on weather, for man is no longer the completely helpless victim of winds or storms. The quarantines that protected the eighteenth century traveler have all but disappeared and are applied only in sudden outbreaks of epidemic.

The dangers that threatened sailors and passengers were infinite in the days of wooden ships and men of iron, from the epic saga of Columbus to the bold adventures of Sir Francis Drake's buccaneers. Along with the so-called fevers—a vague label that covered all infections listed in modern medical textbooks—there were wounds and shock caused by accidents, ship boardings, or naval battles, and malnutrition from insufficient or inadequate food, which was always the same on warships: hardtack and *mazmorra* on Philip II's galleys, and hardtack and salt pork on British and American frigates. There were also *sailor's vapors,* mental disturbances of the neurotic or frankly psychotic type, which beset seamen in long crossings during which they were condemned not only to a vitamin-deficient diet, but also to a monotonous life in hulks like wooden cells wedged between walls of sea-blue and sky-blue, a situation aggravated by the daily official ration of a half pint of rum customary on British ships.

All these threats of pain, sickness, and even death that haunted travelers in former times have been eliminated, thanks to the many physicians who, ignoring the cruel hardships of travel, dedicated themselves to exploring the earth and doggedly spread the art of healing and the science of preventive medicine all over the world. The honor roll of physician-explorers on land, on sea, and in the air is indeed a blazing page in medical history.[1-14]

Among the physician-explorers who bear witness to the perennial fascination of travel for our colleagues we should mention the Portuguese Garcia de Orta, who explored India in the sixteenth century; the surgeon Monkhouse, who overcame scurvy on Cook's expedition to the South Seas in 1769, in which undertaking he was accompanied by Dr. Solander, a physician and naturalist from Upsala; Dr. Walter Russell, *Doctor of Physicke,* who accompanied Captain John Smith on his explorations of the craggy Chesapeake region; the Scottish surgeon James Bruce (1730–1794), who discovered the source of the Blue Nile; the Scottish surgeon Mungo Park (1771–1806), who explored Senegal and Kaarta; Dr. Livingstone (1813–1873), the discoverer of the Zambesi River and the Victoria Falls; and the German doctor, Eduard Schnitzer (1840–1892), the fabulous Emin Pasha, hero of the Sudan.

The most famous explorations of Arabia in the nineteenth century were made by men who had studied medicine and practiced it in

Arabia as the most effective way of winning the confidence of the Arab tribes: Richard F. Burton (1821–1890), the immortal translator of the "Arabian Nights"; W. G. Palgrave (1826–1888); and C. M. Doughty (1843–1926), author of *Travels Through Arabia Deserta* which inspired the saga of Lawrence of Arabia.

It was the naval surgeons who conquered the seas—just as the flight surgeon today shares the credit for the conquest of the skies— naval surgeons such as James Lind, who overcame the scurvy epidemic that had caused ten thousand deaths, according to Admiral Hawkins' reports; Thomas Dover, who discovered on the island of Juan Fernández, not far from the Chilean coast, the man called Alexander Selkirk, who was later immortalized as Robinson Crusoe by Daniel Defoe; Eugene Sue, also famous as a novelist; and last but certainly not least, Tobias Smollett, whose laurel wreath is twined with both medical and literary honors and who "discovered" the French Riviera. Many other naval physicians could be mentioned whose genius dispelled the abysmal terrors once held by the seas.

Having conquered land and sea and loath to remain chained to the earth, man longed for wings to carry him higher than eagles fly. Again physicians were pioneers and heroes in the conquest of the skies. On June 5, 1783, at Annonay near Lyons, the Montgolfier brothers released the first balloon ever to drift through space. The beloved historian, Dr. Victor Robinson, left a brilliant description of this event. The bizarre experiment, forerunner of present-day aviation, was born of the most poetic idea ever conceived in the human mind: What would happen if one of the slow, fat clouds floating through the pale French skies were imprisoned in a bag? Instead of a cloud, the Montgolfiers used smoke to fill their balloon.

A few months later at Versailles, before the astonished eyes of Louis XVI and Marie Antoinette, amid a concourse of powdered wigs and faces and in an aura of scents, there rose a balloon as beribboned and bepainted as a marquise at the royal court. In the basket there trembled a sheep, a cock and a duck, the first living creatures ever to ascend into the air by action very different from that of a bird's wings.

And the first human being to ascend in a balloon, on October 15, 1783, was a physician-apothecary from Metz, Jean Pilàtre de Rozier (1756–1785). He subsequently became the first martyr to aeronautics when he perished in an attempt to emulate a Boston physician named Jeffries, and Pierre Blanchard, the first two men to cross the English Channel in a balloon. And it was Paul Bert, a pupil of Claude Bernard, who founded aeronautical medicine, today a vital part of modern medicine and the key to tomorrow's interplanetary navigation.

What was the moving spirit of these physician-explorers? Men who aspire to rise above their mortal destiny by perpetuating their lives through history are always impelled by two great instinctive motivations: the yearning for truth and the love of power. Truth is sought along the broad paths of science, beauty, or religion. Power must be pursued through the devious channels of money, politics, and war.

But the explorer's soul is different. He desires something loftier though less useful than authentic science, vaguer but less selfish than possession. Perhaps the most genuine way of satisfying an instinct is through the instinct itself. To suffer in order to know, and to know in order to know. That is, to seize the torch of knowledge—*cursu lampada trado,* as Lucretius said—and transmit it ablaze to posterity.[15] That is the clue to the work of the great traveling doctors.

With such precursors it is not surprising that physicians are showing more and more interest in protecting their patients against stress and other dangers of travel.

This symposium will attempt to present a panorama of medicine's contribution to the protection of the traveler's health today, whether the traveler is a man, woman, or child, old or young, healthy or sick, on land, on sea, and in the air, in tropical or polar zones, in great bustling cities or lonely silent deserts, thus crystallizing the dream of making good health as inseparable a companion of the traveler as his passport.

In reality, the objective of medicine as applied to travel is to practice that basic philosophic principle recommended by Claude Bernard as the supreme objective of all vital mechanisms: ". . . to preserve intact the living conditions of the inner milieu . . ." regardless of the means of locomotion used or the new environment to which the traveler is transported.

Let us end by remembering, as a symbol of this symposium, that in Greek mythology Delphi was the center or *omphalos* (navel) of the orb, because, according to the legend, if two eagles soared into the air from the two ends of the earth they would inevitably meet in Delphi. The two eagles of modern preventive medicine and scientific research are today soaring toward a point situated not in Space but in Time. The temple to which their wings will carry them is located in the future.

PADUA AND LONDON:
A HARVEIAN TALE OF TWO CITIES

here is no better way to celebrate this memorable day than by paying homage to William Harvey, supreme symbol of the medical investigator whose entire life is dedicated to the search for truth as the only key to goodness, freedom, and beauty.

Osler said that "history is the biography of the minds of men." His thought was anticipated centuries ago by the great Renaissance physician, Girolamo Cardano, who said that "a man is nothing but his mind." Today, we shall start together on a pilgrimage into the mind of Harvey. Our most distinguished friend and eminent historian, Dr. Douglas Guthrie, will speak with far more authority than I could about the adult years of Harvey and his great discovery.

I shall talk to you about Harvey as a physician and about the cities and the historical period in which he lived in the years prior to his discovery. I shall make a brief sketch of Harvey "seen from the inside," of Padua and London in Harvey's times, of his great teachers, and of the artistic and philosophic trends of the Renaissance and Baroque that influenced his thought and work. In a series of flashbacks we shall see how Harvey came to present in a lecture delivered in London 341 years ago today his discovery of the circulation of the blood.

The occasion was the second of his Lumleian Lectures, the time 10 o'clock one bright spring morning, April 17, 1616, the scene the new Anatomical Theatre of the Physician's College in Amen Street. In the audience there were some 40 distinguished men with highly critical

A lecture delivered at the Harvey Tercentennial Celebration, Charter Day Program, of the New York Medical College, Flower and Fifth Avenue Hospitals, April 22, 1957; published in the *International Record of Medicine 170:286*, 1957.

minds, fellow members, licentiates, and candidates of the College. There were also several illustrious laymen, Digby, Ashmole, and Samuel Pepys, and others, the "curious," as they were called, for whom the anatomy lectures equaled the theatre in attraction. Under the auspices of the president, censors, and fellows of the College, and with an anatomical treatise set on the table, the prosector standing by the skeleton, and the tabulae for the dissection of the arteries, veins, and nerves hanging from the wall, the lecturer began his oration.

"A small, dark man, wand in hand, with piercing black eyes, and a quick, vivacious manner" (Osler), he still had the salt of youth stamped on his face. He was William Harvey, then 38 years old. He talked in Latin interspersed with English words. There was a prolonged break between the morning and afternoon lectures when the company went out for one of those "fine dinners" that Pepys so much enjoyed describing.

Towards the end, after discussing in a novel, modern way the structure of the heart in action, Harvey summed up in a few words that the blood moves in a circle. Few among the audience appreciated the meaning of these history-making words, and a few were actually critical of them.

I shall now endeavor to tell you the story behind Harvey's words and his youthful endeavors, for which I shall have to take you to the Padua and London of three and a half centuries ago.

SPRING IN PADUA

It was spring 1598 in Padua. Stirred by tender breezes, the city unfolded like a flower before the eyes, wide with curiosity and wonder, of students from all Europe. From England and Germany, Switzerland, Spain, France, the Low Countries—from all over in large, noisy flocks the students came. Some arrived on foot, their capes threadbare, their shoes battered and dusty; but their moustaches were smartly curled, and their bearing, perhaps in the futile hope of concealing their poverty, was haughty. Others arrived in elegant carriages, followed by their servants and even their minstrels, their purses bulging with *zecchini*. Some clasped books—then a costly rarity—in their arms, and perhaps between the pages a rose was pressed, a nostalgic souvenir from the faraway homeland. But all of them, rich and poor, had one and the same longing for knowledge and adventure. Padua had beckoned and they had come. For three centuries Padua had shed the purest and brightest cultural light upon Europe. This group of students, the cream of European youth, would later yield, thanks to Padua, some of the most brilliant minds of the old continent.

The arrival in Padua was at first a great disappointment. Those who came from nearby Venice still had before their eyes the image of their lyrical city, as impossibly beautiful as a fantastic dream, sleepily reclining like a fairy tale princess by the lapping waters of its lagoons, where like graceful black swans the gondolas silently glided. Those from the North brought the vision of their home towns, neat and compact, the light from mist-veiled skies transforming the streets into a nostalgic painting by an old master.

But Padua appeared to them to be noisy and far too bright. The sun glared down at high noon; the colors were violent at sunset. The streets were narrow; the houses low, often without glass in the windows. Ankle deep in the mud of the streets, a petulant crowd jostled and chattered, as generous with their gestures as with their quarrels.

Late at night Padua acquired some of the mystery of neighboring Venice. The dark, winding streets were suddenly peopled by silent furtive figures. Knights and ladies wrapped in concealing cloaks, giggling wenches and amorous students, princes and rascals alike, preceded by flaming torches or shrouded in darkness, roamed the streets in pursuit of love, fortune, and adventure. When the stars above the sleeping campaniles began to fade and stillness finally descended upon the city, fresh breezes swept in from the Adriatic, laden with the romantic and picaresque echo of the canals of Venice whose pale waters were to bear the adventurous gondola of Casanova.

And then came the dawn. The limpid sky was rent by the sharp song of the cocks like glass by a diamond. The students, like birds escaped from a cage, flocked down the streets of Padua. It was then that the city unfolded its beauty before their eyes.

From the Prato, radiant with spring, the students beheld Santa Giustina with its eight Byzantine domes glistening in the sun; and the Church of St. Anthony, its pointed spires soaring in the blue, its arches tall and slender, its white marble façade, fashioned like that of a Roman basilica, supported by black marble columns, its balcony like those of a Venetian palace, its exquisite friezes, deep in marble foliage, peopled by horses, fish, cherubs, and swans. There the townspeople prayed to the city's patron saint, St. Anthony, he who in the twelfth century talked with the fish he dearly loved, as St. Francis talked with the birds.

In the Chapel of St. Felix azure cupolas vied with golden canopies, and inside the church the saints and madonnas seemed eager to escape from altars and tapestries.

In the piazzas, the silent aristocracy of arrogant statues stood watch over the city, and everywhere flowering gardens peeped out over walls and fences, enameling the city with polychrome colors.

This was Padua, grave of medieval dogma and cradle of a new knowledge that heralded the Renaissance. The students felt indeed fortunate to be here! Under the spell of beauty and youth, their blood ran warmer in their veins. Their capes bellowed out and the plumes atop their hats fluttered in the breeze. The chimes of bells rolled blithely through the air. Padua was festive and gay.

PADUA TODAY

Padua is no longer like this. I was there not long ago, following the footsteps of Vesalius. Today the city is shabby, dusty, wearisome. The blazing streets are cluttered with traffic, the noisiest perhaps in the world. If one is coming from Venice, as I was, one steps out from the gondola on the mainland and then travels by automobile or bus for nearly two hours through dusty, flat country. The monotonous landscape wearies the eyes, and one remembers with nostalgia the canals, *piazzettas,* and palaces in the magic city left behind, where the wheel is unknown and the only audible sounds are the tolling of bells, the flapping of wings, the gentle lapping of oars, and the mellow chant of the gondoliers.

The pale waters of Venice are replaced by the parched land of Padua. Everything here is old without the dignity of age, ugly without 'the character that ugliness can often attain, and dirty without the picturesqueness that sometimes accompanies dirt.

But let one forget the city and cross the threshold of the ancient, dilapidated university. It is not space one crosses; it is time. Every portal here leads back to the glorious Renaissance. You may sit on the hard benches where the students listened to Galileo expound his theories. You may sit, as I did, on Vesalius' chair, a sacred relic relegated to a corner under the indifferent care of a charwoman. And, above all, you may step into the anatomic theatre, no larger than a doll's house, where Fabricius of Acquapendente unveiled the mysteries of generation and in the flickering candlelight dissected the venous valves. Here are the very same walls that sheltered an English student named William Harvey; here the windows through which he glanced at the Paduan skies.

Padua has now become transfigured, shining forth with the magic light of the past, with the gleaming reflections of history. And in one's heart one feels the glory that was Padua.

THE STUDENTS IN RENAISSANCE PADUA

In Harvey's time the sparkling rivers Brenta and Baechiglioni encircled the city of Padua like two silver bracelets. Padua had been wrested by the Venetian government from the Carrara family, who had long ruled the city. Students loved Padua because the university, like that of Bologna, was governed by the students themselves, whereas in Paris and Oxford the masters ruled.

The University of Padua was organized in 1222 by a group of students from Bologna who, dissatisfied with that city's government, emigrated to Padua, taking with them some of their favorite teachers. The new university was originally set up as an independent community composed only of students and of teachers selected by the students. In those days students went wherever taxes were lower, teachers were better, and life was freer and kinder. Space in some cities was so scarce that, in Paris, for instance, schools shared the same buildings with brothels, much to the students' delight. In Italy the situation was partly remedied by all sorts of barriers contrived between the two "institutions of learning."

Medical schools in those days were called schools of "artists," since medicine was considered one of the seven liberal arts. Students were grouped according to their language and nationality. In 1288 there were four groups of students in Padua: Latins who spoke the *langue d'oïl* (French and Normans); Latins who spoke the *langue d'oc* (Provençals, Catalans, and Spaniards); Germans; and Italians. All the groups, however, were usually designated as *transalpines* or *cisalpines,* according to the side of the Alps they came from. Each group, or *natio,* had its own "councilors" and special privileges. Frequently national pride started many a dialectic quarrel, which often ended in bloody battle.

THE ORIGIN OF THE UNIVERSITIES

The first universities were the fruit of ecclesiastic philosophy. God was the Supreme Educator, and the university was the result of the Church's endeavor to organize education. Medieval scholasticism united the concepts of Plato and Aristotle and the wisdom of Arabian-Jewish philosophers. Monasteries were the first medieval teaching centers. The original curriculum comprised the *trivium,* or grammar, dialectic, and rhetoric, and the *quadrivium,* or arithmetic, geometry, music, and astronomy. The two sections combined constituted the "seven liberal arts." These teaching centers called *scholae publicae* were replaced by the *studia* in the twelfth century, and this name was later extended to the entire educational institution. In the same century the term was changed to *universitas magistrorum* and later to *universitas,* which thereafter encompassed all the disciplines or faculties.

The first European teaching institution to which the term "university" may be correctly applied was Bologna, which in 1156 already had a medical school. Godfathers of anatomy at Bologna were Taddeo Alderotti and Mondino. There, in February, 1302, the first recorded autopsy was performed under the supervision of two doctors and three surgeons on a subject who, it was suspected, had been poisoned. It has been said, however, that in 1281 an autopsy was performed on a plague victim.

In Padua, medical teaching began in the year 1250, and by the fourteenth century the students were well organized into faculties of sciences and medicine. Their teachers, originally selected by the students, were later appointed by the Venetian Senators.

THE TEACHERS OF PADUA

The fame of Padua's teachers attracted students from all over Europe. The golden age of Padua began with the great teacher, Pietro d'Abano, early in the thirteenth century, reached its peak with Vesalius in the middle of the sixteenth century, and ended with Galileo, a contemporary of Harvey. Pietro d'Abano still lives in his philosophico-medical work and in his proud statue on a square in Padua. His noble visage, which resembles that of his pupil Dante, looks down at the curious visitor with the same piercing glance that held spellbound the great crowds of students who flocked from all over to hear him lecture.

Influenced by the Arabian commentators on Aristotle, Pietro d'Abano created an Averroësian atmosphere in Padua that contrasted with the scholastic atmosphere of Bologna. His efforts, however, to reconcile Arabism with scholasticism ended tragically when he was accused of heresy and sorcery—he who had traveled to Constantinople to learn Greek that he might read Galen and Aristotle in the original and who had taught in Paris!—and was condemned to burn at the stake. Mercifully, death overtook him during his trial, rescuing him from the flames. His students succeeded in hiding his body, and the authorities had to content themselves with burning him in effigy in the public square.

Early in the fourteenth century Padua was officially granted by Pope Clement VI all the privileges of a *studium generale,* and it became an epidemiological center. By the end of the fourteenth century Venice had codified sanitary legislation to protect herself from the constant menace of plagues brought to her shores by trading vessels loaded with the silks, metals, and spices vital to her economy.

In the fifteenth century Pope Sixtus IV granted Padua a dissection permit, and Alessandro Benedetti, professor of anatomy, proposed the construction of an anatomic theatre fashioned after the Colosseum of Rome or the Arena of Verona, with ushers to collect a seating charge so that more instruments might be bought with the money. The Emperor Maximilian, the aristocracy of Venice, and the public at large were invited to attend the dissections.

Toward the close of the fifteenth century printing was developed, and the Venetian Republic published more than 1500 books in the last ten years of the century, which greatly contrasted with the scarcity of books in Paris. It now became possible to replace gradually the old medieval anatomic diagrams with those of Leonardo da Vinci, Titian, and the Paduan sculptor Andrea Riccio. The printed word, with its magic power of propagation, inflicted the mortal blow to medieval esotericism, which had been based mainly on the difficulty in transmitting scientific concepts.

THE ENGLISH "NATIO"

Foreign students in Padua steadily increased, as revealed by the ancient books, today kept in Padua's medical school library, in which the *conciliarii* of each nation recorded the most important facts about their group. English students became so numerous that in 1534 the *natio Anglica* split from the *natio Scota*. In 1603 the English, Scots, and Irish were again united in the English nation and had a councilor, a beadle, a secretary, their own library, and special privileges. And while English students flocked to Padua in search of academic freedom and perhaps the radiant Italian sky, Italian humanists traveled to England at the request of the Duke of Gloucester, brother of Henry V, which greatly stimulated learning in England.

In the fifteenth century the University of Bologna also had an English *natio,* the first students of which were Oxonian clergymen. They were followed by the founders of the modern English scholarship, Grocyn, Linacre, and Latimer. Linacre studied humanism in Bologna and graduated in medicine at Padua. Back in England, he became a true *uomo universalis*. Erasmus was one of his pupils at Oxford. Linacre left a fortune to found chairs of medicine at Oxford and Cambridge. Caius also studied at Padua and left the mark of his learning upon Cambridge, whose medical college still bears his name.

THE ANATOMIC THEATRE

And now let us go back to that glorious spring in 1598 with which this narration began. The students in gay, noisy bands repaired to the university. Chattering blithely they entered the beloved *Il Bo* (The Ox) building, so called, according to some, because it was located on the site of an ancient hostelry called the *Hospitium Bovis* (at the Sign of the Ox), or, according to others, because of the ox and wagon tax levied to support the anatomic theatre. The students clambered up the stairs to the anatomic theatre, erected four years before on the initiative of Laurentius Massa, secretary of the *Reformatori* of Venice.

I visited the anatomic theatre last year and I still recall my emotion at seeing the small hall, barely twenty-five by thirty-five feet, in which students must have crowded most uncomfortably. The small oval pit is surrounded by six ascending galleries as narrow as those of a provincial Spanish bull ring. Students must have stood on tiptoe to peer through the beplumed hats of those below them.

More than 300 students elbowed, nudged, and jostled one another, vainly trying to repress their restlessness and discomfort while waiting for the dissection to begin. Voices, curses, and shuffling feet echoed so loudly in the hollow wooden box that was the anatomic theatre that sometimes street musicians were brought in to keep the students quiet while they waited for the teacher to arrive.

Outside, in the piazzas of Padua, the midmorning sun had already set the towers aflame and the sky glared down fiercely. Inside, the window curtains were pulled and darkness descended upon the theatre. Two four-candle candelabras and eight candles were lighted and held aloft by students. Shadows capered on the wooden walls. The air reeked of sweat, the old leather of boots and scabbards, and the dead flesh of the corpse to be dissected.

The entrance of the academic dignitaries was greeted with solemn silence. The rectors of the university and the city, together with high officials from Venice, occupied the seats at one end of the dissecting table. The teachers lined up behind them, and, since the pit was too small for all of them, some were forced to stand in the *luoghi a basso,* the empty space underneath the first tier from which they watched the dissection through small openings. Councilors of the various nations occupied the first tier; behind and above them, students crowded into a human pyramid.

At the other end of the table sat the *Massarii,* or anatomists, who were chosen by the rectors and councilors and who organized the course, purchased the wood for the construction of the theatre, which was dismantled at the end of the course, secured the necessary instruments and the corpses, and, until Fabricius had stopped the practice two years before, in 1596, collected entrance fees from the students.

According to the law, the city allowed the university only two corpses a year, one male and one female; but the *Massarii* or the students themselves did not hesitate to steal bodies whenever possible and even created riots, as when in the previous year they had tried unsuccessfully to steal the corpse of a youth from the Church of Santa Sofia.

Fabricius' entrance always created a moment of drama. The wooden door squeaked like a soul in agony, and all eyes at once turned to it expectantly. The candlelight flickered over the small, dark man, dressed in black, a gold chain hanging from his neck. His beard was short and aggressive, his eyes small and malicious, flashing with impatience and irritation.

The students knew only too well Fabricius' quick temper. Once, angry because a pupil failed to step aside when they passed on the sidewalk, he announced that thereafter he would always carry a dagger, "ready to prove that he could use it for purposes other than dissection." Although he was a true teacher, he nevertheless was forever trying to postpone his classes, which he would have liked to limit to once every two years. His reputation was so great that not only tailors, cobblers, butchers, and shopkeepers, but even street peddlers tried to sneak into his classes.

Trouble also always attended Fabricius' classes. Once, the night before his class, the dissection instruments and the head and limbs of the corpse disappeared. Often the relatives of the dissected subject complained forcibly because the remains after dissection were tossed to the dogs or into the river instead of being given Christian burial. Sometimes the Syndics arrived late at the dissections and the *Massarii* promptly quarreled with them. On one occasion, a *Massari,* an ill-tempered Sicilian, rushed with his dagger upon a Syndic right in the middle of a lecture. Fabricius himself constantly quarreled with the students, particularly those of the German *natio,* the most powerful of all. He so much enjoyed making fun of and mocking them that the Germans finally boycotted his classes.

Fabricius' dissections were so slow that he spent two months on a head while the students grew more impatient every day, fearing that he would not reach the abdomen before summer. He gave lectures on working days and "extraordinary" lectures on holidays. Anatomic demonstrations were given during the winter only and lasted three weeks, three hours daily in the morning, although sometimes they were resumed in the afternoon.

The bells of the University tolled twice daily, in the morning and in the afternoon. The twenty-fourth hour was sundown. In the winter the bells tolled from the fourteenth to the fifteenth hour in the morning (7:00 to 8:00 A.M., our time), and in the afternoon from the twentieth to the twenty-first hour (1:00 to 2:00 P.M.). Fabricius dissected at the hour of *tertia matutina,* the third hour after the morning toll (11:00 A.M., our time).

But let us rejoin the students at the anatomic theatre. Fabricius occupied his place at one end of the table in front of the *Massarii.* His visage, sallow, almost waxlike, was grave as he stooped over the skinned corpse. The flickering candlelight, like the tongue of a compassionate, devoted dog, licked the gaping flesh.

A STUDENT CALLED HARVEY

On one of the tiers, in the group of the English *natio,* there was a youth intently watching the master's expert hands bejeweled with the rubies of gout. The young man was about 20 years old and looked like a Spaniard or an Italian, short, dark, with black, shining eyes like two mustard seeds. His name was William Harvey.

William Harvey was born April 1, 1578, at Folkestone, Kent, the eldest of the seven sons of Thomas Harvey, mayor of Folkestone, and Joan Hawke, related to the counts of Bristol. When William was 10 years old he entered the Grammar School of Canterbury, where Chaucer's winged fantasy still lingered. It was the year when the skies of England echoed with gunbursts of victory over the Invincible Armada of Philip II of Spain.

In 1593, at the age of 15, Harvey entered the Gonville and Caius College, Cambridge, and four years later he received his degree of Bachelor of Arts. It was the year of the Earl of Essex's and Sir Walter Raleigh's expedition against the Spaniards.

The atmosphere of Caius College undoubtedly influenced Harvey's future life and work. The College had been founded in the fourteenth century by Edmund Gonville and enlarged in the sixteenth century by John Keys, also called Caius (1510–1573), physician, humanist, former student at Gonville and Padua, and master of the College from 1559 until his death. In Padua Caius had studied with Vesalius (1539) and, together with Realdo Colombo, had taught Greek physics and Aristotelian logic. It was Caius who, together with Thomas Linacre, encouraged sixteenth century English physicians to import the sun-bathed Italian culture to their misty shores.

His studies at Cambridge over, Harvey's eyes turned to Italy. There art and nature flourished. There humanism and culture lent medicine wings with which to soar to freedom. There the giants of anatomy and science—Vesalius, Colombo, Fabricius, Casserio, Galileo, and Santorio—spread their knowledge. And so, still in the throes of puberty, Harvey traveled to the town that Shakespeare later called, "Fair Padua, nursery of the arts."

PADUA—LIGHTS AND SHADOWS

To understand the forces behind Harvey's discovery it is indispensable to understand various factors neglected by his biographers. They are the burden of our dissertation: the historical crisis in Europe in Harvey's time; the background of the cities where he studied medicine; the rhythm of his own biological development based on a concept that we shall call "of the generations"; the influence upon him of the new anatomy that permeated the atmosphere of Padua and of Galileo's ideas on motion, later intensified by the Baroque era, which was characterized by motion; and, finally, the inner meaning of his scientific vocation.

When Harvey arrived in Padua the air was charged with the *nuova scienza*. Fifty-four years earlier Vesalius' *Fabrica* had burst like a rocket upon the horizon. The illustrations by Titian and Calcar were great windows of light opening onto a new anatomy. Vesalius was now resting beneath pine trees on a remote island, but his creative spirit still lingered in the halls of Padua, where his dissections had set afire the minds of students from all Europe.

Vesalius had left a luminous legend among the students. He was a man of mystery who did much and said little. They still spoke of his noble figure when, on December 5, 1537, amidst great blowing of trumpets, waving flags, towering plumes, cloaks of purple velvet, and glittering swords, he was made a physician at the palace of the Bishop of Padua. The next day he was appointed professor of surgery. The students also recalled the famous trip to Basel across the snow-blanketed Alps, the huge wooden blocks of the *Fabrica* balanced precariously on the back of plodding mules. In Basel they yielded the pages that committed to dust Galen's theories.

But if Padua throbbed with the memory of the heroes of the new science, it also crawled with quacks. There were physicians who earned the freshly minted gold *zecchini* by washing with aromatic vinegar the dead bodies of the rich, wrapping them in linen soaked in essence of aloe, and burying them in lead caskets enclosed in caskets of cypress wood. Other physicians roamed the streets garbed in grotesque costumes devised to protect them from the plague. Some wore long beaks, filled with protective aromatic essences, which gave them the appearance of huge birds. And there were physicians like Tommasso Giannotti Rangone who taught people "how to live 120 years."

Money flowed in Padua. Magic and alchemy were still rampant. Dreaded fevers lurked in the still waters of lagoons and rivers. Typhoid fever, typhus, and plague killed 999 out of every thousand patients. There were more than 100 apothecaries in town, and every one of them featured theriac as a miraculous all-purpose antidote.

On the other hand, Padua had already adopted the Venetian legislation against plague. The dead were buried outside the city, and houses were disinfected with sunlight and sulfur vapors. There were plague physicians easily identified by the small white baton they carried; and a certificate of good health was required from travelers.

THE GIANTS—FABRICIUS AND GALILEO

Such was the atmosphere in which Harvey now moved. He studied under Casserio and Rudio. He learned from Fabricius of the existence of the venous valves, which would later move him to study embryologic and physiologic problems. The venous valves were discovered in 1546 by Canano (by Sylvius, according to Riolan), but Fabricius was the first to describe them in his little book *De Venarum Ostiolis*.

Fabricius observed experimentally that the valves of the great femoral and brachial veins slowed down the movement of the blood from the base of the limbs to the peripheral regions. Fabricius, therefore, almost hit upon the concept of the major circulation. But the Galenic influence upon him was too strong, leading him to conclude that the function of the *ostiola venarum* was "to slow down the blood so as to prevent it from flooding, like a river, now the feet, now all the fingers of the hands, and becoming stagnant in those areas, which might cause two alterations: the upper portions of the limbs would be working, while the hands and feet would be asleep due to perpetual tumefaction."

Harvey was in Padua when Fabricius published his first physiologic works, investigated the formation of the chick in the egg and of the human embryo, and challenged the doctrine of spontaneous generation that affirmed that animals developed from an egg. This triple influence—anatomic, physiologic, and embryologic—had a tremendous impact on Harvey, who was one of Fabricius' favorite pupils.

The controversy that arose in Padua in 1600, when the Galenist, Eustachio Rudio, professor at the university since the previous year, reprinted his work of 1587 describing the lesser circulation and commenting on the texts of Colombo and Cesalpino on that subject, gave Harvey an impassioned vision of the still unresolved problem of the motion of the blood.

To this impact was added that of Galileo's work. In those days Galileo initiated modern physics and the science of dynamics. Galileo had studied medicine and mathematics at Pisa. In the leaning tower of Pisa, that huge paperweight seemingly holding down the landscape so that the strong regional winds may not blow it away, Galileo conducted his famous experiments, demonstrating that velocity is not proportionate to weight. Galileo was appointed professor of mathematics at Padua in 1592, in the same town where Copernicus had studied medicine with Fracastoro, who gave syphilis its poetic name.

While Fabricius demonstrated anatomy, Galileo expounded his theories on mathematics and physics to vast audiences in the amphitheatre of the School of Law. Kings and aristocrats attended, and among the medical students again we discover the eager face of Harvey.

As was the custom then, students boarded with the professors, and in the evening Harvey joined those who lived with Galileo and together they spent many hours either discussing the mysteries of physics with Galileo and the erudite monk, Paolo Sarpi, who helped to discover the venous valves, or observing through Galileo's telescope the stars, brilliant, enigmatic, like the eyes of thousands of celestial cats, in the skies of Padua.

Galileo must have spoken to Harvey often about the movement of the stars and the heavenly bodies, and surely Harvey must have asked him many questions about the laws of motion. How many hours Harvey must have spent also looking through the microscope constructed by Galileo! What thoughts filled his mind on his way back to his lodgings after an evening with Galileo? Perhaps sometimes he stopped at a *trattoria* to sup on the popular porcupine, which was eaten only from

October to January when its odor was less offensive. Was he ever aware of the hot sauce, concocted with garlic, rosemary, mint, wine, vinegar, pepper, and cinnamon, with which they tried to disguise the strong flavor of the meat, or was his mind too occupied with the startling concepts he had heard all evening to notice such trivial things? Back again in his modest room, his head spinning with thoughts of motion, perhaps he found it difficult to induce himself to sleep.

THE HISTORICAL CRISIS OF THE RENAISSANCE

The Renaissance was a great historical crisis.

There are two kinds of historical changes. One affects the whole world; this is normal in every generation. The other affects something in particular in our world; this is a historical crisis. When one system of convictions crumbles down but is immediately replaced by another, there is no room for a crisis. But when no replacement is forthcoming, when man is left without convictions, which is to say, without a world, then man is in crisis. His world has been demolished. There are no new beliefs to replace the old ones. Man then feels lost, disoriented, disconcerted. Often at such times a whole generation may deceive itself by becoming engrossed in doctrines, arts, or politics that are not its own, only to disintegrate if by the time it reaches the age of 40 it has not developed its own convictions. For at that age it is imperative to live by truth.

The Renaissance was a rebirth in general history through a true birth in science. Back in the Middle Ages, in the thirteenth century, there had been a golden age, initiated by Albertus Magnus and fulfilled by St. Thomas Aquinas. This century witnessed the great adventure of the Crusades, a complete military failure but a great cultural success, for stowed away in their battered knapsacks the defeated Crusaders brought back the priceless treasure of classical Greek wisdom, which later would Hellenize Christianity.

In the sixteenth century, man was in crisis, and he did what every man in crisis does: he undressed. When we are in a crisis we shed hat, coat, whatever may hinder action. In a historical crisis man sheds his old beliefs. This is what he did in the Renaissance. He cast off his medieval ideas. The faith he had exclusively given God he now bestowed upon things and himself. Galileo's modern physics provided him with a technical reason; the first European state of Ferdinand and Isabella with the *raison d'état*. Both these reasons were the basis of modern man's thinking. In the fifteenth century, a century without an understanding of which one cannot understand modern history, medieval man vanished like a burnt-out rocket, and modern man rose like a new rocket above the horizon.

Harvey's work was part of this historical crisis. Galenism weighed on him like shot on a bird's wing. Vesalius' anatomy had dealt a mortal blow to Galenism, but it was still a static anatomy. Much had still to be done to give it life, to make it stir and move, to turn it into *anatomia animata*. This became Harvey's youthful endeavor.

It also was his own individual crisis. All of man abhors a vacuum. Just as the human body must promptly fill up with fat and conjunctive tissue any void created by the extirpation of an organ, so must the human mind replace one truncated belief by another. Neither one can abide a vacuum. If Harvey had lived in the years prior to the Renaissance crisis, from a historical standpoint he would have felt no urge to replace the already moribund Galenism by a new scientific doctrine. But his own historical crisis was a fitting parallel to the Renaissance crisis, when the austere medieval concepts were being replaced by a new, passionate concept of life and the world.

To the influence of his teachers, both those absent like Vesalius and those present like Fabricius and Galileo, to the influence of Renaissance Padua, and to the historical crisis of his time—to these three factors must be added the longing Harvey had to create modern physiology. No other place could have offered him more encouragement than Italy.

In every historical period there are "visceral" countries, that is, countries that are the vital organs around which the rest of the world revolves, just as in the body the various organs are organized around the heart. In Harvey's time, at the height of the Renaissance and the Baroque, the "visceral" countries were Italy, England, and the Low Countries.

In one's early youth, longing for personal glory represents not so much the desire to do something great or to be somebody as the desire to *emulate* someone. The young man adopts as model a hero whom he desires to imitate and even surpass. Sometimes a whole generation or a historical period will pattern its entire course after a great figure or a great historical situation of the past. Vesalius' work no doubt was prompted by the desire to emulate Galen or Erasistratus, just as the Renaissance was the result of the desire to emulate classical antiquity in the arts and sciences. Young Harvey's models were Vesalius, Fabricius, and Galileo.

THE HISTORICAL ADVENTURE OF THE DISCOVERY
OF THE CIRCULATION OF THE BLOOD

Every human endeavor in history fits within a "line" and a "situation." The line is the vertical chronology of all preceding endeavors of the same nature; in Harvey's case, for example, everything done on the circulation of the blood prior to him. The situation is the environment in which the endeavor was developed and carried to fruition.

The line of Harvey's discovery, that is, the knowledge available on the circulation of the blood before Harvey, is easy to determine. The circulation of the blood had been a subject of much discussion for many centuries, from the Vedas to Galen. The old ideas on the subject, however, were wrong, and in medicine it is far more difficult to rectify an error than to make a new discovery. Such ideas were based on the fact that dissection revealed two vascular systems: one, the venous, was full of blood, produced, it was assumed, in the liver since the latter contained so much blood; and the other, the arterial, was always empty and therefore must serve, it was believed, to distribute air or vital force throughout the body. Today we know that when parietal tension in the arterioles subsides, these draw blood from the arteries, emptying them and allowing air to enter when they are cut open in dissection.

It was the Spaniard, Michael Servetus, who first described the lesser or pulmonary circulation in his nonmedical, theologic work *De Christianismi Restitutio,* which only earned him the wrath of the Church. Condemned by Calvin for heresy, he was burned alive in Geneva, a sulfur-soaked bramble crown on his brow and a greenwood pyre at his feet that his agony might be prolonged. Not long ago I stood on the hill in Geneva where Servetus was burned. Charitable hands have marked the place with a stone plaque vindicating the Spanish martyr, mercifully omitting the name of his executioner. Should you ever be there at the hour when dusk descends upon the land and shadows lengthen, you will see the mists creep up the hill from the lake, evoking the martyr's shroud. And when the first quivering star appears in the faded sky you may wonder: Is it the soul of Servetus or of his repentant executioner?

Six years after Servetus' death, the Italian, Realdo Colombo, one of Vesalius' successors at Padua, published an anatomic work, filled with much sarcasm and bravado, describing, based on experiments with live animals, the passage of the blood from the right to the left ventricle and its change of color in the lungs. Colombo conveniently overlooked giving Servetus and his predecessors the credit due them.

Colombo was succeeded by Gabriel Fallopius, philosopher, botanist, academician, and personal physician to the Pope, and Fallopius was followed by Fabricius. But before Fabricius there had been one Andrea Cesalpino who came very close to the truth when he asserted that the heart, not the liver, as Galen had said, was the central organ of the vascular system. Cesalpino demonstrated that the blood moves, was the first to use the word *circulatio,* and wrote that the movement of the blood is continuous from the veins to the heart and from this to the arteries, a concept that the Spaniard Valverde would formulate again later. Cesalpino believed that during sleep the blood traveled from the arteries to the veins and thence to the heart; but like Galen he maintained that there was a continuous and direct flow of blood through the interventricular septum.

Later, Fabricius discovered the venous valves, tiny membranous folds or pockets inside the veins, which he interpreted as a confirmation of the concept that the blood moved from the center to the periphery. This physiologic error would later be dispelled by his pupil Harvey.

Day after day Harvey must have watched his master tirelessly demonstrating on the dissecting table his favorite theme—the valves or "the little doors of the veins"—and perhaps at some time or another the thought may have crossed his mind that the valves might very well indicate exactly the opposite of what the master claimed, that is, that the blood coursed through the veins from the periphery to the center. Fabricius' absorbing interest in the valves must have stirred Harvey's interest in the problem of the circulation of the blood, an interest that must have been further stimulated by the anatomic spirit that permeated the University of Padua. To be a student in Padua in those days meant becoming interested in anatomy for life. This is what happened to Harvey.

LINE AND SITUATION OF HARVEY'S WORK

This, then, was the line in the history of medicine of Harvey's work. What was his situation in the history of the human spirit? Harvey was a man of both the Renaissance and the Baroque. His Renaissance spirit explains his interest in anatomy; the Baroque explains his interest in movement.

According to Ortega y Gasset, every historical situation comprises two strata in the life of man: one involves his *principles,* the other his *expressions.* His principles consist in his beliefs and intuitions about God, himself, and the world; his expressions are the ways in which his principles are objectively translated into political, economic, artistic, or scientific realities.

The Renaissance was a time of crisis, of transition from the medieval conception—Christian and Gothic—of the world to a new, modern conception that was naturalistic and Baroque.

Vesalius, primarily a Renaissance man, had a "closed" tectonic conception of the human body that enabled him to represent from the outside what was inside the body. Harvey, who experienced the impact of the new Baroque style, had an "open" conception of the human body. In art, which always heralds new trends in science, these two conceptions were expressed respectively in the massive, monumental architectonic style of the Renaissance and the light, airy, dynamic Gothic and Baroque styles. The vertical and horizontal characteristics of the Renaissance style were changed in the Baroque into the curved line and the circle. Renaissance architecture, St. Peter's Basilica, for example, is organized around a vertical axis; Harvey's anatomy is multiple and is organized around dynamic forces. Vesalius' static and classical morphology became mobile and dynamic with Harvey. The immobile wheels in many Renaissance paintings now began to spin, like the wheel in Velázquez' painting, "Las Hilanderas." This wheel in motion is the artistic symbol of the motion of the blood in a circle that Harvey was to describe.

Such, then, was the "line" and "situation" of Harvey's endeavor. A youth of 20 years spends four decisive years in a town seething with new ideas on human anatomy and on movement. Surely these powerful forces must have exerted a profound influence on his sensitive mind?

HARVEY'S CRUCIAL YEARS

I believe that the greatest moment in any scientific discovery—when it is not a fortuitous accident but the result of determined planning and dogged work—is not that moment when the discovery is made, no matter how spectacular such moment may be, but that other moment when a man conceives a theme of universal importance and decides to devote his entire life to its revelation.

Harvey's moment of greatness, then, was not when he announced that the blood moves in a circle, but when the desire was born in his still adolescent mind not merely to describe the movement of the blood, as his predecessors had done, but to discover why and how it moved and to *demonstrate* the process. Harvey's glory, I believe, lies not so much in his discovery as in his decision to make the discovery, just as Vesalius' glory lies in his decision to rediscover human anatomy and to demonstrate it scientifically.

We can imagine Harvey at the close of his four years in Padua. He has known and listened many times to the great masters. He has shared the youthful enthusiasm and ambitions of students from all Europe. His eyes have basked in the marvel that was Venice when the armor in the palaces was not yet rusting away piece by piece, when the tapestries still glowed with brilliant colors, when tapering candles still burned in the cressets and the pink and ivory façades of the palaces were embroidered in dancing colors by the torches in the passing gondolas. He has visited the wealthy in their homes, veritable fortresses lodging small armies of *bravi,* salaried professional swordsmen and killers of such ferocious visage that even the chatelaines locked themselves in their quarters, receiving their meals through a turnstile. He has shared the tables of the wealthy, drunk their wine brought from Syria and Greece and served in glowing Murano goblets, and had his hands washed by servants in bowls of solid gold. Perhaps he has known the nocturnal Bohemia in the streets of Padua, where students caroused and rioted under a moon livid as the face of Pierrot. And he has also shared the camaraderie in the popular *trattorie* where eels were served in aspic, pork was marinated in garlic and onion, and wine was poured out of leather skins.

He has looked at the human body with scrutinizing eyes, as Leonardo recommended, and has studied the heavenly bodies through Galileo's telescope. Perhaps he has hunted the deer in the 12-mile-long park of the Duke of Ferra Mesola, which boasted of a primeval forest with wolves and wild boar.

And then, saturated with the bright, passionate life of Italy, Harvey shook the sun of Padua off his cape and returned to England to fulfill his destiny.

ENGLAND IN THE SEVENTEENTH CENTURY

Harvey returned to his country possessed of a new intellectual attitude toward the problems of visible nature. The Italy that formed Galileo also influenced Harvey. Aldous Huxley said of Shakespeare that he was an English poet who wrote Italian dramas for German audiences. To a certain extent Harvey was an English physiologist who with great insight elaborated on Italian thoughts and then published his results in Germany. In contrast to the Puritan and isolationist line of Cromwell, Harvey, like Shakespeare, possessed a great liberal European spirit and therefore was a universal Englishman.

Back in England, Harvey found a different London, the early seventeenth century London. This would be the stage for his years of initiation and assertion, just as Padua had been the stage for his early years of youth. This London had witnessed the triumphant onrush of the Renaissance and the slow infiltration of the Baroque.

The history of the seventeenth century is the history of Humanity adapting itself to a new order of things. New political and social institutions were being born. Printing and horse-driven vehicles facilitated communication between men. Gunpowder had defeated feudalism, and the compass had opened new routes overseas. Side by side with the absolute monarchies of Charles I of Spain, Henry VIII and Charles I of England, and the "Sun King" in France, there flourished religious wars and an impressive array of religious reformers and philosophers: Wycliffe, Erasmus, Huss.

The austerity of the Reform contrasted sharply with the fabulous splendor of the court of Versailles. This indeed was a fanciful world, gay, frivolous, mindful only of the trappings of the body. Sumptuous palaces glistened with gold-finished furniture and wall after wall of gilded mirrors. The elaborate gardens afforded a gorgeous setting for the towering powdered headdresses, the exquisitely embroidered tunics, the frothy ruffles of the finest lace, and the voluminous skirts of rich silk, velvet, and satin. Spain lost her place among the world powers, and Russia, under Ivan the Terrible and Peter the Great, became acquainted with the Occidental world. Merchants and industrialists were creating capitalism. The concepts of nation, social classes, state, and balance of power were gradually developing. Great philosophers flourished—Descartes, Leibnitz, Bacon, Locke; and great physicists—Kepler, Newton, Galileo; and great artists—Shakespeare, Cervantes, Lope de Vega, Calderón, Rubens, Velázquez, El Greco. Political power was held first by the Spaniards, then by the French, and finally by the English. Symbols of these changes were the *hidalgo,* the *honnête homme,* and the gentleman, successively.

The severe tensions and contrasts of this period between democracy and absolutism and between reason and the religious fanaticism that sent Giordano Bruno and Campanella to their deaths and forced Galileo to retract his theories, were reflected in medicine. The general practitioner felt bewildered and lost when the old edifice of Galenic doctrines tottered and crumbled down and not one but hundreds of complex theoretic structures sprang up. And since every new faith is reflected first in art, Baroque art expressed far more faithfully than any other field the new dynamic concept of the world and life.

PROFILE OF THE BAROQUE

The term "Baroque," which is derived through the Spanish and Portuguese from the Arabic word *buraq* used originally by jewelers to describe irregularly shaped pearls, designates the style of art and architecture that prevailed in the seventeenth century, characterized chiefly by excessive ornamentation and the tendency to portray movement and expression. The term was later extended to include all the culture of this period. The Baroque style, born in Italy, manifested a preference for curves instead of straight lines. Curves were more dynamic and lent themselves better to the representation of emotion and action. The style had such exponents as the Italian decorative painters and architects Colonna, Mantovano, Algardi, and Bernini and the painters Correggio, Mantegna, Tintoretto, and Paul Veronese; the Flemish painters Rubens and Van Dyck; the Dutch painter Franz Hals; the Spanish painters El Greco, Velázquez, Murillo, and Zurbarán. In this period artists suddenly focused their attention on the world in its infinite mobility. Sculpture acquired a fierce mobility and pillars became intricate spirals. Michelangelo was the greatest exponent of this new style.

Rebellion against Protestant austerity was translated into a display of emotions and ornamentation of flood proportions in art. Figures acquired cyclopean dimensions, every line and fold overtly and even fiercely expressing emotion of some sort. There are many examples of this in Michelangelo's work and in the piazzas in Rome, the Fontana di Trevi, for example. Ceilings were heavily decorated, walls were lined with rich damask, beds were intricately carved, mirrors in heavily gilded frames glistened everywhere, and the façades of churches and palaces became veritable labyrinths of filigree work.

In England, except in literature and drama, the Baroque style failed to grow deep roots. The Roman topiary art (the decoration of gardens with ivy and box trimmed to the shape of animals, persons, or tableaux) was revived and, during the transition from the Tudors to the Stuarts, architecture was improved, although not much building was done during the ten years of Cromwell's protectorate. The great London fire of 1666 destroyed the last remnants of medieval architecture, and lighter woods, particularly walnut, became popular and the new constructions were far lighter.

All in all, the Baroque was synonymous with emotion, ornamentation, and movement. These three trends were reflected in the literary work of Browne, Bunyan, Hobbes, Milton, Lovelace, and Shakespeare, and also in medicine, in the work of scientists like Harvey.

Upon his arrival in London, Harvey revalidated his title of Doctor in Physic, received in Padua on April 25, 1602. He was in London when Queen Elizabeth died and James I ascended the throne. The following year he joined the Royal College of Physicians, and in 1604 married Elizabeth Browne, daughter of Lancelot Browne, physician to James I, going to reside at St. Martins, Ludgate. In the next year his mother died at the age of 50 at Folkestone, and also his father-in-law.

ISOLATION AND CHASTITY OF THE SCIENTIST

The love life of the scientist is generally routinary and uniform. With few exceptions the great artist or scientist, like Velázquez or Harvey, leads a tranquil life even in the love arena. In their lives there is no room for great passions or love adventures. For scientific investigation cannot be conciliated with great amatory activity. Casanova's continuous erotic life, for instance, would have made sustained scientific thought impossible.

There is one other reason. The scientist is often shy sexually. Research is a sexual equivalent of other activities and becomes a passion whose intensity and pleasures equal or surpass those of love. Sexual energy is sublimated into longing for knowledge and to create. This is what happened to Harvey, whose private life is as much a mystery as Shakespeare's and seems to have been dedicated exclusively to research.

His first years in London Harvey spent between research, his childless home, and St. Bartholomew's Hospital, where he attended the victims of the plague. In 1613 he was appointed Censor of the Royal College of Physicians and in 1615, Lecturer, with the duties and salary corresponding to those of a professor of physic, at the Colleges of Oxford and Cambridge.

In these same years there were great historical happenings. In 1609 Henry Hudson anchored the *Half Moon* in the Hudson River; in 1611 King James' authorized version of the Bible was published; the tide of Puritanism was gaining momentum; the friction between the King and Parliament increased. And in April, 1616, exactly 341 years ago, Harvey, at a lecture at the Royal College of Physicians, revealed for the first time his great discovery.

But before we speak further of this discovery, we must consider the historical scene in which it developed, the London of the early seventeenth century, the influence that the Baroque exerted on it, and in what consisted the glory of Harvey.

We often think of a famous scientist as if he had lived in splendid isolation, completely absorbed in the task of creation and discovery. We forget that beyond his worktable the whole world continued making history, and that he as a human being was influenced and moved by the ideas and forces that prevailed in his time. To understand Harvey's achievement, he must be looked at not as a lone figure but as one among the many who peopled the tapestry of seventeenth century England.

Just as one cannot appreciate the painstaking work that went into the making of an embroidered Chinese tunic unless one turns it inside out and observes the labyrinth of threads wherefrom emerged the exquisite dragons and lotuses on the right side, neither can one understand Harvey's achievement unless one knows something about the seething, turbulent London that was the reverse of Harvey's quiet, silent life of research and discovery.

LONDON IN 1602

It is 1602 in London, the year of Harvey's return. The first strains of the Baroque are already subduing the impact of the Renaissance on the city. To understand Harvey's personality and work, we must understand first the ever-changing scene in which his life developed.

These were the great years, turbulent and rich in creation, of England. When Harvey was born Elizabeth was Queen. When he was 10 years old, he must have seen his neighbors in the streets of Folkestone commenting with much excitement on the defeat of Philip II's Invincible Armada by both the elements and the English cannons on the steely waters of the Canal de la Mancha. Harvey's first few years in

London coincided with the relatively peaceful reign of James I, whose court afforded eager shelter to frivolity and sybaritism. Great must have been the contrast between these gay years and Harvey's later years, during the reign of Charles I, when civil war broke out, bringing in its bloody wake great changes in the history of England!

But parallel to the bloody violent changes there could be perceived an intellectual renaissance, a natural sequel to the spiritual greatness of the Elizabethan era. English genius flourished everywhere. Bacon and Newton gave science fresh impetus; Shakespeare and Spenser burnt with the flame of creation; Milton's *Paradise Lost* and Bunyan's *Pilgrim's Progress* were published. Bacon was a patient of Harvey, who employed the Baconian method expounded in *Novum Organum,* although Bacon died two years before Harvey published his immortal discovery.

The major social change in England at that time was the Empire's expansion overseas. It was the great era of iron men and wooden ships. The air was filled with voices urging greater technical progress. The woolen and silk industries prospered, opening a path for cotton. Inventors sprouted all over England, soliciting extravagant patents—"a hydraulic cabinet for sending men to sleep," "an improved fishcall," to mention only two. Meanwhile, the country seethed with ferment and slowly prepared for the next civil war.

What caught Harvey's eyes as he crossed the streets of London on his way to St. Bartholomew's Hospital?

London was shabby and noisy, but the shabbiness was gay like that of the pert urchins who sold fish by the Thames. The streets were lined with pubs and shops, and atop the doors the signboards with their colorful names swung merrily in the breeze. Street corners were provided with water pumps, and for those who refused to stand in line there were "cobs," or water-carriers, peddling water from great barrels.

There were also "stocks, pillory and cage at Cornhill" and "ducking-stools for scolds" along the Thames. Those with a morbid taste could promenade to the London Bridge and watch the heads of traitors swinging in the air, their faces still distorted by the last death spasm. In 1598, the year Harvey went to Padua, 30 heads of traitors swung at once like death bells from the bridge tower.

The women who passed Harvey on the streets had faces like frosted apples, the skin pale, the cheeks pink. The rest of the body was concealed under stiff peaked bodices, adorned with ruffs after the Spanish style, and the monstrous wheeled farthingale, consisting of an enormous circular skirt gathered at the waist and stretched out around the hips over a large hoop reaching down to the ground. Under the enormous beplumed hats, they wore a small French hood to restrain the masses of curled hair. The wives of citizens were obliged to wear white knitted caps of woolen yarn, unless their husbands could prove themselves gentlemen by birth. The men were dressed in trunks, which consisted of very short stuffed breeches and trunk hose, and their shoes had heels. Later, under James I, court ladies wore masks in public, and the men allowed their hair to grow long and replaced ruffs by large lace collars and cuffs. Great whiffs of perfume must have reached Harvey as a woman crossed his path, for perfume was used profusely as a preventive against the plague that devastated London in 1602 and later killed 41,313 persons in 1625. Even men carried pomander-chains of civet and musk and a casting bottle of perfume, as well as a mirror in the hat or elsewhere.

Harvey, a sober man all his life, must have shied away from the large elaborate dinners that were customary in those days. The gentry dined at 11 in the morning, dinner lasting three hours, and they supped at 6 in the evening. Merchants and farmers dined at noon and supped at 7. Meat was consumed in excess, mainly being roasted on the spit. Baking was done in iron boxes placed in the fire or in a brick oven at the side of the fireplace. China was not used. The poor used wooden utensils, which later were replaced by pewter; the wealthy used silver, glass, and delftware.

Sugar was replacing honey, rum was already known, and gin was beginning to be made. The high protein diet—salt fish and salt meat, turkey, venison pasty, whey, hog's harslet (from a pig's inside), chicken, lobster, some potatoes, and salads and asparagus—was the cause of numerous skin and vitamin-deficiency diseases, as well as of gout, which plagued most of the great figures in English history and the rich people.

The men of fashion had adopted the new diversion of smoking, which, then as now, was a subject of great controversy. These fashionable gentlemen lived a life of leisure and pleasure, the lack of physical exercise sharply contrasting with the excess of activities in other fields. They never walked, lest they should soil their highly polished boots in London's mud-padded streets, depending exclusively on horses, carriages, and boats. Much time was spent in having the shoes shined to resemble mirrors and the hair groomed and curled into the lovelocks then so fashionable.

A gentleman's typical day usually consisted of chess in the morning, cards after dinner, then dice to exercise his arms, or tennis to exercise his body, or perhaps backgammon, shuffleboard, or billiards, after which he would repair to the theatre or a social gathering.

One may safely assume that Harvey's life was the antithesis to these useless lives, which indubitably were one of the reasons for the Puritan reaction, and that the sight of these pleasure-seeking, time-wasting creatures must have spurred even further his longing to do something in the field of medical science.

HARVEY AND THE BAROQUE

Harvey returned to England thoroughly imbued with the anatomic teachings of Padua and Galileo's deductions on the movements of the heavenly bodies. Two themes were constantly to revolve in his mind in the years to come: anatomy and movement, which would eventually culminate in his great *anatomia animata*. Thereafter he would be completely absorbed by a third idea: the application of his concepts on movement to the blood. Harvey's one goal, then, was to develop an animate anatomy of the blood, an anatomico-physiologic theory on the movement of the blood.

We have mentioned the source of inspiration for Harvey's concept of movement, basis of his physiology and of modern physiology. Never can one insist enough on the vital influence exerted by the so-called "spirit of an epoch." It is easy to understand today's miraculous progress in microbiology and antibiotic research if we relate it to atomic science, which in disintegrating the universe has equally affected everything else, as borne out by modern art, a fragmentary and disintegrated art, and by modern political philosophy, which has tended to atomize the old concept of nationalities. And so is Vesalius' architectonic anatomy related to the architectonic style of the Renaissance; and detail-loving Byzantine medicine to the precious miniature work on the mosaics of Ravenna and Constantinople; and the flattened anatomy of the Egyptians to their flat and bidimensional reliefs; and the progress in microscopy in the Romantic period to the yearning for infiniteness embodied in their Romantic poetry.

Man's life generally spans one period in history, and his activities, even the meaning of his endeavors, are determined by the cultural currents of his period. Harvey was a Renaissance man straddling on the incoming edge of the Baroque, and if we fail to bear in mind that it was the Baroque period, we simply deprive his magnificent obsession with movement of its historical meaning.

The Baroque was essentially an explosion of movement. Art became dynamic. Spiral columns soared into space, replacing the old classical columns, and the stone of cathedrals and palaces was wrenched from its mystic Gothic placidity and turned into veritable whirlpools. Harvey's mental chemistry must have reflected the spirit of the epoch, the new animated view of nature and life, inducing him to leap from Vesalius' static anatomy to the *anatomia animata,* today called physiology. And it also inspired his embryologic discoveries, which were simply another form of creating animate anatomy in time, just as his physiology did in space. The yearning to impart movement to everything in existence that pervaded the Baroque period was the philosophic inspiration underlying Harvey's discovery that the blood moves and that it does so in a circle.

THE SECRET OF THE CIRCLE

This notion of the circle is philosophically of great importance. In a letter to Dr. Brengger, dated 1608, the physicist Kepler said: "I learned from Wacker that Bruno was burnt in Rome and that he suffered with fortitude, asserting the vanity of all religions and the identity of God with the world, the circle and the point."

This résumé of the thought of Giordano Bruno, the immortal philosopher, symbolizes Unity in the circle, the Eternal Being who is active and immutable against the constant variety in ever-changing phenomena. For Bruno, the circle—as pointed out by Walter Pagel—was the whole and a part, beginning and end, central point and circumference, the root of all other geometrical figures.

Every movement that returns to its point of origin must adopt the form of a circle. Only circular movement is continuous and consistent. Every object of nature is, then, a circle, whose function and activity derive from its center point, which is the soul. From the soul the active principle tends, according to Bruno, to go to the periphery, whence it flows back to the center.

Harvey's discovery, therefore, is bound to a philosophy of circles, and the circular motion of the blood is a microcosmic example of a macrocosmic pattern, it being the cycle that conducts the process of return to its point of departure, a phenomenon that Harvey also identified in his studies on generation.

This cosmologic viewpoint is expressed in a passage by Giordano Bruno that, referring to the air and "spirit" of which the blood is vector, says: ". . . there is no circular or spheric motion outside the body. For the blood which in the animal body moves in a circle in order to distribute its motor, the spirit lies motionless outside the body, is inert and decays, no longer deserving the name of blood." *("Sanguis enim qui in corpore animalis in circulum movetur. . . .")* This extraordinary passage is from *De Rerum Principiis,* published 250 years after Bruno's death, the original manuscript bearing the handwritten date of March 16, 1590. In Bruno's treatise *De Monade Numero et Figura* (Frankfurt, 1591) specific mention is made of the circular movement of the blood.

This is vastly important because Giordano Bruno could have been the philosophical link between Cesalpino, the first to use in 1571 the term *circulatio,* and Harvey. These three men had in common the fact that they used an Aristotelian cosmology. Cesalpino even demonstrated as best he could the path followed by the blood from the veins to the heart and then through the arteries to the periphery. This, however, takes no glory from Harvey. Bruno, with that intuition innate in most artists and philosophers, perceived a scientific truth that he neglected to demonstrate. For Harvey, on the other hand, the essential thing was not that he had discovered the circulation of the blood, but that he could *demonstrate* it. The urge to demonstrate scientifically that which others were content to accept as a mystico-philosophical truth based on the concept of the circle—this urge alone—marks him with a seal of glory.

And now let us examine briefly one other aspect of the times of Harvey that is more than mere coincidence. I refer to the intellectual relations between Shakespeare's work and Harvey's, between the scientific vision of the poet and the poetic conception of the scientist.

THE THEATRE IN LONDON IN HARVEY'S DAY

Love for the theatre was enormous in Harvey's day. The public enjoyed immensely the masques, which were spectacles with music, dancing, beautiful lighting effects, and a wide variety of scene changes. But above all they enjoyed the legitimate theatre. In the 10 years preceding Shakespeare, 1580 to 1590, a group of dramatists called the Bohemians, including such figures as Marlowe, Peele, Greene, and Nash, held sway in London's theatrical world. In Shakespeare's time, 1585 and on, plays were performed in galleried yards of inns, which were also used for bear-baiting and wild beast shows. There were three proper theatres, the Swan, a rather "grubby" place, the Rose, and the theatre in Shoreditch. Shakespeare had his own theatre called the Globe. All the theatres were closed during the plague. The scenery was rather rudimentary and sometimes there was none; there were no actresses, only male actors; plot and action were the most important elements. Hence the reasons that Shakespeare's plays are crammed with action and violence.

It is pleasant to imagine Harvey crossing the Thames on his way to the Globe to see perhaps the opening of *Hamlet* in 1602, of *Othello* in 1603, and of *Macbeth* and *King Lear* in 1606.

SHAKESPEARE AND HARVEY

In no other plays in the entire history of the theatre have the words "blood" and "heart" been quoted as often as in Shakespeare's plays. Shakespeare's dramas are as Aristotelian as Harvey's work. They proclaim the central and basic role of the heart. One can visualize the slight little doctor, his hair black, his eyes deep and dark, his nervous fingers forever stroking the pommel of his dagger, sitting at the Globe many an evening listening to the violent voices that spoke of blood and the heart. "By the soul that guides me and the heart that beats in me, I shall never succumb to doubt," Macbeth said; and Hamlet spoke of the passage of blood through the canals of the body.

In Act I, Scene 1, of *Coriolanus* (1609), Menenius tells the citizens who have complained of hunger a fable comparing the body organs with the State organs, "the belly" being the officers who collect food and distribute it to the needy ones, just as the blood circulates through the body, feeding all parts: "But, if you do remember I send it through the rivers of your blood Even to the court, the heart, to the seat o' the brain And, through the cranks and offices of man, The strongest nerves and small inferior veins From me receive that natural competency whereby they live."

Shakespeare died before Harvey announced his discovery, but once more the poet's marvelous intuition not only antedated the scientist's confirmation, but perhaps also contributed to give meaning to his work.

HARVEY'S EXPERIMENTAL METHOD

Such, then, were the forces that influenced Harvey's restless mind in his London years, filled with patient labor and mercurial hope. We know little of these years of Harvey's life. Anatomy was taught, in a rather crude manner, by barber-surgeons and at the Royal College of Physicians. There were no hospitals or medical schools in Scotland, and physicians traveled to Italy and France and later to Holland to study.

Harvey's daily life in these years (until 1615) was absorbed by his professional practice; but his inner life was absorbed by the memory of Realdo Colombo's doubts of the Galenic concept of the circulation and by Fabricius' discovery of the venous valves. He was not interested, like Galen, in the substance of the blood, but *in its movement in space;* nor was he interested, like Vesalius, in the static form, the anatomic architecture, but in animate architecture, in physiologic movement. He had a Faustian concept of science. Above all, he was the first to apply to medicine two elements completely new in the history of science, having been discovered by Santorio only 14 years before—mensuration and calculation. Harvey successfully introduced the method of quantitative mensuration, which thereafter would replace the old qualitative impression. Although Harvey developed the method in his youth, like many other scientists before him, from Claude Bernard to Cajal, he did not comment on it philosophically until his later years, when meditation replaced experimentation.

Obsessed by the passion for movement of the Baroque, Harvey devoted himself to the investigation of the two movements that persist in the human being from birth until death: the pulse and respiration.

The pulse is an expression of the movement of the blood, which Galen explained by saying that the food ingested was elaborated and converted into blood in the liver, and that it was then carried throughout the body by the vessels in a mysterious ebb and flow, and that the blood passed from the right side of the heart to the left through "pores" in the interventricular septum. According to Galen, the blood was received at three points—the liver, the heart, and the brain—"spirits" that controlled the vital functions, and then went from the heart to the lungs to eliminate therefrom all residues, while the air went from the lungs to the heart to give it pneuma. Since dissection did not reveal the "pores" in the heart, Fabricius investigated this mystery in vain, which Fracastoro admitted was known solely to God.

Harvey used only his senses (did not Cushing say that all that is needed for scientific research is "running water and an idea"?) and some 80 different animals, which he vivisected, studying the heartbeat in vivo. The first problem Harvey wanted to resolve was *how much* blood is pumped by the heart during systole, a question that did not even cross the mind of the old physiologists. This question alone was a stroke of genius.

Harvey reckoned that the amount of blood might be about 2 fluid ounces; since the heart beats 72 times per minute (4320 per hour, more than 100,000 per day, and more than 37,000,000 per year), in an hour it would pump 8640 fluid ounces, that is, three times the weight of an average adult. But where did all this blood come from? It certainly could not come from food and it could not be replenished hour after hour. And where did the blood go? It could not go to the tissues, for these would certainly burst under the pressure of so much blood. There was only one answer. The blood flowed from the heart to the arteries and then back to the heart. But how? There was only one logical way—through the veins.

The next step was to demonstrate that the blood in the veins circulated *toward the heart.* By firmly squeezing a cylinder in the hand and pressing with a finger on the forearm veins it was possible to observe that the venous valves prevented the centrifugal flow of blood in the veins, that is, from the heart outward. Thus Harvey completed the circle. Not only did he discover the circulation of the blood, but, what is even more important, he demonstrated it scientifically by means of mathematical reasoning, a completely new approach in science.

The long years of patient and painstaking dissection of deer, fish, snails, frogs, reptiles, birds, as well as the bodies of executed criminals, were more than amply compensated by the brilliant result, which justifies the words Harvey wrote for a student of his, De Clarges, who collected autographs: *"Dii laboribus omnia vendent"* ("The Gods will sell all for the price of work").

Harvey's great personality is reflected not only in his discovery but also in his method, the famous scientific Harveian method, based on *observation, reasoning,* and *experimentation,* exactly the opposite of the authoritarian, dogmatic method of his predecessors. Harvey's method initiated the mensurative approach in medical science, basis of all modern research.

These ideas were the sum of Harvey's notes, scribbled in an unintelligible handwriting, for one of his lectures in the memorable year of 1616. Later, in 1628, they were comprised in a thin little volume, published in Frankfurt under the title of *Exercitatio de Motu Cordis.* The small volume, teeming with printing errors, changed the face of Medicine.

ON THE EVE OF GLORY

In 1615 the College of Physicians entrusted Harvey with the anatomy course, founded in 1581 by Lord Lumley and Dr. Caldwell, called the Lumleian Lectures. The course consisted in two weekly lectures all year round and one annual public "anatomy" lasting five days, "as well before as after dinner."

Harvey gave his first lecture on April 16, 1616, exactly 341 years ago, one week before Shakespeare's death. The notes he prepared for this *Praelectiones Anatomicae* are preserved at the British Museum in London.

Let us visualize Harvey preparing his notes. Perhaps evening is drawing near and the last rays of the retiring sun sneak through the double arched window and mint the floor with gleaming gold. There is a table and on it a bookstand with a huge book and a bronze candelabra. A man dressed in black, his pale face resembling Shakespeare's, is scribbling some notes. His quill traces strange-looking characters in a mixture of English and Latin. The letters are like ants swarming over a musical pentagram. The man's black garments contrast sharply with the sparkle the late sun draws from the rings on his fingers. His face is angular, his hair short, his beard short and gray, and his moustache sad-looking. His eyes are two black diamonds, the sparkle of which Van Dyck would later capture in a portrait.

What occupies Harvey's thoughts? Perhaps he remembers Padua. Perhaps he sees once more the ill-lighted little room and the hard bed where he spent the nights studying; and he sees the amphitheatre with its wooden benches, where by the flickering light of the candelabras he watched Fabricius dissecting; and there are the star-studded skies of Padua again and Galileo by his side trying to solve their mysteries. The streets of Padua are burning with sun; the capes of the students flare out in the breeze; a beautiful Venetian girl crosses the piazza ahead of him and her graceful torso is silhouetted against the fresh blue of the sky and the time-worn blue of a Byzantine basilica. On its façade the pigeons form a quivering, feathered frieze.

Maybe he also remembers Galen, whom he will mention in his lecture, and Vesalius, the musketeer of anatomy who with his scalpel for a sword fatally stabbed the dogmatic authority of the classics. He thinks of the long years of work, and of Shakespeare's plays, and of the whirling spirals of the Baroque, and the many hearts of animals beating under his pallid fingers. And he feels the beat of his own heart moved by the conquest of Truth. He remembers the title of Doctor in Medicine granted him in Padua, and he can see his *stemma* or coat of arms on the ceiling of the honor hall at the University of Padua, one hand holding a lighted candle with two snakes coiled around it.

His past has filed before his eyes. His future is veiled in hopes. And he pens the immortal lines for his lecture: *"Consta per ligaturam transitum sanguinis ab arteriis ad venas, unde: perpetuum sanguinis motum in circulo fieri pulsu cordis."* The blood moves and it moves *in a circle!* In this hour Harvey crossed the golden threshold to greatness.

THE MEDICO-PHARMACEUTICAL ARTS OF *LA CELESTINA:* A STUDY OF A FIFTEENTH CENTURY SPANISH SORCERESS AND "DEALER IN LOVE"

SPANISH MEDICINE IN THE FIFTEENTH CENTURY

In the history of Spain, the fifteenth century marked the opening of the gateway through which the Spanish people sailed forth to become a decisive factor in the progress of Western civilization. Up to the end of that century, which is to say, until the dawn of the Golden Age in Spain, Spaniards were busy demolishing the last Moorish outposts on the Iberian Peninsula, laying the foundations of national solidarity through the union of the kingdoms of Aragon and Castile, conquering Granada, and discovering the New World.

From a medicohistorical point of view, the fifteenth century was a period of transition attendant to the integration of Byzantine medicine, which was to be re-established in Spain after the fall of Constantinople in 1453, with Arabian medicine.

In this century of the discovery of the New World, against a motley and picturesque scene stirred by the winds of conquest and already lighted by the lamps of new cultures, there prevailed on the Iberian Peninsula a coalescence of the learning of three groups of Spanish physicians: Jewish, Moslem, and Christian.

The medicine of this period was concocted from the varied contributions made by these streams of culture. From the Jews was derived a penchant for Hippocratic principles, a taste for astrology and cabalism, the practice of medical teaching by word of mouth, and a

From *International Record of Medicine* 169:233, 1956.

leaning toward dramatic display; from the Moors—invaders of Spain since the Battle of Guadelete—were imbibed the diehard tendencies of Latinized Hippocratic tradition, a multifaceted culture, naturalistic trends, alchemy, and physiotherapy; and the Christians contributed theologic and mystic strains of clericalism, ceremonialism, and a fondness for anatomy and pathology based on their supernatural concept of the universe.

The lamps of learning lighted in the thirteenth century by the renowned colleges of translators in Toledo, which revived Greek and Roman medicine, were still burning. Spanish, the golden tongue of soldiers, mystics, philosophers, and poets, the beautiful, heroic language of Castile, now became a channel for the conveyance of medical learning.

Universities had been flourishing in Spain since the year 1214. Since 1240 a chair of anatomy had existed in Valencia, and another in Lerida since 1391, one of the first colleges in Europe to sanction the practice of necropsy. Toledo was the hub of Arabic-Spanish culture. It was there that Gerard of Cremona and Michael Scotus were to cement their reputations.

From 1474 onward a printing press was in operation in Barcelona, where, at the beginning of the following century, in 1514, the first polyglot Bible was published by the Theological Faculty of the University of Alcalá; its Greek and Hebrew texts, together with a complete critical appendix, glossary, and grammar, represented in the words of a chronicler in 1844 "the first truly scientific work of the modern age."

The heritage of Seneca, of St. Isidore of Seville, of the Caliphate of Cordova, of Maimonides, the labors of the Benedictines of Cluny and of Alphonso VI, the erudition of the universities of Valencia, founded by Alphonso VIII in the twelfth century, and Salamanca, founded by Alphonso IX in the thirteenth century, the scholarship of the Academy of Medicine founded by Alphonso X in 1255, the results of experiments in the pesthouses and leprosaria established in the time of Rodrigo Díaz, the Cid Campeador, all the abstruse medical knowledge gathered by Arnold of Villanova and Raymond Lully in Catalonia dating from the thirteenth century, the field hospitals established by Isabel II, the College of Surgeons at Valls near Barcelona, the achievements of Gaspar Torruella and Villalobos —all these formed the richly colored warp into which was woven the empirical medical knowledge of the fifteenth century.

As in every period preceding a new age, confusion and disorder were rife. The physician from his watchtower peered at a horizon so wide and crowded that he was distracted from the proper contemplation of the purely medical landscape. The empiricism prevailing in sundry branches of medicine spread to all medicine, particularly to therapy, in the peninsula. As a reaction against the exuberance of Arabian polypharmacy there began a return toward phytotherapy and doctoring with herbs and simples. The masses, however, remained partial to the balms and comfits, pills and sirups concocted by the bounteous hands of the Arabs.

The *Libre apellat Macer,* written by an unknown author, still preserved in the Archives of the Barcelona Cathedral, comprises innumerable references to botanical medicine, grammar, astrology, mystic devotions, and incantations, all jumbled together and topped by a treatise on the art of cooking.

Another folio, author unknown, printed in Burgos in 1495, entitled *Epílogo en medicina y cirugía conveniente a la salud* (*A Sequel on Medicine and Surgery Conducive to Health*), contains a farrago of astrology, pathology, physiognomy, surgery, urinalysis, and bloodletting.

It would appear, therefore, that the fifteenth century, with its protean ramifications, was a "black earth" in which quackery could flourish. In this vast jungle of spellcasting and sorcery there stands out as a pattern for all time the figure of a little old hag, a dealer in love and lechery, a winebibbing go-between, with a full stock in trade of traditional ignorance and wizardry to make her truly typical of the quackery of the period. This bent old woman, whose trotting footsteps still rouse faint echoes in the ancient alleys of Toledo, was the notorious Celestina.

HISTORICAL PROFILE OF CELESTINA AND OF HER CREATOR

The hidalgo Fernando de Rojas (?–1541), the much-discussed author of *Celestina,* was born in Puebla de Montalbán, a small village on the outskirts of Toledo, and practiced as a lawyer in nearby Talavera, where for several years he held the position of mayor. He married, raised a family, and died—all in his birthplace, being buried there in the Church of the Convent of the Virgin. But his monotonous existence was enlightened by one creative period that raised him out of the rut of respectable mediocrity to the dizzy heights of immortality. This period lasted only fifteen days (some say fifteen years), which is what it took him to write his immortal *Tragicomedy of Calixtus and Melibea,* or *La Celestina,* inspired by his readings of Petrarch, Boccaccio's *Fiammetta,* and the works of Juan Ruiz, better known as the Archpriest of Hita.

La Celestina, or *La tragicomedia de Calixto y Melibea,* of which not a single copy of the first edition has yet been found, was reprinted in Burgos in the year 1499. The only copy extant of this second edition is in New York in the library of the Hispanic Society of America.

The original work, in twenty-one acts, is supposed to have been written in 1483 or 1497. *La Celestina* surpasses in tragic strength and realistic conception everything that went before it in Spanish literature of this class; it was the first book in Spanish to spread throughout western Europe and to enjoy universal popularity during the sixteenth century. Rojas' pellucid prose style gave literary embodiment to popular speech and inaugurated the artistic renaissance in Spain. It is a drama of passion in which the youth Calixtus, seeking the favors of the beautiful maiden Melibea, enlists the aid of the aged and crafty go-between Celestina and by such means eventually wins the maiden to his lusty will.

Whether or not the old crone was based on a real person actually known to the author has been a matter of much discussion. The famous Portuguese writer Amato Lusitano (Juan Rodríguez de Castello Branco), who completed his studies at Talavera University in 1529, in his celebrated medical treatise refers to the actual existence of Celestina (this was quoted by Menéndez Pelayo in his *Historical Sources of the Spanish Novel*). Lusitano, in his commentary on Dioscorides (In: *Dioscoridis Anazarbei de Materia Medica Libros Quinque e Narrationes Eruditissimi Doctoris Amati Lusitani. Venetiis, apud Gualterum Scotum*, 1553, lib. III, p. 1907), mentions an animal glue factory located in Salamanca, close to the Tormes bridge, "not far from the home of Celestina, a notorious wise woman appearing in the comedy of Calixtus and Melibea" (*"Non procul a domo Celestinae mulieris famosissimae et de quale ajitur in comedia Calisti et Malibeae"*). Dr. Pedro Díaz also mentioned this quotation in 1895 in his *Archivos da Historia da Medicina Portugueza.*

A later reference to the actual existence of this female quack appears in *El peregrino curioso* (*The Inquisitive Wanderer*), by Bartolomé de Villalba y Estaña (1577), to the effect that certain students showed him Celestina's home near the tan pits.

Sancho Muñón, who plagiarized Rojas' work, in his *Tragicomedia de Lisandro y Roselia* (*Tragicomedy of Lysander and Roselia*) also alludes to Celestina as dwelling in those parts and to the fact that the tomb of this archetype of quacks and bawds is to be found in St. Lorenzo.

SILHOUETTES OF CELESTINA AND HER TEACHER CLAUDINE

When Rojas first presents Celestina, she is seen traipsing through the narrow alleys of Toledo, over which coveys of pigeons are in flight while the church bells are tolling. She is carrying a pitcher of wine in her shaking hands. Inquisitive feminine eyes behind the shutters follow her progress. The convent bells are ringing like the beating of a happy heart. Celestina walks circumspectly, greeting here and there a blushing priest who some while back may have been one of her clients. All the while she pries here and peers there into everything in sight. Sixty years of roguery are heavy on her shrunken shoulders. A crafty smile hovers on her lips, withered and faded like an autumn leaf.

A small boy playing in a doorway shouts *"¡la barbuda!"* (*"Hey, Whiskers!"*), and at the sound of this tribute to her hirsute countenance the old crone threatens to box the ears of the young imp who, however, continues to yell after her until she finally disappears from view. Shrugging her shoulders, she tramps on with the pitcher of wine in her hand, spilling a crimson drop here and there as she stumbles over the stones of the unpaved streets. She is neither good nor evil. She defies all classification. If people call her *satánica* (devilish), it is because they do not know that in her past there is a bitter tale of woe and that the knife slash across her face is a relic from a lovers' quarrel, a scar that all her magic art could not heal.

Meantime, her past life rustles through her mind like leaves in the fall. Her weary feet now follow the slope of the roadway, bathed in the golden glow of a topaz-colored sunset. She remembers how she plied her trade. By the river, near the tan pits and leather yards, is her ramshackle hut, which in itself is sufficient to strike awe into visitors. She goes through the sagging doorway, forever ajar. Her bony hands, glimmering like the bronze of a lamp, move deftly. She shakes off her heavy cloak, drops onto a stool, gets up, thinks back on her past renown and the rewards thereof which are now gone like autumn leaves before the October wind.

Celestina, full of woe and sentimentality, steps outside to take a breath of the fresh evening air laden with the scent of flowers and the pungent odor of drying hay. Her glance wanders toward the river rippling in the distance, seeing in her mind's eye the glossy hides, shining like silver shields in the moonlight, hung out to dry by the placid waters. The cool breeze now caresses her face, wizened and yellowed like ancient parchment. In her boundless solitude, she becomes lachrymose, while the somber poplars near the river's edge lean toward her, their foliage drooping like tresses from the head of a sorrowing woman.*

---

* Celestina, who is first described in the extravagant words with which Sempronius tells his master, Calixtus, of her trade and tricks, is a little old woman whose namesake appears in the play *Libro del esforzado caballero Don Tristán de Leonis* (*The Book of the Brave Knight Sir Tristram of Lyonesse*), where "the tale goes that when Sir Lancelot was parted from the maid, she gathered unto her many people, among whom was her aunt Celestina."

When we meet Celestina she is sixty years of age, she claims, but her crony Parmenus tells that the old dame has already seen "two-and-seventy summers." Despite her senile hairiness, which begot her the nicknames *"vieja barbuda"* (*"Old Mother Bigbeard"*) and *"la barbuda,"* her countenance was probably not unpleasant, for she always wore a crafty but friendly smile. Besides, she was not averse to using on herself the cosmetics that she concocted for her clients, including that antimonial stain beloved by Syrian women that puts a sparkle in withered pupils and dilates their size. This is what Parmenus alludes to when he calls her a "coal-eyed old lady," a pun on *kohl,* Arabic for antimony.

According to her own story, Celestina had been a girl of great beauty, the youngest of four children, but as the result of a dissipated girlhood she had aged rapidly, her wizened face made uglier by a long knife scar.

To the effects of her tempestuous career must be added the influence of her teacher, Claudine, with whom she was hand-in-glove, perhaps united to her by Lesbian ties, a theory supported by her lustful propensities and her statement, ". . . from her [Claudine] I learnt all the choicest there was to know of my trade . . . we ate together, slept together, took our relaxations in one another's company and our pleasures and counsels in common" (*"Della* [de su maestra] *aprendí todo lo mejor que sé de mi oficio . . . juntas comíamos, juntas dormíamos, juntas auíamos nuestros solazes, nuestros plazeres, nuestros consejos y concierto"*).

Claudine, an alcoholic, possessed a virile bearing, which may indicate the manner in which she influenced Celestina's love life. Meaningful are the words Celestina uses when bewailing her friend: "Oh, how sweet she was! How gentle, clean and virile!" (*"¡O qué graciosa era! ¡O qué desembuelta, limpia, varonil!"*).

The aged Claudine practiced sixteen years as a midwife, a profession that cloaked her pandering activities and allowed her to come and go wherever she chose without arousing suspicion.

To her prowess as quack and procuress, Claudine added sorcery, since in those times every medicaster practiced magic in order to acquire supernatural powers and to stand on a pedestal of awe above the people. As a result of all this, the Inquisition hauled her up four times, once together with Celestina. On one occasion she was denounced as a witch—perhaps the deadliest accusation possible in the Middle Ages—because she was caught "gathering earth by candlelight in the dead of night at a crossroad" (in those days a place of execution or a burial ground), and was sentenced to stand in the pillory before the populace with a conical cap on her head. That such accusations were well founded is shown by the words of her disciple:

". . . she went from graveyard to graveyard in the dead of night as easily as by day, seeking the tackle for our trade. There was not a single Christian, Moor or Jew whose funeral she did not attend. She lay in wait for them by day and dug them up by night. With her tweezers she filched seven teeth from a hanged man's mouth, while I took off his shoes. . . . What more for me to say than the very devil's imps themselves were afraid of her? She kept them in awe and terror by the bitter words she flung at them . . ." (". . . *se andaua a media noche de cimenterio en cimenterio, buscando aparejos para nuestro oficio, como de día. No dejaba cristiano, ni moros ni judíos, cuyos enterramientos no visitara. De día los acechaua, de noche los desenterraua. Siete dientes quitó a un ahorcado con sus tenacicas de palacejas, mientras yo le descalcé los zapatos. . . . ¿Qué más quieres sino que los mesmos diablos la hauían miedo? Atemorizados e espantados los tenía con las crudas bozes que les daua . . ."*).

Old Claudine died from her many excesses, particularly alcoholism, for as her follower says, ". . . she never came back without gulping down eight or ten draughts, a pint in the jar and the other inside her" (". . . *jamás bolbia sin ocho o diez gostaduras, un acumbre en el jarro e otro en el cuerpo"*). From her, Celestina got her taste for liquor and the pleasures of the table, as well as her bent for sexual debauchery. She explored all the pathways of erotic excess. In a dialogue with her godson Parmenus, she says: "Do you remember, dear boy, when you used to sleep at my feet?" (*"¿Acuerdaste cuando dormías a mis pies, loquito?"*). To which he replies: "Yes, indeed I do! Sometimes, even though I was then but a child, you hoisted me on to the bolster and pressed me close to your bosom, but you smelt so old I used to run away from you!" (*"Sí, en buena fe. En algunas veces me subias a la cabesera y me apretabas contigo, e porque olías a vieja, me fuya de ti . . ."*).

Great was Celestina's vogue in Toledo. In the story that Parmenus tells his master, we can see, even after allowing for all possible exaggeration, the great fame that the old woman enjoyed, a fact easily explained by the very strait-lacedness that ruled the town and that made every rumor and tale spread like wildfire under the irresistible seal of "it's a secret." In the words of Parmenus: "She is the subject of conversation at all gatherings, meetings, merrymakings, weddings, feasts, burials and occasions of intercourse . . . the woodworkers sing her praises, the woolcombers, weavers, gardeners, field-laborers and vine-tenders rule their daily round by her counsels . . ." (*"En los convites, en las fiestas, en las bodas, en las cofradías, en los mortuorios, en todos los ayuntamientos de gentes, con ella pasan tiempo . . . cantanla los carpinteros, peynanla los peynadores, texedores, labradores en las huertas, en las aradas, en las viñas, en las regadas con ellas pasan el afán cotidiano . . .").*

Her greatest claim to fame, however, was among the priests and clergy, who made up the most important section of the community. She herself said that her trade was "the sale of concubines" to priests. Thus, in her declining years, she is able to recall with zest the days of her prime when her house was crammed full of "old gents and lads, church-folk of all ranks from bishops down to sextons" (*"caballeros viejos o moços, abades de todas dignidades desde obispos a sacristanes"*), who presented her with all kinds of gifts: "many fowls, chickens, geese, ducks, partridges, turtledoves, hams, suckling-pigs, wheat cakes and fine meal loaves" (*"muchos pollos, gallinas, ansarones, anadones, perdices, tórtolas, perniles de tocino, tortas de trigo, lechones, bodigos"*), as well as wine in abundance—the fine red wine of Mondiego, Luque, Toro, Madrigal, St. Martin, and other districts —which she sampled modestly enough to begin with but ended up by gulping down by the bucketful.

THE PASSION FOR WINE

These offerings were a great satisfaction to Celestina, for though in her old age she was circumspect in eating (she could exist for three days on a hunk of bread soaked in wine, reinforced by innumerable swigs from the wine bottle), neither at table nor in bed would she forego her pitcher of wine to warm her blood and sustain her in a condition ever ready for business. Wine for her "drives depression from the heart, puts color into wan cheeks and courage into the coward, comforts the brain, shifts cold from the belly, dispels stench from the breath, sweats out all evil humors, clears out head colds and toothache, and prevents nausea" (". . . *quita la tristeza al corazón, pone color al descolorido, coraje al cobarde, conforta los cerebros, saca el frío del estómago, quita el hedor del aliento, hace sudar toda agua mala, sana el romadizo e las muelas, sostiene sin heder en la mar"*). For all these reasons, she always gulped a dozen draughts at every meal except if invited out, when, of course, she took a double dose.

In her eulogy on wine, we cannot fail to note the empirical equivalent of the cures by alcohol introduced by the Moslems in Spain and popularized there by Moorish physicians, such as Avicenna, who not only recommended such remedies but were themselves great patrons of old wine. All medicine in fifteenth-century Spain embraces this reliance on the curative virtues of alcohol, which occurs in all empirical medicine.

Celestina's passion for drink is a characteristic frequently found

to a greater or lesser degree in all charlatans.* The Dipsas or Pytho-
nesses and go-betweens mentioned by Ovid became what they were
through their unquenchable thirst and not from a lack of water either!
A similar passion afflicted Laena, the doorkeeper of the Cistellaria
in Plautus' *Curculio* (Master Weevil the Parasite). The word "dipsomania" is derived from the name of the inebriated Dipsas. Perhaps
Celestina herself was not many stages removed from this type of
psychiatric disorder. Hence, in the play we find her so frequently, wine
pitcher ever to hand, wending her way with stumbling steps through
the streets of Toledo.

THE POLYFACETIC ACTIVITIES OF A SORCERESS

Celestina owed a great deal of her reputation to her multifarious
activities. Diversity in operations was a characteristic of quacks and
sorcerers, who kept many irons in the fire at one time. Unlike the
physician, the quack needed to create for himself not a science but
an *atmosphere*. What he actually did was not so important as *what
people believed* he could do.

Talking of Celestina, Sempronius said she was "a sorceress
shrewd and cunning in everything relating to the Black Art. I have
been told that the number of spells she has cast or reversed in the
town amounts to well over five thousand. She can awaken lust in
stones if need be!" (*"Hechicera, astuta, sagaz, en cuantas maldades
hay. Entiendo que pasan de cinco mil componendas las que ha
hecho y desecho en la ciudad. A las duras peñas promouerá e prou-
ocará a la luxuria si quiere".*) We then may deduce that she was a
witch—a perilous profession in the days of the Inquisition—and that
she acted as a lovers' go-between, supplying them with aphrodisiacs
to excite their passion (for which purpose she needed only to fall
back on the vast armory of aphrodisiac drugs then in existence) and
afterwards repairing any physical damages resulting therefrom. According to her former retainer, Parmenus, Celestina was "seamstress,
perfumer, past-mistress in the concoction of cosmetics and in patching
up the troubles of maidens, also a procuress and something of a
witch" (". . . *labrandera, perfumera, maestra de fazer afeite e de
fazer remiendos virginales, alcahueta e un poquito hechicera"*).

The profession of seamstress was nothing more than one of the
fronts adopted by all charlatans to evade the eyes of the law and as
an excuse to go everywhere without difficulty. Moreover, such a trade

---

* Shakespeare often praised Spanish wines. His Mistress Quickly, the English
Celestina, remarks to Doll Tearsheet (*Henry IV*, Act II, scene iv): "But,
i'faith, you have drunk too much canaries [wine of Canary Islands], and that's
a marvellous searching wine, and it perfumes the blood ere one can say:
What's this?"

enabled Celestina to leave her door open to maidens, students, and priests, and to enter other people's houses, for though she sometimes called herself a "child doctor," lechery more than pediatrics was her principal means of livelihood. In addition, she spun worsted, wrote doggerel and hymns for the monasteries, concocted perfumes, drugs, ointments, pastes, pomades, rinses, powders, and lyes; she also sold medicinal herbs, cosmetic oils and balms, and possessed, moreover, surgical skills.

THE DWELLING OF A FIFTEENTH CENTURY WITCH

Celestina lived, as was the custom of such soothsayers who paid the greatest attention to the aura surrounding them, on the outskirts of the town (Toledo or Salamanca) where her creator Rojas set the scene. Her dwelling lay "by the riverside," near the leatherworks or tan pits, which in every town were situated in small bystreets on the river banks. Hers was an ancient shack, half in ruins, poorly furnished, "and worse provisioned," all factors of great importance in the art of soothsaying. It would be inconceivable that Celestina should sell her balms or weave her spells anywhere else than in such a shack, crammed full of concoctions and nostrums concealed behind cupboard doors and discreet lattices.

On entering, the visitor's nose was immediately assailed by a bittersweet odor in which the gentle perfume of amber mingled with the pungent scent of musk and civet. Glass retorts and phials and casks of tin and clay of all shapes were strewn everywhere. The tables were littered with pots of ointment, silver pomanders, balls of wax, jars of mercury, storax, philters, musk perfumes, pomades and lotions to put a bloom on the face, bottles of bleaching lotions and essences of roses and other flowers, bits of asphodel root, bladder, senna, goat's horn, oak galls, mistletoe, and various distilled and sweetened liquors. Dressed hides and skins lay about, and preparations such as lime water containing powdered jalap root or marrow from the bones of fallow deer and heron were also on hand, together with pot-bellied glass jars containing sweet-smelling solutions of rose, orange blossom, jasmine, clover, honeysuckle, and powdered cloves distilled in wine or rectified spirit, lyes and dyes made from henna to bleach the hair or restore its color, vine shoots, swamp oak, ergot, and alum. And there were rows upon rows of jars of salves and pomades containing, according to Celestina, extracts from cow, bear, horse, rabbit, camel, hare, whale, fallow deer, bearcat, badger, squirrel, hedgehog, and otter, but which most likely were all of the same composition, although each one was colored differently from the rest.

From the roof hung packets and sheaves of all kinds of herbs for the preparation of medicinal baths: camomile, rosemary, elderberry, marshmallow, maidenhair, melilot, mustard seed, lavender, white laurel, dog rose, couch grass, wildflower, thorn apple, silvertongue, and sepia flake. The study from a pharmacologic angle of this impressive array of herbs should indeed afford a good idea of the state of physiotherapy in that age.

There were also small earthenware pots containing facial oils and essences made of storax, jasmine, lime, violet, benjamin, pistachio, pine kernels, melonseed, jujube, fumagine, lupine, vetches, sea holly, and chickweed, phials of balsam for healing scratched noses, and little boxes containing bits of bladder.

In one corner—and here we follow the detailed "stage directions" in the play—stood a small platform on which lay a painted vessel, some long thin needles such as those used by weavers, and waxed silk thread, while overhead hung roots of spikenard, red sumac, squills, and horsetail—all of which was evidence of her ventures into surgery.

But of all this, the most awe-inspiring and even frightening sight was the room where she concocted her potions for purposes of sorcery and the treatment of love sickness. Here were weird-looking skins and membranes, bones, hearts of stags, adders' tongues, heads of quail, asses' brains, haircloths, horses' hides, cauls, loincloths, black beans, a lodestone, the inevitable hangman's rope, ivy leaves, hedgehogs' quills, badgers' feet, fern seeds, a stone from an eagle's eyrie, and many other items among which, of course, there was no lack of wax hearts pierced with pins and awful little effigies in clay and lead. Examining the symbolism and potentialities of all this gallimaufry of soothsaying, we find the same superstitious usages as were rampant among primitive tribes when the witch doctor claimed to cure pain and even death by the magic virtue of his fetishes.

Perhaps Celestina's infernal apparatus did indeed work miracles. For when the client emerged from that horrendous hovel, he must have delighted in breathing once more the fresh wholesome air and the overriding aroma from the hay fields, and in hearing the whispering Tagus, "Knight and Crusader," while his gaze wandered happily across the cerulean blue of the lofty Toledan skies.

CELESTINA AS A SORCERESS

Despite many allusions throughout the play to Celestina's witchcraft, and Menéndez Pelayo's description of her as "the spirit of evil incarnate in a vulgar and uneducated creature possessing nevertheless intelligence and cunning," and Julio Cejador's observation, "In Celestina there is definite deviltry, she is a true sorceress but no trickster," this does not appear to be her principal activity. The main thing about a witch is that she should believe in her own spells, but for Celestina a spell was merely an adjunct to medicaments or to her panderings to debauchery. True, she did cast a large number of spells, but then charlatans in all ages have done that, either from conviction or to make the most of the credulity of the masses.

In the spell she casts in Act III, before she starts her campaign on Melibea—this being the normal procedure in all performances of magic—she puts herself on a plane of equality with the devilkins she is invoking, using at once threats and cajolery to bring them to heel. But this spell (so different from that practiced in front of the cauldron, where their exotic nostrums are cooking, by the witches in Shakespeare's *Macbeth* (Act IV, scene i)) seems in her case to be more of a play to the gallery and a means of reinforcing her plans than a real spell on whose efficiency she relies.

For Celestina, such a spell is almost a ritual when commencing operations in amorous affairs. In the presence of Sempronius, the servant of her client Calixtus, she purposely calls out to her maid Elicia the whole awe-inspiring list of the magic ingredients she needs, doing this in their presence in order to obtain their greater obedience and to show off her prowess. She therefore instructs Elicia to go upstairs where she keeps her most secret paraphernalia and to bring down "the can of snake-oil, I mean, the compost of adder's venom" (*"el bote del azeyte serpentino o sea aceite compuesto con ponzoña de víboras"*) which, she adds, is next to the hangman's rope she filched from the gallows one dark, stormy night. She bids the girl to open the heddle chest in the attic (which indicates that our sorceress lived in a home formerly inhabited by weavers, who always kept such a chest in the attic) and to take out the sheet of paper written "in bat's blood" lying "under the wing of that dragon from which we pulled the nails" (*"debaxo de aquel ala de drago a que sacamos ayer las uñas"*). And she admonishes the girl while still up there not to upset the May-day rain water that had been brought in for some concoction. All these paraphernalia pertain to witchcraft, and even Pliny in his time mentioned them as popular remedies against all ailments.

She tells the maid to go into the ointment room where she will find what she is looking for "in the black cat's skin, where I told you to fix the she-wolf's eyes" (*"en la pelleja del gato negro, donde te mandé meter los ojos de la loba"*), and orders her to bring down also "the billy-goat's blood and a few of the hairs you snipped from his beard" (*"la sangre del macho cabrío y unas poquitas de las barbas que tu le cortaste"*). Bits and scraps like these show the magical value set in that period on such relics as on certain animal therapy, so common in the Middle Ages, which later became known as "garbage pharmacy" (*"botica de las inmundicias"*). In all her activities, we recognize in Celestina a clever woman who knew how to exploit to the full the rich vein of popular superstition.

CELESTINA'S COSMETIC, PHARMACOLOGIC, AND MEDICAL KNOWLEDGE

Generally a quack's wisdom had roots different from those of the true man of science. The former based his knowledge on direct naturalistic observation of the symptoms displayed before him. If several persons affected by the same disease were cured by a drug or nostrum, he immediately inferred that that drug or nostrum would cure all similar cases. The quack therefore proceeded by personal induction, and his methods gave rise to a system of therapeutic abstractions stemming from the purely visual facts of the case.

The scientific method, on the other hand, was just the opposite, procedure and performance being by deduction. The physician arrived at the facts through contemplation from the heights of his abstract knowledge. In treating disease, the cure was performed through a chain of abstractions. Concrete action in a particular case grew out of an abstruse concept of illness and some scattered ideas on therapy. Science was not individualized, and the fifteenth-century physicians, hidebound by inflexible dogma, treated their patients by rule of thumb, forcing them to fit into the framework of their abstruse theories on medical practice. Today, the empirical methods, after careful examination by medical historians, appear to be more practical and effective than the accepted "official" medical system of the fifteenth century. The former was an artless and rudimentary therapy based on a pseudoscientific and popular medicine; the latter was a species of medical metaphysics in which the prevailing notions on body fluids and temperatures canceled the physician's intuition.

The basis of Celestina's character as a healer was a profound self-confidence and the trust she inspired in her patients. Sometimes she reached the heights of blatant showing off and theatrical braggartism, for this sort of byplay was an indispensable factor in the success of any self-respecting charlatan. The medieval physician considered himself completely trained once he had swallowed up the indigestible medical science of the Moslems. The quack, on the other hand, realized that he had to shape his personality to fit his clientele, and he therefore forged an inner core of flamboyance and tempered it in the light of his own immeasurable self-conceit. As noted by Liek Danzing, that was the element lacking in many physicians, who, despite their learning, were unable to heal because an excess of criticism damped their own personal initiative.

Celestina placed no reliance on science nor on drugs or incantations. She was as devoid of confidence in her own science as she was full of faith in her own power of suggestion and in the power of every living being to cure himself. Celestina was, in fact, as much a born psychologist as a quack.

Her poor opinion of surgeons, who were gaining importance in this period as anatomy gained scientific recognition, is evident in her words, "I rejoice at this news as much as a doctor does at fractures, and in the same way that he first makes the sores worse in order to increase his fees for the promise of recovery, so also do I reckon to work on Calixtus" (". . . *me alegro de estas nuevas como los cirujanos de las descalabraduras, e como aquellos dañan en los principios las llagas e encarecen el prometimiento de la salud, asi pienso yo hacer a Calisto*"). Celestina is well aware of the tricks employed by any back-room physician of the time to exaggerate the gravity of a wound and thus increase his social renown and his financial rewards.

Deep in Celestina's medical conscience throbbed a complete lack of faith in the medicine of the time: "There is no greater clog on good health than abundance and variety in victuals . . . and a sore will never heal when so many remedies are there to be tried out" (*"No hay cosa que más la sanidad impida que la diversidad mundanza e variedad de los manjares . . . e nunca la llaga viene a cicatrizar, en la cual muchas melecinas se tientan"*). The following words summarize her complete disbelief in the effect of remedial cures: "as they say of the dipping-pool of Bethesda, where out of every hundred who go in, only one comes out properly cleansed" (". . . *como se escriue de la probática piscina que de ciento que entrauan sanaba uno*"). At the bottom of this skepticism lies an unshakable belief in her own healing powers.

For the rest, Celestina possessed not only the empiric culture of the period but also a knowledge of sex determination in plants and of the habits of beasts: of the "unicorn who cringes when he spies a virtuous maiden" (*"unicornio que se humilla ante cualquier donzella"*), a fable already mentioned by Pliny and repeated in more modern times by Huerta and other writers; "of the dog that out of pity will not bite him who kneels in front of him, and the pelican that pierces her breast to feed her young" (*"del perro que por piedad no muerde a quien ante él se hecha al suelo, del pelícano que se rompe el pecho por mantener a sus hijos"*), which facts are confirmed by Valdecebro in his treatise titled *Birds*.

CELESTINA'S ACHIEVEMENTS IN SURGERY

To her theoretical knowledge Celestina added the surgical activities already mentioned. All Toledo (or was it Salamanca?) knew that she trafficked in maidens and then "restored their virginity in more than five thousand instances," as we are told in the play.

The whole practice of quacksalvers in the fifteenth century was built up on shady sexual intrigues, as was to be expected in an era when aphrodisiacs and love philters were the mainstays of libidinous dealings. An age of prudery always produces persons whose mission is to make a mockery of the harsh moral austerity surrounding them. Celestina or Don Juan never could have existed in ancient Greece or during the Renaissance, for they are the offspring of periods of intense sexual repression, such as existed in fifteenth century Spain.

Celestina herself on a certain occasion alluded to "the impotency I am able to bring about" by means of her charms and to the recoveries she could similarly effect. She was therefore past mistress in all the secrets of the complicated medieval control of sexual powers.

Her surgical stock in trade was limited but adequate for her requirements. A colored skillet, a few slender needles like those used by leatherworkers, and bits of waxed silk thread and catgut were all she needed for repairing the damages of illicit love affairs. She had roots of spikenard, bloodwort, red sumac, squills, and horsetail, styptic herbs and other astringents for stanching the flow of blood. This tackle was all she required for getting away with the most audacious impositions on her clients, as, for instance, "on the occasion of the French Ambassador's visit" (*"cuando vino el embajador francés"*) when, three times running, she sold as a "virgin" a lusty, buxom lass already well versed in the arts of harlotry.

THE PHARMACOLOGIC ARSENAL OF CELESTINA

It was, however, in the business of cosmetics and pharmacology that Celestina's greatest success lay. The entire medieval pharmacopoeia, as well as the purely empiric, was at her disposal. Celestina, however, suspicious of drugs, shared in the new tendency to resort to plants and more natural remedies.

Characteristic of this reaction was a book published sometime during the first three decades of the fifteenth century under the title *El menor daño de la Medicina* (*The Least Mischief in Medicine*) by the learned physician Alphonso Chirino, "professor of medicine and physician extraordinary to His Highly Illustrious, Enlightened and Powerful Majesty, John II of Spain, mayor and supervisor of physicians and surgeons in His Majesty's Realms and Dominions" (*"profesor de medicina e físico del muy alto, esclarecido, muy poderoso Rey Don Juan el segundo, alcalde e examinador mayor de los físicos e cirujanos de sus Reigno e señorios"*). This work shows a naturalistic reaction against the writings of the Moslem colleges, the *praxis medicinalis,* and other medical works based on alchemy and chemistry popularized at the beginning of the fifteenth century by Arnold of Villanova. In this work, phrases such as the following occur: "Be assured that it is better to cure without medicines than with them. There is no shadow of doubt but that it is nature herself and not the artificial remedies that effect the cure" (*"Sabe siertamente que es mejor sanar sin medicinas que con ellas . . . Tener sin duda que natura ha de sanar las enfermedades e no las melesinas"*).

Celestina, the great disbeliever in drugs, nevertheless kept handy the whole vast and varied battery of them, for she was well aware that common folk have a strong fancy for the mysterious concoctions in bottles and jars.

Like the soothsayers in their mansion mentioned in Apuleius, she kept in her shack a varied stock of perfume and cosmetic liquors, ointments, and creams such as those often mentioned by Pliny and Dioscorides. To all this she added herbs for medicinal baths, so much in vogue among the Arabs. In another room she stored remnants of woodland creatures such as beaks, claws, skins, and hoofs, as well as blood and fats from wild beasts, all brought to her by sundry peasants and others who, at her bidding, clambered up the thyme-scented mountains to hunt such birds and beasts.

Sometimes she resorted to black magic and stuck needles and pins into hearts made of wax. That such wonder-working practices coincide in various parts of the world and periods, as pointed out by Frazer in *The Golden Bough,* is confirmed by the practices of the witches in *Macbeth,* which corroborates Bastian's contention that there exists a common universal practice among peoples of different races but of a similar level of intelligence.

Skeptical though Celestina was about the power of her incantations, yet when her maid suffered from monthly pains, she advised her to first sniff some friendly odors and then, instead of the more usual course of devotions and prayers, to undergo a violent and erotic type of treatment. On the other hand, against toothache she prescribed a prayer to St. Apollonia, and here it is curious to note that the sufferer in question tells of trying to alleviate the pain by drumming out tunes with his fingers. Cure by music was already known to Hippocrates, who prescribed Corybantic songs as a remedy for melancholy. At a later date, Christopher Hufeland treated St. Vitus' dance by making his patients listen to Handel's oratorios, while Hunter in his turn treated cases of neuralgia with sonatas and fugues.

Celestina must be considered from all angles. Only then is it possible to understand her peculiar mental make-up and manifold activities so full of contradictions. She was no blind adherent to one particular dogma, nor was she tied down to some particular way of healing. She was aware of the effects obtainable with botanical medicines and cosmetics; she was completely amoral in her lecherous dealings; she practiced witchcraft while keeping one foot within the Church—as a sop to the religious atmosphere of the times—among whose priests she had enough friends to assist her with prayers, and even she herself did not boggle on odd occasions to tell a rosary, though she did so rather as a matter of good business than from any true sense of devotion.

To appreciate Celestina's high repute, we must consider her environment and times, as well as her own particular personality. The fifteenth century in Spain represented a period of transition from the high-flown science of the Moslems to the more rationalized and scholastic learning of the sixteenth century, when people, hitherto accustomed to medicine padded out with the lyricism and fantasy of the Arab physicians, first came in contact with scientific anatomy.

The people's appetite, however, was not to be easily satisfied. They hankered after something else. They wanted their physicians (too busy in their thirst for scientific knowledge to do more than peer down at their patients from their ivory towers) to stretch out the hand of understanding and set working again those spiritual resources that might have been battered down during the course of their sickness. But the physicians of the period could not do this without endangering their professional prestige, and only practitioners of the falser arts, like Celestina, would undertake such a task.

The atmosphere of the times played a big part in Celestina's success. In the lascivious underworld surrounding her, she had entry into all homes and all minds, enabling her to learn their secrets, which she could then use discreetly in her cures, applying herself more to the treatment of the ailing mind than of the body. Two further factors in her success were self-conceit and the knack of winning the patient's full confidence.

Nowadays, when biochemistry and microscopic research have somewhat mechanized the art of medicine, such an overrating of the personality of the healer may be incomprehensible. But, as Stefan Zweig said, "The desire for a guide and master lives and stirs inextinguishably in the human mind, eternally athirst for some miracle to happen."

Celestina, expert in lechery and artful in physic, appears on the transitional stage of the fifteenth century as a true sorceress who goes about rooting with bony fingers into the treasure house of popular tradition and comes out with a few of those nuggets of psychologic gold so vital to the art of healing. Celestina, in her complex character and multitudinous activities, crystallizes that empirical practice of medicine which was the historical subsoil underlying the hidden spring from which issued the first trickles that became, in time, the majestic river of medicine in the Golden Age of Spain.

In the eyes of history, the greatest merit of Celestina—direct descendant of that Dame Trot who romps through the earthy pages of Juan Ruiz's *Libro del buen humor* (*Book of Good Humor*)—is that she became a timeless model for all later witches, soothsayers, and quacks, for instance, those in Goya's *estampas* or in the pages of Théophile Gautier. And, above all, that she was the model for the famous witch-queens of Andalusia, "La Cañizares" and Camacha de Montilla, immortalized in the *Coloquio de Cipión y Berganza,* a tale of two wise talkative dogs, by the masterly quill of Cervantes.

Note: All bibliographic references have been integrated in the text of this paper. The edition of *La Celestina* consulted by the author was published by La Lectura, Madrid (Spain), in 1926.

The author highly recommends the translation into English, with magnificent and scholarly annotations, of *La Celestina,* by Mack Hendricks Singleton, published under the title of *Celestina* by the University of Wisconsin Press (Madison, 1958), in which generous mention is made of this article.

MEDICINE IN THE SPAIN OF DON QUIXOTE

I. SPAIN IN SPACE: THE COUNTRY AND THE PEOPLE

The Spain of Don Quixote was the Spain of the late years of Philip II and the early years of Philip III, or the latter half of the sixteenth century and the first decade of the seventeenth. It was still the Spain of the Golden Age, but already turning to silver, and at that somewhat tarnished. It was in this period of Spanish history that Don Quixote rode across the fields of Montiel, leaving the imprint of his romantic whimsies on the face of Castile, at that time the face of the civilized world.

The Spain therefore portrayed by Cervantes was the Spain of the Golden Age, which covered two centuries of Spanish history and summed up the history of Renaissance Europe. For some time Spain had yearned to shed its touch of Africa and become European. This yearning was translated into such an explosion of the will to conquer that Spain ended by being truly universal. Once this cycle was completed, Spain, exhausted by the effort, regressed in the seventeenth and eighteenth centuries and has remained so to this day through its unhappy fate in our time.

In space, as seen on the map, Spain is like a massive head that Europe grips by the hair. African by its geographic position, i.e., its position in space, European by its history, i.e., its projection in time, Asian by its anthropologic origin, American by virtue of its conquests, Spain geographically is the most Occidental and spiritually the most

From *International Record of Medicine 171:277, 1958.*

Oriental of all the countries in the European continent, a continent so crowded that sometimes it must erupt in order to release the mighty forces constantly bubbling inside it.

Such an eruption was the conquest of the New World, the greatest, most heroic venture in Western history. In that undertaking, a handful of semiliterate men, impelled more by their dreams than by the winds that billowed the sails of their vessels, embarked upon the navigation of alien waters until then known only to the stars in the American skies.

In Spain the spirit of Africa is alive in the blazing—honey and wax—paintings of El Greco, while that of Europe throbs in the subtle wonders of Velázquez pastorals. The spirit of Africa blazes also in the very personality of the Spaniard, an Arab at heart, with all of the latter's delight in startling colors and outlandish meals and his propensity for violent rages and wild passions.

On the other hand, Spain is a lamp shedding light over Europe with her art: Cervantes' influence is noticeable in the French and English literature of the seventeenth and eighteenth centuries; Calderón de la Barca's poetry gave inspiration to Shelley, and Goya's paintings to Whistler and to modern surrealism. In its great epoch of American colonization, from 1516 to 1700, Spain was the spiritual creator of twenty nations and her influence was their mainspring, as Greece was of Egypt and Asia Minor in classical times.

Spain's geographic position has been both her might and her misfortune. The Pyrenees, the Atlantic, and the Mediterranean isolate her from the rest of the world. Bristling with mountains and riddled with rivers, she nevertheless suffered innumerable processions of invading races: the Iberians, a Hamito-Semitic race of North African origin, Cro-Magnon in type; Afro-Semitic races; Tuaregs; Copts; and Kabyles from the Sahara. Spain was in the beginning an African country peopled by Africans, from whom the Spaniards themselves are descended. These were followed by Celts, Phoenicians, Greeks, Carthaginians, Romans, Vandals, Visigoths and Swabians, Arabs, Berbers, Almohades, Almoravides, Jews, and, at long last, the Spaniards themselves when Spain became an independent nation upon the union of Aragon and Castile in 1479 with the marriage of Ferdinand and Isabella.

The geographic situation of Spain in the extreme west of the Mediterranean and the extreme south of the European continent has been, at least to a certain extent, a determinant factor in her historical destiny. Spain was the last refuge for people emigrating from the Orient by sea, for beyond Spain there was nothing but the *mare incognito,* the frightening *ne plus ultra.* For emigrants from the North, Spain was the extremity of the continent, the last point at which they could replenish their strength before jumping into the fearsome mysteries of the African mainland.

Since ancient times Spain, with that prodigious faculty to absorb intruders she has always had, accepted and absorbed Phoenicians, Greeks, Carthaginians, Romans, and Visigoths. In the dawn of the Middle Ages, with the Moslem invasion in the eighth century, the exclusiveness of the Mediterranean was broken and thereafter new routes and new ways of life were adopted.

For seven centuries Moslems and Christians lived side by side in Spain, and, what is more important, they lived for the most part in peace and harmony. From this union was born the social class of the Mozarabs, or Moslems, living in accordance with Christian laws. For seven centuries periods of intolerance alternated with periods of collaboration, which is not difficult to understand if we recall that in the thirteenth century the three religions, Christian, Mohammedan, and Jewish, held services in one and the same place of worship, the Mosque of Santa María la Blanca in Toledo.

II. THE GOLDEN AGE

It was toward the end of the sixteenth century, at the time when Cervantes was an adventurous soldier, that Spain became a decisive factor in Western history. This burgeoning was determined by the destruction of the last Moorish outpost in Spain, which together with the conquest of America led to a remarkable rise in Spain's influence on the European continent.

Spain's Golden Age lasted almost two hundred years, but no two historians agree on the actual beginning or end of this period. As far as we are concerned, we may say it stretches at least from the birth of Charles V in 1500 until the Peace of Westphalia in 1648. During that period the Spanish monarchy became a token of world hegemony to which was added the idea of the spiritual universality of Roman Catholicism.

Spain's Golden Age, the setting for Cervantes' life and the exploits of Don Quixote, included the reigns of Charles V and the three Philips. Within this period there took place the unification of Castile, León, and Aragon; the conquest of Granada by Ferdinand and Isabella; the epic of Columbus and his ships; the victories of the Duke of Alba in Flanders; the conquests of Mexico and Peru by Cortes and Pizarro; and the battle of Lepanto in 1571 which halted the Turkish invasion. With El Greco, Velázquez, Lope de Vega, and Calderón, Spain reached the pinnacle of glory, just as its decline and fall began with the politics of Philip III.

During the Golden Age Spain continued the wondrous process of integration initiated at Toledo in the thirteenth century, when, in the greatest example of tolerance ever known in history, Christians from all parts of Europe met with Arabs, Jews, and Castilians at the College of Authors in Toledo. In that epoch of Byzantine Spain, Toledo could boast that all three religions, the Jewish, the Mohammedan, and the Christian, officiated in the same place of worship and dispensed to their respective faithful what each believed to be the True Word. This integration process ended toward the close of the fifteenth century with the expulsion of the Jews and the Moors and the persecution of heretics.[A]

In the sixteenth century the King of Spain was still the principal arbiter on earth. A Spaniard could go practically anywhere throughout the civilized world without treading alien ground. In Europe one language, Latin, and one faith, the Catholic, were supreme. This period of Spanish predominance was, however, more the reward of chance and the fruit of inheritance than of legitimate effort. In contrast to the great armies and the powerful circles of the Court, the common people were in great poverty. Inflation was on the increase. The Golden Age was in fact an age of copper, the coin of base metal being more abundant by far than the gold doubloon.

But the Spanish nation was living in the full bewitchment of a legend. A fabulous navigator was conquering a new world; the galleons kept returning laden with treasure, spices, and befeathered Indians resplendent as birds of paradise; ragged but invincible hordes of Spaniards were overrunning Europe; a chairbound monarch overcame the legendary Ottoman at Lepanto on the silver and blue waters of the *mare nostrum,* and erected in the Escorial marvels wrought in stone.

This atmosphere of enchantment finally destroyed the spirit of Don Quixote. For from the bowels of the bold vessels plying the American waters were born the fops, drones, and rogues who later plagued the Spain of Don Quixote.

The atmosphere was a mixture of excessive national pride, laziness, collapse of the spirit of idealism, bigotry and fanaticism, sexual license, cruelty, frivolity, arrogance, and, to a certain extent, indifference to universal principles.

More than half the population of Spain consisted of nobles; the rest were beggars and vagabonds. Fanaticism ran cheek by jowl with sorcery. The wanton flirtation of the nobles often ended in bloody brawls that embroidered in red the silks and satins of their ladyloves.

Brigands, cutpurses, and students made it impossible for respectable people to venture abroad at night without an armed escort and blazing torches. Religion, sadism, and licentiousness frequently formed an unholy trinity, as in the mysteries of the sect of *Alumbrados* at the convent of St. Placidus. Lovers presented their sweethearts with souvenirs of linen soaked in the blood shed in their brawls. And Don Juan, kissing his inamoratas between wrangles and corpses, covered his victims' tombs with roses of passion.

III. THE SPAIN OF DON QUIXOTE

The Spain of Don Quixote was a veritable Renaissance stage but with Gothic cathedrals all over. It was a period of wandering, when even the Royal Court moved from place to place as if it were a mere encampment of soldiery.

The rich, sonorous Castilian tongue already vibrated in the clear Renaissance prose of Castile. Garcilaso's poems found their way into the pockets of Spanish soldiers throughout the empire and were sung to the strum of guitars. Mystic imperialism was now opposed to the humanistic and humanitarian tradition of the Middle Ages. The realist tradition was imposing itself in great strides. And one day the filigree verse of Góngora, the ornate architecture of Churriguera, and asceticism would take the place of Cervantes.

Two worlds were already fighting each other in the Spanish conscience. Calderón would maintain that life was a dream; Góngora would affirm that nightingales were nothing but "music of the mind." Cervantes himself before them would say, through the lips of Sancho Panza, that windmills were not giants; and Don Quixote would finally end by calling an inn an "inn," after having called it a "castle" to compensate for those prosaic souls who would make even a castle into an inn.

The picture of the Spain of Don Quixote, the Spain of the beginning of the sixteenth century, was sad and somber. Despite the galleons from America, creaking under the weight of the gold they carried, poverty and hunger reigned throughout the Iberian peninsula. The lack of food and refreshment at the places where Don Quixote stopped, where there was nothing to eat "except what the traveler himself carried," the proverbial meagerness of the saddlebags of the ever-hungry Sancho, are tokens of the misery of the period. Even the nobles, living apparently in luxury and ostentation, like the dukes portrayed in *Don Quixote,* were actually riddled with debts and constantly confronted with starvation. Castile at the end of the sixteenth century was impoverished, and the needs of the clergy and the nobility exhausted all the gold arriving from the Indies. The nobles dissembled their misery with traditional Spanish pride, maintaining ever a haughty face to the greatest misfortunes, covering their famished bodies with threadbare cloaks and darned habiliments, fasting through sheer will power, like the *hidalgo* described in Mendoza's *Lazarillo de Tormes.*

But if the Spanish belly was empty, the Spanish mind was filled with dreams. Foreign ambassadors commented in letters to their sovereigns on Spanish splendor and extravagance. Don Quixote himself neglected the management of his estate and sold many acres of glebeland to buy books on chivalry. As soon as the bugle blew, the hungry nation jumped to arms, forgetting their troubles in their eagerness to embark upon another great adventure. Meantime, the monarchs ground the nation down with new imposts and neglected the only flourishing industry that remained, vine growing, on which in 1604 the Duke of Lerma imposed outrageous taxes not without considerable protest from the people, which event perhaps is symbolized allegorically in Don Quixote's battle with the wine skins.

At other times, as under Philip III, the king's agents took possession of the gold and silver at the moment of unloading from the galleons for delivery to private individuals, leaving in exchange receipts not worth the paper they were written on despite the solemn promises to pay inscribed therein.[B]

The general abandonment of agriculture and all the useful arts and trades contrasted with the pinnacle reached in the fine arts. Youth was devoted solely to the exercise of arms and to seeking its fortune in the New World. Others sought shelter within the easy existence of the Church, and the ecclesiastical concourse increased so, that Brother Luis de Miranda delivered Philip III a memorial suggesting ways of impeding the waxing growth of the clergy. The same was done in Toledo by the lawyer Geronimo Ceballos and other illustrious men. Don Quixote alludes to the enormous number of friars, monks, and priests in chapter 8, part 2:

"Ah," replied Sancho, "but I have heard that there are more monks in heaven than knights errant."

"That is so," answered Don Quixote, "for the number of clerics is greater than the number of knights."

With the expulsion of the Moors, Spain lost the hands most useful in agriculture and the only ones successful in trade and industry. The number of Moors expelled was one hundred and fifty thousand, according to some authorities, and one million five hundred thousand, according to others.

The depopulation of Spain took on alarming proportions in the times of Philip III and Philip IV. The city of Burgos, which had more than seven thousand inhabitants during the time of Philip II, had barely nine hundred in the year 1624. León went from five thousand to five hundred. In Toledo more than a third of the residents were gone. Spain, in fact, became semideserted, so much so that the resultant lack of soldiery was the greatest obstacle in the carrying on of warfare.

The administration of justice was corrupted in the highest degree. The admirable laws that Spain had always possessed now no longer held valid even for the judges themselves. No one was safe even in the most important places. Cervantes' description of the notorious brigand Roque Guinart, who foraged under the very noses of the armed forces in Barcelona and mingled with highly placed personages in the city itself, confirms the gravity of the prevailing situation. In 1602, the very date when Don Quixote and Sancho came up against Guinart and his band of brigands, the Viceroy of Catalonia declared that the government was powerless to suppress banditry.

The Duke of Lerma[c] was blamed to a great degree for the disasters suffered by the nation during the reign of Philip III, just as the Duke of Olivares was blamed for those during the reign of Philip IV.

So bad was the situation that in 1590 Cervantes begged in vain for a government post in Guatemala. Had he been granted it, Cervantes might have ended up as just another government bureaucrat buried in some obscure American mission, and Don Quixote would never have deployed through the landscape of La Mancha.

IV. GRANDEES, KNIGHTS, HIDALGOS, BURGUESES, AND LETRADOS

The structure of Spanish society was based on an intricate system of hierarchies. The *grandees* of Spain (dukes, marquesses, and counts) were the highest rank, being appointed by the king from among the most ancient lineages of the aristocracy. From a mere twenty-five grandees at the end of the sixteenth century, the figure increased to more than a hundred, all endowed with coronets on their shields and the right to remain covered in the presence of the king, to be called "cousin" by the monarch, and to make the queen stand up when they entered her quarters. The grandees of Spain were in the beginning valiant leaders in battle and later patrons of the arts and sciences, but in the end degenerated into a gang of favorites and flatterers.

After them in rank came the *knights,* members of the orders of chivalry of Alcantara, Calatrava, Montesa, and Santiago, who were conferred their right to arms by the king in the ritual of the accolade. One of these knights of the Order of Santiago was Calderón de la Barca, the immortal author of *La vida es sueño.*

The lowest class of the nobility were the *hidalgos* (the word *hidalgo* derived from the Spanish term *"hijo de algo,"* somebody's son, or a "somebody"), scions of men raised to the nobility for their doughty service and merits during the *Reconquista,* the overthrow of the Moors. One of these hidalgos, living "in a certain place in La Mancha," was Don Alonso Quijano, later known as Don Quixote.

During the Reconquest a class of *burgueses,* or middle class, commenced to arise, whose privileges were later suppressed by the kings of the House of Austria. In contrast, the immigrants to Spain from all over Europe benefited more than these middle classes from the rich booty arriving from the New World. In turn, the indivisibility of the great estates owned by the Crown, the aristocracy, and the clergy, and the rights granted to these classes, particularly that of pasturage, which authorized their cattle to graze on the fields along their route, made the existence of a well-to-do agrarian class impossible. This lack of a middle class and husbandmen was one of the causes of the economic decline of Spain's Golden Age.

Finally, the *letrados,* that is, the nobles and *burgueses* devoted to humanistic studies through love of literature or as an apprenticeship to obtaining administrative positions at Court, increased in number as university instruction increased.

At the beginning of the seventeenth century there were in Spain some thirty-two universities in existence, the oldest being that of Salamanca (founded in the year 1243), "a forum of all the sciences and virtues," at which in 1566 more than sixty professors were teaching and seventy-eight hundred students were registered. It was a bulwark for freedom of education: not only were women allowed to study there, but also to teach and even to bear the title of *docente.* It was also one of the few centers in the world where the dissection of corpses for the teaching of anatomy was permitted.

In the University of Alcalá de Henares,[D, E] next to Salamanca in prestige and standing, according to Cervantes in his *Coloquio de los Perros* (*Colloquy of the Dogs*), two thousand of the five thousand registered students were studying medicine, which, commented Cervantes, was "a bad omen, since either every one of these two thousand students finds patients to heal, which implies a great misfortune for the country, or they all die of hunger."

V. EMPIRE AND INQUISITION: THE "BLACK LEGEND" IN SPANISH HISTORY

In order to understand Spanish medicine in the Golden Age, that is, in the times of Don Quixote, it is necessary first to consider some of the problems—brilliantly discussed by Marañón—which, like dark clouds, have obscured from times of old the firmament of history and prevented our obtaining a clear view of this epoch.

For many, too many, years the so-called "Black Legend" of the Inquisition has hung like a cloak of infamy on the shoulders of the Spain of the Golden Age. This black story was woven out of two basic ingredients: the Spanish imperialism of the period, looked upon as a military juggernaut which, with the aims of oppression and profit, bound the whole world in an iron belt; and the influence and power of the Inquisition, looked upon as the age-old enemy of spiritual and scientific progress.

That fable has been scattered to the wind as historical research has shown that the Spaniards were neither more nor less demanding than any other European empire; that they fostered to a remarkable degree the advance of literature and the sciences; and that, after the begored days of the Conquest, they granted the natives of what we nowadays call Latin America a social rank and human respect never granted before by any other colonizing power in history.

Moreover, the Inquisition, a mere political instrument which paradoxically had a "unifying" mission, in view of the decision of the kings of the period to unite a Spain until then disunited, was not really an obstacle to scientific progress. Many works today prohibited in Spain received the fiat and approbation of the Inquisition, which seldom blocked the way to any scientific contribution of real merit.[F]

VI. LACK OF PEACE AND PROSPERITY AND THE BACKWARDNESS OF SCIENCE

Science in the Spain of the Golden Age never achieved the same progress as the arts. For art can coexist with poverty, but science, particularly pure science, needs the wherewithal to clothe and feed itself. In poor countries or in periods of want and penury, poets, writers, philosophers, mystics, painters, musicians, and saints have flourished and blossomed, their inspiration, clothed in the florid tunic of words and idiom, needing nothing more to fly than the wings of their own genius. On the other hand, the researcher and the scientist, though occasionally succeeding in penurious surroundings, as a rule require the support of their country and their times in order to be able to do their work.[G]

This is why in sixteenth-century Spain, whose power and wealth contrasted so with the dire poverty of the common people that the country was, so to speak, a mart of mendicants loitering on benches of gold, only those physicians in the service of the rulers, as we shall see in due course, made important discoveries or clinical advances of real merit.

Art in Spain was at that time of more interest than science, perhaps from reasons of race and temperament. In the Spaniard, imagination always prevailed over logic and intuition over perseverance. Tenacity was a quality he lacked while impatience he had in abundance. All of this made scientific progress difficult.

To that must be added the notorious individualism of the Spaniard, which makes of every Spaniard a pinch of salt and pepper: one pinch would be enough to season his entire surroundings; but if more than one, like any excess of seasoning, it would ruin everything. This is what happened in the actual compass of the Iberian peninsula.[11]

Spain knew only one hour in history when she worked as a team, and that was hundreds of years before the Golden Age, when King Alfonso the Wise gathered together Christian, Moslem, and Jewish scientific investigators and gave them the watchwords of simplicity and clarity, which is the pennon of true science in all ages and countries.

Although the Spanish monarchs of the Golden Age favored a discreet patronage of arts and sciences, they were in fact, as Marañón has pointed out, collectors rather than patrons. Philip II erected the Escorial as a temple, a museum, and a permanent exhibition of science and geography, but he did nothing to stimulate scientific research.

In Spain research had to be carried out at the cost of personal sacrifice. Science, however, cannot advance unless it is backed by peace and prosperity, which is the same thing as saying tranquility of mind and financial support. This is borne out by the fact that in periods of war, depression, great explorations, conquests, or colonization, entailing misery, penury, unrest, or a lack of mental peace or of general interest in anything but the great issue of the moment, scientific progress is practically paralyzed. On the other hand, it is frequently at such instances of great collective disturbance that progress in art is attained, for a state of agitation and unrest always stirs artistic genius.

In the Spain of the Golden Age the air was filled with the unrest characteristic of times when great new lands are being discovered, and minds were filled with a blind belief in the marvel of America and with pride for the greatness of their country, which in a single century had attained the foremost position in the world. All this fitted poorly with the spirit of modesty and intellectual sobriety so necessary for concentration on scientific tasks.

Only in universities and convents, the only two centers of learning in the Spain of the Golden Age, do we see the dawning of scientific conquests. Unfortunately, universities such as Alcalá and Salamanca were dedicated more to theology and philosophy than to science, while the convents were brewing centers of political intrigue as well as of all sorts of news and rumors.

VII. ROYAL PROTECTION OF MEDICINE

The only thing that favored the advance of medicine was that only worthy doctors were appointed personal physicians by the monarchs of the House of Austria. This meant that thereafter they could count on the financial assistance of the king and the benevolent eye of the Inquisition. Furthermore, since they had to accompany the monarchs in their warring expeditions, these physicians became men with a universal outlook, which explains the many-sided and humanistic direction of their work.

This same direction brought it about that even pedantic physicians, who at first sought to keep their science enwrapped in the mysterious cloak of the Latin language as a protection against the curiosity of the public at large, ended by accepting the clear language of Castile, which finally became the vehicle for the transmission of scientific knowledge throughout Spain.

It must be acknowledged, at all events, that the Spanish monarchs of the Golden Age contributed largely to molding that age according to their own idiosyncrasies.

Charles V was extravert Spain "stretching outward," devoted to war and the cultivation of humanism, which paradoxically enough are two ways to make an impression upon the rest of the world, that is, by force of arms and by force of mind.

Because of his incessant warmaking, Charles V had time for nothing else beyond selecting the Gobelins and pictures for his own palaces. But his royal decrees were sometimes favorable to the progress of medical thought. In his *Constitutio Criminalis Carolina* he laid down certain rules regarding physicians, creating the ranks of "Latin surgeons" for those who had completed full studies, and "five-year surgeons" for those who were excused from learning Latin. Ferdinand and Isabella had already authorized the practice of medicine and surgery in certain special cases by "practitioners," who obtained their diploma merely upon payment of four gold escudos.

Philip II was Spain once more retired within itself and austere, a Spain that believed more in serried battlements and the mausoleum of the Escorial than in fine prows and flaunting banners; a Spain of strife in the universities, a Spain in which the soldier and the courtier predominated.

A protector of the arts and sciences, Philip II organized scientific expeditions to the Spanish possessions in America, founded an Academy of Mathematics in the Escorial as well as a magnificent library, and drafted a plan for the historical and geographic description of Spain by sending out numerous questionnaires.

In his proclamation of 1588 he extended the powers of royal physicians, requiring them to enter and leave the royal bedchambers or those of the royal children "always by the main door," to taste the wines at the royal table—as Dr. Recio de Tirteafuera did at the table of Don Quixote—and to use bezoar stone against skin eruptions. He also set down that the starting salary of a doctor should be sixty thousand maravedis and that great physicians like Valles should get an extra twenty thousand maravedis.

Under this ruler, Spain began to react against the obscurantism still rampant in Europe. The Cardinal of Seville himself condemned in a written work all superstition and sorcery. The "Divine" Valles dared to purge Philip II one day when there was an eclipse of the moon, remarking sarcastically: "Let's shut the window so that the moon won't know." Father José Sigüenza in 1580 described Philip II's sickness at Badajoz (viral pneumonia), scoffing at the astrologer Juan de Meletio because "until the last days of this year he failed to inform us of the colds and unnatural humors that would attack the inhabitants of the earth."

Philip III missed his opportunity for greatness by failing to exalt himself sufficiently to reach the heavens with the mystics or the ends of the earth with the explorers and colonizers. *Don Quixote,* written during his reign, was his only claim to glory—a reflected glory, at that.

Although Philip III showed little interest in the intellectual life of his country and in politics, which he left in the hands of his favorite the Duke of Lerma, during his reign the Escorial library increased notably, for in 1612 two Spanish sea captains captured several vessels belonging to the sultan of Morocco which were carrying more than three thousand Arabic manuscripts on poetic, philosophic, theologic, and medical themes, all of which were taken to the Escorial. A large portion of these manuscripts were destroyed by fire in 1671.

Spain's preoccupation with the health of her vassals is borne out by the statute signed by Philip III in 1560, stating: "Desirous that our lieges may enjoy long life and perfect health, we are taking the precaution of providing them with doctors and experts who shall direct and instruct them and cure their illnesses, and to this purpose Chairs of Medicine and Philosophy have been established in the more important universities of the Indies as shown by their articles of title. Furthermore, recognizing how much benefit will result to all our realms here and overseas from the discovery of and trade in certain plants, herbs, seeds and other medicinal substances which may lead to the healing and good health of human bodies, we have resolved to send at certain times one or more of our personal physicians to the provinces of the Indies and their adjacent islands."

In this last proclamation, Philip III fostered the study of therapeutics by counseling doctors to observe and report "all medicinal herbs, trees, plants and seeds there may be in their provinces . . . how they are cultivated, whether they grow in dry or damp places, and they shall write notes and indications of any trees and plants of different species . . . they shall conduct experiments and make tests of everything possible, of all medicines and herbs that there may be anywhere and that may seem remarkable to them, sending specimens to this Kingdom if they do not exist here." (*Digest of the Laws of the Kingdoms of the Indies,* Madrid, The Hispanic Council, Volume III, 1943, p. 139.)

In the same proclamation, another rule was aimed at quackery: ". . . the same rules and provisions shall apply in the Indies regarding those prohibited from acting as doctors, surgeons or apothecaries under the laws of Castile, and no one shall take the title of doctor, master or bachelor without having been examined or having graduated in an approved university."

Legal requirements for the practice of medicine and the duties of viceroys and governors in inspecting drug stores and medicines for the natives were also laid down.[1]

Philip IV, great patron and protector of the arts and literature and particularly of the theatre, is worthy of sympathy. On the other hand, Charles II, with whom the glory of the Golden Age came to an end, deserves only pity for his many illnesses and for the hardening of the arteries which with him invaded the political body of Spain.

VIII. SPANISH MEDICINE AND MAGIC

Spanish medicine in the Golden Age inherited the magic of the fifteenth century, transforming it into an art in the seventeenth century, a century replete with superstition, witchcraft, astrology and chiromancy, which bred the decay of Spanish scientific medicine.

Spain then was isolated from the rest of the world, more than by her formidable geographic barriers, the Pyrenees and the Mediterranean, by her arrogant imperialistic spirit, by the pride of being Spanish, which to the Spaniard was the same thing as being ruler of practically the whole of the known world. Scientific trends from abroad barely reached the country through those physicians who went to pursue their studies at Bologna or Padua.

Spanish medicine was mainly transmuter and transmitter. It tried to improve the healing methods inherited from the Moors when they were driven from Europe, and at the same time it Europeanized the ancient therapeutics, which had been Arabianized.

From America there was a considerable influx of knowledge of natural sciences. And from Italy, with Vesalius, there came in the middle of the sixteenth century an anti-Galenist impulse, which ultimately overcame the rigid influence of classic dogma. This great step forward toward modern physiology with the acceptance of

Vesalius' teachings was made in Spain by Valverde (about whom we shall speak in more detail later) whose treatise, published four hundred years ago, in 1556, was more modern and morphologically advanced than Vesalius' own famous *De Humani Corporis Fabrica*. Valverde's revolt against scientific conservatism was supported by Vives, Pereira, Sánchez, and Servetus.

Once past the decisive decade from 1550 to 1560, Spanish medicoanthropologic research, following the natural process of counterreformation, became more metaphysical and theological than physiological. The animal aspect—body and motion—of human "nature" was ignored; instead attention was concentrated on personal existence and personal moral freedom. Thus, while Harvey was creating modern physiology in England and Galileo, physics at Pisa, Spain was developing the rights of man and the theologic doctrine of medical science. While Harvey was arguing physiology with Riolan, Spanish Jesuits were arguing about *auxiliis* and human liberty.

From 1556 to 1648 (the Peace of Westphalia) physics and physiology in Spain were at no time of the same stature as her art, explorations, laws, and metaphysics. Against the expansionist European policy of Charles V, there arose like an insurmountable wall the defensive and "Escorialist" policy of Philip II, who "anchored the monarchy to the writing desk," and condemned Spanish medicine to empiricism, to renounce almost all scientific endeavor in favor of magic.

IX. THE DISEASES OF THE GOLDEN AGE

The diseases most frequent in Spain in the time of Cervantes were gout, exanthematous typhus, diphtheria, plague, intermittent fevers, and "buboes" or syphilis.[J, K]

Gout was so common as to give rise to the idea that Spain was the "cradle of the disease," an idea borne out by the menus for the banquets of the period. On the occasion of his forthcoming marriage with the Marchioness of Alcaudete, the Count of Oropesa, in May, 1636, gave a great banquet consisting of "thirty appetizers, thirty desserts and ninety main courses." One of the meals planned by Martínez Montiño, the King's chef, included at one single sitting hams, capons, stewed mutton, pies, chickens stuffed with beans, trout, legs of mutton, custards, jellied veal pasties, small pies made of sweet dough, cold fowl in pastry blankets, ham stuffed with artichokes, fruits, pastries, cheese, preserves, jams, wafers, puddings, and junkets.

The treatment for gout was in fact very queer. Philip II's gout was treated even on Fridays, by virtue of a special papal dispensation, with meat, which because of the beef purines must have increased the monarch's uric acid. Philip II had, moreover, an allergy to fish, which gave him hives, especially in Lent, and later he suffered also from dropsy, ascites, and cirrhosis of the liver. The last was probably syphilitic in origin and was somewhat checked by his rich meat diet.

This period was rife with badly treated syphilitic infections and purulent mouth lesions. There were also many fevers diagnosed as malarial which were probably suppurative fevers caused by oral focal infections, as well as numerous cases of erysipelas. Disease and death occurred frequently and prematurely in the Spanish dynasties, probably because of consanguinity resulting from the practice of intermarriage over many centuries. Certain external characteristics, such as the Hapsburg underlip, a melancholy disposition, and renunciation of worldly pomps, were frequent in these dynasties. In contrast, the three children of Joan the Mad were extremely intelligent and well fitted for life.

Charles V was pale and taciturn from boyhood, had exaggerated cravings, suffered frequently from fever and heart attacks, became easily tired, and had dizzy spells and fainting fits. It has been impossible, however, to verify whether he was an epileptic. His Milanese doctor and companion devised the sovereign's motto, *Plus Ultra*. He had a huge outjutting lower jaw. Later he was tormented with gout, after which he contracted tertian fever, from which he eventually died.

Philip II, shortly after his marriage with his cousin Mary of Portugal, suffered from "pustulant dampness" of the skin. He also suffered from gout and tumorous swellings of the feet, leading later to acute dropsy and abscesses. Some people deemed him a schizophrenic because of his aloofness and constant withdrawals from the world. It is impossible to overlook the tragic picture, described by the Austrian ambassador, of this king when he summoned his children to show them, in the ambassador's words, "his malodorous body riddled with ulcers and infested with lice," that it might serve them as a warning on the transience of human glories.

Philip III was sickly and melancholic; Philip IV suffered from paralysis of the right side contracted three years before his death; and Charles II was a degenerate, with whom the famous dynasty that ruled in the Golden Age came to an end.

X. CHRONOLOGY OF THE GREAT

When considering the various aspects of medicine in the Spain of Don Quixote we shall split the vast panorama thereof into various groups of physicians, more for the sake of clarity than of discrimination, since all these physicians after all shared the same love for the humanities and general knowledge. First we shall study the anatomists, then the surgeons, the nosologists, the epidemiologists, and those who worked on what we now dub medical specialties, specifically psychiatry, pediatrics, therapeutics, urology, ophthalmology, obstetrics and gynecology, and social welfare; and finally the humanists and the philosophers.

Let us consider first some famous events in Spanish history from the years 1545 to 1571. In that quarter of a century the following events took place, the mere reading of which sounds like the electrifying flourish of trumpets.

In 1545 El Greco was born. In 1547 Cervantes was born. In 1548 Andrés Laguna described the method of excision of vesicourethral caruncles. In 1549 Pedro Gimeno wrote his *Dialogus de Re Medica*. In 1550 Montaña de Monserrate published his *Anatomy*. In 1551 the universities of Osma (Castile), and Lima (Peru) were founded, and Lobera of Avila published the first Spanish contribution to pediatrics. In 1552 Las Casas issued reports on the cruelty of the Spaniards toward the Indians. The year 1553 saw the foundation of the universities of Oropesa in Peru and Almagro in Spain, and also the University of Mexico; and in the same year Servetus gave a description of pulmonary circulation. In 1556 Valverde published his treatise on "Anatomy"; and in the same year Philip II commenced to reign. In 1557 Huarte de San Juan completed his *Examen de ingenios para las ciencias,* one of the earliest attempts to show the connection between psychology and physiology. In 1552 Lope de Vega was born. In 1565 the University of Baeza was founded, and in 1568 that of Orihuela. In 1569 Monardes published his *Materia médica de las Indias*. In 1570 Francis Bravo gave a description of spotted fever. And in 1571 Philip II attained victory at Lepanto.

XI. ANATOMISTS IN THE SPAIN OF DON QUIXOTE

The passion for anatomy.

The roots of Spanish anatomy in the Golden Age are buried in the cultural subsoil of Italy, since it was in Italian universities that Spanish physicians studied.

At that time the mysteries of the human body were being opened to popular and scientific curiosity, just as overseas a vast and mysterious new portion of the planet was opening to the *conquistadores*.

The yearning to explore unknown lands ran parallel with that to explore the mysteries of the human body. Anatomy was taught on pure theory, but inquisitive physicians bolstered their scant theoretical grounding by keen observation of the wretched creatures who in interminable lines filed past them, mangled by the executioner or suffering from horrible diseases and plagues of such violence that in a few days they could turn a whole city into a charnel house.

Clinical teaching in Spain prior to the Golden Age was theoretical, and instruction in anatomy was reduced to a cursory study of the human body. Luckily, four years before Columbus' first journey, His Most Catholic Majesty King Ferdinand authorized (1488) the dissection of corpses at the hospital of Saragossa, whose motto was *Urbis et Orbe*. The schools of Valladolid and Guadalupe followed. In Valladolid the first complete anatomy courses, of twenty months' duration, were given by Alonso Rodríguez de Guevara. These were published in book form in Coimbra in 1559. Gout-ridden though he was, like so many of his contemporaries, Professor Bernardino Montaña de Monserrate attended the classes in a litter, alleging that "anatomy is the alphabet with which anyone who wishes to be a physician must commence."

Modern anatomy, as is well known, was born in the sixteenth century from the work of Vesalius, who prior to being a physician at the Spanish Court from 1543 to 1564 crystallized in his *De Humani Corporis Fabrica* the point of view already foreshadowed during the decline of the *Quattrocento* by Berengario da Carpi and Leonardo da Vinci. Vesalius replaced the traditional dynamic descriptive method of the Galenists by a somewhat static but new method, which described the human body as a "workshop" or building, thus giving impetus to the development of "pure" anatomy.

Anatomists before Vesalius (Laguna, Lobera de Avila, Montaña de Monserrate).

There was in Spain a group of writers, prior in time and ideas to the work of Vesalius, among whom the leading ones were: Andrés Laguna (whom we shall study among the humanists), whose *Anatomica Methodus* pertains to the sphere of classic anatomy; Luis Lobera de Avila (whom we shall also consider later) whose *Libro de Anatomia,* though of small importance in itself, is the illustrative complement of the philosophic "dream" interpolated in his work; and Bernardino Montaña de Monserrate.

The latter owed his name to having been born, during the last decade of the fifteenth century, on the historic mountain Montserrat, a wild, steep sierra a few miles from Barcelona, where there still exists a ninth-century Benedictine monastery with its famous *Moreneta,* the "Black Virgin," scene of the romantic legend of Parsifal and the Holy Grail, and where Ignatius of Loyola held vigil over his arms laid on the holy altar.

Montaña de Monserrate studied at Valladolid and possibly at

Montpellier. He practiced in Valladolid and exercised an active mastery of his profession both in his professorial chair and in his book.

At the age of seventy, with forty-five years of professional practice behind him, he wrote his famous work, which already evinced, as against the architectural idea of anatomy current in the Renaissance, the first trends of the dynamic anatomy of the approaching Baroque period. His work was the second (Pedro Gimeno's in 1549 was the first) written by a pupil of Vesalius.

The title of Monserrate's work reads like a modern publisher's blurb: *Book of the Anatomy of Man, recently compiled by Doctor Bernardino Montaña de Monserrate, physician to His Majesty. A most useful and necessary work for physicians and surgeons desirous of perfecting themselves in their art, and available to other discreet persons interested in learning the secrets of Nature. Wherein is shown the structure and reparation of man, the way in which he is engendered and born, and the causes wherefrom he inevitably dies. Together with an interpretation of a dream occurring to his Most Illustrious Worship Luis Hurtado de Mendoza de Mondejar, etc., which appears at the end of the present volume. Which dream, under a very elegant design, deals succinctly with the said structure of man, and everything else contained in this work. Addressed to my said Lord Marquess . . . Valladolid . . . Sebastián Martínez. In the year 1551.*

This lengthy, pompous title, beautifully printed together with the coat of arms of the Marquess on the cover of the book, epitomized the solemn and theatrical spirit of the age. It indicated also the author's worthy endeavor to point out clearly the new path his anatomy was following.

Ten of the plates in this work were taken from Vesalius, and the text follows closely the pattern set by Henri de Mondeville's *Anatomy.*

This was the first work on anatomy published in the Romance tongue (just as Valverde's was the first in the common tongue), so that anatomic vocabulary was enriched with terms taken from this tongue, which in turn acquired great importance together with scientific recognition.

The work contains, as an appendix or supplement, a curious and delightful story or "dream," in which the composition of the human body is represented by strange architectonic forms.

That "dream," like the one that appeared later in Valverde's work, held a double historical meaning, since it was both an expression of the urge to spread in medicine, which until then had been a closed science, and a genuine example of the literary style of the Renaissance. Although the writer's ideas on human morphology were Galenic, his metaphor was of Renaissance origin, that is, he looked upon the organism as a tower, a fortress, or a palace.

It would be interesting to consider how the historical moment was projected into the author's dream, for no idea blossoms forth on the spur of the moment without some backthread or forerunner in the human mind.[L]

In this sense, the dreams of Montaña de Monserrate revealed his concern—a reflection of the feeling of the times—in the problem of morphology, which at that time obsessed artists as well as anatomists, and his paradoxical method of clothing the Galenist classic conception in such Renaissance symbols as the tower and the fortress forestalled the notions of Vesalius.

Other anatomists (Gimeno, Collado, Sánchez Valdés).

Other anatomists of less renown were the already mentioned Pedro Gimeno, who studied at Louvain, Paris, and Padua with Vesalius and wrote *Dialogus de Re Medica* (Valencia, 1549); Luis Collado, who published a commentary on the Galenic work *De Ossibus* (Valencia, 1555), and who defended Vesalius against Sylvius; and Juan Sánchez Valdés de la Plata, who wrote a general anthropology including a long chapter on anatomy.

Anatomists after Vesalius (Valverde).

The second third of the sixteenth century is the Golden Age of Spanish anatomy, and during that period a number of great anatomists flourished. Among them Juan Valverde de Amusco stands out. He was a native of Palencia, took his general courses in philosophy and the humanities at the University of Valladolid, after which he went to Italy to study anatomy under the aegis of Realdo Colombo in Padua, and later at Pisa, being a witness of the revolution in concepts initiated by Vesalius.

The finest fruit of his anatomic studies was his work entitled *Historia de la composición del cuerpo humano* (*History of the Composition of the Human Body*), first published in Spanish in Salamanca in 1556, being widely read for practically a hundred years. Pope Paul IV granted the license for its publication and imposed the penalty of excommunication and a fine of one hundred gold ducats on "anyone selling it without the author's permission."

After the first Spanish edition, two editions in Italian were published in Venice in 1560 and 1586, another in Flemish at Antwerp in 1568, and two others in Latin in 1589 and 1607.

In the bustling Renaissance atmosphere, Valverde could have

bowed to the prestige of Galenist ideas and servilely adopted the classic view of Sylvius. He could also have allowed himself to be carried away by the whirlwind of Vesalius' personality when it struck Padua. Instead, because of his own forceful personality, Valverde adopted Vesalius' work only to submit it to a profound intellectual scrutiny, personally checking Vesalius' findings and rectifying his errors.

Valverde made no mere rehash of Vesalius' *Fabrica,* but conscientiously labored at remodeling the Vesalian monument. "Whom [Vesalius] I shall always follow in this history," said Valverde, "except in the order of description, in which he is slightly confusing (through not wishing to diverge from Galen) and in certain things in which verily he used less diligence than was properly due (perchance leaving off in the middle of a long labor), which things I shall deal with at their proper time. . . . " Therefore, Valverde corrected the order of description and improved the morphology of the *Fabrica;* on the basis of his great experience in dissection, he corrected many of Vesalius' errors and expounded clearly the minor circulatory system.

Valverde was therefore no plagiarist but a fit re-creator of Vesalius' work. He described man as a building or a statue, and his anatomy was basically static. His text amended and completed Vesalius' work, and his anatomic illustrations were superior scientificomorphologically and artistically to those of the *Fabrica,* being founded upon his anatomicopathologic necropsies and his wide clinical experience.[M]

In his *History,* Valverde introduced anatomic figures after the style of Vesalius but greatly improved upon them both artistically and in their exactness. He entrusted their execution to the Spanish painter Gaspar Becerra, who belonged to the schools of Alonso Berruguete and Michelangelo. One can clearly perceive the influence of the Italian master as one studies the magnificent plates. The general nature of the composition, the clean-cut relief, the effect of motion in the figures are characteristic of the art of Michelangelo. They are tense forms, overflowing with vitality and athletic energy.

In Vesalius' illustrations the background of fine Italian landscapes animates and softens the whole, counteracting the doleful impression of skeletons and bodies in the raw. In Becerra's plates, the background of bare arid land, of the jagged hills typical of the bleak wastelands of Castile, dramatizes the dissected bodies with their contorted muscles and limbs.[N]

Valverde pointed out in the explanations to his plates the corrections he had made of mistakes in Vesalius' *Fabrica.* He acknowledged withal the value of his predecessor's plates, as shown in the warning he gives the reader at the beginning of his *History:* "Although some of my friends," he said, "opined that I ought to make fresh drawings instead of using Vesalius', I preferred not to do so in order to avoid confusion, it not being known so easily how far I agree or disagree with him, and besides his drawings are so well made that it might have looked like ill will or envy had I not used them. In fact, it has been as easy for me to improve on them as it would have been difficult for anyone in disagreement with them to make new ones. But since mine are cut out on copper and cannot be inserted within the text of this History without a great deal of confusion, I have put at the end of each book those which belong specifically to it."

In the eulogy Valverde made of Vesalius' drawings, he pointed out as one further reason why he did not discard the illustrations of the *Fabrica* that in this way he was better able to show wherein he was at variance with them, thus indicating his belief of having done an original work.

It is of importance to point out that Valverde (who from his portraits appears to have been a gaunt, bearded, shrewd type of man) used Spanish in his writings, sprinkled with terms borrowed from the common vernacular.

The Renaissance witnessed the birth of national states. The great mass shiftings of population caused by the Crusades created an economic phenomenon that demanded the creation of new states. With political freedom, monetary economy, credit, bureaucracy, and a new social system made their appearance. National consciousness then sought footholds in local tongues, in opposition to the abstract internationality of Latin. The Renaissance dignified a vernacular language for political reasons, so that the language might be the first foundation stone of the legal structure of the new nations, and the "new" languages acquired decisive importance.

Vesalius' *Fabrica* was published in Latin because its author was saturated with the universalist unity of medieval Europe, which was being dismembered under the cudgeling of the Reform, and because he was dedicated to Charles V as the last representative of political unity in Europe; while Valverde on the other hand gave his work a purely vernacular style and spirit.[o]

Even if the sole merit of Valverde's work were no more than its rich, expressive Castilian language, that would still be sufficient to make it immortal.[p]

Artistic anatomy and ascetic anatomy (Arfe, Fray Luis de Granada).

Two other famous Spaniards, not physicians, wrote about anatomy at this time. The first was Juan de Arfe y Villafañe, an artist in whose

Varia commensuración para la pintura y arquitectura (*Variable Proportion for Painting and Architecture*) was contained a whole book on artistic anatomy.

Arfe, the "Spanish Cellini," belonged to a family of artists of Teutonic origin who had settled in Spain. A talented sculptor and goldsmith, his work graced many churches and cathedrals, including the famous monstrances of Avila, Valladolid, and Seville. After learning his craft under his father and grandfather and attending the anatomic expositions of Cosme de Medina, he wrote in his mature years the aforementioned work (Seville, 1585), which he dedicated to Pedro Girón, Duke of Osuna and Viceroy of Naples.

Arfe divided his work into four books: Book I, dealing with geometric figures; Book II, dealing with the individual dimensions and proportions of the members of the human body, and their bones and arm muscles; Book III, dealing with the statures of birds and beasts; Book IV, dealing with architecture and church ornaments.

Anatomy, therefore, was for this artist a subsidiary sphere of knowledge necessary for the perfection of his art.

The Spanish monk, Fray Luis de Granada of the Order of Preachers, attained a fame as an orator that reached out to all the confines of the Iberian peninsula. In his last years he wrote a basic apology on faith, *Introducción al símbolo de la fé* (*Introduction to the Symbol of Faith*), a singular milestone in the ascetic literature of Spain.

According to Fray Luis, contemplation of the world invokes a series of fundamental principles on the existence of God as the Arranger of created things that may be reduced to: arrangement of the cosmos or inanimate world; the marvelous organization of nature in the service of man; and the wonderful structure of man himself forming a lesser universe within him.

Fray Luis briefly described the anatomy of the organs, starting with the liver. Although he never mentioned them, he was probably aware of the works of Montaña de Monserrate and Lobera de Avila, particularly of their anatomic descriptions in the form of "dreams." These probably helped him to arrive at his comparison of the stomach and liver. The liver, he said, is "like the butler in a great household, who distributes the food and gives something to eat to all its members. If the stomach is the cook, the liver is the butler and the one who deals out everything." Fray Luis ended his work with a brilliant eulogy of the hands, "servants and ministers of reason and wisdom." His is probably the most remarkable work on ascetic anatomy ever written.

The meaning of Renaissance surgery.

Renaissance surgery is an adventure in the etymologic meaning of the word, as Laín Entralgo has commented. It is *ad ventura,* "come what may," risk, original insight, or technical mastery of things.

Some phases of history incite man to adventure. One of these was the Renaissance, when European man, coming out of the medieval age though not yet quite at the modern stage, felt himself at a turning point and sought adventure as a plain seaman, a conqueror, or a pirate. At his side stands the surgeon.

Two new concepts of reality were born in the Renaissance, according to one of which nature was a combination of geometric shapes, and according to the other the universe was an organism of living forces and beings. Paradoxically enough, the chief work of the Renaissance was Vesalius' *Fabrica,* which is modern only in the dynamism of its anatomy and Galenist in its physiology.

The story of the new surgery, however, was in itself an adventure. The professional distance between physicians and surgeons was much greater in France, England, and Germany than in Spain and Italy. The growing importance of the post of hairdresser at the Royal Court placed all surgical activities in the hands of the barbers, or rather of the master barber. In the latter half of the seventeenth century, the barbers and surgeons joined forces *against* the "professional" physicians.

In England, "long-robed" surgeons strove against "short-robed" surgeons or barbers until well into the sixteenth century. Henry VIII, at the request of Thomas Vicary (1495–1561), Barber-Surgeon to the King and writer of the first text of anatomy in English, brought the long-robe and short-robe surgeons all into one guild.

On the other hand, in Spain as in Italy chairs of surgery had already been established. Vesalius, Fallopius, and Fabricius of Aquapendente were at once surgeons and anatomists. Francisco de Arceo depicted the academic surgeon as a lesser and empiric type of quack.

Firearms, which had recently been invented, posed fresh problems for the surgeon, and the new anatomy and its techniques made surgery a stimulating adventure.

Spanish surgeons of the Golden Age revised their treatment of old cold-steel wounds and new firearm wounds, and made advances in amputation, skull trepanation, ruptures, grafting and urologic operations, obstetrics, and ophthalmology. The union of medicine and surgery was finally reached in Spain under the enlightened auspices of Ambroise Paré.

Fragoso, Arceo, Hidalgo de Agüero, Daza Chacón, López de León, Vigo.

Juan Fragoso, a resident of Toledo and physician to the Royal Chambers of Philip II, was a classic surgeon with wide experience gathered on the battlefields of Europe. Among other treatises, he wrote an excellent *Cirugía Universal* (*Universal Surgery*) (Alcalá, 1601), containing many a contribution to forensic medicine and references to the ligature of arteries and the treatment of aneurysms.

Fragoso defended the mercurial treatment of syphilis as against fumigations recommended by Agüero. He practiced intestinal suture. He became the father of Spanish forensic medicine with his *Second Treatise on the Statements to be Made by Surgeons Regarding Various Illnesses and Many Ways in Which Death May Customarily Take Place,* which to this day would well serve as a guide to surgeons in the formulation of legal opinions as to possible causes of death.

Born at El Fresno (1493), Francisco de Arceo studied at Alcalá de Henares, and was physician to the monastery of Guadalupe (Spain), attending surgical patients from even France and England. He was a fellow-student and intimate friend of the noted theologian Arias Montano, who edited one of Arceo's surgical treatises. Arceo continued to perform operations with success even in his eighties.

In 1574 Arceo published at Antwerp his *De recata vulnerum curandorum curatione,* written in Latin so that only the truly learned physicians might make use of it. His basic surgery principles were simplicity, cleanliness, and humility. His *Treatise on Wounds and Their Healing,* translated into English, Dutch, and German, covered forty-five years of practical experience. Arceo developed a balm that bears his name and a method of rhinoplasty antedating that of Tagliacozzi.

Andrés Alcazar, of Guadalupe, invented an apparatus for draining the fluids from carbuncles.

Juan Calvo, a graduate of Zaragoza and professor of medicine at Valencia, established a surgical academy in his own house and published textbooks on surgery, syphilis, and internal medicine.

The first surgeon in Spain to teach first aid for wounds was Bartolomé Hidalgo de Agüero (1530–1597), who was born and educated at Seville. His so-called *Tesoro* is the first Spanish treatise on the human eye. He was aware that the "dry cure" was a round-about method in the treatment of wounded and traumatic cases, which, prior to Agüero, had an eighty per cent mortality rate. His axiom "interfere the least possible with a wound" is the basis of modern traumatology.

The Spanish venerated him as a god and whenever they became involved in a fight, they would say: *"En Dios me encomiendo y en las manos de Agüero"* (In God I trust and in the hands of Agüero). He was the Spanish Ambroise Paré and, like Paré, did not believe in the value of suppuration.[Q]

Agüero was, moreover, a forerunner of medical statistics when he stated that "in the past year, 1573, four hundred thirty-six cases entered the hospital and twenty died, and in two and a half months in which head wounds were recorded separately, fifty-seven came in and only seven died, and during the years in which I and my predecessors have practiced cures in the common way, the number of deaths was smaller than the number of survivors."

The humanitarian surgeon Dionisio Daza Chacón (1503–1596) was born in Valladolid, studied philosophy there and surgery at Salamanca, and was an army physician during the wars of Charles V and in the fleet of Don Juan de Austria at Lepanto. It is said that on that "the most memorable occasion to be seen for centuries" he treated the wounds of a soldier called Cervantes. A precursor of vascular surgery, he rejected the boiling oil treatment of wounds, and was the first to recommend ligature of the tumor in the treatment of nasal polyps.

A true Castilian, he lived for more than ninety years and was both soldier and courtier during two great reigns. He was a conservative surgeon and a merciful one, devoting time and attention to both the victims of the executioner and the wretched slaves on the king's galleys. A great faultfinder among his colleagues and a glutton for globe-trotting, he was greatly mortified when he was pensioned off on his seventieth birthday. After this enforced retirement, he wrote *Practice and Theory of Surgery* (Valladolid, 1609).

Daza Chacón disagreed with Vesalius regarding the cure of the heir apparent, Don Carlos. Vesalius thought that the abscesses and erysipelas from which Philip II's son suffered were affecting "the membranes" (the meninges) and he advised trepanation. Daza Chacón held that the meninges were not affected, basing his opinion on the patient's very slight symptoms. Trepanation was performed, being started by Vesalius and finished by Daza Chacón, upon the orders of the Duke of Alba. During the operation no pus was observed below the cranium. Many participated in the consultation, with the King seated in the middle, and there was great flaunting of medical erudition by all parties concerned.

As affirmed by Daza Chacón in one of his writings, the Spanish and Flemish physicians "killed" Don Juan de Austria, the hero of Lepanto, when they lanced his hemorrhoids and bled him to death. Daza Chacón said that he "would have used leeches." "Had I been present," he added, "such a mistake would not have been made."

Daza Chacón had much military experience. He commenced his military practice under the orders of one of Charles V's surgeons, and ultimately participated in all the Mediterranean campaigns of Don Juan de Austria aboard the Spanish galleys. In the removal of nasal polyps he used injections of sour pomegranate juice as a cicatrizing agent.

The reputation of Pedro López de León extended from Seville in Spain to Cartagena in Colombia, where he practiced and published a treatise on surgery containing a description of the treatment of aneurysms and the application of the methods devised by his master, Agüero.

One of the greatest Spanish authorities on surgery in the seventeenth century was Juan de Vigo, who rose to the position of physician to Pope Julius II. He wrote *Técnica práctica en cirugía* (*Technique and Practice of Surgery*) (Perpignan, 1627), referring to internal illnesses, particularly gout.

Sickness and death on the royal galleys.

Medical practice on the galleys of Philip II has been brilliantly described by Marañón, whose work should be consulted in any study of Spanish medicine in the times of Don Quixote.

The galley was an oar-propelled vessel symbolizing will power, against the sail-propelled vessel symbolizing chance. The galleys were floating hells, oar-driven by slaves chained together and lashed to their seats, their sore-infested backs bent under the flogging of the whips applied incessantly by the brutal gangmasters. The gyves were removed from their feet only upon death, and often they had to endure the howls and ravings of the last agonies of their dying companions.

They slept in the open with nothing more than a sackcloth, exposed to the rain, the sun, and extremes of cold and heat, rowing without surcease, the *anguila* or whiplash forever playing on their backs, days upon days, without a moment's respite.

Their diet consisted of hardtack, that is, half-fermented bran bread baked twice in order to eliminate the moisture, which made it so hard that it was necessary to soak it in sea water and even then the teeth stuck into it at the first bite and were torn from gums softened by the scurvy with which all galley slaves were afflicted. To the piece of hardtack, a mash of *habas* or dried beans boiled in plain water was added once a day. On rare occasions a little oil, vinegar, or wine was added. With the leavings of hardtack a miserable soup called *mazmorra* was concocted and served at night. Weevils and mold frequently rendered the food and water unfit for consumption. Filth, excreta, vermin, rats—this was the environment of the unfortunates condemned to the galley chains.

Punishments included starvation diet, flogging, amputation of nose and ears, and quartering of the convict by four galleys. Galley sentences were usually limited to a year or two, since any longer was—as Don Quixote said—"living death"; but lack of men for the oars caused sentence to be passed on ordinary vagrants, on poor souls who "stole ten ducats," as is mentioned in *Don Quixote,* and on gypsies.

The most frequent diseases in the galleys were avitaminosis, rickets, scurvy, beriberi, pellagra, enteritis, and infections. Medical attention was in the hands of barbers and "wound surgeons" who bought their diplomas for four gold escudos. Galley slaves were sometimes attended at port hospitals such as Santa Marta and Cartagena in Colombia. On important naval expeditions, court physicians, such as Lobera de Avila or Pérez de Herrera, accompanied the fleet. These positions preceded appointment to the coveted post of personal physician to His Majesty. Amputations were done by hot iron, scraping knife, and saw, while the galley slave bit on a rag clenched between his teeth. Medical treatment was elementary if not entirely lacking.

López Madera and Daza Chacón, as previously mentioned, were physicians on the flagship at Lepanto. Daza Chacón was well acquainted with hackbut wounds and did not customarily extract the bullet unless it happened to have lodged in some vital organ. Instead of using white-hot iron for amputations and to stop bleeding, Daza Chacón used bandages, effecting the final healing with a mixture of egg whites, dragon's blood, Armenian bole, and aloe. In cases of the cutting off of a hand, a common punishment for thieves, Daza Chacón first stretched the skin upward, bound the arm tightly where the skin had been stretched, and drew the line for the ax blow; later he covered the stump with the retracted skin, sewed the skin edges together, and then plunged the stump into the belly of a live chicken in order to prevent hemorrhage.

Twenty-five thousand Turks and eight hundred Christians died at Lepanto. Cervantes was among the fighting Christian soldiers and was very likely treated for an arm wound by Daza Chacón. Only during battle did wounded galley slaves receive medical attention and a double ration of vegetables, white bread, and wine.

The galleys and their human drama were indeed the dark side

to the glittering story of the Spanish conquests in the times of Don Quixote.

XIII. NOSOLOGISTS AND EPIDEMIOLOGISTS (VILLALOBOS, VALLES, MERCADO, TORO, PORCELL)

At a time when infection, besides death in armed combat, was the most frequent cause of death, it is logical that epidemiology was more important than it is today when, thanks to antibiotics and chemotherapeutics, it promises to become a preventive science.

In the Spain of Don Quixote, "the plague," as all contagions were then called, was the subject of special attention by physicians.

The first book on medicine printed in Spain—and this fact is of utmost significance—was the *Tratado de epidemias y pestes* (*Treatise on Epidemics and Plagues*), by Velasco de Taranto, translated into Spanish by Juan Villa (Barcelona, 1475). Ten years later came *Medicinas preservativas y curativas de la pestilencia* (*Healing and Preventive Medicines Against Pestilence*), by Diego de Torres (Salamanca, 1485), which was the starting point for the epidemiologic literature of the following century.

Although all the physicians of that period were nosologists and epidemiologists from sheer necessity, the most outstanding among them were Villalobos, Valles, Mercado, Toro, Porcell, Lobera, and Laguna. The last two will be discussed under another heading.

Francisco López de Villalobos, a native of Old Castile, probably from Zamora, and perhaps of Jewish blood, was born in 1473 and lived in the glorious epoch between the end of the fifteenth century and the beginning of the sixteenth, when an extraordinary queen performed the feat of lifting Spain back on its feet. A born builder possessed of great vision and a miraculous faith, Isabella the Catholic erected the sturdy political scaffold that provided Spain with a new glowing façade of glory.

Villalobos was physician at three great courts: Ferdinand and Isabella's, Charles V's, and Philip II's, being present as personal physician at the deaths of both Ferdinand and Isabella. He wrote scientific treatises of the highest order, particularly a *Sumario de medicina en uso mayor y Tratado sobre las pestíferas bubas* (*Summary of Medicine in General Usage and Treatise on Pestilential Buboes*) (Salamanca, 1498). He was a poet, an astrologer and astronomer. One of his works bore the extraordinary title *Book of Problems Dealing With Natural Bodies and Ethics and Two Logbooks on Medicine; the Treatise of the Big Three: Babbling, Buffoonery and Brangling; with a Song and an Amphitryon's Feast* (Zamora, 1543).

When he was near the end of his life, Villalobos joined the Franciscan order. Humorist, skeptic, and master of the Castilian language, Villalobos became famous for his work in verse entitled "Dr. Villalobos on the Contagious and Accursed Buboes, Their History and Medication" (Salamanca, 1498).

The most famous practitioner of his times in Spain was Francisco Valles (1520–1592), a native of Covarrubias, near Burgos, who obtained his doctorate at the University of Alcalá where he afterwards taught. Through his erudition and knowledge he became known as the Spanish Galen. He published many versions of and commentaries on Hippocrates, Aristotle, and Galen, became Court Physician of Castile, and standardized the requisites for securing medical degrees and licenses.

Valles was a great commentator of Galenic tradition and mentality and a pioneer of pathologic anatomy. Boerhaave, speaking of Valles' commentaries on Hippocrates, said that "if one believed in the transmigration of souls, then Valles was the reincarnation of Hippocrates himself."

Valles anticipated Bacon in proclaiming the excellencies of the experimental method, and he was a "Cartesian" even before Descartes since he advised methodical skepticism as a method of trial and error, advice that he stressed in his medicoanthropologic exegesis of the Bible (Lyons, 1588) entitled *De Iis Quae Scripta Sunt Physice in Libris Sacris, sive de Sacra Philosophia Liber Singularis*. As a reward for this work, Philip II appointed him, together with Ambrosio Morales and Arias Montano, to organize the Escorial library.

Valles assuaged the gout pains of Philip II with tepid water footbaths. Grateful for the relief thus afforded, Philip II bestowed upon him the title of "El Divino." It was to Valles that the tragic and beautiful one-eyed Princess of Eboli, confined for life by order of Philip II for complicity in the murder of the Duke of Escobedo, appealed without success to certify that her health depended on her liberty being restored.

Of his many works, we mention as worthy of distinction the *Comentarii de Urinis Pulsibus et Febribus* (Alcalá, 1565) and the *Methodus Medendi Francisci Valesii* (Madrid, 1588).[R]

Valles' portrait shows him as a man of noble countenance, with that expression of skepticism and melancholic cynicism worn by the greatest spirits of the at once melancholy and merry, mundane and monkish epoch of the Golden Age.

More versed than Valles in clinical practice was Luis Mercado (Valladolid, 1520–1606), personal physician to Philip II and Philip III, and teacher of Avicenna's Canon of Medicine at Valladolid.

Looked upon as the Saint Thomas Aquinas of Spanish medicine

because of his predilection for the scholastic style, Mercado in his writings was as classical in content as he was Renaissance in clearness and balance. He was Physician to the King's Council and Auditor of the Treasury. Among his works, his *Institutiones Medicae* stands out. He inquired especially into intermittent and malignant fevers, women's complaints, and diseases of the liver, spleen, kidneys, and bladder. In his work *De Veritate et Reta Ratione Principiorum, Theorematum et Rerum Omnium ad Medicam Facultatum Spetantium* (1604) he showed himself to be a philosopher of the highest rank. For the curing of gout he advised lukewarm baths and a minimum of opium, cupping, and purges, thus ranging himself against the bloodletting "vampirism" of the times. He was the first Spanish physician to describe the "garrotillo" or agranulocytic angina, recommending that it be treated with copper salts and boiling gold caustics, a method immortalized later in Goya's famous painting "El garrotillo." [8]

Together with Antonio Pérez, physician to Philip II and to Don Juan de Austria in his final illness in the Netherlands, and Luis de Toro (Palencia, 1522), who gave a description of the Great Plague (exanthematous typhus)[T] that scourged Spain from 1557 to 1572 (probably in its second epidemic wave, there having been a previous one during the siege of Granada by Ferdinand and Isabella) we must mention Juan Tomas Porcell from Sardinia (which at that time belonged to Spain), who was famous for his bravery as well as for his scientific curiosity, which in the famous plague of Saragossa in May 1564 moved him to perform autopsies on five of the ten thousand victims of the epidemic, thus ascertaining that it was the bubonic plague.[U]

Porcell was the greatest Spanish epidemiologist in the sixteenth century and the originator of medical statistics. He once wrote: "I carried about with me my large notebook, divided alphabetically, in which I noted down details about those who had succumbed and how many days elapsed in the sickness and the opening (of the abscesses), or if they had died through their having burst prematurely, and why and how this had occurred . . . and everything else that was necessary."

XIV. THE "SPECIALISTS": PEDIATRISTS, OBSTETRICIANS AND GYNECOLOGISTS, UROLOGISTS, PSYCHIATRISTS, AND HERBALISTS (SORIANO, VELAZQUEZ, CHIRINO, MONARDES, ACOSTA, CARBON, VALDES, DIAZ, LEIVA Y AGUILAR, PEREZ DE HERRERA, VEGA, HERNANDEZ)

The roll of physicians specialized in certain branches of medicine was so very long that we shall mention only a few as part of the main tableau of medical practice in the Golden Age of Spain.

Jerónimo Soriano, born in Teruel in 1575, so worthy and good that he was called "San Jerónimo," published a remarkable work on children's illnesses, the *Mejor modo y orden de curar las enfermedades de los niños* (Saragossa, 1600), which is one of the first treatises on pediatrics in the world.

A contemporary of the great Huarte of San Juan was Andrés Velázquez, who published *Libro de la melancolia* (*Book of Melancholy*) (Seville, 1585), of great psychiatric interest.

Alfonso Chirino published *Menor daño de la medicina . . .*, wherein we may note the curious mixture of superstition, magic, empiricism, and rudimentary science that characterized the therapeutics of Spain in the Golden Age.

Nicolás Monardes (1493–1588), a Sevillian and a brilliant business man besides being a physician and herbalist, published two famous works, one dealing with "everything brought from our Western Indies" (Seville, 1565), and the other entitled *Treatise on the Effect of Various Herbs* (Seville, 1571), whereby he imparted considerable impetus to the application of medicinal herbs. In another article[v] I have written about Monardes' botanical garden, where among other curative plants from the Indies he cultivated curare and tobacco.

Cristóbal de Acosta, nicknamed "the African," was a Portuguese settled in Spain who wrote in Castilian and published *Tratado de las drogas y medicinas de las Indias Orientales* (*Treatise on Drugs and Medicines from the West Indies*) (Burgos, 1578).

Besides to botanists, naturalists, and mathematicians of standing, credit must be accorded to those friars devoted to the study of medicine, such as Friar Bernardino of Laredo (1542), a Franciscan of Seville; Friar Agustin Farián, a Sevillian who practiced in Mexico; Pedro Barba of Valladolid (1541), who investigated the effect of cinchona; and the Benedictine Pedro Ponce de León (1520–1584), who conceived an original method of teaching deaf mutes.

The Majorcan, Damián Carbón, published *Libro del arte de los curadores . . .* (Book on the Healers' Art) (Majorca, 1541), one of the first treatises written on obstetrics.

Benito Daza Valdés published his *Uso de los anteojos* (Use of Eyeglasses) (Seville, 1623), in which lenses were described for the first time.

Francisco Díaz, physician to Philip III, published (Madrid, 1588) *Treatise . . . on All Diseases of the Kidneys, Bladder and Fleshy Growths in the Penis and Urinary Tract,* wherein he expounded his method of urethral catheterism, praised in sonnets by both Lope de Vega and Cervantes, which throws an intimate and revealing light upon the secret medical history of these two writers. He described the "Spanish operation" of lithotomy, and originated the first medical specialty in Spain.

Francisco Leiva y Aguilar published a book on the evil use of tobacco entitled *Desgano contra el mal uso del tabaco* (Cordova, 1634), which was typical of the florid literary style of the period.

The Salamancan, Cristobal Pérez de Herrera, established in Madrid, with the aid of Philip II, the great asylum for the poor which later became the general hospital. He was both physician and soldier. His works appeared in the seventeenth century. He published one book in which he advised the use of "bland" remedies against epidemic "garrotillo" or diphtheria rather than painful cauterization with sulfuric acid, which was then the customary cure. He recommended "shaving the bulls," since three hundred people died in one year alone "on the bulls' horns." He was the archetype of the medical and humanistic adventurers of the sixteenth century. As attending physician on the galleys, he devoted many years to alleviating the lot of the poor, and in his immortal book *Discourse on the Protection of Real and Pretended Poor and on the Establishment of Housing in These Kingdoms and the Shelter of the Soldiery Pertaining Thereto* (Madrid, 1598) he studied the then appalling problems of the poor.

The poor were numerous due partly to the rapidly improvised social structure of Spain, which gave rise to a fearful misery side by side with magnificent institutions, and partly to the great number of vagrants who followed begging as a profession and thrived in the shadow of that grandiose but disorganized social structure. The boundary between true and false beggars was difficult to establish because of the Spanish love for a vagabond life, which suited their lack of discipline, their love of freedom, and their few material needs. Perhaps the age-old habit of religious pilgrimages had intensified the desire to wander under the shelter of a mythical prestige and organized charity along the wayside.

The joy of Don Quixote and Sancho Panza on abandoning the soft, luxurious life in the palace of the Dukes and finding themselves, without food or shelter but with their freedom, marching on the open road, is one of the truest literary symbols of the psychology of the Spaniard.

Cristóbal de Vega, physician to the Royal Chambers of Don Carlos, was perhaps the first Spanish psychiatrist, and in his works, published in 1576, there are detailed descriptions of melancholy and certain maniacal affections.[w] Spain at that time was far above the rest of Europe in the care of the insane, there being an insane asylum in Valencia as far back as 1409.

Francisco Hernández, physician to the Royal Chambers of Philip

II, made a survey at the King's behest through New Spain, now Mexico, during which he studied the curative action of Mexican plants in the hospitals established by the Spaniards and tried out the effects of medicinal plants upon his own person. He was one of the foremost scientists Spain has produced. On his return to the Peninsula, he produced a twenty-six volume work.

The materia medica of the New World was described by Diego Alvárez de Chanca, who accompanied Columbus on his second voyage.

Considerable botanical research was carried out on the plants of the New World, and among the more famous botanists we may mention Gonzalo Fernández de Oviedo, García de Orta, and José de Acosta, as well as the aforementioned Francisco Hernández.

Travelers returning from America and the East Indies introduced quinine and four types of sudorifics: guaiacum, sarsaparilla, cinchona, and sassafras.

XV. THE HUMANISTS (LAGUNA, LOBERA DE AVILA, SERVETUS, PEREIRA, SABUCO DE NANTES, HUARTE, SANCHEZ)

The philosopher-humanist-physician represented Spain's greatest claim to glory in the Golden Age.

Medical humanism originated with Boccaccio and Petrarch in the fourteenth century, the word "humanism" deriving from Cicero's *humanitas* and from Dante's "humanistic spirit," interpreted by Ariosto in the sense of Terence's *homo sum; nihil humani a me alienum puto.*

Humanism was born out of Europe's dissatisfaction with its immediate past and present conditions, and from the general pining for the good old days then revived in three forms: the translations of ancient literature by *philologist-physicians,* the instructive exposition of knowledge by *humanist-physicians,* and the philosophic commentaries by *philosopher-physicians.*

Among the humanists we shall consider the seven greatest, all of them spiritual heirs and successors of Juan Luis Vives: Andrés Laguna, Luis Lobera de Avila, Michael Servetus, Gómez Pereira, Miguel Sabuco de Nantes, Huarte, and Francisco Sánchez. These are the greatest medical humanists of the Golden Age of Spain.[x]

Andrés Laguna (1499–1560), a native of Segovia, was a redoubtable humanist, Hellenist, polygrapher, traveler, translator, and philosopher. He studied at Salamanca and Paris under Sylvius and at Padua with Colombo, and taught in the universities of Paris, Alcala, Toledo, and Bologna. He was physician to Charles V, whom he accompanied on his campaigns through Italy and Germany, to

Popes Paul II and Julius II, and to Philip II, executing many religious and diplomatic missions in Europe. Laguna was one of the first great Spanish physicians of universal repute, and he belongs in the honored company of Villanova and Servetus.

Famed at the Spanish Court, Laguna spent many years traveling all over Europe in attendance on royalty and in the retinues of great personages. He had the pride of his class and the awareness of his mission; and he let fly without mercy at those unqualified people who presumed to lift the veil of mystery surrounding the human being.

His work *Anatomica Methodus, seu de Sectione Humani Corporis Contemplatio* (Paris, 1535) was representative of the anti-Vesalian phase of Spanish anatomy, which was still drawing its nourishment from medieval learning. His treatise, a short text of some seventy pages, included a dedicatory epistle to the Bishop of Segovia, his father's patron and protector. His anatomy started with the mouth, "where food undergoes the first process of digestion," and ended with the brain, "where the final and most absolute transformation of the mind takes place."

Laguna also published a treatise on the plague entitled *Short Discourse on the Curing of and Preservation from the Plague* (Salamanca, 1546), wherein he put forward his mercurial friction treatment, dietary rules for impoverished students, and a critical commentary on Galen.

In his *Enfermedades de las articulaciones* (*Diseases of the Joints*), he described a method of treating ulcerous arthritis or suppurating tophi in the secreting stage with poultices of lard and fermenting cheese (*casei ad modum inveteratum*), thus anticipating by four hundred years the empiric use of penicillin for the treatment of infections.

He investigated the dispersion of pollen and plant physiology and was a noted botanist, making a particular study of sassafras, guaiacum, and sarsaparilla.

Laguna was called upon to control and study the plagues that decimated the cities of Antwerp and Metz. He attended patients of the highest rank, including Queen Elizabeth, together with Villalobos, though in this case he was unsuccessful. He created the first botanical gardens in Spain, at Aranjuez, the idea coming to him from his botanical studies at Cologne. He contrived an apparatus for turning sea water into drinking water, and made an excellent translation of Dioscorides.

In his famous political speech solemnly delivered at Cologne in 1543 under the title *Europa Sese Discrutians,* he spoke with deliberate pessimism regarding the breaking up and death of nations on the continent and the mortal danger of their internecine warfare to the future peace of Europe.

Laguna's bones are preserved at Segovia, enclosed in a modest wicker hamper.

Luis Lobera de Avila was born sometime between the 1470's and the end of the century. His main work appeared in November 1551. He was a follower of Galen, and accompanied Charles V on his warring campaigns. He studied at Salamanca and other European universities, and was active as physician and traveler through Europe and Africa with the Emperor's armies. He wrote commentaries on the classics (Aristotle, Hippocrates, Galen, and Avicenna) and produced much work on anatomy, plague, and syphilis. We may mention here his *Banquet of Noble Knights and Rules for Living from the Time of Rising until That of Retiring* (1530); *Garden of Health* or *Gentlemen's Banquet* (Alcalá, 1542); *With Two Treatises on Spanish Travels by Land or Sea* (*Precepts on the Sea* and *Precepts for Land Travelers*); and *Book on the Four Genteel Diseases, Namely: Catarrh and Gout; Arthritis; Gallstones, Renal Calculus and Colic; and Buboes* (Toledo, 1544).

Michael Servetus (1511–1553), whose home town was Villanueva de Sijena in the province of Huesca, studied the humanities at Saragossa and law at Toulouse, and upon reading the free commentators on the Bible lost his Catholic faith. He took refuge at Basle and Strasbourg, leading a lonesome and tormented existence, writing his *De Trinitatis Erroribus* (1531), which resulted in his being expelled from all reform churches.

Setting up at Lyons under the name of Michel de Villeneuve, he studied medicine in Paris as a pupil of Fernel and a classmate of Vesalius, assailing the Arabian system of using sirups in his *Syruporum Universa Ratio* (Paris, 1537). He resided afterwards in Lyons, Charlieu, and Vienne (Dauphiné), practicing as a physician for several years; but led away by his zeal for religious reform, he undertook a ridiculous exchange of polemics with Calvin, the theological dictator of Geneva. In 1553, Servetus clandestinely published his *Christianismi Restitutio*. Arraigned by the Catholic authorities of Vienne, he was imprisoned but escaped. Victim, however, of his obsession, he went to Geneva, where he was subjected to a lengthy trial and, in October 1553, at Calvin's command, was burnt alive slowly over green wood.

Though Galen had mentioned the passage of blood from the pulmonary artery to the pulmonary vein, Servetus was the first to describe the lesser or pulmonary circulation, even *prior* to Valverde and Colombo. His was an anatomic and theological physiology. In his writings genial intuition was mingled with secret experimentation, but his mentality was still of the Galenic school. Servetus was the martyr of Spanish free thought, a Quixote in ideas who never attained his Dulcinea of fame.

Antonio Gómez Pereira, born in Medina del Campo in 1500, a Jewish philosopher and physician to the royal chambers of Philip II, was one of the doctors attending the prince Don Carlos in his final illness, when that illustrious patient, suffering probably from catatonic schizophrenia alternating with bulimy and negativism, was seized by a gastroenteritis aggravated by a purge that brought on a choleriform syndrome.

Long before Sydenham and in opposition to the school of Galen, Pereira established the value of fever as an expression of nature's effort to restore normality, and he identified body heat with fever heat. He had patients from all over Spain, in Burgos and Segovia.

His famous work *Antoniana-Margarita Opus Nempe Physicis, Medicis ad Theologis Non Minus Utile Quam Necessarium* (Medina del Campo, 1554), the name of which is a tribute to his parents Anthony and Margaret, was a reasoned revolt against the tyranny of the doctrines of Aristotle and Galen, which formed the basis of the medical dogmatism ruling at the time. Fanatical Galenists nearly destroyed the whole of this work.

Pereira belongs to the same great tradition as Luis Vives, Raymon Lull, and Suárez on the one hand, and Seneca, Averroës, and Maimonides on the other. A born enemy of the authoritarian principle in science, in physical matters he accepted only the sanction of experience. Endowed with considerable dialectic force, he was the champion of the anti-Galen school and of direct observation of nature. He was a century ahead of Descartes in his realistic concept of life. In his book, he expounds the original idea of automatism or involuntary action in animals, later amplified by Descartes. On the question of the immortality of the soul, he adduced, before Descartes was even born, the Cartesian proof based on the dualism of humanity.

In experimental psychology in his time he was more advanced than either Bacon or Descartes were later. He denied that animals could feel, since if they had feelings they would have to form judgments and he held them to be no more than machines. He was the originator of the syllogism, "I know that I know something. Everyone who knows *is;* hence, I am."

Miguel Sabuco de Nantes, another humanist, had a daughter "endowed from head to foot," in the words of her contemporary Sotomayor, "with a thousand divine gifts." Sabuco de Nantes published, under his daughter's name, a passionate, intuitive, long-winded, and arbitrary book, dedicated to Philip II, entitled *Nueva filosofía de la naturaleza del hombre no conocida ni alcanzada de los filósofos antiguos* (*New Philosophy on the Nature of Man, Unknown and Unattained by the Old Philosophers*), in which the classic dogmas of the past were vigorously attacked.

Sabuco promulgated the theory of a "cerebral or neural juice" which it has been believed was an intuitive anticipation of the cerebrospinal fluid, or a harbinger of the basic role that is given nowadays in the vegetative and affective life to the diencephalon area and the adjoining pituitary gland, i.e., the hypothalamic-pituitary system. Here are his own words: "The cause and factory of every disease is the brain; there the emotions, passions and motions of the mind have their seat; there feeling or sensation is rooted; there lies the root and nature that causes vegetation; there life and cravings spring from; there disease originates; and there death comes from." We should note that he attributed "vegetation," i.e., origin and control of vegetative life, to the diencephalon.

The cause of disease was to Sabuco "the drawing or flow of moisture from the brain, damaging the parts where it stops; or cessation of the functions of the brain."

Juan de Dios Huarte y Navarro (1529–1589) studied medicine at the University of Huesca, where he obtained his diploma upon writing his *Examen de ingenios para las ciencias,* in 1557, of which Marañón has said: "If I were to be asked what is the most important work on medicine in Spain up to the eighteenth century, the work most worthy of being placed permanently in the great bibliography of the universe, I should answer without hesitation that it is this one, the only book written by a humble doctor born in a village, San Juan de Pié de Puerto in Navarre, who studied in a provincial university, the University of Huesca, who practiced in sundry places of Spain, and who was far from all academic and official honors and posts."

Starting with Galen's *De Temperamentis,* Huarte made his way through the works of the physiognomists and established the basis for subsequent phrenologic, constitutional, and psychosomatic studies. His treatise is a splendid instructive psychology, a perspicacious and clever work that establishes connections between the ethical and the physical, and shows how the cranial and cerebral structures affect the professional aptitudes of every individual. The natural temperament of a man, Huarte claimed, is what predisposes him for the exercise of a particular technical or intellectual activity. Thus Huarte originated the theory of professional aptitude. Huarte established the thesis of the native equality of spirits and the correlation of temperament and talent, denying the effects of apprenticeship, habit, and vocation on intellectual aptitude and efficiency. On this subject of aptitude, he also took into account such features as the hair, the smile, and temperament and ingenuity.

This genius of a man, reared at the foot of the age-old oaks of Roncesvalles, wrote a singular book from which despite his protestations of orthodoxy the Holy Office deleted several pages. As against the professional guidance practiced today, Huarte recommended the "investigation of aptitude"; as against today's technical aptitude, he advised personal inclinations and vocation, that is, enthusiasm for the job chosen, a sincere and efficient enthusiasm. Huarte recommended that instruction be preceded by university training of the teachers, without which teaching is like "drawing water into a basket."

Francisco Sánchez (1551–1623), literary forerunner of Montaigne, of Jewish descent, was born in Braga and studied medicine in France and Italy, becoming a professor at Montpellier where he had graduated at twenty-four years of age, practicing subsequently at Toulouse. Like Juan Luis Vives, Sánchez was a standard-bearer of sixteenth-century Spanish skepticism and criticism. A skeptic regarding the science of his age, he started a rebellion with his medical works, his commentaries on Galen and Hippocrates, and his philosophic writings. In his famous book *De Multum Nobili et Prima Universali Scientia, Quod Nihil Scitur* (*On Many Worthy Universal Principles of Science of Which Nothing Is Known*), written in 1576 and published in 1618, he displayed his enthusiasm for the physical sciences and natural philosophy, and formulated the methodical questioning that is the basis of Cartesian philosophy some sixty years before the *Discours de la Méthode* made its appearance.

He based his philosophy on the dissections he was able to perform as a member of a secret society in Toulouse which provided him the corpses. It was his idea that metaphysics had to give way to the experimental science that studies all phenomena according to a scientific criterion. He was a nominalist in opposition to the essentialists. "Our philosophy," he said, "is a Cretan labyrinth in which it is impossible to avoid the Minotaur."

EPILOGUE

Spanish medicine, as Spain itself, in the Golden Age was a vast multicolored tapestry woven out of passionate contradictions. If Spanish individualism hampered the progress of scientific research, on the other hand encyclopedism, humanism, and the avid curiosity of the physicians widened the clinical horizon of medicine and speeded its progress.

The yearning to explore new worlds was also translated into the urge to unveil the mysteries of the human body, thereby stimulating anatomy. The endless wars and military campaigns fostered the progress of surgery and traumatology, and forced medical attention to focus on epidemiology and nosology, as "fevers" and "the plague" were national scourges. The national diseases—gout, *garrotillo,* urinary tract stones, and *tabardillo*—also spurred the study and treatment of these diseases.

But the greatest glory of the Spain of the Golden Age were its humanist-physicians, who integrated science and conscience, thought and belief, medicine and philosophy, scientific spirit and professional humanitarianism. These men performed feats in psychiatry and medical philosophy, and they established the foundation upon which it would be possible to build the future Spanish medicine.

They made ideals of to serve and to heal. Their dedication to these ideals is the proudest heritage handed down by that passionately quixotic country which was the Spain of Don Quixote.

NOTES

A. The great epoch of tolerance extended from Juan de Valdés to Michael Servetus, whose last words on being burned at a green wood stake in Geneva were, "Mercy! Oh Lord! Mercy!"—noble words full of pleading, not to the Trinitarian clemency of Calvin, but to the concept of the Supreme Being. After the burning of Servetus by Calvin's henchmen, the followers of Erasmus gathered around the remarkable figure of Sebastian Castello Castigliani and issued the first European proclamation regarding tolerance.

B. In Chapter 17 of *Don Quixote* the peccancy of Spain, at that at once grandiose and miserable moment of her history, is described with a keen, almost clinical eye.

C. One device of the favorite, the Duke of Lerma, who thought he had found a universal panacea against inflation, was to raise the value of the currency in order to make good the difficulties of the exchequer and turn all Spaniards from poor to rich! This madness was symbolized in the cure-all or balm of Fierabras described in *Don Quixote.*

D. The first polyglot Bible in the world was published in 1514 at the Theological University of Alcalá, complete with critical and grammatical appendix and glossary, being probably "the first scientific work printed in the civilized world."

E. Spain took enthusiastically to the art of printing. The first Spanish book was printed at Valladolid in 1464. Up to the end of the fifteenth century, seven hundred twenty books were printed in twenty-five Spanish cities, as against three hundred fifty-eight books printed in England. Because of the world-wide importance of Spanish at that time, books were printed in that language as well as in Latin.

F. Though the "Black Legend" was not historically justified, we must on the other hand recognize that the Spaniards of yore, just like their descendants today, possessed a racial tendency toward violence and theatricality, exaggerated then by the feeling that they were the leaders on the universal stage of history, with the whole world hanging breathless upon their actions and pronouncements.

G. While art is a flower capable of blossoming on the sterile ground of poverty, science requires wealth and well-being as well as a universal idiom. The arts have their own language, namely, melody, color, rhythm, or harmonious shape. Science on the other hand requires a linguistic instrument with which to raze all barriers and guarantee itself an indispensable universality. All discoveries become universal as soon as made. The laws of gravity, the refraction of light, the microbial origin of infection, vaccination—all these discoveries became universal from the very moment they were announced.

H. Individualism, because it goes hand in hand with a spirit of rebellion, has often given birth to artistic genius or has accompanied it, but it has always been a stumbling block to scientific progress. Individualism frequently embraces encyclopedism, as occurred among the physicians of the Golden Age, each of whom individually presumed to embrace the whole of the scientific knowledge of his time.

Science, however, advances only by teamwork, which is the same as saying the proper combination of specialized labors. Science, except for cases of geniuses who by intuition make great advances in a scientific field, requires teams, that is to say, specialization instead of individual encyclopedism, which is the best grounding for the arts.

I. While in Spain quackery was being attacked, in Italy Vesalius' efforts to revive the Hippocratic tradition were failing, since even Paracelsus was beset by the superstitions of the age, as proved by his famous "homunculus" in a bottle.

J. The most ancient Spanish work on syphilis appeared in Venice in 1502, under the title *Libelus de Morbo Galico*, written by Juan Almenar of Valencia, who recommended the mercury treatment.

K. Among the writers on syphilis we should mention Francisco López de Villalobos, of Valladolid, who published (Salamanca, 1498) the poem entitled, "Dr. Villalobos on the Contagious and Accursed Buboes"; and Rodrigo Díaz Ruíz de Isla, whose treatise published in 1542 propounded the theory of the American origin of syphilis.

L. "History," said Ortega y Gasset, "is perfect continuity. . . . The historian must seek the origin of any idea arising at any particular date, which is to say, he must look for some other idea arising at some date prior in time."

M. One feature of Valverde's nomenclature, typical of the Renaissance, is the use of numbers in anatomic denominations. The number, which in antiquity was an expression of a magnitude, a length, or a quantity, that is, of something sensorial, measurable, or tactile, became thus something figurative, a symbol of size and rank, a metaphor. The ancient number represented magnitude; the modern number, relation. Ancient anatomists called a particular part of the gut the *duodenum* because it measured the breadth of *twelve* fingers. Valverde used the numerical classification in the muscles in order to denote their mutual relationship.

N. The exact representation of the reality of the form goes hand in hand with the personal interpretation given to it by the artist. When, in Book Three, he wanted to show a pregnant woman, he sketched the rotund shape of a Venus. Artistic inspiration and scientific objectivity knit well together in the illustrational work of Gaspar Becerra.

O. As the *word* is the sensorial expression of a *concept* within whose limits we confine abstract ideas, to name an object, as Valverde did, is to bring it within the ambit of our world, for "through men and numbers, human intelligence gains power over the world," as Spengler said.

P. Valverde incorporated a large number of colloquialisms in his work, thereby establishing them as technical terms—for instance, *tolondrones* (bumps) for condyles, *nudos del espinazo* (spinal knots) for vertebrae, *atajo del pecho* (chest partition) for mediastinum, *tripa docena* for duodenum, *tripa del cagalar* for rectum—and compared the nerves and their sheaths to the "bark of a tree."

Q. A Galenic text in which the Asiatic or "dry" method was extolled over the Roman or "soft" method with suppuration gave Agüero his inspiration for the dry cure and cicatrization *per primam*.

R. Suárez de Rivera told in the eighteenth century the following story about Valles: "His Majesty Philip II being ill at Badajoz, and in such straits that it was feared he would die within the week, his physicians held a consultation together and Dr. Valles' opinion was contrary to that of the others. The King, however, followed Valles' advice, took the purge he recommended, and was delivered from danger. For having saved his life, the King granted Valles three great honors: first, the title of 'El Divino,' calling him 'my divine Valles'; second, there being no Office of the Royal Physician in a form worthy of Spain, His Majesty entrusted him with the establishment and disposition of such Tribunal; and third, the Divine Valles entering mournfully one day into the presence of the recovered King, His Majesty enquired of him what the matter might be. He replied that there was nothing, but being ordered to answer truly, he obeyed, saying to the King: 'Sire, what hurts me so greatly is that the Admiral (who was present) told me that if your Majesty were to die from taking the purge, he would have to place the rope around my neck.' Upon which the King told the Admiral that men like him came by the dozen but that men like Valles were difficult to come by, since it required extraordinary qualities to become a doctor. At this point, the Admiral devised how to exculpate himself with the King, saying: 'Sire, what I told Valles was that if he did actually cure your Majesty, I would place a rope around his neck, but the rope I had in mind was the cord of this order of the Golden Fleece, whereof he is more worthy than I am.' " (*Universal Medicine,* by Francisco Suárez de Rivera, Madrid, 1748, pages 37 and 38.)

S. The treatise on "garrotillo" by Nicolás Gutiérrez Angulo (1444–1522) is probably the most ancient Spanish work on diphtheria.

T. The first report on spotted fever or endemic typhus came from the New World in Francisco Bravo's *Opera Medicinalis* (Mexico, 1560). There were six diphtheria epidemics in Spain from 1581 to 1638, and the disease was first described by Casales, Fontecha, and Villa Real in 1611.

U. During the sixteenth and seventeenth centuries there were epidemic outbreaks of bubonic plague in Barcelona, Seville, Valencia, Saragossa, and Valladolid, all entailing tremendous mortality. They were described by Luis Lucena (1523), Laguna (1542), and Lobera de Avila (1542).

V. See MARTI-IBAÑEZ, F.: Three enigmas in the history of curare before Sir Walter Raleigh, Internat. Rec. Med. *164*:700, 1951.

W. Andrés Velázquez in 1585 wrote on melancholy and epilepsy.

X. Other humanists were the Portuguese Amato Lusitano and Isaac Cardoso.

THE FORTUNES OF CERVANTES
AND THE ENDEAVOR OF DON QUIXOTE

Some four hundred years ago, in a certain place in Castile whose name "I do not wish to remember" except with pride, a boy called Miguel was born, the son of a humble surgeon.

Miguel grew up in that critical period when the sun was beginning to set on the Spanish empire and the somber attire of the Philips became throughout the Iberian peninsula a sign of mourning for the dire poverty that was descending upon the Spanish people, leaving them nothing but the legacy of heroism inherited from the past. The only treasure they now knew did not come by galleon from the New World, but from the pens of the great writers of the Golden Age. The public treasury was exhausted; great fortitude was necessary to withstand the ravages of impoverishment; there were too many nobles and not enough wise rulers, though her Christian knights still fought to uphold Spain's proud position in Europe, and her great commanders continued to hoist the flag of universal empire over the Americas.

The youth of Miguel de Cervantes Saavedra remains a mystery. In his life story, as in that of Christ, there is a period of fifteen years "lost" in the shadows of the unknown, and, as with Christ also, there is no iconography to tell us what he looked like in childhood or youth. He studied at Alcalá de Henares, taught school in Madrid, contrived a few verses before the catafalque of Elizabeth of Valois, served as a waiter in Italy, and weapon in hand fought five years as a soldier, until, ploughing the limpid waters of the Mediterranean at the battle of Lepanto, he lost his left hand. Then came his captivity in Algiers, the

This paper was written to commemorate the four hundredth anniversary of the birth of Cervantes and is included here to supplement the previous article.

embittered return to Spain, years of bohemia in Seville while collecting taxes for the Invincible Armada, debts and imprisonment in Seville, Valladolid, and possibly Argamasilla del Alba. Prison bars, however, could not clip the wings of the soldier now in full command of his literary craft. Like Chaucer, Bunyan, Silvio Pellico or the Archpriest of Hita, Cervantes was to achieve immortality from within prison walls where he wrote his masterpiece *Don Quixote*. Stifled by poverty, military discipline, conjugal ties, and bureaucracy, he petitioned the king to exile him to America, but his pleas were in vain. What he craved to be in real life—scholar, knave, actor, gypsy, shepherd—he became only on the pages of his immortal book.

In 1605, when Cervantes was already in his sixties, the first part of *Don Quixote de La Mancha* made its appearance, and in 1615 the second part. The triumphal arch of Cervantes' literary labors was complete. A year later, a few days after the death of Shakespeare, he too died. We have his likeness in a portrait painted by Juan de Jáuregui —a Cervantes neither impulsive like Quevedo nor petulant like his detractor Lope de Vega, but sardonic and generous, with melancholy veiled eyes gazing out at us "slightly lopsided," an hidalgo who, in the words of Ortega y Gasset, has sat patiently four hundred years waiting "for the birth of a 'grandson' capable of understanding him."

Don Quixote (yes! just plain "Don Quixote," simply as we say "the Bible") is the novel of novels. It is as classical in style as Montaigne and as modern as Marcel Proust. It is as realistic as a tale by Boccaccio, as mystic as a page from *Las Moradas,* as African as an El Greco, and as European as a Velazquez. It tears down with salvos of laughter the make-believe tin walls of King Arthur's castle, and it builds upon a foundation of robust prose a new and ardent chivalry of ideals. With "difficult simplicity" it weaves across its pages a new art of graphic description of scenes and people and a new technique of flashbacks with all the subtle tricks of our modern writers; and in its diversity of universal experiences it anticipates the unity of eternal things of the literature of tomorrow. The entire Spain of Philip III marches boisterously across the sun-drenched green-shaded pages. Country wenches and swaggering troopers, merchants and duchesses, humble hidalgos and village clerics, strumpets and shepherdesses, actors, barbers, beggars, and pilgrims—all these and others file past our eyes, on foot or riding sorry nags, in fancy coaches or mean carts. On a stage more vast than Tolstoy's, more profound than Dostoyevsky's, warmer than Stendhal's, and more humane than Balzac's, the joys and woes of all mankind are depicted. It is more idyllic than Virgil's *Georgics,* more rending than St. Augustine's *Confessions,* kaleidoscopic as a passage from Homer, rebellious as one of Goya's *Caprichos,* and harmonious as Beethoven's *Ninth Symphony.* It has been acclaimed by the great—Hegel and Goethe, Turgenev and Saint-Beuve —and mankind will continue to read it as a source of study, solace, and inspiration *in aeternitas*. For this book has provided man with a symbol to help him in his misery in the face of imperfection—the symbol of Don Quixote, a martyr sacrificed to save the world from a destiny of vulgarity and ill-breeding. Christ Quijano is transfigured by his passion and death into Our Lord Don Quixote.

Don Quixote's journey begins in Argamasilla and ends in Toboso, traversing in universality all of our planet and in spirit the whole immensity of time. *Don Quixote* is Bible, missal, sword, and guiding star; it is also compass, scapulary, banner, and standard anointed with humanism and universality. In contrast to his squire, "the mad" Sancho Panza, who sacrifices the ideal for the material and ignores the eagle's mighty flight in order to clutch at a sparrow, Don Quixote "the sane" grasps the eternal truths hidden behind the false illusions of the "material." Sublimely sane in a world of ignorant lunatics, Don Quixote rejects reality as imperfect, transmuting it in his mind prior to reforming it with his lance. Rucio, Sancho Panza's donkey, noses out barley and fresh water from the gullies; but Rosinante, Don Quixote's own sorry mount, prefers to graze in the starry meadows of the heavens and to drink from the pools into which the moon pours all her silver. Don Quixote (more universal than Faust or Hamlet)—who with Don Juan and La Celestina forms the great trio contributed by Spain to world literature—laughs at "practical" people, the poor in spirit who are incapable of seeing castles because at heart they are nothing but innkeepers, who, because they lack nobility of mind, call princesses wenches and cravenly shout, "Fight not! Those are only windmills!" merely to hide their fear at the legend of the giants.

Don Quixote begins his travels in Argamasilla, which symbolizes imperfect reality, and rides towards Toboso, where Dulcinea embodies the perfections of the Ideal. Four hundred years later he is still riding in the heart of man whether in Arabia, France, China, Oklahoma, or Mexico. The "Ingenuous Knight" sees deeper and more clearly in his peculiar sanity than the "practical" lunatics who, munching their fare round the fire, sneer at the chaste sober knight, who, a Holy Grail in his heart, keeps vigil over his arms beneath the night sky. With ardor and clarity stamped in his soul and pride and nobility blazoned on his shield, Don Quixote still lives in those who practice "the worship of the fairest," who still tilt at windmills, who seek the road to Toboso in their life and in their soul, who even in the shadows still see "the sun shining on the vine-draped fences," who like Don Quixote himself still set out at dawn across the sun-scorched plains to engage with courage, idealism, and dignity in the wondrous adventure of life.

THE HISTORY OF ENDOCRINOLOGY AS SEEN THROUGH THE EVOLUTION OF OUR KNOWLEDGE OF THE ADRENAL GLAND

THE THEORY OF THE "TIME-AXIS" IN HISTORY

Karl Jaspers, psychiatrist and philosopher, applied to research in history the theory of the "time-axis," designating that supremely important moment in the evolution of nations when modern humanism and culture began to flower. As Jaspers has shown, it is not possible to understand the structure of a cultural problem unless it is placed within the over-all framework of universal history, since only by viewing history as a whole can we understand our individual destinies. We must therefore make of history something contemporaneous, changing it from a matter of mere aesthetic curiosity into the often painful task of understanding ourselves.

It is not possible to evaluate the progress and goals of any branch of medicine except in the light of its origin and development, factors that also allow us to study its future tendencies. Only by conceiving the history of medicine as a unit and by perceiving its meaning can we give it an architectonic structure.

The beginning of the most powerful cultural forces of man took place, according to Jaspers, in the year 500 B.C., a time-axis when man as we know him today appeared. In three regions entirely independent from each other—China, Greece and India—a gigantic spiritual movement developed in which man became conscious of himself, aspired to self-liberation, and asked himself profound spiritual

A lecture delivered at the Thirteenth International Congress of the History of Medicine, Nice, France, September 7–14, 1952; published in *International Record of Medicine 165:*547, 587, 1952.

questions which became the bases of the philosophic and religious categories that guide our thought today. What happened then was so fundamental that everything that came before it was mere preparation and everything that came after was mere sequel.

The strange chronologic parallelism in the time-axis of those three cultures, with which the historicocultural evolution of modern peoples began, was probably due to the sudden appearance of horsemen from Central Asia, who introduced the horse in these areas. The invaders knew how vast the world was for they had "conquered and ruled ancient cultures, were conscious of the problems of living, and were responsible for a crucial turn in history." They had reached the Mediterranean and Europe at the end of the third millennium B.C.; by 1200 B.C. they had reached India; and they had invaded China and Iran at the end of the second millennium before Christ. Finally they came face to face with the ancient, matriarchal, cattle-breeding, sedentary cultures.

In medicine, time-axes also exist. They are basic periods during which the seeds of medical progress are planted and tremendous leaps in science are made. Among those time-axes in medicine, we distinguish the periods of: Hippocratic medicine, which was naturalistic and observational; the liturgical, psychotherapeutic, and hypnotic cult of Aesculapius; the school of Alexandria; Galen; Vesalius; Paracelsus; Harvey and the experimental method; and Thomas Addison, marking the origin of modern endocrinology. The years running from 1849, when Addison made his first report on the adrenal gland, to our day constitute a time-axis, a fertile century for the development of endocrinology, which, although the youngest of medical sciences, offers the greatest promise and perhaps holds the secret of the medicine of the future.

In those two half-century periods, the first of which brings us to the beginning of our century and the second to the present date, the bases not only of endocrinology but also of a new view in medicine were laid.

PRELUDE TO THE HISTORY OF ENDOCRINOLOGY

The history of endocrinology[A] is still to be written. Our sole aim here is to present its basic stages as seen through the evolution of our knowledge of the adrenal gland. Just as we would have to review the entire history of psychiatry in order to trace the history of ideas on schizophrenia; just as we would have to review the entire evolution of neurology in order to write the history of epilepsy; so must we review the philosophicohistorical evolution of all endocrinologic ideas in order to study the development of ideas on the adrenal gland.

So far as our study is concerned, the last half of the nineteenth century was highlighted by only a few events, but these are of monumental importance because they are the foundations on which modern endocrinology was erected. The dates are: 1849, when Addison published the first written report in the history of medicine correlating a clinical syndrome with a lesion of the endocrine glands; 1891, when Murray in England treated a myxedematous patient for the first time with a thyroid extract; and 1899, when Brown-Séquard propounded his notion of the existence of a mechanism of endocrine integration in the organism different from that of nervous integration. Perhaps the first date—1849—should be considered as marking the birth of modern endocrinology, since Addison's brilliant work was responsible for the development years later of a new view and a new method, if not in research in endocrine diseases at least in tackling the problems of medicine and biology.

The history of the ideas concerning the adrenal gland embraces not only the history of all endocrinology, but also much that is valuable in the study of the evolution of modern medical thought, especially the introduction in medicine of the new philosophicobiologic concepts related to the adrenal cortex, concepts that may hold the key to the medicine of the next half century. We shall study these ideas rather than the men who formulated them, sacrificing the anecdotal to the substantive. Thus we shall situate the ideas in space and time: that is to say, on the scene and at the historical moment in which they evolved.

It has been said that medicine is entering an "Adrenal Era." Although this may be an exaggeration, we must recognize the fact that the biography of the "adrenal idea" contains the germs of many modern methods of medical experimentation.

This task of reviving the endocrinologic past is one of the most fascinating a scientist can undertake, for he cannot only resuscitate the past, but also anticipate what is yet to come. In reviewing the ground covered by endocrinologic thought, he may find that at certain points he can soar from the plane of thought to the horizons of the future.

History is a tremendous attempt at resurrection. And to resurrect is not to expose the bones of the past to the light but to restore the vitality of that past and divine the forces that impelled it when it was alive. To understand the endocrinologic bridge that is now under construction is to project into the future its dynamic curve and surmise where on tomorrow's shores the rest of the arch will end.

The history of endocrinology is of enormous importance at the present moment, when the endocrine system and its nervous correlations have opened fresh paths for research into the problems of health and disease. It offers a valuable lesson in methodology: it teaches us not to disdain theoretic and interpretive thought, a notion revindicated by Hans Selye when he affirmed that such thought is of supreme importance in endocrinologic research because endocrine correlations, the basis of modern endocrinology, can be elucidated only after sketching a plan coordinating related facts theoretically on the basis of available knowledge.

THE GREAT NEGLECT: BIOGRAPHY OF AN IDEA

The adrenal gland was for a long time neglected in the history of medicine. A curious combination of factors delayed the incorporation of adrenal physiology and pathology into the sum of medical knowledge. Some of these factors are: the hidden anatomic location of the gland; the effects that the delay in performing dissections (done clandestinely for many centuries) had on this gland, converting its inner tissues into an amorphous mass as a result of the autolytic process; proximity of the gland to the kidneys, which made it resemble an excretory gland; the lack of correlation between this gland and the clinical syndrome it produced; and the extraordinary difficulties in clinically isolating its hormones. However, when adrenal physiology was finally understood, it revolutionized a great number of medical, diagnostic, therapeutic, and biologic concepts, and initiated a philosophicoscientific revolution in modern biology.

"Writing history," Ortega y Gasset has said, "is an enthusiastic attempt at resurrection." Here we shall attempt to write an introduction to the biography of the "adrenal concept" in medicine, presenting the evolution of the idea of the adrenal gland along with the thoughts of some of the men who tried to solve its clinical, physiologic, chemical, and biologic secrets. As we do that, we shall also be tracing the panorama of endocrinology, for the history of the study of the adrenal gland—its failures, its victories, and the brilliant work being done now as a result of the triumph of experimental thought over authoritarian tradition in medicine—summarizes the eternal conflict between clinical experimentation and intransigent dogmatism, which in turn summarizes the *entire* history of science.

AGE-OLD ORGANOTHERAPY

It is highly significant that when in 1849—the date we have chosen as signifying the beginning of modern endocrinology—Thomas Addison discovered lesions in the adrenal glands of a corpse and related them to the clinical syndrome he had observed when the patient was alive, very little was known about the ductless glands.

The majority of these glands had already been described, but until then no one had pointed out the importance of their functions in the organism. Anatomists were accustomed to looking for glands with an excretory duct, the morphology of which provided them with the key to the function of those glands. They had no conception of glands without an excretory duct. The unanimous tendency therefore was to consider the latter simply as ontogenic survivals, relics of atrophied organs, or mere organic formations with insignificant excretory functions.

Man discovered the therapeutic use of these glands before he understood their function. Empiric organotherapy historically precedes scientific endocrinology by more than a millennium.[B] Scarcely half a century has passed since the function of all the endocrine glands was understood, but we have been aware from time immemorial of the correlation that exists between the form of our body, the mechanism of our emotions, and the actions of certain endocrine glands. Primitive warriors ate the heart, liver, and other innards of their enemies killed in combat so that they might assimilate the warlike virtues that they believed were immanent in said innards. In the *Ebers Papyrus,* the medical bible of ancient Egypt, glandular extracts are among the seven hundred medicaments cited.

The most ancient mystical insight into the existence of the adrenal glands and the physiologic role they play may be found in the ancient metaphysics of the *Chakras.*[C] The first trace of the theory is to be found in the book *Yogasikhu* of the Hamsa Upanishad, whence, after several centuries, it passed to the Tantras or sacred books of the *Shaktas.* These books expounded the idea of the spiritual power inherent in the body in the form of a *Kundalini* that lies "curled like a serpent" at the level of a "vital center or *Chakra*" called the *muladhara,* situated "at the bottom of the spinal column." From this center, when the power is stimulated by ascetic discipline, it ascends "through a series of seven centers" or *chakras* (a word meaning "wheel," "that which turns" in Sanskrit). This theory was revived in the yoga of Patanjali and Vyasa and in later Indian philosophies. The strange part of all this is that the location and functions of these centers of energy or *Chakras,* not only in philosophic descriptions but also in ancient Hindu mystical iconography,[D] coincide exactly with the ductless glands. We may conclude, therefore, that the ancient mystical books of India have contained for more than three thousand years descriptions of the location and functions of the adrenal gland, identified by them as the "sacred center" or *svadishthana.*

The most ancient reference extant to an endocrine disease is to be found in the Atharva Veda, a collection of Hindu religious rites written in India before 1500 B.C., containing an enchantment recited by the Buddhist bonzes to cure goiter patients. In the Ayurva-Veda of Susruta (1400 B.C.) a case of goiter is described.

Aristotle (384–322 B.C.) recommended organotherapy. Pliny the

Elder (23–79 A.D.) dedicated books XXVIII to XXXII of his *Natural History* to *materia medica,* and studied the medicines derived from animal and human organs. Hippocrates was the first to make a nosographic study of hypo-orchidism, a disease of the Scythians, and of climacteric hypo-ovarism, connecting certain symptomatic complexes with endocrine alterations. The Alexandrian physicians in the third century B.C. described the gonads and the liver. Aretæus of Cappadocia (A.D. 150) described diabetes, although he attributed it to renal poisoning of the bladder caused by the bite of a poisonous snake. The Greeks and Romans knew of diabetes mellitus, and Celsus, the elegant Roman physician (1st century A.D.), knew of polyuria, polydypsia, and emaciation of the diabetic patient. In his autopsies on monkeys, Galen found the thymus—he compared it to a bunch of thyme leaves, which accounts for the name he gave it—the thyroid, the pituitary, and the epiphysis glands. For him the pituitary acted as a sieve for humidity and for the fluids discharged from the brain into the nasopharynx. In his work *De Voce,* he vaguely described the thyroid as part of the vocal apparatus. Juvenal, Pliny, and Paracelsus also described it. In 1180 Roger of Palermo treated goiter with marine sponges and seaweed rich in iodine, a method already used in China (1600 B.C.) thousands of years before iodine was discovered.

Paracelsus (1493–1541), the father of pharmaceutical chemistry, justified opotherapy with his *similia similibus curantur;* he felt that the best method of curing a diseased organ was to administer another similar organ, thus initiating therapy by substitution.

In 1755 Théophile de Bordeu, of Montpellier, in his *Analyse médicinale du sang* expressed the opinion that all organs produce specific substances that pass into the blood and are useful to the organism; that the deficiency symptoms of castrates may be caused by a lack of the humoral substances produced by the sex glands; and that the anomalies of humoral secretions play an important role in pathology. (*"C'est au médecin à suivre et à classer les divers reflux qui surviennent par la faute de chaque organe en particulier."*)[E] But the predominant opinion that integration of the activities of distant organs was performed in our organism by the nervous system, solidly established by Descartes in the seventeenth century and then confirmed by the Viennese physiologist Prochaska (1784), impeded the recognition of endocrine activity as a process of organic physiologic correlation.

Berthold de Göttingen (1849) indicated that the testicles contained an internal secretion, and proved that it was possible by castration to destroy secondary sex characteristics in cocks and to develop them through testicular implantations.

Before Addison, the adrenal gland, as well as the other endocrine glands, had already been described by ancient anatomists who, however, were incapable of attributing any important function to it. Ancient anatomy was a static branch of medicine, and working on corpses increased that staticism, for it was thought that the only organs important to life were those whose anatomic configuration pointed to some vital physiologic function. Glands for which no duct could be found were considered—as occurred with the endocrines—unimportant anatomic vestiges. In the case of the adrenal glands, their position and exiguous size made them unimportant in the eyes of anatomists. When we consider this attitude in the light of the new theories on the all-important role played by the adrenal cortex in all the phases of human life, we come to the conclusion that it is time to write a *true* adrenal interpretation not as part of the history of medicine but as part of history in general, and to revindicate not so much the role of this vital gland in the history of the diseases of mankind, as its influence on the actions, decisions, and vicissitudes of man, that is, on the destinies of nations.

Two centuries after Bartholomeus Eustachius (1520–1574)[F] described the adrenals (1563), these glands—which he called *"glandulae renibus incumbunt"*—were still catalogued as mere anatomic curios.

In 1607, Jean Riolan (1577–1657), professor of anatomy on the Faculty of Medicine in Paris and a follower of Galen and Descartes, referred to them as *"capsulae suprarenale."* But the secret to the functional role played by these glands lay dormant in the copper plates engraved by Eustachius for his *Tabulae Anatomicae,* which he completed years before the publication of Vesalius' *De Humani Corporis Fabrica.* These *Tabulae Anatomicae,* because of economic and other difficulties, did not appear during the lifetime of the author. For one hundred thirty-eight years, until they were rediscovered by Lancisi in the Vatican Library, these plates were unknown. Unfortunately, Pope Clement XI did not permit his physician Lancisi to publish them until 1673. By one of those ironic paradoxes of history, the mysterious disappearance of the copper plates, whose illustrations, although less artistic, were more exact than Vesalius', determined their publication after the *Fabrica.* Otherwise Eustachius would have been considered with Vesalius cofounder of modern anatomy.

In 1627 Spigelius had mentioned these glands as *"capsulae renale."* In 1687 Malpighi stated that the name of *"capsulae suprarenale"* should be rejected because it expressed only the aspect of central liquefaction produced by autolysis in the corpse.[G]

Significant proof of the close relationship existing between historical events and the progress of medicine is contained in the ancient secular terror at touching dead bodies, not to mention performing autopsies. That terror, increased by the religious persecution of those who dared to defy the prohibition against dissection of corpses, retarded the progress of anatomy and medicine, which were limited to animal dissection for thousands of years. Later, when impatient anatomists clandestinely used corpses dug up from cemeteries, autopsies were carried out with great caution, often several days after death, when autolysis had already transformed the adrenal medulla into a dark viscous liquid (*atrabilis*) contained within the cortex. Hence, it was thought that the adrenals were capsules (*capsulae suprarenale*) full of liquid, which testifies to the close tie existing between the historical *ambiance* of each period and the evolution of medicine. A religious taboo retarded the knowledge of the anatomic structure of the adrenal glands for hundreds of years!

One century after the publication of the *Tabulae Anatomicae,* the Academy of Sciences of Bordeaux offered a prize for the best essay on *What Do the Adrenal Glands Do?,* but the prize was never awarded, further proof of either how unimportant the problem was considered at the time or how little was known about the gland.

In 1841, Magendie said that no value should be set on the *"atrabilis negra,"* since the adrenal glands *had ceased being* secretory agents. Other scientists, misled by the small dimensions of the gland, believed that they were fetal kidneys whose function ceased with birth.

Thus ends the first morphologic period in the history of the adrenal gland, a period that yielded only an anatomic description of that organ. When in the year 1849 Addison published his paper, the unimportance of the adrenals was an article of faith among physicians.

An anatomic dogma therefore impeded the development of a scientific truth. Until that time, all important glands had excretory ducts; *ergo,* ductless glands did not excrete anything important. Medical research methods proceeding from the organ to its function proved to be erroneous and harmful. The description of the organs, based on the dogmatic authority of the ancient anatomists, prevented the development of research methods based on clinical observation and the study of functions.

The next event represented a revolution in the methods of clinical study. For the first time a brilliant mind presented medicine not only with the description of the first endocrine syndrome, tying it up with the causal gland, but also with an extremely original method that, ignoring anatomic dogma, came face to face with clinical truth and only then—no earlier—tied it up with its anatomicopathologic basis. The patient and his symptoms from then on became the guide to the corpse and its lesions. Such was Addison's great contribution.

THOMAS ADDISON AND THE BEGINNINGS OF CLINICAL ENDOCRINOLOGY

Modern endocrinology was born on March 15, 1849, when Thomas Addison made his first report to the South London Medical Society concerning "a remarkable form of anemia" invariably associated with lesions of the suprarenal capsules.[11]

Addison's paper is the first report—succinct but so perfect that today we can add but few details—on the illness that today bears his name. The importance of this paper lies in the fact that for the first time such diseases as diabetes mellitus, exophthalmic goiter, and cortico-adrenal tumors were connected with endocrine affections.

At the time he presented his report, which marked the beginning not only of the scientific study of the adrenal glands but also of endocrinology in general, as well as the transition from the morphologic to the clinical study of the internal secretion glands, Addison was a man of fifty-six and had been a physician for twenty-five years in Guy's Hospital in London. That quarter of a century spent in anonymous work in such a splendid institution sharpened his powers of observation and made of him an excellent clinician and a learned pathologist.

Addison led a life as circumscribed geographically as it was broad in thought. He was born near Newcastle-on-Tyne in 1793, won a reputation as an outstanding student—he took notes of his teachers' lectures in Latin—and was graduated in Edinburgh as a physician in 1815. Later he went to London where he practiced in Hatton Garden and was the first surgeon at Lock Hospital. In time he became assistant to Dr. Bateman, a famous dermatologist in Snow Hill. However, this fashionable professional life held no attractions for him. Loyal to his individual bent, he entered Guy's Hospital as physician in 1824, remaining there until shortly before his death in 1860, five years after he made the report that immortalized his name.

At Guy's Hospital, Addison collaborated closely with Richard Bright, another giant of his time. Fate, it seems, was pleased to unite two men representing two human opposites. Bright was rich, handsome, worldly, popular; Addison was poor, stern, unsociable. Bright spent long periods of time traveling in Germany, Austria and Hungary; Addison had to struggle to make ends meet. These two men, united only by their intense and sincere interest in clinical problems, were appointed co-professors to the chair of medicine. It is possible that close contact with Bright increased Addison's timidity, badly concealed beneath a mask of gruff haughtiness.

The History of Endocrinology 221

Basically, Addison was a man of exaggerated shyness and sensibility, perhaps a psychoneurotic, who tried to compensate for the social vacuum in which he lived by devoting himself entirely to his pupils and the hospital. Those who knew him said that he had an outstanding personality, an impression created perhaps by his imposing physique, abundant beard, and penetrating eyes. He was gifted with great powers of clinical observation which, aided by his persistence, sought out the hidden causes of disease.

Let us note what his contemporaries and disciples, Wilks and Bettany (1892), had to say: "For many years he was the leading light of Guy's Hospital, so that every Guy's man during the 30 or 40 years of his teaching was a disciple of Addison. . . . He was dogmatic in his teaching and thus the pupils accepted as pure gospel every word which flowed from his lips. The force of his words was enhanced by his mode of delivery and by the presence of the man himself. . . . His penetrating glance seemed to look through you and his whole demeanor was that of a leader of men enhanced by his somewhat marked attitude. . . . As a teacher, it is difficult to conceive a better. . . . The clinical lectures were most excellent, as he never failed to thoroughly unfold the case which he was discussing. . . . His examination of the patient was of the most complete character; possessing unusually perceptive powers, being shrewd and sagacious beyond the average of men, the patient before him was scanned with a penetrating glance from which few diseases could escape detection. He never reasoned from a half-discovered fact, but would remain at the bedside with a dogged determination to trace out the disease to its very source for a period which constantly wearied the class and his attendant friends. . . ."

The same words were used by the writer of the obituary notice in the *Medical Times and Gazette* in 1860 when Addison's body was laid to rest near the priory of Lanercost, where his father had been the owner of Banks House.

During his period of private practice in London, Addison's principal interest was dermatology. This was fortunate, since later it focused his attention on the dark pigmentation of adrenal patients. At Guy's Hospital, Addison supervised the preparation of fine clay models of pathologic areas, which are still the pride of that institution. In the years that preceded his epoch-making monograph on adrenal lesions, Addison published several works of clinical interest, among which must be mentioned the *Elements of the Practice of Medicine,* which he wrote together with Richard Bright and which contains an excellent description of appendicitis and other clinical descriptions unsurpassed even today; a report, *On the Pathology of Phthisis* (1845), in which he differentiated between lobar pneumonic inflammation and the tubercular process as such, which was inspired by his great admiration for Laënnec. Addison modified Laënnec's concept concerning the destructive process of consumption of the lungs, and he described the *xanthoma diabetorum,* which he called "vitiligoidea," in a work entitled *On a Certain Affection of the Skin: Vitiligoidea: a. Plana, b. Tuberosa.* Perhaps because of the retiring nature of the author, these works did not win the fame they really deserved. Perhaps for that very reason when he published the clinical picture that he called *melasma suprarenale,* which again called attention to the mysterious little glands that are enveloped in perirenal fat, his report was "a comet in a starless sky." His contemporaries, who had none of his qualifications or his insight, failed to appreciate the importance of his study. To be able to correlate the aspects of the disease intimately connected with its pathogenesis, it was necessary to be at once, as Addison was, a dermatologist, a surgeon, a clinician, and a pathologist. All of which further proves that medical discoveries, especially in endocrinology and psychiatry, must be backed by the weapons of experimentation in their struggle against authoritarian dogmatism.

Addison was not discouraged. We know that he continued his clinical research with the same fervor as before. Probably the only thing he had in mind when he wrote his valuable report was to perform his duty by communicating what he had observed in the clinic and the autopsy room, without expecting recognition or applause. Since he never had many patients, he could devote a great deal of time to each one. He thus proved that it is much more important to study conscientiously a few cases than to skip through thousands just for the sake of piling up statistics.

Addison was the first to use (in 1837) static electricity in the treatment of spasmodic and convulsive diseases. In collaboration with John Morgan he wrote the first work in English on the action of poisons on the living organism. Some of his favorite medicines, like the pills that bear his name—calomel, squill, and digitalis for dropsy—were widely used in his time, although Addison set so little value on medication that he frequently forgot to prescribe anything for his patients. This reveals not his indifference to the patient as a human being but rather his acceptance of the therapeutic nihilism then in fashion among many doctors.

Such an attitude contrasts sharply with his all-absorbing desire to establish an ultra-accurate diagnosis. His scientific virtuosity carried him to unbelievable extremes. Deaf in one ear, he walked around the patient's bed many times in order to auscultate him in all positions, exhausting the patience of both pupils and friends. Often after visiting a patient he would repair to his home to reflect on the case, and if there were any doubts in his mind, he would return to re-examine the patient even if he lived miles away. This obstinacy in obtaining an exact diagnosis made him spend many hours at patients' bedsides and in the autopsy room, comparing his findings in the living patient with the lesions observed in the necropsy. We owe his great discovery to that persistent curiosity.

His psychologic make-up reveals a man tortured by doubts, scruples, uncertainty, inferiority complexes and frustrations. His timidity, his sternness, his deliberate rejection of worldly pomp, his late marriage at the age of fifty,[1] and his crises of anguish which forced him to go out into the streets late at night seeking nocturnal companionship indicate a psychotic personality.

It is possible that Addison compared his personal fate with that of colleagues like Bright or Gull (the first to describe myxedema) who was knighted and left a fortune of three hundred and forty-four thousand pounds sterling at his death. In contrast to them, Addison lived a sad solitary life. He sought neither honors nor fortune and was not even made a fellow of the Royal Society, let alone a baronet. His greatest honor was to be elected president of the Medical and Chirurgical Society of London. In 1860 he retired from public life and his beloved Guy's Hospital because he was obsessed by the idea that younger physicians coveted his post. He went to live in Brighton, the proverbial retirement place of his time, which Samuel Johnson had praised as the "most ideal spot in the world." There, despite the fact that he was watched by two nurses, he took his own life by jumping out of the window.

The period during which he earned his glory comprises the six years between 1849, when his original report on the syndrome of adrenal insufficiency appeared (London Med. Gaz. *43*, p. 517), and 1855 when, urged by his friend the surgeon John Hilton, by his disciples, and especially by Samuel Wilks who would later be the compiler of his work, he published his authoritative clinical monograph on the constitutional and local effects of lesions of the adrenal capsules.[1]

In his monograph, Addison described eleven cases of lassitude, bronze-colored skin pigmentation, loss of weight and death, in which necropsy invariably revealed a bilateral destruction of the suprarenal capsules, to which Addison attributed the disease, suggesting that they mainly influenced the red blood cells. In his description he confused two different diseases: pernicious anemia, today called the Addison-Biermer disease, and the affliction that was later called Addison's disease. In addition to these two diseases, keloid or localized sclerodermia also bears his name. It is a strange paradox that this timid man, who felt defeated in his greatest ambitions and finally committed suicide, should, after death, have had his name immortalized in three medical eponyms and should have opened a radiant path to endocrinology.

Addison published eleven works. No more, no less. But his work gained in scientific quality what it lacked in quantity.

In his monograph, Addison differentiates between anemia in which no organic lesion can be detected, which later would be called pernicious, and anemia associated with bronze-colored skin pigmentation and lesions of the suprarenal capsules. His little book is *in quarto* and contains only eleven cases, of which only those in which one suprarenal capsule was lesioned have been questioned. Sir Samuel Wilks accepted only four of the eleven cases. This once again indicates that observation of a few rather than of many patients has been the basis of great discoveries in endocrinology. We do not mean to belittle the importance of statistics, but we insist that had modern statistical methods been applied in the analysis of the earliest endocrine cases, it would have immediately inhibited some of the most important scientific discoveries. The history of the knowledge of the adrenal gland has proved that the thorough study of a single clinical case, such as performed by Addison, can provide, in endocrinology as well as in psychiatry, the key that opens a new door to scientific investigation.

CRITICAL ANALYSIS OF ADDISON'S MONOGRAPH

Addison's monograph, which placed him above the other three clinicians and anatomopathologists (Richard Bright, William Gull, and Samuel Wilks) who along with him were the "four greats" of Guy's Hospital,[K] was a little brochure of forty-six large-type pages, richly illustrated with colored lithographs. Let us analyze its importance in the light of the state of medical science in Addison's time.

First, the title: *On the Constitutional and Local Effects of Diseases of the Suprarenal Capsules.* Addison did not give a timid or hesitant title to his work. He decisively established an endocrine etiologic implication. For the first time in the history of medicine, a physician took the revolutionary step from the purely morphologic to the clinical stage in endocrinology. Without the help of laboratory facilities, Addison, like Pasteur in bacteriology, showed how much the clinician can do by using a neo-Hippocratic method of observation and the importance of describing and correlating with clarity and concision the discoveries made in the clinic and the necropsy room.

Second, Addison described not one but two new diseases, since he revealed pernicious anemia—for which he found no explanation on the autopsy table—by way of introduction to the fundamental theme of his work. In his search for new cases of the disease that preoccupied him, he "stumbled upon" another discovery of greater importance, to which he devoted his monograph. It is quite possible that at first both diseases appeared identical to Addison, since anemia, lassitude, and death were common to both; however, when he published his little book, he already clearly understood that they were different diseases, and his purpose was to describe what he called "bronzed skin," or "melasma suprarenale," which is altogether different from the "idiopathic anemia" he describes in his introduction. His clinical description of both diseases is so perfect that even today, a century later, there is no need to add anything else except some symptoms observed with instruments unknown in his time. Sir Henry Dale said that had Addison examined the bone marrow of deceased idiopathic anemia patients, he would not have failed to observe its anomalous aspect even macroscopically. In any case, he was the first to describe that type of anemia, the endocrine factors of which, with its dramatic treatment, were disclosed not long ago.

In the third place, we must stress the fact that Addison based his discovery on only eleven cases, just as Pierre Marie in 1886 would base his description of acromegaly on two cases of his own and five reported by others. This proves, as F. G. Young pointed out, that "the world of biology, and particularly of medicine, rarely displays the mathematical regularity and platonic perfection that allow a statistician to assess the significance of the result of the small number of observations that alone are often impossible."

We must bear in mind that Addison's work was carried out at the end of an observational period and when the experimental period was about to begin. Forgotten were Harvey's demonstrations that the experimental method might lead to almost anything in medicine, including the description of the circulation of the blood. English physicians had relegated experimentation to the position of an amusement for capricious surgeons, like Hunter or Bell. Addison did not experiment. It is therefore historically important to emphasize that he went as far as anyone could go, relying only on observation at the patient's bedside and in the autopsy room. Experimentation came later, beginning in the Old World, and it initiated a new era in endocrinology. Addison represents the end of two thousand years of observation of the endocrine glands. He is the link between the clinic and pathologic anatomy. His is a triumph of observation, but a triumph limited by the natural boundaries of the Hippocratic method.

Finally, Addison was the first to emphasize that the nature of the symptoms of adrenal patients—to whom he was first attracted, no doubt, by the bronzed pigmentation of their skin, a carry-over of his first love, dermatology—does not depend so much on the lesions found in the suprarenal capsules as on an interference in their function.

When Addison made these statements, he was going against the grain of the times, because reflexology—correlation and integration by purely nervous mechanisms—was still fashionable among physicians, and biochemical and endocrine correlations had not yet made their appearance. Nerve coordination had prevented the development of any concept of a humoral regulation and had therefore held back the progress of chemistry.

In a discussion at the Royal Medical and Chirurgical Society, Addison said: "We know that these organs (suprarenal) are situated in the direct vicinity and in contact with the solar plexus and semilunar ganglia, and receive from them a large supply of nerves and, who can tell what influence contact of these diseased organs might have on those great nerve centers and what share that secondary effect might have on the general health and in the production of the symptoms presented?"

Addison introduced into the study of the adrenal gland the holistic principle that today dominates endocrinology. Following that principle, the patient is examined clinically in the light of neo-Hippocratic criterion: he is considered as a whole, and then a detailed examination of his parts is made. Finally, a study is made of the relation among the parts in order to arrive at a final synthesis, in which there reappears the totality of the endocrine patient and his disease. Addison's was the dialectical method—introduced by Plato as the supreme road to knowledge, and applied by Hippocrates to medicine—which proceeded from the knowledge of the whole to a knowledge of the parts and then returned to the whole. Addison was the first to view the hypoadrenal patient as a clinical whole and then to relate the disease to the disturbance of one of the diseased organs: the adrenal glands.

Addison initiated the clinical and physiologic phase in the history of the adrenal glands.

THE EXPERIMENTS OF BROWN-SÉQUARD: THE PHYSIOLOGIC STAGE

The next stage in the history of our knowledge of the adrenal glands started across the channel from England, on continental soil. In England, the experimental method in medicine had been gradually abandoned, but in France, the naturalistic and experimental method enjoyed a new renaissance, manifest not only in medicine but especially in art, literature, and philosophy. It seems that the great medical movements through the centuries have followed the evolution of the dominant philosophic tendencies; they have been epicycles linked, like beads on a necklace, to the development of the great historical processes.

In the second half of the nineteenth century, men of science, as well as men of letters, in France and other European countries were drawn into the vortex of "naturalism." *Fin de siècle* novels became ill-disguised clinical histories and had their counterpart in a wave of experimentation in European medicine. Physiology appeared to European minds to be the most philosophic of sciences because its objective was to investigate the functions of life.

The new physiologic phase in the history of our understanding of the adrenal glands began in France in the wake of a report made by Trousseau, who suggested that the "bronzed disease" be called "Addison's disease." In his paper, Trousseau criticized some of the methods of Brown-Séquard; he said that these methods had to do with examination of animals, whereas the problem was mainly of a clinical nature. Once more the clinician and the physiologist clashed in the scientific ring without realizing that both were dealing with the same problem but from different points.

When Addison published his monograph in 1855, Charles Edouard Brown-Séquard, the passionate research scientist whose romantic life and dazzling experiments in the field of nerve physiology had earned him world-renown, was a man of thirty-eight with a restless mind constantly seeking new scientific fields to conquer.[L] When Brown-Séquard read the effect that, according to Addison, adrenal lesions had on the human being, he immediately tried to reproduce this effect experimentally, thus taking the decisive step—from observation of the disease to its experimental reproduction—in endocrinologic research. In his laboratory, Brown-Séquard removed the adrenals from fifty-one rabbits, eleven pigs, dogs, cats, and rats, and observed that all of them died after twelve hours. When we try to interpret the experiments of Brown-Séquard historically, we see that what he set out to do (he was a physiologist, not a clinician, and the animal in the laboratory, not the patient in the clinic, was his working tool and the object of examination) was to show that these neglected organs played an all-important role in the life of mammals. He himself was perhaps unable to appreciate fully the tremendous significance that his discovery would have in endocrinology.

In his epoch-making report, presented to the Academy of Sciences in Paris on August 25, 1856, Brown-Séquard pointed out that the symptoms observed after removal of the adrenal glands were progressive muscular debilitation, accelerated, irregular, and gasping respiration, debilitation and acceleration of the heart beat, dizziness, and convulsions. If the blood of a healthy animal was injected into the veins of an animal without adrenals, the latter lived a few hours longer.

Brown-Séquard was convinced that the cause of death was not hemorrhage, peritonitis, lesions of the surrounding organs, or interference with the fibers that the great sympathetic nerve sends to the adrenals. The blood of adrenalectomized animals was probably charged with a toxic principle, since when an animal with only one adrenal was injected, his death was speeded up. His final conclusions were that those organs were essential for the life of dogs, cats, rabbits, and guinea pigs; that their removal produced death more rapidly than the removal of both kidneys; and that they were intimately related with the cerebrospinal centers.

Brown-Séquard presented three papers to the *Académie des Sciences,* in which he summarized eight months of work on the adrenals of laboratory animals. To what has been already mentioned, he added that, contrary to the then prevalent opinion, the suprarenal "capsules" were not simply embryonic structures, but that in both man and animals they increased in size from birth to maturity. He also affirmed that their removal caused the death of the animal because of a toxic principle in the blood, which either was neutralized by the adrenals or these invested the blood with a "disintoxicating" property that disappeared with their removal. In addition, he pointed out the strange parallel between the rabbits then dying in Paris from a certain fatal epizootic disease—which showed symptoms analogous to those of adrenalectomized rabbits, presenting an inflammation of the adrenals in autopsy—and patients suffering from Addison's disease.

Brown-Séquard's work was a milestone in the history of endocrinology; it initiated the physiologic and experimental stage in the investigation of the adrenal gland, and established the latter's "antitoxic function." This concept would be extended to the other endocrine glands during what we might call the "antitoxic" stage in the evolution of endocrinology. Brown-Séquard was so impressed by the results obtained that from then on his individual philosophy seemed to change. He, who had been a pure physiologist, became an applied physiologist.

As was to be expected, Brown-Séquard's colleagues criticized his work, for in medicine innovations are nearly always criticized out of sheer habit and envy. Trousseau, on the other hand, faithful to his clinical education, insisted that he had examined a case of Addison's disease and that, after the autopsy, he had sent Brown-Séquard the patient's adrenals so that he might examine them under the microscope. Brown-Séquard found in them tubercular deposits and a "cretaceous material," a humorlike pus, as well as very few leukocytes, which confirmed Trousseau's findings and joined the hospital and the laboratory in a harmonious synthesis.

The History of Endocrinology   229

To his colleague Bouillard, who called his experiments an "amusing sort of physiology," Brown-Séquard answered with great dignity that criticism of his work was "a negation of the value of a great scientific method." He thus broke a lance in the cause of the experimental method in endocrinologic research.

Brown-Séquard was a pioneer in endocrinology. Although he probably knew only superficially the speculations of Théophile de Bordeu,[M] he broadened the concept of the existence of an internal secretion in the ductless glands, thus anticipating neurohumoralism on the basis not only of experimentation but also of imagination.

The major criticism that can be directed at his experiments is that Philippeaux in 1857 showed that it was possible to remove the adrenals in rats and yet to keep them alive for many months. Philippeaux explained that the deaths reported by Brown-Séquard were the result of traumatic lesions of the tissues contiguous to the adrenals, especially the sympathetic nerves. Probably many of the deaths during the experiments were caused by traumatic shock and sepsis, since those deaths caused, according to Brown-Séquard, by the removal of a single adrenal gland were later, when a good surgical technique was used, shown to be due to other causes. Tizzoni (1886) and Abelous and Langlois (1891) confirmed the fatal effect of double adrenalectomy. Whatever was responsible for the result of Brown-Séquard's experiments, physiologically his concept was correct and, biologically, it was brilliant.

Brown-Séquard's contribution to the knowledge of the adrenals was completed on June 1, 1899—another memorable date in the history of endocrinology—when he presented to the *Société de Biologie* of Paris a paper on autorejuvenation. Although the quantities of testosterone that he injected into himself exercised no notable effect except psychologically, his thesis on the mechanism of endocrine integration, independently of nervous integration, established the bases of modern endocrinology.[N]

"We admit," Brown-Séquard said on that occasion, "that each tissue, and more generally each cell of the organism, secretes for its own account products or special ferments which are poured into the blood and which come to influence, through the mediation of this liquid, all other cells which are thus separated one from the other by a mechanism other than that of the nervous system."

If Addison made the first clinical interpretation of the role played by the adrenals, Brown-Séquard represented the beginning of experimental and physiologic research into these organs. With him began the antitoxic stage in the history of the "concept" of the adrenal glands, an interpretation that was abandoned later but that has been revived in Selye's investigations into the "defensive" role of the adrenals. All of which once again indicates the eternal *ritornello* of medical theories in the unrolling panorama of history.

Suddenly the concept of the adrenals took a gigantic step forward. Instead of studying the anatomy of the adrenal glands, research scientists proceeded to study their secretion. Interest no longer centered on the organ, but on its functions.

As the nineteenth century drew to a close, technical progress stimulated interest in the problems of physics and chemistry. Research, aided by new instruments and a new concept of science, buttressed laboratory work and eased out philosophy. The result was a notable progress in organic chemistry. The study of internal secretions gradually replaced the anatomic study of the endocrine glands.

We cannot consider this stage, in which facts were more important than men, without citing the series of links that led to the discovery of adrenal hormones and prepared the way for what may be called the metabolic stage in the history we are sketching.

In 1856, Vulpian, a physician at La Salpêtrière, had discovered that in the adrenals the medulla cells differed from the corticals in color—only the medulla acquired a green tint in a solution of ferric chloride—and that their blood contained a chromogene related to the secretion of these glands. Henle, in 1865, observed that certain granules of the medulla cells gave a cloudy red precipitate, the chromaffin reaction, in diluted solutions of potassium bichromate.

Perhaps the most important historical factor in the trend to study internal secretions chemically was a new interest in the until then neglected branch of medicine—therapeutics. In the early part of the nineteenth century therapeutics was in exactly the same state as it was fifteen hundred years earlier; it was still based on the idea that disease was something foreign that had entered the body and that had to be expelled. All therapy therefore was of the eliminative type. True, diuretics, emetics, diaphoretics, laxatives, and bloodletting were used instead of exorcism and other ancient measures intended to expel the "demon" from the patient's body, but essentially they sprang from the same philosophic process: to eject from the body whatever was making it ill.

At the beginning of the nineteenth century, the new diagnostic methods of auscultation and percussion stimulated the interest in diagnosis, but they did not help therapeutics. At the end of the last century, new developments in immunology and endocrinology awakened a universal medical interest in therapeutics, leading to a passionate search for serums, vaccines, and hormones comparable only to the relentless search of medieval alchemists for the philosopher's stone.

Forty years after Addison's great accomplishment, the adrenal glands seemed to have fallen into oblivion. This contrasted with the impressive cavalcade of clinical and physiologic discoveries that were leading to the integration of certain ideas concerning internal secretions. Because of technical difficulties, the adrenals were set aside, and the progress of scientific knowledge about them was interrupted. The idea that Addison's disease was a sort of "autointoxication" because of an "insufficiency of adrenal excretion" still prevailed. Under these circumstances, two English physicians made a contribution that marked the next milestone in the history of endocrinology: the discovery of an active adrenal extract.

In the summer of 1894, there was practicing in the English town of Harrogate a physician by the name of George Oliver, who was interested in the measurement of pulse rate and blood pressure in man. Oliver observed with amazement the beneficial effect produced when he injected into patients suffering from hypertension watery extracts from the adrenals which *raised* their blood pressure. He then decided to inject these extracts into his own son. When he observed a contraction of the radial artery, he consulted his friend Professor E. A. Schafer of University College in London. His incredulous friend injected the extract into an anesthetized dog whose blood pressure he had been measuring and noticed with great surprise that the mercury column rose until it almost burst out of the tube. That was unheard of, since all the work done up to then with tissue extracts had revealed that the latter *lowered* blood pressure.

Later studies revealed that that active principle was not produced in the cortex but in the adrenal medulla,° and that, when animals whose adrenals had been removed were injected, the aforementioned symptoms were not relieved. It was thus arrived at the important conclusions that the adrenal was a gland with two anatomic parts performing two distinct functions, that the medulla produced a principle capable of *increasing* blood pressure, and that the cortex probably produced other vitally important secretions. These experiments (1894–1895) paved the royal road that led Abel in 1899 to isolate the adrenal (medullar) active principle in the form of insoluble benzoylate; it also led Furth (1897–1903) to obtain amorphous compounds purified to the highest degree from Abel's "epinefrine"; and finally it led Takamine and Aldrich—independently of each other—to obtain in 1901 a pure crystalline compound of natural levo-adrenalin which was called "suprarenin" by Furth and "adrenalin" by Takamine.[P]

The importance of the discoveries of Oliver and Schafer lies not so much in the fact that they led to the first isolation of a hormone, as in the fact that they opened a path to new conceptions concerning endocrine dynamics. These were the beginnings of the confirmation of the law that the pathologic importance of an organ is the function of its physiologic importance, and the physiologic complexity of the adrenals indicated their vital importance. When it was perceived that multiple tissues and different secretions existed in this gland, thought was also given to the multiplicity of its physiologic functions. Today we know that the functional and hormonal division of the adrenals corresponds, to a certain degree, to the clear division of its cortical or epithelioid tissues and the medulla or nervous and chromaffin tissues. It has even been said that the adrenal is made up of two different glands wrapped up in the same capsule. That there was a great deal of truth in this assertion has been proved, since from that point on in the evolution of our knowledge of the adrenals it became necessary to consider separately the adrenal medulla and cortex, the physiologic and philosophic synthesis of which is again, at least partially, being carried out today.

In 1905, Stolz and Dakin simultaneously prepared a racemic adrenalin. Friedman established in 1906 the structural formula of the hormone. Flacher obtained in 1908 two optic isomers from this formula. Thus for the first time—the history of the adrenals is crammed full of facts that happen for the first time in endocrinology—a pure crystalline hormone was obtained, isolated, and synthetized. The concept of the adrenal function had crossed another decisive threshold: it was possible to reproduce in the laboratory the natural hormone in which lay the mysterious adrenal function.

TECHNICAL PROGRESS CONTINUES: THE LABORATORY AND THE CLINIC

For years—ever since 1867 when Stockman made the first fruitless attempts at adrenal hormonotherapy—scientists had been using adrenal glandular products, obtained through different and rather rudimentary techniques, such as the entire gland fresh or desiccated and dry glycerinated extracts, which were applied through different organic channels. In 1903 Adams published a statistical report of ninety-seven cases treated with these extracts, most of which, because they contained marrow, raised the blood pressure. Quite a few patients improved under this therapy. In 1904, Raven used pure adrenalinic hormone on a patient suffering from Addison's disease, and for the next fifteen or twenty years this was the principal therapy for this disease. In conjunction with whole extracts and general tonics, this therapy brought about a rise in the number surviving that mysterious illness. The case cited most often in medical literature was that of Muirhead, professor of pharmacology, who diagnosed and treated himself successfully with large quantities of adrenalin and total adrenal glandular extracts, initiating a wave of popularity for this therapy.

A revolutionary advance then took place in the techniques used during this historical stage in the chemical investigation of the adrenals.

For many years, all active endocrine extracts—including the original preparation of insulin by Banting and Best—had been obtained by aqueous extraction starting from the glandular tissue. This method was based on the conclusion that if a hormone were liberated in the blood, then it must be soluble in an aqueous medium; ergo, an aqueous vehicle was the best method of glandular extraction. In 1927 Rogoff and Stewart reported that they had prepared unpurified saline adrenal extracts that were active in prolonging the life of adrenalectomized animals, but this was not quite confirmed. Two other scientists, Swingle and Pfiffner, eighty years after Addison's description, had the brilliant idea of extracting adrenal tissue with alcohol, after breaking it up with several types of lipid solvents, including benzene, and injecting it in an oil suspension. These extracts were found to prolong the life of adrenalectomized animals and they were pure enough not to cause abscesses. Today this method of extraction with lipid solvents is still the basis for the industrial manufacture of these hormones. According to Young, the success of these scientists was due to the following facts: they used an enormous amount of experimentation material (three hundred and fifty cats in the preliminary experiments); they surmised that aqueous adrenal extracts contained a certain quantity of adrenalin that made them dangerous and toxic if given in great quantities; they used fat solvents for a gland as rich in lipids as the adrenal cortex; on the basis of the great amount of cholesterol in the blood, they destroyed the point of view that a hormone cannot have the structure of a lipid; and they administered enormous hyperphysiologic quantities of the extract. As Vogt pointed out (1950), normal adrenal secretion would exhaust in six to twelve seconds its stored-up active material, since it was evident that this gland stored up very little of the hormone in a form capable of being extracted. Later, Swingle and Pfiffner also described a method of extraction in aqueous solution, and another method for eliminating the adrenalin by filtering it through permutit which utilized the interchange of ions for biologic purposes.

The laboratory, in happy association with the clinic, thus brought to a close another stage in the historical evolution of the concept of the adrenal function.

HORMONES AND NERVE FIBERS: NEW ORGANIC CORRELATIONS

The next stage would be of enormous biologicophilosophic importance in the evolution of the concept of adrenal hormones.

Up to then, the notion that had been taking shape, as a result of years of research and theorizing, was that the hormones in general were chemical messengers carrying physiologic orders through the blood to the different organs of the body. One of those brusque shifts so frequent in history swung the pendulum radically from the concept of organic regulation by the nervous system to the concept that this function was carried on by internal secretions. The following events showed that this organic regulation is not exercised unilaterally by the hormones, but that it is a function of both the hormones and the nervous system.

In 1902 Lewandowsky and Langley showed that a notable similarity existed between the action of adrenal extracts and that produced by stimulation of the sympathetic nerves. Two years later, Elliot made the same observation, using adrenalin. He propounded the hypothesis that adrenalin might be the chemical excitant that was liberated when the sympathetic nerve impulse reached the periphery at the level of its nerve endings. In 1921, Loewi showed that by making a Ringer solution circulate through a heart removed from a frog, the solution acquired sympatheticomimetic properties (and increased the frequency and amplitude of the cardiac contractions when applied to another heart) if the sympathetic fibers of the vagosympathetic nerve were stimulated.[Q] This *Acceleransstoff,* or Loewi's accelerating substance, hypothetically liberated during sympathetic stimulation, was later (1931) called *sympathine* by Cannon and his collaborators. It was then shown that stimulation of the sympathetic nerve liberated a substance, in the nerve endings of the organs innervated by fibers, of the type called adrenergic because they imitate the adrenalinic effect. So another new concept was introduced in endocrinology: that the effects of all nerve impulses emanating from peripheral nerves are caused by the liberation of certain chemical substances.

Doubt about whether the transmitting adrenergic substance was always and totally adrenalin was allayed years later when Cannon dubbed it "sympathine." It was thus established that the effects of adrenalin, when applied artificially, are similar but not absolutely identical to the effects of the sympathetic nerve impulses and the chemical transmitter that is released into the blood—at the point where the endocrine gland producing it liberates it—to be carried a great distance.[R]

The History of Endocrinology

The endocrine function of the adrenal medulla, as Cannon would show, was thought to strengthen the actions of the sympathetic nerves in emergencies, in sudden requirements of activity, or in cases of emotional tension, and its hormone or adrenalin was considered the peripheric transmitter of the adrenergic impulses. At first, it was thought that a lack of this hormone in the adrenal medulla played an important part in Addison's disease. Afterward it was discovered that the principal symptoms of this disease—weakness and languor, muscular asthenia, high blood pressure, alterations of the normal balance of inorganic salts in the humors and organic tissues, disposition to attacks of hypoglycemia, and general lack of normal resistance to infections and intoxications, thermic changes, and other influences —are always or almost always contingent on a deficiency of the hormones produced by the adrenal cortex, that is, on the collapse of a vast endocrine arch of functional structures the keystone of which is the adrenal cortex.

A NEW CONCEPT IS BORN: PERIPHERIC HORMONES

Following on all these discoveries, the conceptions of endocrinology varied radically. Endocrine diseases ceased being mere problems of glandular hyper- or hypofunction that could be cured in the manner of moves in chess—by removing one piece or replacing it.

It was proved that both the adrenal internal secretions and the other hormones were not "chemical messengers," and that when they were released into the blood their chemical structure was changed and did not change back until they acted on the end organs.

Elliot, Dale, Loewi, Cannon, Bacq, and others proved that, as soon as it is released into the blood of the adrenal vein, adrenalin becomes oxydized and disappears, reappearing by reduction in the sympathetic nerve endings in the smooth muscular fiber, and that it is this nascent adrenalin that makes the vascular and visceral muscular fibers contract. Adrenalin is not found in the blood because it is not a chemical messenger, but rather the beginning and end of a chain of chemical actions that begins in the adrenals and ends in the adrenalin of the end organs. Covering its course through the blood it passes through innumerable intervening links that do not exhibit the characteristics of adrenalin.

The same happens with the other hormones. They do not pass through the blood in the same form they are produced by the organs; instead, they become separated into temporary atomic complexes until they reach the points where they must act, and it is there that they are recomposed. It is like machinery shipped from the factory disassembled to be put together again at the place of destination. Therefore, contrary to the beliefs of Gley and other physiologists of the old school, it is *not* possible to find adrenalin in the blood, except when it has just been released into the adrenal veins.

Another notion that was destroyed was that endocrine diseases were caused by glandular hyper- or hypofunction, since the main thing is what happens in the end organ. There may be adrenalin insufficiency, even with sufficient adrenalin production in the gland, if the "terminal" tissues where the adrenalin is resynthesized and acts function badly. This explains the cases of Addisonian syndrome with adrenals apparently intact, as well as the absence of this syndrome, even though in the autopsy the adrenals may be found to be totally destroyed. Sometimes, the "terminal" tissues are incapable of reacting to the hormones. Like situations of peripheral humoral-hormonal "resynthesis," this condition may cause endocrine disturbances. If the hormones that are not used up in their specific tissues accumulate in the blood, they may give the appearance of an auto-intoxication or an endocrine hyperfunction that does not really exist. Insufficiency may be caused by an excessive consumption of normal hormones, as in puberty, and intoxication may be due to the presence of normal but inactive hormones.

Organic functional unity is not established therefore by the vegetative and hormonal or chemical systems alone. The hormones function in the nervous system as batteries, with their fluids distributed through the system of nerve networks. Only one organic correlation exists, and that is neurohormonal. Electric stimulus of the sympathetic nerve (Langley) makes its nerve endings segregate adrenalin, which in its turn stimulates the sympathetic nerve and provokes a new secretion of that substance. These intermediary substances are probably peripheral hormones segregated by the nerves at their point of contact with the tissues, so that the nervous impulse changes to chemical action, since the chemical "language" into which nerve commands are translated is what the tissues understand best.

THE SEARCH FOR THE HORMONES OF THE ADRENAL CORTEX

In ontogeny, the hormones precede the endocrine glands. In the history of endocrinology, after centuries of studying the glands, scientists began to study the hormones only.[8] In what we might call the chemicometabolic stage of the history of our knowledge of the adrenals, research into the hormones of the adrenal cortex sprang from the intimate conviction that the adrenal cortex and not the medulla contained the secret of Addison's disease. Sir William Osler, with his usual insight, had already used an adrenal extract to treat Addison's disease, but not until twenty years ago were cortico-adrenal preparations of constant activity compounded.

Rogoff and Stewart in 1925, Hartmann and others in 1928, and

The History of Endocrinology

Swingle and Pfiffner in 1931 demonstrated that it was possible to maintain adrenalectomized dogs and cats alive almost indefinitely by administering cortico-adrenal extracts continuously. Later work led to the isolation—from the adrenal cortex principally of cattle—of several crystalline compounds of high corticoid activity (Grollman and Firor, 1935; Kendall and others, 1935; Wintersteiner and Pfiffner, 1935). Several of the crystalline fractions were perhaps mixtures, but they were pure enough to be identified as steroids or substances closely related to ovarian and testicular hormones.

Until 1930 it was a rule, to which the only exception was the pituitary gland, that each endocrine gland secreted only one hormone. This law, like the law of the specificity of certain tissues within a gland to produce a certain type hormone, was to be destroyed when new research into the cortico-adrenal hormones got under way. Once again, investigation of an adrenal problem would be all-important for endocrinology and would force a change in the methods of chemico-endocrinologic research.

The quantities of hormones existing in the adrenal gland were minute in comparison with the quantities produced by the gland and used by the organism daily. That inefficiency of the extractions with a glandular base as a means of obtaining the hormone led to the development of new methods of chemical synthesis. And that particular historic moment marks the beginning of a series of discoveries that would lead to the isolation of cortisone and similar compounds —the gate to a new phase in the history of the adrenal gland.

CORTISONE: A CHEMICAL FEAT

From 1935 on, several groups of scientists, especially Kendall and Wintersteiner in the United States and Thaddeus Reichstein in Switzerland, began to isolate a series of crystalline substances endowed with great power to keep animals alive without adrenals. The chemical nature of these substances slowly began to be clarified. It was indeed a great feat to identify pure cortico-adrenal hormones, because for years it had been a Utopian dream. The task was facilitated by the recognition of the different physiologic activities of the substances formed, adding various lateral groups and chains to the common carbohydrate skeleton or nucleus of the cyclopentenophenanthrene that forms the central structure of sterols, bile acids, certain glucocides, steroid vitamin D, sex steroids, and adrenal hormonal steroids. Kendall isolated several of these hormones taken from animal adrenals and Reichstein synthesized them artificially.

In 1936 Kendall, Mason, and others isolated compounds A and B, which are identical with dehydrocorticosterone and corticosterone respectively, while Reichstein showed that several cortical steroids may also be transformed into adrenosterone, an androgenic compound normally present in the adrenal cortex. Since then a great number of cortico-adrenal steroids have been isolated, some of which are mere hormonal metabolites and others have pharmacologic, corticoid, testoid, or luteoid properties.

In 1937, Steiger and Reichstein, starting from a phytosterol (stigmasterol),[T] synthesized desoxycorticosterone, which would later be the basic treatment, with sodium chloride, of Addison's disease. It is of historical interest that the isolation of this compound directly from the gland, which proved that it was a natural hormone, was not carried out until some time after its synthesis was made.

There have been prepared recently from desoxycholic acid, 11-dehydrocorticosterone (Lardon and Reichstein, 1943), corticosterone (by v. Euw and two others, 1944), and 17-hydroxy-11-dehydrocorticosterone or Kendall's compound E (Sarett, 1945). The multiplicity of steroids would lead to the inference that there may be a selective increase in mineral corticoids during adaptation and defense against harmful agents.[U]

Kendall has recalled on several occasions the years of silent work culminating in the discovery of cortisone, which, like a magic seed, has bloomed into a tree with many promising ramifications. In his own words, the adrenal cortex "is the last of the endocrine glands to have yielded its secret to the scientist." The total time required for the investigation of the adrenal cortex has been, according to Kendall, twenty-one years, of which six-sevenths were spent in the chemistry laboratory, the ratio of the chemical to clinical work having been approximately the same as the ratio between that part of an iceberg that is submerged and the glistening peak that juts above the water.

The first investigations were made by two groups of physiologists: Hartmann and his collaborators at the University of Buffalo, and Swingle and Pfiffner at Princeton University. Cortisone was isolated for the first time in 1945—its chemical structure was determined in the three years that followed—simultaneously with the work done along the same lines by Wintersteiner and others at Columbia University, and Reichstein and his collaborators in Switzerland. The total number of sterols isolated from the adrenal cortex was twenty-eight, and four compounds (A, B, E, and F) capable of restoring normal characteristics to animals were developed. From this series of compounds, the least complicated of the pregnene or desoxycorticosterone series had already been developed by Steiger and Reichstein in 1937.[V] In Switzerland, Lardon and Reichstein prepared from desoxycholic acid the first sample of compound A, which later, in 1944, Kendall produced through a simpler method and which was followed by the manufacture of cortisone (compound E) in May of 1948 and the manufacture of compound F. We must mention the technique of Dr. L. H. Sarett, without which this magnificent result would not have been obtained. Several North American laboratories, especially Merck Sharp & Dohme and The Upjohn Company, contributed notably to this splendid accomplishment.[w]

In 1925, Herbert Evans reported that the pituitary extracts administered to hypophysectomized animals prevented atrophy of the adrenal glands. Research was done on the separation and purification of the adrenocorticotropic hormone in animals (ACTH), which could then be tried out quantitatively by Sayers through a biologic method, and in 1947 preparations were obtained that were strong and pure enough to be tried out in human beings. Later it was confirmed that the secretion of ACTH by the pituitary gland stimulates the secretion of cortisone.

Of the twenty-eight crystalline steroids of the adrenals, it is today estimated (Young) that seven are active in maintaining the adrenalectomized animal in good condition, and that the amorphous fraction is very active in this direction. When corticosterone was discovered in 1937, it was thought that this might be the adrenal hormone, since it was much more active in the maintenance of life than cortisone or compound E discovered by Kendall the year before; it was later proved that the different steroids possess different properties depending on the position of their oxygen atoms or hydroxyl groups, or of their hydrogen atoms.[x]

These steroids are liberated under the control of the nervous system. According to G. W. Harris (1948), the stimulation of the hypothalamic centers leads to the liberation of the humoral transmitters from the infundibulum, these substances being carried away through the pituitary portal system to the anterior lobe of the pituitary where the liberation of the adrenocorticotropic hormone is stimulated. ACTH is then carried in the blood stream to the adrenal cortex where the production and secretion of two or more active steroids is stimulated. The adrenalin segregated by the adrenal medulla may also stimulate the secretion of adrenal steroids from the adrenal cortex, acting directly or indirectly through the hypothalamic centers on the anterior pituitary lobe to stimulate the liberation of ACTH; this theory reconciles nervous coordination with humoral.[y]

CORTISONE—THE THERAPEUTIC MIRACLE

The next stage in our knowledge of the adrenal gland starts when Hench and his collaborators begin to try out cortisone on different clinical diseases. The history of the development of cortisone and its clinical application represents another fascinating chapter in the development of clinical endocrinology and in the history of the adrenal gland.

On September 21, 1948, in Rochester, Minnesota, 100 mg. of a cortico-adrenal hormone (designated as compound E) were injected intramuscularly in a rheumatoid arthritic patient. The pain and stiffness in the joints that had been torturing him for five years disappeared as if by miracle after a few days of treatment. For ten years, Hench had been seeking out the nature of a hypothetical "substance X" that might be capable of alleviating rheumatism and had discussed the cause of rheumatic arthritis with Kendall; it was finally decided to use cortisone as soon as that hormone was available.[z]

On May 31, 1949, I heard Dr. Phillip S. Hench, of the Mayo Clinic, read in New York his historic report explaining the clinical application of cortisone in the treatment of rheumatism.

The history of this research work is extremely interesting. In 1941, in the beginning of World War II, rumors circulated in Europe that the pilots of the *Luftwaffe* could fly without oxygen at a height of more than forty thousand feet without suffering the violent reactions that Allied pilots suffered under similar circumstances, and that the magic key to their incredible resistance was a mysterious extract from the adrenal cortex.

This false rumor inspired a vast program of investigation, in which Kendall, who had earlier discovered, isolated, and partially synthesized several adrenal hormones, participated. Using great quantities of desoxycholic acid in a process that required twenty-nine stages, to which twelve more stages were added in another laboratory, Kendall produced a steroid: Compound E or cortisone. Some American laboratories (Merck) helped notably in this work, and other laboratories (Upjohn), which since 1933 had been manufacturing cortico-adrenal extracts to treat Addison's disease, proved the increase in survival time among rats, and developed the Cartland-Kuizenga unit to measure the power of steroids. They also identified the three compounds: corticosterone (Kendall's compound B), cortisone (Kendall's compound E), and hydrocortisone (Kendall's compound F). The Upjohn Company, together with S. B. Penick & Co., sent an expedition to Africa, and for six months they looked for the mysterious "lost" liana of the strophanthin that was thought to contain a steroid from which cortisone could be manufactured. The Upjohn Company also developed a process to make cortisone by biosynthesis and later by enzymatic fermentation, using a Rhizopus mold that can introduce oxygen at position C-11 in a great series of steroids, from progesterone to plant steroids, like yeast ergosterol, soy stigmasterol, and diosgenin from Mexican yam.

Cortisone, with ACTH or corticotropin discovered at Yale in 1943, has been used since 1950 to treat rheumatic fever and thirty-six other diseases. Hydrocortisone seems to be fifty per cent more efficacious than cortisone in many cases. For some years now cortisone has been increasingly used in a vast number of diseases—from rheumatic arthritis and ocular inflammations to pemphigus.

When the "adrenal concept" reached this stage, it blossomed into any number of therapeutic possibilities. The tiny endocrine gland and its mysterious hormones were to become one of the most precious weapons in the modern endocrinologic arsenal.

A BRIEF PARENTHESIS CONCERNING THE PHILOSOPHIC IMPLICATIONS OF THE ENDOCRINE GLANDS

We have seen how our knowledge of the adrenal gland passed through a series of phases that culminated in the clinical application of the cortico-adrenal hormone to a great number of diseases. This chapter has barely begun. It represents the widening of the role played by the adrenal cortex, which has proved to be one of the most important vital centers in the human body.

From a philosophic point of view, the interest in the ductless glands has meant a revolution in modern biologic thought. Classic biologists of Darwinian evolutionism made of life a gigantic process of adaptation, classified the vital functions in series of separate acts, each one of which was an operation carried out by an organ perfectly equipped for its function, with life as the end product of this series of functions.

In contrast with this notion, the growing science of endocrinology nourished the idea that the essence of life does not lie in fixed and specialized structures endowed with secondary vitality; the essence of life does not depend on the functions of adaptation but on that very inner power that later became specialized and mechanized in those secondary and peripheral functions.

Evolutionism was a biologic mechanism rather than an authentic biology, since it fixed its attention on the organs that life creates for itself rather than on the organs of primary creative activity. Modern biology considers internal vitality primary and its external manifestations secondary. The living being has ceased to be the sum of his organs in movement to become the creator and origin of concrete specifications in cells, tissues, and organs.

The internal secretion glands are the organs that take care of secreting the hormones that spread all over the organism, and their mission is to stimulate the peripheral functions. Through the centuries, it has been gradually discovered that the hormonal function, especially in the case of the adrenal cortex, is internal and regulatory and does not come in contact with the world except when it becomes exhausted in the integral maintenance of the functional unity of the body. Endocrinologic study of the functions of organic regulation has been bringing medicine nearer to the real core of life and alienating it to a certain extent from the idea of the external functions of adaptation or peripheral functions of the other visceral organs.

The evolution of the concept of adrenal function served to open a path to the new endocrinology and, in medicine, to the idea, already adumbrated by Claude Bernard, that life is a movement from within outward. The organism does not adapt itself to the environment but rather becomes integrated with it; it absorbs it and closes off possible escapes to another ambiency that is not its own. Every organism creates its own environment which becomes its natural dwelling, since it is but a prolongation of its organic individuality. The description of the living being must therefore begin with a description of the milieu that it formed, developed, and incorporated into itself. In that tremendous biologic task in which the living being has to rebel against and dominate the milieu, the endocrine glands are its most powerful weapons.

THE "DEFENSIVE" PHASE IN THE HISTORY OF THE ADRENALS

When it appeared that everything was already known about the anatomy, physiology, chemistry, pathology, and clinical aspects of the adrenal gland, a new theory appeared on the historical scene, a theory that later became a basic branch of modern medicine and revolutionized endocrinology through a new concept of the function of the adrenal cortex and the other endocrine glands related to it. I refer to the theories of Hans Selye, which chronologically preceded the discovery of cortisone, but were not fully developed until after that discovery, and which initiated the "defensive" phase of the concept of the endocrine functions.

This theory was preceded by the notion of the integration of the endocrine system, which owes so much to the concept of Sir Walter Langdon-Brown, to wit, that this system is like an endocrine orchestra the conductor of which is the pituitary and the composer the hypothalamus. Thanks to him, it was shown that the adrenal cortex, the hypothalamus, and the anterior pituitary functionally form a single organ that, through the corresponding trophic hormone, can transform nervous energy into chemical energy and provoke the secretion of hormones, which, in their turn, stimulate other endocrine glands. Then the endocrine glands may, by the same route but inversely, influence the state of our emotions. This interrelationship between the endocrine and nervous systems has been of great value in the application of endocrinology to psychiatry and has introduced in medicine certain notions that have culminated in the so-called psychosurgery, which attempts to break certain resistances prevailing among nervous association cells by separating the receptor and emotional genesis zones from those zones that are purely the seat of intellectual functions in the brain. With psychosurgery, endocrinology has developed a concept of enormous value in modern medicine.

The "defensive" stage in our knowledge of the adrenals (and at the same time of all endocrinology, since this gland has once more had the historic privilege of serving as a vehicle for the introduction of new endocrinologic concepts) therefore starts with the concepts of Hans Selye, an Austrian doctor today living in Montreal, who picked up the germ for those ideas from his teacher Cannon and, through the latter, from James, the father of modern psychosomatic physiology.[AA]

In synthesis, Selye's theory holds that the mission of the ductless glands is to adopt adequate functional measures, so that the body may not perish from the unspecific aggressions that bombard it incessantly. The directive action that the endocrine system wields over metabolism erects an organic defense against the environment. This defensive reaction is a biologic concept, much broader, philosophically, than the former antitoxic concept which held that the endocrine function exercised a specific defense against organic poisons by fighting each toxic with an endocrine antidote and each toxin with its specific antitoxin.

This endocrine defense, which begins at birth and ends with death, guarantees the survival of the human being faced with an environment to which he does not adapt, as Darwin claimed, but over which he triumphs owing to his capacity to withstand attacks. It is an unspecific general defense against all types of attacks and abuses to which the body may be subjected, including excessive smoking, drinking and eating, overwork, worries, heat and cold, emotional exhaustion and setbacks. Tensions and traumas create in our organism a permanent state of defense, an effort at adaptation that Selye has called "stress," a word that is acquiring currency in all the languages of the world. Against this endless gamut of harmful stimuli, physical or mental (stress), the organism can count on its generic defenses located in the ductless glands.

This concept has revolutionized the idea that the greatest danger for the human being lay in infectious or allergic attacks, an idea that motivated the search for agents miraculously endowed with the specificity necessary for fighting each germ with its corresponding serum and each allergen with its specific antiallergen. What kills us, according to Selye, is not hypersensibility or infection, which are relatively rare in human life, but continuous unspecific aggressions (slight infections, intoxications, excessive effort, great emotional tensions) that progressively wear us out until we are brought to old age and death. In an enormous constant effort we defend ourselves against these onslaughts by processes of defense and adaptation determined by the endocrine glands. These glands work continuously, resisting daily attacks, but if the latter are excessive in intensity and duration, the process of adaptation and organic defense is impaired and "diseases of adaptation," as Selye calls them, develop. These diseases have no determined etiology; they are excessive reactions of the general defense process of the body brought on by the bankruptcy of the defensive apparatus of the body.

The defensive processes are located especially in an endocrine axis: the anterior lobe of the pituitary and the adrenal cortex, to which Marañón and others would add the thyroid and even the other endocrine glands. However, we know for certain that the adrenal cortex reappears again as the basis for the most revolutionary concept not only in endocrinology but in modern medicine.

When the body is attacked, it at once marshals the organic part relating the cosmos to our internal reactions, that is, the pituitary-hypothalamic block—the hypothalamic vegetative centers that form an anatomico-functional unit with the anterior lobe of the pituitary—which segregates its specific hormones, especially the so-called corticotropic hormone or ACTH. This hormone lacks metabolic action but it stimulates the adrenal cortex, thus producing a series of steroids or hormones including the so-called cortisone group. The cortisone then releases all metabolic resources, promotes the liberation of antibodies, alters electrolytic, protein, lipid, and carbohydrate metabolism, and permits the organism to defend itself against all environmental attacks. These generic defenses are sometimes sufficient to prevent disease even if the specific internal etiologies, e.g., septic foci, or external etiologies, e.g., infections, or other etiologies, e.g., excesses of all kinds, are in action. The endocrine defensive axis—the anterior pituitary lobe and adrenal cortex—protects us against all those attacks. But if the axis is broken, the germs lodged in the infectious foci (a tooth, a tonsil, the gall bladder), poisons, excess work, worry, or emotional upsets, cause rheumatism, high blood pressure, and other illnesses of adaptation which may even cause sudden death through exhaustion. Therefore, even though they are a generic system, the adrenal cortex, and perhaps the other endocrine glands, may protect us against all specific attacks.

With these notions, endocrinology upset the old concepts of allergies and infections, which ascribed everything to the specificity of the causal germ or allergen and to the low resistance of the body and its generic defenses. Thus was started a new and brilliant chapter in the study of the adrenal cortex.

According to Selye, the general syndrome of adaptation is the "sum of all those general unspecific reactions of the body following upon a prolonged stress, and is characterized by hypertrophy of the adrenal cortex with increase in the secretion of corticoid hormones, involution of the thymus and other lymphatic organs, gastrointestinal ulcers, metabolic modifications and variations of organic resistance." If an individual is continually exposed to stress, the general adaptation syndrome passes through three different periods: reaction of alarm (sometimes subdivided into phases of shock and countershock), the resistance period, and the exhaustion period.[BB]

Selye arrived at this idea through a series of previous concepts among which we may mention as having the greatest historical importance: Cannon's homeostasis or the tendency of the living organism to maintain its internal balance constant (Claude Bernard[CC] would have said: *maintaining its internal milieu invariable*); tachyphylaxis or nonspecific resistance developed by the injection of toxic extracts from tissues, vasopresin, or renin; Dustin's karyoklastic crisis or the sudden moment of the number of pyknosis in the thymus and lymphatic ganglia of animals treated with karyoclastic poisons; the hemoclastic crisis of Widal observed in acute infections; the polypeptidetoxic syndrome of French medical literature that occurs in hepatic insufficiency; the theory of the serous inflammation of Rossle and Eppinger; the *maladie postopératoire* (postoperation disease) of Leriche; and other syndromes described in the past which were only phases or aspects of the general adaptation syndrome.

Selye's concept grants that the adrenal gland as one of the poles of the endocrine axis plays an all-important role as a directive element in human biology, perhaps as the intermediary element between the psyche and the soma and between Darwin's external milieu and Claude Bernard's internal milieu.

THE ADRENAL GLAND AND PSYCHIATRY

Then the adrenal gland suddenly turns up in the field of psychiatry to initiate the present-day neuroendocrine stage.

The close connection among the hypothalamus, cerebral cortex, anterior lobe of the pituitary, and adrenal cortex was to lead scientists studying the latter organ—and the other endocrine glands—to do research into its correlations with the nerve organs, its role in organic physiology, and its relationships with mental pathology.[DD] Thus was started the last and perhaps the most extraordinary chapter in our knowledge of the adrenal gland, the one concerned with its role as a possible etiologic agent in psychiatry and its use as a therapeutic agent in a series of psychiatric diseases.

The work done by Pincus, Hoagland, Hoskins, Holmes, Hemphill, Reiss, Altschule, and others has shown the importance of the adrenal gland as a possible causal factor in certain psychoses. The adrenals of schizophrenics, unlike those of normal persons, do not react to the stimulus of ACTH [EE] in situations of stress. This led Hoagland to formulate the hypothesis that schizophrenia may be the result of the incapacity of certain individuals to react through their adrenals to situations of stress because of disturbances suffered by the enzymatic balance which prevent them from carrying out the synthesis of adrenal steroids.[FF]

The new theories concerning the adrenal function have transcended the limits of clinical medicine and have launched a new biochemistry of individuality, a concept that is already having far-reaching philosophic and medical repercussions.[GG] The idea of an endocrine individuality has led to the belief that a metabolic and biochemical individuality exists. R. J. Williams has advised that that biochemical individuality be studied instead of the simple normal biochemistry. Several discoveries have reinforced this concept, such as the fact that schizophrenics excrete a larger amount of magnesium (Young, Berry, Beerstecher, and others) and of all the amino acids except histidine, which would indicate that there exists in these patients a metabolic pattern different from the normal one, and that it probably is not the consequence but rather the cause of certain mental diseases.[HH] Hoskins and Pincus have connected these discoveries with endocrine alterations, especially of the adrenal gland. Other scientists, particularly A. M. Sackler, M. D. Sackler, R. R. Sackler, Co-Tui, and La Burt, all of the Creedmoor Institute, have demonstrated in their outstanding contributions the immense therapeutic and etiogenic possibilities of the adrenals in psychiatry. In another paper we shall study their historical contribution to the use of adrenal and sex hormones in psychiatry.

The new concepts derived from the study of cortisone establish that this hormone depresses the reactional capacity of the organic cells to toxic stimuli. Claude Bernard's idea of the importance of the "constancy of the internal milieu" of the organism has been of the greatest importance in interpreting the function in complex organisms. Today it is felt that adrenal steroids confer upon cells the capacity of resisting abnormalities of the inner milieu, which seems to be more important in the preservation of cellular functions than the constancy of the internal milieu. In this way even the basic ideas of the Father of Physiology have been revolutionized.

A NEW NEUROENDOCRINE PHILOSOPHY

The endocrine system develops from the tissues that form part of the barrier between the external and the internal milieu of the organism, and it is related to the regulation of the passage—inward and outward—of the components of the primitive external milieu to the internal milieu. Among these components are sodium, chloride, potassium, and other mineral ions. The adrenal hormones seem to be related to the passage of substances through the barrier between the internal milieu and the interior of the cell. Perhaps the hypothalamus, whose centers regulate and coordinate endocrine activity, contains tissues in which the interior of the cell is exposed *directly* to the effect of the internal milieu. The beneficial action of cortisone on the myocardium during rheumatic fever is another fine example of the general process of regulation of intracellular conditions, even if the internal milieu is seriously damaged, and a proof of the fact that the study of the part of the internal milieu most accessible to analysis, the blood, is not an exact pattern of intracellular structure.[11]

If we summarize this historical cavalcade, we see that behind the synthetic concept of the endocrine glands before the seventeenth century, there appeared the analytical concept that in certain tissues there are isolated cells that specialize as incretory cells and fall into groups of diffuse endocrine organs or authentic glands. The next step was to accept the integration of the endocrine system and its role as regulator of metabolism in the body. Harvey Cushing and W. Langdon-Brown demonstrated the role of the pituitary as an organ conducting the endocrine orchestra. It was also thought that it acted as a system of organic chemical integration and regulation, parallel to the system of nervous regulation. The following step was that of synthetic endocrinology and the creation of the neurohumoral concept. Anatomic discoveries proved that the nerve fibers end around the secretory cells; that there is a relationship between the hypothalamus and the pituitary; that the influence of nerve stimulation on humoral secretion and the intimate diencephalopituitary connection; that the demonstration that certain endocrine diseases are due to nerve lesions which act on the hypothalamus and, through the nerve fibers, on the pituitary and other endocrine glands; that the nerve impulse acts through a hormone liberated in the terminal nerve fibers; and that the nervous function is neurohumoral—all these opened new horizons in endocrinology.

The notion expressed twenty-five centuries ago by Alcmæon of Croton, Greek philosopher and a disciple of Pythagoras, that the entire body was integrated by cerebral hegemony, was confirmed by Gaskell's studies on the integrating role of the vegetative system and by Sherrington's studies on the nervous system.

CONCLUSION

The history of our knowledge of the adrenal gland culminates in the recent discoveries of its hormonal functions. The high points of the progress of this history since Addison's clinical findings and Brown-Séquard's physiologic experiments are: the discovery of the adrenal hormones (adrenalin, medullar, and cortical hormones); that the portion of the gland necessary for life is the cortex and not the medulla; the intervention of the adrenals in the metabolic and electrolytic balance and the importance of the disturbance of both equilibriums in adrenal insufficiency; the intervention of the cortical hormones in sex life; and the beginning of a therapy based on saline medication and cortical hormones.

The biography of this idea reveals a concept that has become one of the most important in modern medicine: the concept of internal secretions and their tremendous importance as supreme directive factors in biology and in the clinic.

It is also the story of how the efforts—at first isolated and today harmoniously combined—of physicians, surgeons, physiologists, pathologists, clinicians, chemists,[JJ] and psychiatrists have succeeded in creating a concept that is changing the entire outlook of medicine today. The history of the adrenal gland synthesizes the history of endocrinology. The hundred years from Addison's first clinical description to the present—but especially the first half of our century—have been the most fertile in the history of medicine. Addison established for the first time the correlation between an endocrine gland and a clinical syndrome; the studies made by Oliver and Schafer started the collaboration between clinicians and chemists in the study of medical problems; Kendall's cortisone created a new endocrinologic view in medicine; with Selye, brilliant philosophic ideas have been introduced in biology; the use of steroids in psychiatry initiated neuro-endocrinology.

This is an experiment in writing the biography of an idea, the function of the most mysterious ductless gland, and in tracing its evolution through a century aglow with brilliant medical history. The study of the adrenal gland has only begun. We are living at the beginning of a neuroendocrinologic era in medicine heralded by the study of the adrenals. We have but barely listened to the crow of the cock announcing the dawn of a new day in modern endocrinology.

NOTES

A. The word "endocrinology" was introduced by Nicola Pende (Italy) in 1909 to designate the science of "internal secretions" (Claude Bernard, 1855), which Starling (England) was to call "hormones" (1905).

B. There are ancient traces of organotherapy in the Homeric legend of Achilles who, as a child, was fed lion's marrow, and in the Biblical legend (Book of Tobias) about the Archangel Gabriel, the divine master of organotherapy.

C. Report of the Tenth International Congress on the History of Medicine (Martí-Ibáñez F.: Historical Evolution of the Indian Theory of the Chakras, Madrid, 1934).

D. Martí-Ibáñez, F.: Mystical Psychology and Physiology of India in its Relations to Western Psychology, Madrid, Ediciones de la Universidad de Madrid, 1935.

E. De Bordeu's work was, to certain extent, continued by the French physiologist Gley.

F. A fierce Galenist and an enemy of Vesalius, whom he attacked in his *"De Renibus Libellus"* for "having represented in his *Fabrica* the kidneys of a dog instead of a human."

G. Bernardo Houssay suggested that they be called not "suprarenals" but rather "adrenals," because they may not always be *above* the kidneys but they *are always next to the kidneys.*

_ H. It is of the greatest interest to note that the earliest empirical report on what would later be known as Addison's disease was found by Gregorio Marañón in the work *Fundación del Monasterio de El Escorial* (Foundation of the Monastery of the Escorial), written by Father José de Sigüenza who personally witnessed it. In the year 1577, when Philip II reigned in Spain, a flash of lightning hit the Monastery of El Escorial, which was then under construction, and set the west tower on fire. The monk who took care of the tower clock suffered an accident the consequences of which the illustrious historian of the Order of St. Jerome relates: "A young man who was in orders three or four years, and took care of the clock in the tower, was awakened by its premature ringing. While he was thinking about this, the lightning struck and threw him to the floor in a faint; when he came to, he shouted: 'Fire! Fire in the bell-tower!' He went up and began to ring the bells immediately; at that time he felt nothing; but then, slowly, he was overcome by a heavy melancholy; his color changed from white to a sad brown; black freckles appeared; he lived about three more years and died an unexpected death. It was understood that a humor had entered his body, that night, which caused this."

"There is no doubt," Marañón commented, "that an adrenal insufficiency was involved; this is borne out by the emotional antecedent which plays a part in many clinical histories of this illness; the 'heavy melancholy' which expresses the deep psychic depression of those afflicted with Addison's disease; the change in color which is defined by the very exact phrase 'sad brown'; the innumerable 'black freckles,' that is, the freckles which characterize this melanodermia; the three years which is the average duration of chronic adrenal insufficiency, and finally, the 'unexpected' death which certainly means sudden death: they probably found the monk dead in his cell."

I. Addison's marriage took place in a church the dome of which fell on the altar during a storm a few moments before the ceremony. He interpreted this as an omen.

J. Half a century later, Bulloch and Sequeira (1905) would correlate the suprarenogenital syndrome of virility with the tumors of the adrenal cortex. Later there was established the association of the tumors of adrenal chromaffin cells (pheochromocytomas) with the paroxistic crises of hypertension.

K. At the same time, another giant, Thomas Hodgkin, was curator of the Anatomical Museum of Guy's hospital.

L. To Claude Bernard (1813–1878), whose fame precedes that of Brown-Séquard, we owe the concept (1875) that aside from the *"sécrétions externes"* of the ordinary glands, all organs produce a *"sécrétion interne"* through which they influence the *"milieu interne,"* the composition of which they help to keep invariable, this being a basic law of endocrinology. His concept was too wide, since it did not differentiate between internal secretions and excretions in the blood of metabolites, blood cells, and nutritious substances, and since he included among the endocrine glands the adrenals, thyroid, thymus, spleen and lymphatic ganglia, and among the "partially endocrine" the liver "which pours glucose in the blood," and "the lungs which supply oxygen."

M. Théophile de Bordeu in his *Analyse Médicinale du Sang* pointed out that each organ manufactured substances, of great importance for organic integrity, that penetrated the circulatory system: his famous "specific emanations." His intuitive genius was matched only by Claude Bernard and Brown-Séquard.

N. Years later, when already in his seventies, Brown-Séquard crowned his extraordinary life with his sensational experiments in rejuvenation. He injected himself for two weeks with six testicular emulsions from dogs and guinea pigs with extraordinary results in so far as recovery of his juvenile vigor was concerned, he said. Commenting on this experiment, Olmstead pointed out that Brown-Séquard carried his efforts at rejuvenation so far that shortly after he completed them he was sick with whooping cough.

O. The multiplicity of adrenal hormones served to clear up the confusion that existed between "internal secretions" and "hormones," which until then were considered synonymous. *One* internal secretion, it was discovered, may be composed of several *hormones*.

P. Twenty-two years later Bernardo Houssay (Argentina) and Lewis were to show that the cortex, not the medulla, of the adrenals was the portion necessary for life.

Q. These fibers run through one single nerve in frogs.

R. More recently, Young and others proved that the primary amine corresponding to adrenalin (noradrenalin or arterrenol) is the principal component, and adrenalin the residual component, of the mysterious chemical transmitter of the sympathetic system, extracted from the sympathetic chain, from a purely adrenergic nerve or one which goes out through the splenic veins during stimulation of their adrenergic nerves. Another notable experiment consisted of stimulating the splanchnic nerve and studying the secretion released into the blood by the adrenal medulla; it was observed that it consisted mostly of noradrenalin and after repeated stimulations it may contain only this primary amine.

S. In the lamprey we can observe cells that secrete adrenalin before they gather and form an adrenal gland. Biedl in 1910 demonstrated that in Elasmobranchii, such as the torpedo, it was possible to prove that, because the adrenal cortex forms a separate organ, adrenalin is not the only adrenal hormone, and that the substance indispensable for life is formed in the cortex. If the cortex is removed from these fish without harming the adrenal medulla, signs of adrenal insufficiency appear and death follows.

T. In 1933 Loeb introduced the treatment of Addison's disease with sodium chloride, which had been established experimentally and physiopathologically for years, a measure carried out (Wilder and Kepler, 1937) with diets low in potassium.

Desoxycorticosterone later constituted the basis of therapeutics together with sodium chloride. Thorn proposed (1939) the subcutaneous implantation of desoxycorticosterone compresses. The production of soluble derivatives of this hormone, with the possibility of injecting them intravenously, and the injection of suspensions of crystalloids of retarded absorption (Meier and others) opened up new therapeutic possibilities.

Future progress will depend on the synthesis of other cortical steroids with effects on the carbohydrate metabolism, which will allow completion of desoxycorticosterone. The amorphous fraction that remains after having obtained the crystalline fractions is much more potent in its effect on the distribution of electrolytes than desoxycorticosterone itself. This fraction may hold a new therapeutic possibility.

A number of scientists have experimented on the treatment of adrenal insufficiency with synthetic compounds, the chemical characteristic of which is that it contains oxidized C 11 in the form of COH or CO, that is, the 11-oxy-corticosteroids. The tests involve 11-dehydro-corticosterone (compound A) and 11-dehydro-17-hydroxy-corticosterone (compound E), (Perera, Blood, Forsham, Thorn, Hamburger, Abels, Randall, Sprague, Gatineau, Power, and others, 1946–1948). These hormones, unlike desoxycorticosterone, exercise experimentally a marked activity on carbohydrate metabolism; on the other hand they have little influence on electrolytic balance (compound A), or else they have a contrary action with a paradoxical increase in the elimination of chloride and sodium (compound E). The 11-dehydro-17-hydroxycorticosterone (compound E) has a comparable action on carbohydrate metabolism, but it provokes an increase in the renal elimination of sodium chloride.

U. Mineralo-corticoid steroids act on the regulation of the electrolytic balance; they provoke the retention of sodium and water and increase urinary excretion of potassium and phosphorus but have no important influence on glucide metabolism. They represent a small group with two components: 11-desoxycorticosterone and 17-hydroxy-desoxycorticosterone. The glucocorticoids affect glucide metabolism, avoiding the fall of hepatic glycogen.

V. In desoxycorticosterone there are three atoms of oxygen, and in chemical complexity it is followed by compound A, which has one atom of oxygen in position 11, and compound E, which has a fifth atom of oxygen in position 17.

W. In 1940 it was generally accepted that the twenty-eight steroids isolated from the gland could be divided into four groups: the sex hormones (androgens, estrogens, and progesterones) which were not characteristic of the adrenal cortex; the group of physiologically inert cortico-adrenal steroids; the six derived from the 4-pregnene, which possess physiologic activity; and the residuum after the separation of the crystalline compounds, an amorphous fraction of intense action on the electrolytic metabolism. The work of Kendall and Sarett prepared the way for the development of 17-hydroxy-11-dehydrocorticosterone, compound E or cortisone (Sarett, 1948), which followed compound A by Kendall in 1940–44. In 1950 (Wendler et al, Merck, 1951) 17-hydroxycorticosterone, compound F or hydrocortisone, was developed.

X. Pincus' experiments, isolating the adrenal by perfusion, showed that the potent enzymic system of its tissues may catalyze the introduction of a hydroxyl group at position 11 of the steroid nucleus.

Y. The quantity of hormones segregated normally by the adrenal gland in a dog, according to Vogt (1943–47), is more than 5 mg./Kg. daily; in a human being it would be about 350 mg./Kg. daily.

Z. In 1951 Kendall was still wondering if "substance X" was cortisone or not.

AA. Selye formulated his theory after having injected ovarian hormone extracts into rats for the purpose of finding a new hormone. What he found when he performed autopsy on the rats was not the ovarian hormone but signs of poisoning similar to those observed in the necropsy of rats intoxicated with laboratory poisons. Despite the fact that the injection consisted of a biologic substance that exists in rats, the little adrenal glands were enlarged, the thymus was destroyed, and the stomach ulcerated. At that moment it occurred to Selye that the rats had not died from poisoning. The autopsy revealed a condition in the body similar to that in rats that had died from tension and fatigue. Selye published his discovery, explaining that fatigue and tension had killed the rats; but his work was ignored by the scientific world, and with the rats was buried the concept that fourteen years later would cause a great scientific revolution.

BB. In the course of the general adaptation syndrome, body heat decreases, glycemia increases, the adrenal cortex suffers hyperplasia and cellular disintegration. According to Selye, during stress there prevails a state of relative cortico-adrenal insufficiency and the lack of corticoids increases the production of pituitary corticotropin, thus starting the defense reaction. During the countershock phase of the alarm reaction, general resistance increases, which implies a mobilization of the organism's "adaptability." On the other hand, after the organism develops resistance and becomes adapted to a stress agent, it becomes especially vulnerable to other harmful stimuli, which suggests that it has a limited degree of adaptive energy. The stress starts a chain of reactions through a channel as yet unidentified, and then brings into action the mechanism of pituitary-adrenal defense, acting first on the pituitary by inducing it to increase the production of corticotropin and warding off the production of the other pituitary hormones. This causes a cortico-adrenal hypertrophy with hyperproduction of corticoids, which produce organic metabolic alterations and atrophy of the thymus and lymphatic organs, also affecting the cardiovascular apparatus, kidneys, articulations, and blood pressure.

CC. Claude Bernard was interested in studying organic adaptation to slight stimuli by metabolic variations of the internal milieu; Selye concentrated on adaptation to excessive and unspecific stimuli. The hormones segregated by the adrenal cortex to carry out this unspecific adaptation are: the glucocorticoids (of which cortisone is the main one), which have the property of transforming proteins into glucose; and the mineralo-corticoids, among them desoxycorticosterone acetate (DOCA), which regulate the retention of minerals like sodium. Some factor, as yet unknown, determines the first phase of the general adaptation syndrome; cortisone acts in a second phase; and DOCA in the third. The ACTH hormone causes the liberation of cortisone, but the pituitary hormone that liberates DOCA is not known. It is believed that the external stimulus causes the secretion of adrenalin which is followed by the pituitary ACTH which, in its turn, induces the adrenal cortex to secrete cortisone. Another pituitary hormone, somatotropin, activates the mineralo-corticoids of the DOCA type, like desoxycorticosterone.

DD. One of the important modern contributions to psychiatry was the incorporation of the adrenals by several scientists, especially Gregorio Marañón in Spain, into the group of endocrine extragonadal glands of sexual action, or, in other words, glands that favor the upsurge of sex in a general sense and act in a specific sexual sense by favoring the development of virile and feminine characteristics. The masculinizing group is represented principally by the adrenal cortex and the pituitary, which exercise said function in both sexes; and the feminizing group is represented by the thyroid.

EE. ACTH acts on the adrenal cortex as its only stimulant, since only the adrenal medulla has nerves.

FF. Interest in the study of the adrenal function in schizophrenics was born of the consideration that such patients, when threatened by external stress, react by withdrawing into their inner world. This led scientists to subject normal and schizophrenic subjects to tests of emotional stress to induce corticoadrenal stimulation.

The History of Endocrinology   253

GG. Selye has shown that the human body responds in a stereotyped way to numerous agents of different specific effects (infections, intoxications, traumatisms, emotional tension, heat, cold, excessive physical fatigue, or radiations), the common denominator of which is that they place the organism in a state of stress. The first manifestations of response to stress are cortico-adrenal enlargement, thymo-lymphatic involution, gastrointestinal ulcers, and shock. While other organs show degenerative changes, the adrenal seems to spring into activity, sending out a "call to arms" to the organism and its defensive forces (alarm reaction). These reactions do not occur in animals whose adrenals have been removed unless cortico-adrenal hormones are injected into them. When it was discovered that hypophysectomy prevents adrenal response during alarm reaction, it was deduced that stress stimulates the adrenal cortex through the pituitary ACTH hormone.

The mechanism is supposed to be the following: the agent of the stress acts directly on the organic cells, producing lesions in them. The lesioned organ—through humoral or nerve channels, we do not yet know which—stimulates the anterior pituitary which produces ACTH and sometime STH, that is, the somatotropic hormone. The ACTH hormone stimulates the production in the adrenal cortex of glucocorticoid compounds like cortisone, which have an inhibiting effect on the lesioned organs. The STH hormone stimulates defensively the conjunctive tissue of the organs attacked and increases the production of mineralo-corticoids.

HH. Chromatography on paper has been of great value in studying the elimination of amino acids, just as flame photometry has aided in discovering an important feature of schizophrenia. Schizophrenics do not respond to situations of stress like normal people, in whom this situation normally provokes a flow (started by the pituitary ACTH) of steroid hormones of the adrenal cortex. In schizophrenics, this adrenal response does not exist even if the patients are injected with ACTH. As the function of the steroid cortical hormones is, among others, to regulate the electrolyte and aqueous balance in the body, especially of sodium and potassium, the changes in the concentration of these two salts are one of the most useful indices in the investigation of the level of the cortico-adrenal hormones; flame photometry is used as the most rapid and exact method of determining the organic content of sodium and potassium.

II. In his essay on "The Humanization of Man," L. Bolk, Professor of Anatomy in Amsterdam, points out that the essential characteristic of man as an organism is the slow *tempo* at which he develops. He calls this the "principle of retardation in the humanization of man" and considers it the result of a "fetalization" to which man owes the historical humanization of his form. ("Man," said Bolk, "is a primate fetus which has come to sexual maturity.")

This delay—according to Bolk—is the result of the action of the endocrine system directing the constitution of form and its preservation, which are based on metabolic processes. The hormones accelerate or retard growth, since any organic property can be accelerated or rejected. The maximum of retardation is the biologic stop, or in other words, the repression of the birth of a property, which explains the fact that certain human characteristics, such as lack of hair on the body, or loss of pigmentation, present a negative character in comparison with similar states in monkeys.

The causal relationship between endocrine action and the historical evolution of the human form throws light on some atavisms that bespeak the pithecoid nature of the human being. The endocrine influence on evolution was retarding. The retarding hormones repressed certain properties in a state of latency. Hormonal normality guarantees that latency; its abnormality gives free rein to retarded or deadened properties (hirsutism, pigmentation, acromegaly) when certain hormones are altered. The endocrine system holds back sexual life; but if it is altered, sexual precocity follows, as happened with our ancestors. For Bolk, endocrine symptoms are pithecoid characteristics, and innate deformities are the result of arrested development and endocrinopathies. The historic evolution of the form of our body is directed by endocrine chemistry; the endocrine system divides the entire organism and forms an *imperium in imperio*. For Bolk, the human being consists of soma, germa, and endocrinon. The germa regulates the genesis of the species; the endocrinon, the genesis of form in the individual and its preservation. The decadence of the species indicates that the germa is insufficient; individual senilization indicates insufficiency of the endocrinon.

JJ. The services of organic chemistry have never been as important as in endocrinology. Methods of endocrine research include: (1) correlation of the clinical features with anatomopathologic alterations in the endocrine gland, which was the method used by Addison; it may be associated with observation or the substitution treatment, that is, the clinical effect of the administration of an extract of a lesioned endocrine gland and the removal of a gland considered hyperactive, like the adrenal in the suprarenogenital syndrome; (2) the experimental removal of the normal endocrine glands, and, when the symptoms have been produced, the insertion of the same gland in the animal or the injection of its extracts; (3) extending in successive generations of animals the excision of the endocrine organ or the administration of its extract; and (4) the isolation, crystallization, and synthesis of the hormones by organic chemicals, a recent historical event of supreme importance.

THE MIND AND THE WORLD OF
PAUL EHRLICH

TIME AND SPACE IN HISTORICAL BIOGRAPHY

hne Hast, ohne Rast. Without haste, without pause. The Goethean* motto of Paul Ehrlich, father of modern chemotherapy, whose centenary physicians the world over are celebrating this month,† is still an inspiration to the scientists of our time. There are two kinds of great men in history: men of action, whose great deeds exercised an enlightening influence on their contemporaries and became a source of encouragement and inspiration for the generations to come; and men of thought, who handed their great knowledge down to posterity in their written word.

In the history of medicine, men of action were Boerhaave and Paré, who are remembered more for their personalities than for anything else; men of thought were Avicenna and Vesalius, whose *Canon* and *Fabrica,* respectively, were of such importance that they almost eclipsed the men who penned them.

But there are also men who leave behind them both great actions and great written works, men who soar to towering heights leaving in their wake a glorious scar on the face of the earth. Such a man was Paul Ehrlich, of whom it can be said—as was said of Claude Bernard in connection with physiology—that he was not a chemotherapist but chemotherapy itself.

From *International Record of Medicine* 167:143, 1954.
* Goethe's motto was similar: "Without haste, but without pause, like the stars."
† March, 1954.

Our interpretation of the history of medicine is no longer based on a conception of genius as an isolated phenomenon. Today we realize that the man of genius can be thoroughly understood only if we place him against the background of his time and his milieu. By projecting a life in time and space, we can uncover the meaning of the psychologic motives behind the man and his scientific development. The scientist is also a man, a human being who lives in a certain country at a given time, and these two factors condition the genesis and significance of his work. The brain of the investigator is not a point isolated in ether; it is an organ that is subject to the influences of space and time—milieu and epoch—and it reflects the cultural complex of the age in which it lives.

THE WORLD OF PAUL EHRLICH—A GLIMPSE INTO NINETEENTH CENTURY SCIENCE

Paul Ehrlich was born in the middle of the nineteenth century (in Strehlen, Silesia, March 14, 1854). If our own century has been shaken by the portentous advances made in therapeutics, the last half of the last century truly trembled beneath the firm tread of notable advances in the art of diagnosis. The laboratory played the all-important role then, just as the clinic does now. The late nineteenth century physician lived in an atmosphere galvanized by philosophic theories. Europe was still agitated by a tidal wave of political upheavals. The governments of France and Germany had just suppressed several revolutionary movements. England, under the iron hand of Queen Victoria, tried to stanch the wounds caused by the war in the Punjab. There was a renaissance of cultural and religious interests. The technologic revolution was making rapid headway, but the horse was still a very important means of transportation and railroads had scarcely begun to embroider the planet with cobwebs of rails.

In the middle of that century, medicine was still encyclopedic and the physician aimed at competence in all fields of his endeavor. A professor of medicine still tried to teach all phases of medicine. In 1848 a professor at Rostock taught clinical medicine, surgery, ophthalmology, and obstetrics! The scientific panorama was dominated by the work of Virchow, cellular architect, Pasteur, magician of ferments, and Claude Bernard, cartographer of physiology. The importance of anatomy in a physician's education had already been recognized, but medicine was not yet a science. By 1850 the use of chloroform, ether, and nitrous oxide had been discovered. The discovery of antiseptics twenty years later made possible scientific surgery. The theory of the conservation of energy dominated the universe of the physicist, while Darwinian evolutionism pervaded the world of the biologist. There was a general acceptance of the supremacy of the nervous system as rector of the organism, and the old Platonic concept of the unity of the soma and psyche was reborn. Physicians were beginning to specialize, and the year of Ehrlich's birth saw the recruiting of nurses for the Crimean War.

In the forty-six years that elapsed between Ehrlich's birth and the turn of the century, amazing progress was made in medicine, thus providing a historic parallel to the scientific development of Ehrlich himself. As Ehrlich grew from adolescence to youth and then to maturity, he witnessed the experimental confirmation of the bacterial origin of infections and the change from active immunization by vaccines to passive immunization by serums. The imperialistic ambitions of some nations were, paradoxically, to stimulate notable advances in tropical medicine. Since the jungle held back the ambitions of Germany and England, it became necessary to defeat the jungle in the laboratory. That was the beginning of the victory over recurrent fever, dysentery, malaria, filariasis, and trypanosomiasis.

After fifteen hundred years of stagnation, the last quarter of the nineteenth century witnessed the birth of modern therapeutics. In 1874 antipyrin was synthesized, while the introduction of the first thyroid extracts in 1891 marked the beginning of modern endocrinology. Such therapeutic resources were soon followed by the use of radiation, vitamins, immunobiology, and psychoanalysis.

Into this medical world in ferment, Paul Ehrlich was born. We must, however, bear in mind that not until Ehrlich reached maturity did the world realize that the true objective of medicine was to heal, and that although the art of diagnosis was of transcendental importance, it was not—philosophically speaking, at least—an indispensable requisite for curing the sick. This helps us to understand young Ehrlich's anxiety to go beyond his time and discover the cure for some of the age-old plagues that scourged mankind. Ehrlich's scientific optimism challenged the ebbing strength of that therapeutic nihilism emanating from the famed medical school of Vienna. Almost from childhood, the budding genius was gnawed by an obsession to find a pharmacologic panacea to cure all illnesses.

EHRLICH'S YOUTH—THE SPELL OF THE BRILLIANT DYES

Paul Ehrlich was an absent-minded child and later an unsatisfactory student. It is interesting to observe how often the childhood of a genius is characterized by apparent backwardness. The superior mentality of the child prevents him from adapting himself to the absurd routines and rigid disciplines that govern the school life of his so-called "normal" companions.

Ehrlich studied medicine at the universities of Breslau, Strasbourg, and Leipzig. His lack of concentration and excessive slovenliness caused his teachers to despair. Like Ramón y Cajal, who failed in anatomy only to receive the Nobel Prize years later for his anatomic discoveries, Ehrlich failed in chemistry, the very field in which he was to make his name.

When he was graduated, the laboratory assistants heaved a sigh of relief at being rid of the absurd young man who was forever dabbling in dyestuffs, bespattering not only all his clothes but the walls of the laboratory. Indeed, when Koch once visited the laboratory someone pointed out to him Ehrlich's table, all smeared with dyes, and remarked that "he would never get to pass his courses."

From adolescence on, Ehrlich had been fascinated by the complicated architecture of the cell and bewitched by the modern alchemy of the laboratory. Histology and chemistry were the springboards for his future accomplishments. Day after day his curious little myopic eyes peered through the microscope at the manifold cellular formations; then, in the laboratory, he tried to ascertain the composition of the mysterious substance that filled the pale cellular profiles.

One day his cousin Carl Weigert, the indefatigable histologist from Silesia, taught him the technique of dyeing bacteria with coloring anilines. At that time researchers were beginning to stain sections of tissues from the various organs on a large scale, availing themselves of special dyes to study the different affinity of each dye for given organic cells. Histologists were intrigued by the mysterious preferences of a given coloring agent for certain tissues and thus arrived at an all-important method for differentiating one tissue from another.

During Ehrlich's student years, German industry produced an amazing number of new coloring anilines for use in textile factories. In the laboratory, the young student, his fingers and clothes forever stained with brilliant greens, blues, yellows, and reds, dyed one tissue after another, then placed them under the microscope and discovered a magic world of vivid colors and brilliant irisations.

Like Ramón y Cajal, whose childhood dreams about remote unexplored lands led him years later to call the brain "a matted jungle" and to enrich histopathologic terminology with an arsenal of words related to forests and fields, Ehrlich escaped from the gray monotony of his prosaic environment into the multicolored world revealed by his microscopic slides. With the passion of the lover and of the fanatic, he fused into one his two great scientific interests: histology and chemistry.

Ehrlich's doctoral thesis was on histologic methods involving anilines. When he was granted his degree in 1878, he began work with

Frerichs, with whom he spent seven years followed by a few years with Gerhardt. His first scientific undertaking was concerned with the use of his beloved coloring agents on blood and led to the discovery that different types of blood corpuscles have affinities for different staining agents. This helped him to study the variable ratio of the different blood cells in infections, a method of immense diagnostic value. Ehrlich's very first venture into the scientific arena already modified and enriched Virchow's work in cellular morphology.

His next step was to study the staining of *living* tissues. At this stage he began his research with methylene blue,* another one of his precious atoxic dyes which, as it was absorbed in the tissues, revealed what happened to oxygen inside the human body. In 1885 Ehrlich published his book *Das Sauerstoffbedürfnis des Organismus,* in which he studied the need of the organism for oxygen and developed a method for studying intimate cellular functions in vitro.†

WORK IN HEMATOLOGY

It is at this point that Ehrlich's genius shot over the horizon like a star-crested rocket. His method of intravital staining provided the cornerstone for modern chemotherapy and ushered in a new era in the study of immunity. Using the "trial and error" method, Ehrlich plunged into what he called *Spiel-Chemie,* or play-chemistry, and like a first-rate prestidigitator, he pulled out of his sleeve a series of

* Ehrlich was the first to use methylene blue as a bacteriologic staining agent. It has been pointed out that Ehrlich did for aniline dyes what Mayer would do ten years later for carmine and hematoxylin.

† It is not our purpose to study here the work of Paul Ehrlich so much as his thought and the philosophic meaning of his life. The scientific harvest of Ehrlich's mature years was rich and abundant. Let us mention here but a few of his contributions: his methods of dyeing and fixing hematic corpuscles with heat; his classification of leukocytes into acidophils, basophils, and neutrophils on the basis of their granulations; his differentiation of leukemias and of myeloid and lymphoid tissues; the distinction he drew between normoblasts and megaloblasts; his demonstration that leukocytosis is a function of the bone marrow; his study of aplastic anemia; his staining of the tubercle bacillus with fuchsin; his diazoreaction of urine used in the diagnosis of typhoid; his sulfodiazobenzol test for bilirubin; his investigation of the microchemical reactions of tissues to coloring substances; his studies of the requirement of oxygen by the body, which was the seed that blossomed into his theory of side chains; his perfecting of Behring's diphtheria antitoxin; his studies on immunity in cancer; his use of methylene blue as a chemotherapeutic agent against the quartan form of intermittent fever; his use of trypan red against cow pyroplasmosis and of arsenophenilglycene in trypanosomiasis. And especially his philosophic conception of the "side chains" based on the hypothesis that the molecule of living protoplasm contains a central stable nucleus and unstable peripheral side "chains," which he called "chemoreceptors," capable of combining chemically with nourishing substances and of neutralizing toxins or poisons by throwing the loosened side chains into the circulatory system.

spectacular discoveries. His "chemical imagination," or the power to conceive new paths of investigation in several different fields of chemistry, made him the greatest biochemical philosopher in history.

When Ehrlich's name is mentioned we generally think of the discoverer of salvarsan, but we should not forget that he was also the founder of modern hematology, that he converted what was previously descriptive cellular pathology into experimental intracellular chemistry, and that he laid the foundations for chemotherapy.

When Frerichs died and Ehrlich realized that his successor Gerhardt was not interested in furthering his research, he resigned his post at the Charité Hospital in Berlin. This decision, however, was not really motivated by the lack of funds for further work. There was another reason. As a result of years of work with the tuberculosis bacilli, Ehrlich's lungs became infected. The terrifying disease suddenly threatened to cut short his career. Never is the lesson of humility given us by the failings of the body as tragic as when it is experienced by a great man. Realizing that if he stayed in cold misty Berlin he was lost, Ehrlich decided to journey to Egypt in an attempt to regain his health.

Ehrlich remained in Egypt from 1887 to 1890. The hot sun, the dry air, and physical rest—we cannot talk of mental rest, since for genius it does not exist—produced the desired effect. A cured and eager Ehrlich left the hot honey-colored African lands and returned to the mists of Berlin to continue his scientific adventures in the iridescent world of stained cells.

A NEW PHILOSOPHY OF IMMUNITY AND A
NEW CONCEPT OF THERAPEUTICS

Ehrlich was thirty-three years old when he returned to Berlin. He knew that a medical practice would not leave him sufficient time for research. He decided therefore to sacrifice his financial security rather than to give up his dreams. He rented a tiny apartment in a remote neighborhood of Berlin and—again like Cajal in his Madrid home—turned it into a laboratory, alternating between his work as *Privatdozent* (he later became professor) and the search for new scientific horizons.

Once again Ehrlich's life was characterized by the originality of his scientific undertakings. I believe that, philosophically, a human being lives by creating his own life at every step and expressing it in each one of his thoughts, words, and actions. That is why to be a *person,* in the true psychosocial meaning of the word, is to be *original,* a quality conditioned by two factors: the inner germ of originality that exists in every human being, and the historic situation— milieu and time—that surrounds the person, which may encourage the development of that originality or may paralyze it. The essence of genius has always been to impose the creative force of originality on external conditions and, if such conditions be adverse, to rise above them, just as the great poet forges lovely verses even from his agony.

Ehrlich threw himself with characteristic enthusiasm into his study of the problems of an embryonic scientific discipline: immunobiology. At that time scientists were beginning to give more consideration to bacterial toxins than to bacteria, just as years later in endocrinology hormones would be considered more important than the endocrine glands. The discovery of the diphtheria antitoxin had revolutionized the cathartic theories of ancient therapeutics, for it was established that we come closer to the processes of nature itself if instead of supplying the organism with exogenous medication we provide it with the instruments required to bolster its natural defenses, whether through phagocytosis or the action of organic fluids. It was more effective to provoke active immunization through vaccines or passive immunization through serums than to attack the pathogenic germs chemically. Scientists learned then that, in legitimate defense against any bacterial toxin, the organism created its own antitoxins. By analogy, certain poisons, like ricin, provoked a similar reaction of immunity in the organism.

Ehrlich studied the laws of immunity and developed various methods of encouraging active or passive immunity in infections. His studies culminated in the concept—so basic to immunology—known as the theory of "side chains." That theory, originally formulated to explain the formation of antitoxins, led Ehrlich to conceive the possibility of completely overcoming a toxin by *using a drug* instead of an antitoxin. In that sense, chemotherapy was later born in Ehrlich's brain as a concept philosophically destined to complete—and compete with—immunobiology.

Ehrlich's masterly contribution, then, was the idea that drugs could do what antitoxins did. A synthetic organic compound could, theoretically speaking, bear a side chain that would adhere to a bacterial poison or neutralize the microbe and thus destroy it. Nowadays, the word "chemotherapy" is used to designate the treatment of parasitic diseases through chemical control of the infecting agent without any marked toxic effect on the patient. But originally "chemotherapy" meant the treatment of any illness by means of a chemical agent of known composition.

Ehrlich's philosophic concepts were responsible for an immense leap forward in the historical evolution of therapeutics. For fifteen centuries, first witch doctors and then physicians had considered disease to be the result of a foreign body, e.g., demon, miasma, or germ, entering the organism, which therefore had to be expelled by exorcisms, enemas, diaphoretics, or bloodletting. The new concept of immunobiology maintained that the important issue was to stimulate and reinforce natural organic defenses. Immunobiology thus represented the historical transition between curative magic and modern chemotherapy.

ON THE THRESHOLD OF CHROMOTHERAPY

Ehrlich's work attracted the attention of Robert Koch, who was already at the peak of his fame. In 1890 Koch placed Ehrlich in charge of an observation room at the Moabit Hospital containing patients experimentally treated with tuberculin. The following year, when the Institute for Infectious Diseases was founded, Koch furnished Ehrlich with fresh opportunities for work. Genius never fears genius. A great man is never afraid to surround himself with other great men.

Since serotherapy was making huge strides in a Germany that was leading the world in scientific progress, Althoff, the Prussian Minister of State, decided to establish an official institute for serum research. The *Institut für Serumforschung* was opened in Steglitz. It had two rooms, one had formerly been a bakery, and the other a stable. Ehrlich was appointed director of the institute and was provided with facilities for work. Thus his genius was "officially" recognized. Three years later the *Institut für experimentelle Therapie* was established under Ehrlich's supervision at Frankfurt-am-Main; in 1906 it became affiliated with the Georg Speyer Institute for Chemotherapy. (Ehrlich's loyal wife was responsible for the foundation of the Speyer Institute, for it was she who persuaded Speyer's widow to establish an institute in memory of her husband.) And so it came to pass that Ehrlich finally saw the realization of an investigator's most cherished dream: to have a laboratory of his own and the tools vital to the fulfillment of his dreams.

It is a characteristic of the great researcher to deviate suddenly from his original ideas. Such changes may be incomprehensible to the contemporary observer, but when examined in the light of final results they seem not so much deviations as a broadening of the original horizon. Ehrlich at this point decided to concentrate his efforts on therapeutics, although he never abandoned his work with coloring dyes which were as much an integral part of his soul as of his hands and clothes.

The original philosophic concept that provided Ehrlich's point of departure was that if certain chemical staining substances possess a special affinity for given organic tissues, it might be possible to find dyes that would adhere *only* to bacteria without affecting the cells invaded by those bacteria. And if the amount of nontoxic coloring agents applied to the invaded organism was strong enough, it might be possible to destroy *with colors* the invading microbes without harming the invaded cells. Thus, Ehrlich focused his research upon the vast problem of finding staining chemical substances with a strong affinity for bacteria and little affinity for organic cells.

His initial results were not too encouraging. The compounds that seemed capable of killing parasites were too organotropic, while the others were not sufficiently parasitotropic.

Ehrlich was then forced to work within the narrow limits of tolerated and toxic effects, and he found it necessary to discover some means of expressing the chemotherapeutic activity of the compounds for purposes of comparison. He therefore determined for each new substance the ratio between the minimal therapeutic dose and the maximum tolerated dose and called it the chemotherapeutic index.

That was the beginning of the decisive stage in Ehrlich's life. His laboratory became a beehive of activity. As soon as German industry brought out any new dyestuffs, Ehrlich tried them out on his laboratory animals. The fact that when he injected mice with methylene blue only the nervous system was dyed in blue led him to the idea that he could probably inject colorants into a living animal or human being, color the invading microbes, and thus kill them *with dyes*. Modern chemotherapy really started as a true *chromotherapy* or therapy by means of dyes.

Ehrlich's laboratory, where Jews, Prussians, and Japanese fraternized and worked happily, became an amazing center of experimentation with dyes. Every day Ehrlich and his loyal collaborators, Bertheim, Hata, and Kadereit, tested hundreds of dyes with no greater result than the conversion of papers, books, and walls into samples of the rainbow. And as the days went by, their hands and everything around them were smeared with bright gay colors, but their hearts remained dark and gloomy under the pall of discouragement.

AND THE MAGIC BULLET

It was at this juncture that Ehrlich noticed that some dyes, like the trypan red he introduced as a therapeutic agent for trypanosomiasis in mice, had a strange quality. He observed that the trypanosomes dyed with trypan red, instead of dying, swam merrily in a drop of blood; they, however, lost this infecting capacity when inoculated in mice. The reactions between chemotherapeutic agents and parasites were quite often produced *within* the human body but *were not* produced in vitro. This indicated that dyes tended to prevent reproduction of the germs within the human body, and the germs were therefore devoured by the phagocytes or were swept out by the broom of organic defenses. Thus, Ehrlich achieved the first chemical interference with bacterial reproduction and provided what is today one of the basic principles of chemotherapy.

When Ehrlich learned that atoxyl was more efficient than other arsenicals in experimental trypanosomiasis, he tried to modify its chemical structure by making it more specifically toxic for certain microbes.

In 1905, the same year that Schaudinn and Hoffmann discovered a pale undulating parasite, which they called *Spirochaeta pallida,* Ehrlich studied the effect of atoxyl on sleeping sickness. To his disappointment he discovered that besides being toxic it was ineffective in vitro. He then decided to modify atoxyl and make it atoxic for living beings and lethal for microbes. His objective was to find an efficient treatment for sleeping sickness, the African *nagana* and the South American *mal de caderas.* One after another he developed modified compounds of atoxyl which he tested in his laboratory without success. In contrast with other scientists who are only too ready to publish the results of even their failures, Ehrlich remained silent and continued to live like a monk.

Those were trying days for Ehrlich. It was a strange man his neighbors saw: small, thin, absent-minded, simple, often impatient with people and even more so with himself, his clothes forever spotted with dyes and tobacco ash for he was always smoking ominous-looking black cigars imported from a Broadway drugstore in New York. He never had a free hour, nor did he allow himself any amusement except the occasional perusal of a detective-story magazine to which he subscribed. He scribbled formulas everywhere —on the menus of beer halls where he sometimes supped with his collaborators, on the walls of his bedroom, on any blank surface. His scientific imagination burned like a light bulb that never goes out.

On the other hand, he hated to expound his theories or write papers. But since he could not avoid such tasks and was often compelled to write scientific monographs, he would shout his words incoherently while striding up and down his laboratory, and his assistants would try to put together a coherent text. In that form the work was delivered to the printer and finally published with few, if any, corrections.

Six hundred and five times Ehrlich failed. In 1907 he developed compound 606, which became a spectacular cure for trypanosomiasis and spirochetosis in chickens and mice as well as for *mal de caderas* in horses. What was even more amazing, compound 606, later called salvarsan or arsphenamine, could cure syphilis in monkeys and rabbits.

Compound 606, or diaminodihydroxyarsenobenzene dihydrochloride, did not kill the protozoa causing the illness in vitro, but only *within* the living organism when the body cells liberated the arsenic from the product injected, after ionizing it into the pentavalent form. Two years later, in 1909, the final step was taken and 606 was tried with complete success in human victims of syphilis. In a single year (1910) sixty-five thousand injections of salvarsan were given. The whole world rejoiced. Paul Ehrlich, who had once said, "We must learn to make magic bullets which, like those of the ancient fable, will not miss the mark and will destroy only those pathogenic agents they are aimed at," had carried out his magnificent dream. The age-old disease, which the Renaissance poet-physician Fracastoro had named "syphilis," was at last curable, thanks to the genius and perseverance of Ehrlich.*

Salvarsan did not turn out to be in the fullest sense the *therapia sterilisans magna* for syphilis that Ehrlich had hoped it would be, but it served to cure recurrent fever, yaws, certain forms of angina, Aleppo boil, and many epizootics.†

Two years later Ehrlich developed a much more soluble and less toxic form of salvarsan, compound 914 or neosalvarsan. A new "bullet" was added to his arsenal of magic weapons against syphilis.

Three years later, on August 20, 1915, Paul Ehrlich died. As was said when Wagner died, that day the world lost some of its value.

AN EVALUATION OF THE RESEARCHER OF YESTERDAY AND THE RESEARCHER OF TODAY

When we try, thirty-nine years after Ehrlich's death, to evaluate his work and thought, we are faced with the contrast between the Ehrlich of the first half of his life and the Ehrlich of the final years. At the end of the last century, Ehrlich stands out as the prototype of the individualistic and romantic scholar, still common at that time.

But with the years, scientific research has become "de-individualized"; it has become a collective undertaking, a matter of teamwork. The scientist has rearranged the compartments of his mind and has become a good organizer, capable of managing the powerful instruments put in his hands by industry, official organizations, or university centers; he has become the captain of a team of collaborators.

---

* Paradoxically, Paul Ehrlich was awarded the Nobel Prize, together with Elias Metchnikoff, for his work in immunobiology before achieving this great victory.

† My friend and teacher, Gregorio Marañón, was studying with Ehrlich in Berlin during the year of his great discovery. At Ehrlich's special request, Marañón took back to Spain some of the rare golden powder to fight smallpox and typhus, which in those days were causing many deaths in my native land.

He is no longer the individual explorer drawing the map of a *terra incognita*. Today, he is the leader of a scientific expedition, methodically supervising the cartography of unknown lands. The old-style scientist made his very home a laboratory and workshop. Ehrlich, like Cajal and Freud, was both captain and soldier of his own personal crusade. Heir to the noble tradition of Pasteur, he did research on his own because he was compelled by a passion for knowledge. To his work he sacrificed his personal well-being and economic security.

EHRLICH'S "ERRORS"

Nowadays, we frequently hear about Ehrlich's "errors." But Ehrlich's "errors" were fruitful. His theory of side chains has been criticized, yet that theory has been a heuristic principle behind immunobiology for a quarter of a century. His 606 was not the final solution to the problem of syphilis, but it cured many other diseases. Ehrlich may have overevaluated the idea that a disease is the effect of a germ and neglected the fact that the characteristics of an infection are specially determined by the reaction of the host and not by the nature of the parasite. But because of this concept, he sought a method of destroying parasites and converted his erroneous concept into a glorious truth. Perhaps he was too fond of complex theories and complicated hypotheses to refute his adversaries, thus repeating Galen's mistakes; and he was fond of quoting Duns Scotus and St. Thomas Aquinas in his addresses to his scientific enemies, thus overwhelming them with Latinisms. But perhaps this was pure mischief— a child's mischief that age had not overcome.

If Ehrlich was fond of complex theories, he was equally addicted to simple instruments. He reminds us of the advice Harvey Cushing once gave to a young researcher who was compiling a long list of expensive equipment for a new laboratory: "All you need to do research is running water and one idea." In Ehrlich's laboratory there was an enormous table piled high with test tubes and bottles and a lonely Bunsen burner, whose tiny flame seemed to symbolize the ever-incandescent mind of its owner. The simplicity of his methods reflected the simplicity of his manners and his person. And greatness is simplicity.

THE PHILOSOPHIC THOUGHT OF EHRLICH

Ehrlich's philosophic thought is a continuation of Paracelsus' thought. If the *médecin maudit* was the father of medicinal chemistry in the Renaissance and if he entertained the idea of replacing Arabic polypharmacy by a few but select and powerful drugs, Ehrlich was the father of chemotherapy and he replaced *perscrutamini scripturas* by *perscrutamini naturas rerum.* In other words, he preferred observing nature to interpreting books in the Aristotelian fashion.

It has not been sufficiently emphasized that Ehrlich's philosophy represents the revival of Paracelsus' philosophic spirit in an age of scientific materialism. At the end of the nineteenth century, Paracelsus' spirit walked abroad, again impelled by the old obsession to find "specific remedies for specific illnesses." Ehrlich applied this philosophy in his search for a *therapia sterilisans magna,* a sovereign remedy that with one injection would destroy invading bacteria. The result was his side chain theory.

This historic relationship between Paracelsus' and Ehrlich's thought is important for another reason. If antibiotics descend historically from primitive phytotherapy, once called Galenic medication, modern chemotherapy—started by Ehrlich and continued by Domagk (1932) —descends directly from the heavy metals or non-Galenic medications (iron, lead, mercury, arsenic) that Paracelsus used.

The supreme lesson we derive from Ehrlich's thought is the necessity of understanding in time—as he did, and before him as Paracelsus and Descartes did—that in science it is vain to accumulate facts and data unless one is guided by a philosophy that integrates such information rationally, interprets it, and later translates it into practical conclusions.

True science, as Claude Bernard illustrated in his *Introduction à l'Étude de la Médecine Expérimentale* (1865), experimentally establishes a given relationship between phenomena and their immediate cause. "Therapeutics," he said, "will be a science only when it has established the relationship existing between the remedy used and the cure of the sickness." That principle governs research in chemotherapy today just as it did in Ehrlich's work.

Paul Ehrlich was able to reconcile religion, philosophy, and science. He believed. He reasoned. He experimented. He sought God not in the bright light of the stars in the heavens but in the cold, pale gaslight of his laboratory. As time wears on, Ehrlich still holds out to us the *opera omnia* of his scientific discoveries, the supreme lesson of wisdom implicit in personal simplicity, and the grandeur of philosophic ideas. He observed natural phenomena and tore from them the secret of their immutable laws, which he then proceeded to control. Didn't Bacon say *Natura parendo vincitur?* To obey Nature is to learn how to conquer her.

AS I REMEMBER HIM:
SANTIAGO RAMÓN Y CAJAL

I remember seeing him often in the early nineteen-thirties, a pale, pensive, silver-bearded old man, slowly crossing the cool green shades of the patio at the Medical School of San Carlos in Madrid. On the occasion of the centennial of his birth, I want to recall Santiago Ramón y Cajal.

Thanks to him, Spain, which had slowly declined to a state of scientific indigence in sad contrast with the Golden Age of Spanish medicine of the fifteenth and sixteenth centuries, again joined the vanguard of medical progress. Gimbernat in the seventeenth century and Casal in the eighteenth century partly redeemed Spain from her scientific sterility, but it was Cajal who put her back in the scientific hall of fame.

Cajal was born to the gloomy untamed earth of a dusty village in the province of Navarre, on May 1, 1852. His father was a rural doctor. An indifferent, even poor, student, Cajal gave up school to work as apprentice first to a barber and then to a shoemaker. "Reforming," he resumed his studies and gravitated toward medicine. Cajal began his career as a physician, became interested in anatomy, then in histology, and finally concentrated on the study of nerve tissues. His efforts won for him the post of Professor of Anatomy, and later of Histology, in Saragossa, Valencia (1885), Barcelona (1887), and Madrid (1892).

Cajal's work, after half a century, is still a source of true knowledge. When we review today those works on pathology, therapeutics,

From *Journal of Clinical and Experimental Psychopathology*, 13:131, 1952.

and psychiatry which fifty years ago—when Cajal was first beginning—were the medical bibles revered by the doctors of the time, we are amazed at the great number of facts that were then considered solidly established and that today we regard ironically, unless we keep in mind their importance as forerunners of modern scientific truth. But Cajal's works have endured.* Their basic structures are still valid today, and his discoveries in the field of neuronal anatomicophysiology are constantly reconfirmed by new advances in neurology and psychiatry. Experimental thought in medicine will always have the supreme advantage over discursive and dogmatic thought, since it is based on facts and not on speculations. Cajal refused to accept the dogmatic authority of the classics, which he replaced with observation and experimentation. That is why the luster of youth still clings to his work.

Cajal was a poor man. His only capital was ideas. Unable to find channels through which to reveal his discoveries, Cajal created his own journal, the quarterly *Revista trimestral de histologia normal y patológica,* which, when it first appeared in 1888, was entirely written and illustrated by himself. He could publish only sixty copies per issue, which he sent to scientists in other countries, perhaps because nobody is a prophet in his own land. With a monthly salary of two hundred and sixty pesetas (about twelve dollars at that time), plus a small income derived from private teaching, he managed to support his family, his journal, and his research laboratory; in addition, he created a school and made an outstanding place for himself in the fields of philosophy and literature! But his *Revista* did not secure him the recognition he deserved. Only when Cajal was made a member of the Anatomical Society of Germany, whose Berlin convention he attended, did he start the climb to immortality.

Cajal established the anatomic individuality of the neuron and

* Cajal published more than four hundred scientific works and innumerable literary works, ranging from short stories to philosophic treatises. By the end of his life, in addition to the Nobel Prize, he had accumulated more than two hundred decorations and more than one hundred academic titles from all over the world. He was appointed member of more than twenty academies and scientific societies and made doctor *honoris causa* of the Universities of Cambridge, Würzburg, Clark, Stockholm, Munich, Louvain, Barcelona, Mexico, Cadiz, Strasbourg, Guatemala, Vienna, Philadelphia, Paris, Santiago de Chile, Coimbra, Valladolid, Turin, and New York. He was also honorary member of the Psychiatrie- und Nervenkrankheiten Society of Berlin, the Philosophical Society of Philadelphia, the Reale Istituto Lombardo di Scienze e Lettere of Rome, and the American Neurological Society, the Neurological Society of Philadelphia, the Coninbricensis Institut Societas of Coimbra, the Royal Irish Academy of Dublin, the Academia Scientiarum Ulisiponensis, the Neurological Society of Kazan in Russia, the Academia Regia Scientiarum Neerlandica, the Academia Regia Scientiarum Suedica, and many others.

promulgated the neuron doctrine. He described for the first time the true relation of the nerve fiber to the nerve cell, illustrating it with his description of basket structures around the Purkinje cells. His technique made possible the definition of isolated nerve elements in detail, their ramifications, arborizations, fibril nets, and synapses. His work neatly rounded out the anatomic arch running from the impression-receiving organ to the effect-producing organ. His chromosilver and reduced silver nitrate staining methods made him a true miniaturist of the nervous system, a water-colorist of the neurons. Not content with lighting up the night of the nervous system, he colored its component parts with his dyes and engraved its cells into the history of medicine. In 1906, he was awarded the well-merited Nobel Prize in conjunction with Golgi. The anatomic discoveries of Vesalius and his followers were succeeded in the history of medicine by the physiologic discoveries of Harvey and his successors. Cajal, however, was able to succeed *himself* and to proceed from his morphologic preoccupation with the *what* of the nervous system to the *why* of its physiologic functions. His contributions to the knowledge of neuroanatomy form the permanent basis for present-day concepts in neurology and psychiatry. He belongs with His and Forel, Nissl and Weigert, Alzheimer and Bielschowsky, Vogts, Spielmeyer, and Jakob. His chapter on the doctrine of the neuron in the *Handbuch der Neurologie* of Bumke and Foerster (published posthumously as a sort of scientific last will and testament) was eulogized by Bielschowsky: "in ihrer Art bewunderungswürdig" (a marvel). In that essay he objectively demonstrated his doctrine of neuronism, which was the supreme historical rectification of the Galenic doctrine of a morphologic-functional continuity in the nervous tissues. He also added the conclusive proof to the cell doctrine of Schleiden, Schwann, and Virchow when he demonstrated the anatomic, genetic, functional, and trophic unity of the neuron, along with the unity of pathologic reaction and the polarization of nervous stimulation.

Adolf Meyer, commenting on Cajal's lectures on his investigations into the visual and other regions of the cortex, said: "The very remarkable accuracy of description and the sober, critical presentation, free from hypothetical flights, displayed principles of work which unfortunately are abandoned by too many today; it was not an attempt to prove a preconceived hypothesis, but aimed primarily at the accumulation of data. That patient and steady work will, as it has in the past, lead to more valuable results than a mere elaboration of ideas is strongly proved by the entire history of Cajal's career. It is only fair to say that Ramón y Cajal was the greatest champion of neurology that Spain has ever produced. No one discovered and demonstrated more well-defined details in confirmation of the views of Forel and His than this indefatigable Madrid histologist. He did what neither His nor Forel did conclusively: demonstrate the blind arborizations or end-brushes of so many kinds of nerve fibers and the connection of the latter with cell bodies in the cerebellum, the medulla, olfactory bulb, retina, optic centers, the great sympathetic, the cerebral cortex, that the concept and the detailed data in its support are established beyond doubt.

"Cajal demonstrated that: (1) There is no substantial continuity between the processes of different nerve cells. The nerve elements represent cell units, for which he accepts Waldeyer's term 'neuron.' (2) The protoplasmic processes are those parts of a neuron with which the arborizations of other neurons most likely come in contact and that the contact with the cell body itself is exceptional, being found only in those cells where there are no protoplasmic processes (spinal ganglion, retina). (3) The spreading of received impulses is cellulipetal in the protoplasmic processes and centrifugal in the axis cylinder (law of dynamic polarization).

"In his work, Cajal maintained three *laws* he himself established: (1) The law of economy of time. In the spinal ganglia the cells are attached to the fibers so as to form a T. The conductors are thereby placed in the very axis of the ganglion and in the direction of the shortest way between periphery and posterior root; and the current need not pass through the eccentric cell. (2) The law of economy of matter. In the midbrain of fish, batrachians, reptiles, and birds, there are certain fusiform cells, the axon of which originates from a dendrite. In this way the axon spares the whole distance between the cell body and the point of the dendrite from which it originates. (3) The law of economy of space. The body is occasionally placed in regions poor in dendrites of final arborizations of axons: for instance, Dogiel's cells of the internal granular layers of the cortex. The cell body presents the convergence of the protoplasmic expansion towards the origin of the axon, enlarged by the presence of the nucleus."

Cajal's popularity is an interesting historic phenomenon. In Spain, during his lifetime, "Don Santiago" had already become a legendary figure, and when he died, his myth continued. The fame of this man, who was as modest as he was humble, rests on his way of life. His entire existence was made up of study and research at the university and long nights of work at his home until he would fall asleep from sheer exhaustion. All those who knew how Cajal lived admired this learned and good man, who had a goal in life and never swerved from the path he had chosen. Even when famous at home and abroad, he had no wish to be minister or ambassador; he would not accept any public post. Like Pindar, Cajal wished only "to become what he was." This consecrated authenticity of Cajal's life, this fidelity to himself, is the secret of his legend.

Cajal's vocation derived from romantic inclinations of his boyhood when he wanted to be a painter. Psychologically, Cajal was a visual type. His thought was of chromatic texture, which stimulated his interest in coloring the drab gray structure of the nervous system. His work is written with the pen of a man who had the eye of a painter, the mind of a colorist, and the soul of a romantic. His early frustrated desires to be an explorer of unknown lands prompted him to explore the human brain. But he was not satisfied with examining the brain under the microscope; he also wished to scrutinize its most recondite structures. Psychologically, he sublimated his desires to explore the earth's jungles (this explains the romantic vegetable terminology he always used when describing the structures of nerve centers) by exploring the anatomic jungles of the nervous system.

Cajal was a great teacher. For him the university was not simply a means of obtaining a diploma, whose yellow creases years later hide the lost illusions of an ambitious student. For him the university was a true *civitas hippocratica,* where technique must be subordinated to thought. On his lecture platform, he dedicated his brilliance to clarity and to lucidity. Cajal created a school of Spanish histology that was continued by his disciples, many of whom later did their most important work in exile. After he died, his contribution—which during his lifetime was extolled by the masters of medicine all over the world and by philosophers like Bergson—was continued in the physiology of Pavlov and Sherrington.

Gregorio Marañón, in his speech on Cajal before the Real Academía de Medicina in Madrid (1950), said: "We are conscious of the abyss that separates a book on neurology written prior to 1880 and one written today; the contrast between a treatise on psychiatry published in the last decades of the nineteenth century and one published today is even greater. The progress that has been made is due in great part to Cajal. Cajal, Sherrington, and Pavlov are the three men who have done most to provide a rational explanation for the mystery of the nervous system." Cajal, like Sherrington, was a philosopher of the nervous system who did his research with the brain of a scientist and the pen of a poet.

Ehrlich once said that the three fundamental requisites of a scientist are: *Geld, Geduld,* and *Geschick* (money, patience, and luck). That was not the case with Cajal, who always worked in humble attics and basement laboratories. He had instead the three qualities that Pavlov enjoined upon the young people of his country who wanted to devote themselves to science: "First, *consistency.* Study, compare and accumulate facts. No matter how perfect a bird's wings, they could never raise the bird aloft if it were not supported by air. Facts are the air of the scientist. Second, *modesty*. Never think that you know everything. Third, *passion*. Remember, science requires your whole life. Even if you had two lives to give, it still would not be enough. Science demands of man effort and supreme passion. Be passionate in your work and in your quests."—All that was Cajal.

THREE ENIGMAS IN THE HISTORY OF CURARE BEFORE SIR WALTER RALEIGH

*t*he historical origin of the "flying death" is today as much a mystery as was for centuries the preparation of poisoned arrows by primitive Indians in the impenetrable jungles of South America.

Almost every scientific study on curare is introduced by a historical sketch, and most authors use as their point of departure a reference about curare supposedly made by Sir Walter Raleigh in the account of his 1595 voyage *The Discoverie of Guiana*. When this romantic figure of English history (1552–1618) wrote about the Arora Indians, who lived on the plains of the Orinoco and were "as dark as Negroes, but with straight hair," he mentioned their poisoned arrows and expressed the desire to find an antidote for "the winged death" inflicted by the Indians on the white men with blond beards and greedy blue eyes. When he returned to England (there were no medical men with him on the trip), it is said that he brought back, hidden in a chest in his stateroom, samples of curare. Yet not until two hundred years later did curare become one of the most precious weapons in the modern therapeutic arsenal.

The fact is that, although Sir Walter Raleigh did say that the Spaniards used garlic juice as a cure for arrow poisoning "that caused thirst" (curare?), it has never been proved that he brought curare to Europe or even that he mentioned it in his writings.

After quoting Sir Walter Raleigh, writers generally refer to the

A paper presented at the Thirteenth International Congress of the History of Medicine, Amsterdam, Holland, 1950; published in *International Record of Medicine* 164:700, 1951.

reports of Alexander von Humboldt (1769–1859), the first European to witness the preparation of curare in the town of Esmeralda on the banks of Upper Orinoco. Humboldt has described this experience in his immortal *Voyage aux Régions Équinoxiales du Nouveau Continent*.

Humboldt's book takes us back to the steaming jungle, where the "master of curare" distilled the poison from plants using an earthen caldron as a crucible and rolled plantain leaves as a filtering funnel, while the Indians who had brought the plants from a certain place near the Paramo River celebrated their return with feasts and drunken orgies in the midst of a forest vibrant with mystery.

After Humboldt, writers usually quote the works of Waterton, Schomburgk, and Quelch; they refer to the contributions of Virchow, Böhm, and Claude Bernard, precursors in the modern use of curare in therapeutics; then they relate the great adventure of the American, Richard C. Gill, who brought to the United States the first samples of curare, which were to open a new horizon for medicine and surgery.

But this method of presentation gives only a partial history of curare. It neglects the contributions made by pre-Columbian Indo-America and by Spain in the fifteenth and sixteenth centuries. And it fails to point out three great enigmas in the history of curare: the aboriginal culture of poisoned arrows; the use of curare by the primitive peoples of the American continent; and the Spanish contribution to the knowledge of curare *before* Sir Walter Raleigh.

This article will outline these three enigmas, and then end where most other papers on the history of curare would begin, that is, with Sir Walter Raleigh. This is therefore in the manner of an introduction to that other familiar introduction—like the tuning up of the orchestra before a concert begins.

THE CULTURE OF POISONED ARROWS

The study of ancient maps of the world reveals that the so-called "culture of poisoned arrows" * once embraced almost all of Africa, Central and Southern Europe, plus the entire Mediterranean basin. It spread to Asia and included the Pacific Islands, from Suez to the Bering Sea, from New Zealand to the Gobi desert, forming a belt all around the earth that comprised a wide variety of peoples: Greeks, Romans, Celts, Dacians, Dalmatians, Scythians, the peoples on the shores of the Caspian Sea and in the Caucasus, the Medes, and the Persians.

---

* The reader interested in the history of curare is advised to consult the splendid book, *Curare,* by T. S. McIntyre and the excellent article by W. Naumann, published in 1941 in *Ciba Symposia.*

Certain tribes of Africa and Asia used arrows poisoned with substances causing inflammatory reactions. In Moorish Spain, some parts of Asia, Nepal, Burma, and Yunnan, the poisons used were of the aconite type affecting the respiratory system. Arabic Spain, Togoland, Bagana, Bonga, Somaliland, and Wataita, as well as certain tribes of Africa, Cochinchina, Malacca, Sumatra, Bali, and the Philippines, used poisons affecting the heart. The Bushmen and Basutos in Africa and the aborigines of the Solomon Islands and New Hebrides used poisons causing convulsions, and, of course, there was the paralyzing type of poisons used by tribes in South America.

As time went on, the range of the poisoned arrow began to shrink as it was replaced by other weapons. Today, the areas where poisoned arrows are still used to kill man are limited to Maganja and other African territories, Burma, Yunnan, and some Asian zones. In South America the use of poisoned arrows is now confined to less than half of the northern part of the continent. Nevertheless, there are still about a million and a half South American Indians who use blowguns and poisoned arrows.

One of the main difficulties in tracing the present-day geographic boundaries of curare on a map lies in the infinite variations in names used by the Indians of South America for their towns and rivers.

Still another difficulty is presented by the fact that in ancient times the name *curare* was applied indiscriminately to all arrow poisons, whether of the convulsive type, the heart-paralyzing type, the aconite type affecting respiration, or the type with inflammatory effects. Only in the last half century has the word "curare" been used to designate a certain chemically identifiable poison, the predominant effect of which is paralysis of the voluntary muscles. Paradoxically, a curarized arrow is lethal to a quadrumane, only slightly so to a batrachian, and has no effect whatsoever when introduced in the fat of a pig or the horn of an animal.

In his excellent study of curare, McIntyre states that the word *curare* is a generic term applied without distinction to all South American poisons used on arrows, although only some of them are really curares in the strict sense of the word and others are not even muscle-paralyzing agents. There are those who even claim that curare is a poison similar to strychnine, whereas curare is not a convulsant, but a muscle-relaxing agent that may be fatal because of the cardiorespiratory paralysis it induces.

The word *curare* is not of Indian origin, nor did the Jesuit Acuña coin it as it has been claimed. According to the Brazilian naturalist Barbosa Rodríguez, the Indian word for poison, *uiraery,* derives from *uira,* bird, and *eor,* to kill. The word used by Humboldt to imitate the indigenous sound meaning poison was *uirary,* which subsequently underwent numerous phonetic changes, including *urare, avara, kurari, worali, woorara,* and so on, until it became *curare,* the word universally used today.

It has been pointed out by McIntyre that the connection between the word *curare* and the idea of poisoned arrows is apparent when we consider that the word employed today to refer to the science that treats of poisons, i.e., toxicology, and its derivatives derive from the Greek *toxon,* meaning bow. People fond of archery are still called "toxophilites." The ancient idea of bow and poisoned arrow therefore had one and the same root, *toxon.* When in the year 60 Dioscorides for the first time applied the word *toxos* specifically to poisons, the original meaning of bow and arrow was forgotten, only to be dug out again later by the probing hands of the archeologists of language.

To the geographic difficulties encountered in tracing the profile of the culture of poisoned arrows must be added the difficulties in tracing its historical roots.

We know that poisoned arrows are among the most ancient weapons in history. It is an indisputable ethnic truth that our civilization is based on lethal instruments, one of which is the "flying death," still the favorite weapon of certain primitive peoples. But the use of poisoned arrows goes back to paleolithic times. In 1857, in a cave in the Pyrenees dating back to the paleolithic era, Fintan discovered human fossils, in addition to the fossilized bones of animals now extinct. Among the latter he found arrowheads made of bone and deer horns, some of which contained grooves to hold poison. Later the Celts, Vandals, Gauls, Germans, Dacians, and Dalmatians of the Adriatic and the Danube used hunting weapons poisoned with vegetable juices and snake poisons.

Reference to poisoned arrows in mythology, literature, and history, as well as in the Bible, are as abundant as they are colorful. The poet of the Psalms (91:5) wrote, "Thou shalt not be afraid for the terror by night; nor for the arrow that flieth by day; nor for the pestilence that walketh in darkness; nor for the destruction that wasteth at noonday." In the Book of Job we find, "Because the arrows of the Almighty have pierced me and my soul is drinking their poison."

According to Greek legend, contagious diseases and other types of sickness were caused by invisible arrows shot by malign gods and destructive demons. It was an angry Apollo who, with his bow, shot an arrow "causing pestilence" among the Greeks. The Scythians, in hunting and warfare, used animal poisons mixed with human blood. Homer (*Odyssey* I:260) mentioned that Odysseus traveled to Epirus in Corinth to obtain a salve or ointment, fatal to man, with which to poison the heads of his arrows, but Ilos would not give it to him because he feared the wrath of the gods. Aelianus said that man learned the terrible art of poisoning from wasps that filled their stings with poison from dead snakes.

Horace, Theophrastus, Vergil (*Aeneid* IX:772), and Ovid mentioned poisoned arrows, and these weapons are also mentioned in German epics of chivalry. Verse 3259 of *Tristan and Isolde* reads: "Suddenly a frightening knight appeared with a poisoned arrow and pierced Tristan only once, but Tristan knew that he was fatally wounded. . . ."

CURARE AND THE PRIMITIVE INDO-AMERICAN

The psychology of primitive man is like that of an infant, in that aggressiveness precedes self-defense in the disposition of his instincts. It follows that curare must have been used as a weapon of aggression before it was used as a means of protection against illness and death.

We do not exactly know how the aboriginal American Indian stumbled onto the idea of increasing the effectiveness of his weapons by poisoning them. According to Richard C. Gill, it happened in any one of four ways: (a) the ancient Indians first became conscious of and then tried to imitate the poisonous stings of snakes; (b) when they tried to cure their wounds with the sap of plants and trees, they accidentally discovered toxic substances in the sap; (c) they noticed that wounds caused by weapons smeared with dried blood developed septicemia, which prompted them to use animal poisons and later vegetable poisons; (d) they noticed that animals perished after eating certain plants, and used the juices of these plants to poison their arrows. Certain plant names currently used in England, like *cowbane, sowbane, wolfsbane,* contain the suffix *bane* derived from the Anglo-Saxon *bana* which means *killer.*

Poisoned arrows have been used down through the centuries. Until recently the natives of New Hebrides used arrowheads fashioned of human bone and smeared with a certain type of mud containing tetanus bacilli. Hakluyt, ghost writer for Sir Walter Raleigh, mentioned a similar type of arrow poisoning which, to judge by the symptoms, must have been of the tetanus type.

There are definite indications that curare existed in the pre-Columbian therapeutic arsenal of the American Indian. These aborigines, who lived in huts of straw and mud and spent their time either hunting and fishing or in orgiastic religious festivals; who knew nothing of the wheel or iron, wheat or horse; who sat before their huts grinding corn or preparing manioc; who shared the vast green prairies with the buffalo, which they hunted on foot with the simplest of weapons; who at night gathered under the stars to smoke their pipes and tell tales of hunting expeditions and ghosts—these aborigines developed their medical science by imitating animals and learning empirically from their experiences.

It was a boon for the medicine man to discover the medical virtues of plants and flowers, and he gradually sought a specific remedy for each illness. To extract poisons left in the flesh by the bite of a snake or a poisoned arrow, he used a hollow tube to suck out the dangerous fluid. His medicine was a mixture of magic, ritualistic mysticism, and a practical sense of curative measures. He stressed the overcoming of disease rather than the tending of the sick person.

It is possible that curare was also used as a therapeutic agent among these primitive Indians. With their empiric knowledge, the Indians of Patagonia and the Orinoco, and the Ticunas, who lived on the shores of the Marañón River, may have conceived the idea of utilizing curare in their medical concoctions. According to La Condamine, the Ticunas sprinkled salt and sugar on their wounds or took them orally as antidotes against curare. The *urari* of the Makushi, studied by Schomburgk in his travels, may have been used as a curative in cases of tetanus type convulsions. In the empiric mind of the medicine man, the gourds containing the dark sirup may have figured as a source of life as well as of death.

It is highly unlikely that once the aboriginal Indians discovered the deadly powers of curare they probed no further. We know that in the Upper Orinoco and in the vicinity of the Rio Negro the Indians swallowed curare, claiming to be immune to its toxic effects. This legend, now disproved, seems to point to the desire of the medicine man to try the curative powers of curare, since he was already acquainted with its lethal effects. Such experiments must have caused many deaths, but perhaps during these tests the primitive medicine man, bent over his vegetable alembic, watching the dripping of the deadly juice, may have perceived some of those very properties that the modern scientist has discovered in his laboratory.

Richard C. Gill relates that the flesh of any animal killed in the hunt by curare is perfectly edible. According to the Indian folklore of Ecuador, moderate quantities of curare taken orally are not harmful. Gill actually saw some Indians lick off small quantities of curare sticking to their fingers, which they asserted had a stomachic effect. He himself frequently tasted drops of curare and ate any number of animals killed by curare. The only precaution he saw the Indians adopt was to cut off the area in the animal's flesh where the poisoned arrow had struck.

The first confirmation we have that the aboriginal Indians of America used poisoned arrows comes from Pietro Martire d'Anghera, native of Lake Maggiore and "citizen of the universe." Pedro Mártir, as he was known in Spain where he went to meet his adored Queen

Isabella, was the first to publish for his astonished contemporaries the news of the new world on the other side of the ocean. His *De Orbe Novo,* published in Spain in 1516, was the first history of the New World from Columbus' first trip to about twenty years later. In this work he refers several times to poisoned arrows. He relates, and McIntyre quotes him, that in Santa Cruz thirty Spaniards observed a canoe coming toward them with eight men and eight women. When the Spaniards attacked the canoe, a rain of arrows fell upon them and before they could protect themselves with their shields, one of them had been killed and another gravely injured by the arrows. Later they discovered that the arrows contained a liquid which oozed out when the arrow was broken. This is supposed to be the first lay description of the existence of poisoned arrows in the American continent.

In a letter addressed to Pope Leo X, the same author mentioned the fact that the natives smeared their arrows with the juice of a "poisonous herb of fatal effect," and that no remedy was known until the natives of Hispaniola discovered an herb that contained an antidotal juice. He also said that the cauterization of wounds might be a cure and that the Indians manufactured their arrows from certain kinds of palms and poisoned them with an ointment compounded of ants' heads, scorpions' stings, and vegetable juices prepared by old women who were locked away for two days to fulfill their task. After two days, if the women were not found half-dead from the vapors of the poison, they were severely punished.

This means that less than half a century after the discovery of America, it was known that several types of poisoned arrows existed; that the poison was obtained by distilling certain plants; that the arrows were made of palm; that the savages knew of antidotes; that wounds were cauterized; and that the poison was prepared by mysterious old women.

It should also be noted that references are made to poisoned arrows in the writings of Fray Bartolomé de las Casas, Oviedo, Cristobal de Acuña, Gumilla, and the Jesuits, Herrera and Gomara. The latter (1510–1560) in his *Historia General de las Indias* mentions several types of poisons whose effectiveness depended on their ingredients: snakes' blood, ants' heads, certain types of rubber, and other plants.

According to the *Historia de las Indias* of Fray Bartolomé de las Casas, written in 1561 but not published until 1875, when Amerigo Vespucci reached the New World he was met by a dozen canoes carrying warriors and sixteen maidens. After they had climbed on board, the old women of the nearby Indian village began to shriek, whereupon the girls jumped into the water, and their companions shot poisoned arrows at the Spanish crew. The author says that the antidote used was seawater, which coincides with the Indians' use of plain salt.

The historiographer Oviedo y Valdés, a friend of Columbus, was the first to describe the structure of the arrows. He says that in 1535, when Rodrigo de Bastidas was near the mouth of a "great river" (the Orinoco?), he observed that the Caribbean Indians smeared their arrows with a lethal poison made from an herb. The wounds inflicted were fatal, "no matter how little they bled."

The Italian Antonio Pigafetta, who circumnavigated the globe with Magellan, wrote in his *Il Viaggio fatto dagli Spagnuoli,* published in 1539, that one of his soldiers landed in Patagonia in June, 1520, and was killed by a poisoned arrow.

Antonio de Herrera, official chronicler of Philip II and Philip III, in his narration of Francisco de Orellana's journey across the Amazon from Quito to the Atlantic, mentions that Orellana came across Indians with poisoned arrows, and a certain García de Soria was killed although the poisoned arrow "penetrated only about half a finger deep."

The portentous Inca, Garcilaso de la Vega, describing the tragic expedition of Gonzalo Pizarro to the land of cinnamon, speaks of poisons used by the Indians.

And then, of course, we must not neglect the fabulous expedition of the Marañones, who crossed the Amazon from west to east and finally reached Trinidad and the Island of Santa Margarita. It was on this expedition that the Machífaro tragedy occurred, when the mad Don Lope de Aguirre had Don Pedro de Ursa, the expedition leader, assassinated. During this trip the Spaniards were shot at with poisoned arrows by Indians hiding in the jungle foliage.

THE CONTRIBUTION OF THE SPANIARDS
TO THE KNOWLEDGE OF CURARE

It is gratifying to vindicate the Spanish contribution to the knowledge of curare.

Bored with sailing their ships on the Mediterranean, which they knew by heart; lured by stories of the Vikings, who had reached uncharted lands, by pieces of wood found floating in the route eastward which bore strange carvings done by mysterious hands beyond the Atlantic, by legends of Marco Polo, and by the *Laurentium Portolono,* a masterpiece of Italian cartography which showed the so-called "Atlantic Isles"; impelled by the dream of reaching Cathay by sailing westward; and guided only by the stars, the Spanish sailors set sail for strange lands and one night anchored their ships under the virgin stars of the American sky. And, on an all-important day for American civilization, men with long beards, pale faces, and shining armor, mounted on fabulous animals never before seen on this continent, entered the dense American forests. It was the beginning of Spain's exploits in America.

In a letter written by Columbus' doctor, the Sevillian Don Diego Alvarez de Chanca, to the municipal authorities of Seville—the "great happy port" of Spain in the sixteenth century—concerning the flora, fauna, anthropology, and ethnology of the Americas, no mention is made of curare. But long before Sir Walter Raleigh, the Spanish *conquistadores* were fighting their way with pick and lance, horse and banner, through the thickets and brambles of the New World. On many occasions poisoned arrows struck them down. And since the Spaniards of the time were men possessed not only of a tremendous urge for adventure and power, but also of a great curiosity and a genius for observation, there were those, like Diego Alvarez de Chanca and Bernal Díaz, who wrote about everything they saw, including poisoned arrows.

Alvar Núñez Cabeza de Vaca, that Estremaduran of superhuman courage and fortitude, who set foot on American soil thirty-five years after Columbus and sixty-eight years before Sir Walter Raleigh, led his troops of farmers, soldiers, merchants, and sailors in the most fabulous undertaking of the Conquest. Starting from Tampa Bay, he covered almost all of North America, from ocean to ocean, crossing Texas, Sonora, and Chihuahua, fording the Mississippi, the Colorado, and the Río de la Plata, crossing Paraguay, and meeting Pizarro's Indians on the Igualú River in Bolivia, thus uniting two Spanish expeditions that had started from the opposite coasts of South America.

In his book *Naufragios,* published in 1542, Cabeza de Vaca describes the Indian tribes that he encountered in detail: "I exchanged commodities I obtained inland for hides and ochre, which they [the Quevenes, who lived near the Mississippi Delta] use for smearing and staining their faces and hair, flint arrowheads, paste and stiff reeds used in the making of their arrows. . . . They threw lumps of mud at us and pointed arrows at our hearts every day, saying they would like to kill us." (Part I, "Relacion," Chapter XVI.) "They [the Aguenes and Guevenes, who lived in the Charruco Mountains] are the readiest people with a weapon I have ever seen, and if they suspect enemies near, stay awake the whole night with their bows by their sides and a dozen arrows; they sleep with their fingers on their bows, and if they cannot feel the string, turn around until they touch it again. . . . When day breaks they slacken the strings until ready to go hunting. The bowstrings are made from deer tendons." (Part I, "Relacion," Chapter XXV.)

In both parts of *Naufragios* ("Relacion" and "Comentarios"), there are many references to poisoned arrows that were deadly simply because of the mechanical trauma they caused. In Chapter XLII, "Comentarios," the author refers to some "Christians" wounded in skirmishes with the Indians of Tabere and Guazani. He says: "They [the wounded Christians] were sent to the city of Ascensión to be treated, and four or five of them died because of the excesses they committed, since their wounds were slight and not at all dangerous or fatal. One of them had been scratched on the side of the nose by an arrow, and he died *because the arrows had been smeared with the juice of grass.* Those who are wounded in this way should not indulge in excessive intercourse with women; otherwise, there is no reason to fear the herbs of that land."

The book abounds in allusions to poisoned arrows. After all, these Spanish expeditions took place in the heart of the geographic zone of curare. Cabeza de Vaca also refers to the preparation of poison in clay pots by the Indians, which they later smeared on the arrows they shot at the *conquistadores.*

The most basic contribution of the Spaniards to the knowledge of curare was the work of a physician, Nicolás Monardes (1493–1588), a graduate of the University of Alcalá de Henares, who, without ever leaving his native Seville, devoted himself to collecting specimens of plants and herbs—sarsaparilla, resins, guayabo, sassafras—brought by ships returning from the West Indies. He wrote the first Spanish pharmacopoeia containing a study of curare. In 1554 he founded a museum where he exhibited everything produced in the West Indies. This museum was considered a section of the Museum of Natural Sciences and contained a botanic garden including a parcel of land alive and fragrant with American flora that had been brought over, plant by plant, by Spanish ships.

Nicolás Monardes was the first doctor anywhere to write about poisoned arrows in his medical history of the New World, entitled *Simplicium Medicamentorum ex Novo Orbe Delatorum . . . Historia.* His first work, published in Seville in 1565, was entitled: *Historia Medicinal que trata de las cosas que se traen de nuestras Indias Occidentales* (History of Medicine Dealing with Things Brought from Our West Indies), and bears the following subtitle: *"Dos libros. / El uno trata de todas las cosas que traen de nras. Indias Occidentales, / que sirven al uso de Medicina, y / como se ha usar de la rayz del / Mechoacan purga excelentissima. / El otro libro, trata de dos medi / cinas maravillosas que son contra to / do veneno, la piedra Bezaar, y la / yerua Escuerconera. Con la cura / de los Venenados, o veran mu / chos secretos de naturaleza y de / medicina, con grandes esperiencias. / Agora nueuamente compuestos por el Doctor Nicu-*

loso Mo / nardes, medico de Sevilla. / Con el priuilegio de su Magestad / 1565. / " ("Two books. One dealing with all things brought from our West Indies which can be used as Medicine and how the root of Mechoacan an excellent laxative is to be used. The second book deals with two marvellous medicines which are against all poison, the Bezoar stone and the Escuerconera grass. The cure of those poisoned, and many secrets of nature and medicine, with great adventures. Now compiled by Doctor Nicolás Monardes, doctor of Seville Privileged by His Majesty 1565.")*

The above work is concerned with American medicinal herbs, among them tobacco, used by the Indians as curatives and introduced in Europe by Monardes in 1558, when Raleigh was still a child. It was reprinted in 1569, and two years later Monardes brought out a complementary work. Much later he combined both parts in one volume and added a third part. The complete work was published in Seville in 1580. A Latin translation was printed in Antwerp in 1580, an Italian translation in Venice in 1585, and a French translation in Lyons in 1619. An English translation was done in Antwerp in 1579, bearing the title: *Joyfull Newes out of the New founde worlde.*

In the last work we read that some people who were sailing to San Juan, Puerto Rico ("cartaine wilde people goynk in their boates to Saint John on Depuerto Rico, for to shoote at Indians or Spaniardes, if that they might finde them"), wounded several Indians and Spaniards and, as they had no sublimate to treat them with, applied tobacco

---

* The treatment of curare poisoning is described on pages 34 and 35 of Part One, entitled "De las cosas que traen de las Indias que sirven al uso de Medicina," of the edition of the book by Nicolás Monardes that is now in the collection of the Botanical Garden in Madrid. Among other various uses for tobacco described by Nicolás Monardes, such as in the treatment of toothaches, carbuncles, and several types of poisonings, the author tells of its use as an antidote to poisoned arrows—the poison is certainly curare—with which the Caribbean Indians wounded the conquistadores. "The Cannibalistic Caribbean Indians shoot arrows poisoned with an herb or a composite of many poisons which they aim at everything they wish to kill, and this poison is so harmful and so pernicious that it is fatal beyond hope, and the wounded die in great pain and convulsions . . . and no remedy has been found for this terrible illness." And later he adds, "Some time ago, some Caribbean Indians set out in canoes for San Juan de Puerto Rico to wound any Indians or Spaniards they could find, and they came to a plantation and killed a few Indians and Spaniards and wounded many. Since the foreigners did not have corrosive sublimate to cure them, it was decided to treat them with tobacco juice or the skin of pressed grapes, and God willed that, as these remedies were applied, the pains, ravings and fainting spells, from which they used to die, were relieved. Thus the power of the poison was removed, and the wounds were cured, and everyone was amazed and the islanders, being acquainted with this cure, are now using it for wounds received when fighting the Caribs. And they are no longer afraid, for they have found such a great remedy for such a desperate menace."

juice and ground tobacco leaves to the wounds as antidotes, thus saving them from death. Earlier in his own work, Monardes alludes to the fact that "the Indian savages smear on their arrows some herb or concoction made of many poisons, which they shoot at any thing they wish to kill, and this poison is so pernicious that it causes great pains, accidents, madness, and is irremediably fatal."

Monardes' monumental work provided the inspiration for the eminent Toledan and personal physician to Philip II, Francisco Hernández (1514–1587), who, in his capacity as *Protomedico* or head doctor of the Indies, tested the effects of the medicinal herbs of New Spain (Mexico) not only in the Spanish hospitals of the New World but also on himself. When Hernández returned to Spain, he devoted nine years to preparing his manuscripts and drawings for the press; in all, they made up twenty-six volumes. Philip II had the work bound in sixteen green leather deluxe volumes with corner brackets of gold and silver, and they were made part of the library of the Escorial Monastery in 1577, where they were destroyed in the fire of 1671.

A later *conquistador,* Bernardo de Vargas Machuca (1557–1622), whose *Milicia y descripcion de las Indias,* Madrid, 1600, is practically contemporary with Raleigh's book, mentions that an expedition commander must be ready to tackle rattlesnake, cayman, poisonous fish, and poisoned arrow wounds. For wounds made by poisoned arrows, the surgeon should be instructed to raise the injured flesh with a hook and slash it off with a razor. Then the wound should be plugged with a pellet of corrosive sublimate in tallow to neutralize the poison, and the whole plastered with a paste of flour, salt, gunpowder, and ashes to arrest the flow of blood. Other "useful remedies" are theriac, ground clams, and St. Martha's amber. The patient should not be given any water to drink, and Vargas points out that, if he is not treated promptly, he will die in delirium.

Finally we must not forget another Spaniard, Hipólito Ruiz (1754–1816), who made a scientific expedition to the Americas and studied the Menisperraceae plant (which he baptized *Chondrodendron tommentosum*), from which we get curare today.*

SUMMARY

The use of curare as a poison for arrows is a historical fact that must be considered within the anthropologic and ethnic scope of the

---

* On page 132 of *Florae Peruvianae, et Chilensis Prodromus, sive Novorum Generum Plantarum Peruvianum, et Chilensium Descriptiones, et Icones,* there appears a description of the genus *Chondrodendron.* An illustration of this plant may be found in *Flora Brasilienses,* by Martius, in the collection of the Botanical Gardens of the Bronx Park in New York.

culture of poisoned arrows; curare was used not only as a poison, but also therapeutically by the aboriginal Indians of America. Sixty-eight years before Sir Walter Raleigh was supposed to have introduced curare in Europe, poisoned arrows had been described by the Spaniard Alvar Núñez Cabeza de Vaca; the plant from which curare is extracted had been described by another Spaniard, Hipólito Ruiz; and curare itself had been studied by the Sevillian physician, Nicolás Monardes.

A more thorough study of the three enigmas of curare might provide the missing links in the history of this drug, which now stands like one of those old, discarded stone bridges we come across in the country, one end torn down, the other still tracing half an arch in the air; with our mind's eye we can trace the missing half and reconstruct the whole bridge.

The rest of the story of the "flying death," from Sir Walter Raleigh on, and how the scientists converted it into a fountain of life, is well known. Here we have merely attempted to cut through the age-old jungle of the history of curare to get closer to the mystery of its origin.

TOWARD A HISTORY OF MEDICAL THOUGHT

A STAINED-GLASS WINDOW

*t*he stained-glass window has played an important role in the history of mankind. Man has always derived great pleasure in decorating the windows of his churches and dwellings with varicolored glass through which the sun pours streams of gold, purple, and indigo. Late pre-Constantinian art produced the famous glass panes with gold designs, like the disc with three portraits against a dark blue background in the silver cross at the Brescia Museum. Medieval Christian art is a long series of scenes from the Passion in the windows of cathedrals. Both believer and artist have always delighted in watching the sun light up with blazing rubies and sparkling gold coins the flowing robes of the madonnas and saints who dwell in stained-glass windows. Thus man added to the stone, incense, and silver of his churches all the jewels of the rainbow.

There is a magnificent stained-glass window in the Mayo Brothers House in Rochester, Minnesota. It was installed in March, 1943, on the east wall of the third floor hall where scientific societies convene. This window has twelve panels tracing the entire history of medicine in its threefold aspect of clinical practice, medical teaching, and scientific research. On these panels the physician, the teacher, and the dedicated research worker live side by side.

A lecture delivered at the Honor Halls of the Universities of Lima (Peru), Santiago de Chile (Chile), Buenos Aires (Argentina), Rio de Janeiro (Brazil), Bogotá (Colombia), San José (Costa Rica), and Havana (Cuba) in October and November, 1946; published in *International Record of Medicine 165*:484, 523, 1952.

On one panel, tracing scientific research from 500 B.C. to 1500 A.D., a medieval alchemist is shown at work in his laboratory, extracting medicinal juices from plants and seeking the philosopher's stone, the elixir of life, and the universal panacea, the triple goal of the astrologers and the medical men of the time.

Another panel in blue, silver, and vermillion glass symbolizes the theories, systems, and experiments from 1500 to 1800 in the figure of Harvey demonstrating the circulation of the blood to Charles I of England. The shadows of Bacon, Hunter, Galvani, and Volta surround him, and the legend is Claude Bernard's injunction: "Put off your imagination, as you take off your overcoat, when you enter the laboratory; but put it on again, as you do your overcoat, when you leave the laboratory."

On another panel—1800 to 1900—Pasteur, surrounded by his assistants and favorite domestic pets, carries forward the work of reorganizing scientific methods, pioneered by Bernard, Koch, and Beaumont.

The era of preventive medicine from 1900 on is the subject of another panel. Two students are shown using the electronic microscope. Physics, chemistry, biology, and roentgenology are united in the field of preventive medicine. Several books scattered about the laboratory suggest the continuity of knowledge in time and space. On this window appear the words of W. J. Mayo, symbolizing the unity of the real and the fantastic in the history of medicine: "Take of my experience but give me of your dreams."

The next scene, portraying the art of healing, has been divided into practice, teaching, and research. It is these branches we wish to discuss: the historicocultural evolution of modern medicine as a "science of integration, summing up the other sciences," with the specific purpose of understanding disease, preventing it, and curing it.

THE CONCEPT OF MEDICAL CULTURES

The evolution of medicine is the history of a gigantic conflict between creative and experimental thought and traditional dogmatic authority. Of what interest is its study to the physician? Not only does it help him to avoid the risk pointed out by Santayana—"Those who forget history, will have to repeat it"—but it also is of value in that it is not enough to be a good physician; a physician must also be a man of culture. He must view the world historically, biologically, and philosophically, as Ortega y Gasset said. If he lacks such knowledge, he cannot be even a good physician, and if he does manage that, it is at the risk of being a man unable to cope with the exigencies of life in general.

It is essential, then, that the physician have an idea of the time and space in which he lives, reconstructing in his own mind the work already done by about five thousand years of human civilization. Professionalism and specialization have bred an astounding specimen of a man who is only a fragment or one dimension of himself. It is necessary to combine several of these fragments to create the complete man and reconstruct the vital unity of the modern scientist.

The problem, therefore, is to revise critically the history of medicine, to present it as the integration of a series of living medical cultures, not as a succession of dead epochs. Spengler and others accepted certain fundamental cultures in human history: Egyptian, Chinese, Hindu, Greek, Roman, Babylonian, Arabian, Mayan, and Mexican. Let us accept a series of medical cultures that are born, develop, reach their zenith, begin to decline as they are crystallized into a large metropolis, and then die, leaving traces to be picked up by a succeeding culture.

Thus, we observe a titanic advance of medical culture from the Orient to the Occident, following the rivers and seas, the paths of the sun and stars. In this advance toward the West, in this expansion of civilization, there is a metropolis for each medical culture, to wit: Egypt, Alexandria, Athens, Rome, Salerno and Monte Cassino, Cordova, Montpellier, Padua, Vienna, Leyden, Oxford, Cambridge, and the Americas.

Medical culture was born in the Orient at the confluence of two rivers of biblical memory, the Tigris and the Euphrates in Mesopotamia. It flowed on to the West, to the shores of the Nile, and from there to the coasts of Greece, following the course of the Mediterranean, whence, in ever-westerly direction, it leaped to Rome; then, by way of Byzantium, the universities of Salerno, Padua, and Bologna, and Moslem Spain, it jumped to Montpellier and Paris, then to Leyden, and from there to Oxford and Cambridge. And finally it crossed the Atlantic to the American shores. From here it may some day continue on to the West across the waters of the Pacific.

MAGIC THOUGHT AND WITCHCRAFT IN PRIMITIVE MEDICINE

We are familiar with only some six thousand years of civilized man, hardly a hundredth part of the half million years of his history. However, although the good condition of the teeth in the most ancient human fossils found attests man's rational feeding habits, we know that disease antedates man. Bone tumors have been found on the remains of dinosaurs, which preceded man by millions of years, and when prehistoric man appeared, he already suffered from disease. Egyptian and Incan mummies exhibit signs of tuberculosis and rheumatoid arthritis.

On the subject of the origins of medicine, many historical errors have been committed, among them that of considering the modern physician as the descendant of the primitive medicine man or magician. Primitive man, like prehistoric man, held disease to be a magic phenomenon, a demonic influence exerted by an enemy or an irate god. In order to combat it, the medicine man or witch doctor surrounded himself with an aura of mystery and pretended to expel the devils by means of trepanation, emetics, amulets, and spells. This view of disease as something supernatural, which persisted until Hippocrates, made of it a separate entity with a life of its own, like storm or fire. But to his magic rites the witch doctor added phytotherapy, massage, and hydrotherapy, the oldest treatments known.

In studying primitive medicine, it should be borne in mind that all living matter, be it man or microbe, grows and forms colonies. The main social problems that then arise are personal ailments affecting growth and social situations that interfere with the development of the individual. Responses to stimuli are identical. Plants on a window sill bend their leaves to the sun, responding to the stimulus of light and heat; the branches of a mountain pine grow less to windward; mountain cattle by nature consume the grass and salt they need. There is a spontaneous wisdom in nature. By the same token, primitive peoples often had biologically correct habits. Their taboos and rituals were aimed at protecting their food sources, their reproduction, and their social relationships. Aggregations of human beings likewise respond biologically by seeking such things as can help them to avoid disease, pain, and death. In the primitive mind, such things were associated with benevolent gods or with devils. Witch doctors therefore constitute the most ancient professional class in the evolution of mankind. Their original task was to intercede by means of magic with the gods and evil spirits, and by their great power they became chieftains, priests, and physicians. One must therefore look to primitive medicine for an understanding of the origins of the double path of philosophy and faith, that is, of science and miracle followed by medicine up to modern times.

When we say "primitive medicine," we refer to a body of ideas apparently antiquated and erroneous by comparison with our modern ideas. But this lack of development is not a function of the biologic but rather of the cultural state of the group, which, in its turn, is a function of its history as a social group. Primitive man is primitive because of his isolation from the cultural currents of the West. It would be more correct, as suggested by some, to call him "isolated" man instead of primitive man, since in order to compare the culture of two groups, one must think in terms of opportunities for intellectual development. The knowledge any group accumulates represents a harmonious segment of its mode of life and an integrated part of the social structure as a whole. Its medicine should be studied as a social phenomenon if it is to be understood. Science is not fully derived from magic. Magic is the manipulation of the supernatural by ritual acts. Science has been defined as verifiable and communicable, not esoteric, knowledge, based on observation, experiment, and meditation. Magic and science treat supernatural and natural causes respectively, and both are mechanical procedures. Science studies the causes and effects of the natural world, *experimentally determined*. Magical cause and effect are products of the human mind operating in the imaginary world of the supernatural and are based on analogies; whereas science is based on the confirmation and verification of real experiences. Primitive peoples admit to a universe influenced by natural *and* supernatural causes and effects. In order to act on the latter, one must exercise special powers; in order to deal with the natural world, natural techniques that act on the environment are resorted to. In this regard, the material culture of isolated peoples attests their ingenuity and inventiveness. Science is derived from technology acting on nature; magic from magic techniques that influence the supernatural.

Among primitive peoples both practices are at once parallel and different. If a man breaks his leg, it is splinted empirically by the tribe's medicine man. If he complains of intense cephalalgia, he is trepanned until cured or dead. This is his rational medicine, which, as in the use of medicinal plants, lacks magical content. Primitive man's thinking therefore was not illogical but rather excessively logical; it led him to discover quinine, curare, opium, and digitalis, to splint fractures, and to practice surgery.

Isolated man recognized three causes of disease: the natural, the human--through sorcery—and the supernatural. He believed in animism, or the view of the universe as imbued with a mysterious, powerful spiritual force (the *orendam* of the Iroquois, the *manitou* of the Algonquians, and the Melanesian *mana*), personified in superhumanly endowed beings or in disembodied superhuman qualities, such as the powers of objects.

Primitive religion is the technique of supernaturalism. Magic tries to control demons by sorcery; religion seeks to obtain the favor of the gods by means of prayer or worship. Prayer surrenders; incantation imposes. In animistic societies the unknown was explained in terms of spirits, and white magic was employed for good ends and black magic for sinister purposes to force the spirits to obey.

Among the treatments used by primitive doctors are venous punctures, bloodletting, wound drainage, the extraction of foreign bodies, sutures, the cauterization of ulcers, trepanning, hydrotherapy, dieting, enemas, massage, fumigation, and suction.

The medicine man came by his profession through inheritance, or manual dexterity, or because he suffered from epileptic convulsions or hallucinations on account of being schizophrenic, or through special talents, as in the case of primitive midwives. Sometimes a medicine man specialized in a particular disease because he had cured himself of it. Among the North American Indians, a secret society still exists which preserves the medical knowledge of its members from generation to generation.

Primitive medicine was a rational system, and its medical practices were the result of spiritualistic beliefs representing a logical body of thought based on the data available to primitive man.

MEDICAL THOUGHT IN BABYLONIA

Four thousand years before Christ, the Sumerians inhabited the "Land of the Two Rivers" in Mesopotamia, between the Tigris and the Euphrates, which is today Iraq. About two thousand years before Christ, the ancient kingdom of Babylonia was founded which, under King Hammurabi, organized all the small states of Mesopotamia, only to be destroyed in turn by the Persians.

Babylonian thought was orderly and scientific, and tended to systematize. The Babylonians used to bury their sovereigns with their entire court of wives, concubines, and warriors, as well as with their horses and chariots, so that their life in the hereafter might be pleasant. At the same time, they placed God over mortals, not only spiritually but also physically, raising great ziggurats which, besides being towers of worship, served also as astronomical observatories, since God was identified with the stars. The Babylonians organized their earthly existence; hence their legal codes written in cuneiform characters on blocks of diorite, and their code of Hammurabi, which marks the beginning of the systematization of medicine. Only the surgeon was truly looked upon as a physician, although his science moved in the direction of magic. Livers sacrificially dissected from sheep were used to foretell the future by hepatoscopy.

In the Zend-Avesta, three classes of physicians are cited among the Persians: *knife-doctors, grass doctors,* and *conjuring doctors,* who were the equivalent of our surgeons, internists, and psychiatrists.

Seven centuries before Christ, surgery was making notable advances because of the wars waged against Egypt by the Assyrians who ruled the Empire after the destruction of Babylon. Good proof of how systematic they were lies in the fact that "conjunctival icterus" (jaundice) was already included under the heading of biliary diseases, and the dualism of humoral and pneumatic pathology was established.

But the dense clouds of astrology and necromancy darkened medical thought in Babylonia.

MEDICAL THOUGHT IN EGYPT

A thousand years after the Assyrian civilization, when its backwash reached the valley of the Nile, medical schools were founded in ancient Egypt, where, according to Richet, all was God but God himself. Through five thousand years and thirty Egyptian dynasties, seven hundred and fifty million corpses were prepared for embalming; yet in Egyptian papyri not a single allusion to pathologic anatomy can be found. Opotherapy was practiced and hygiene received attention, as attested by Ebers' papyrus. In Egypt also appeared the figure of Imhotep, the first physician known as an individual in History.

Egyptian thought was devoted to the compiling of data during the long period of Persian, Macedonian, Roman, and Arab domination over Egypt. Medical pedagogy was created. If, according to Pharaonic papyri, medicine was based on magic at the beginning, in Edwin Smith's papyrus giving exact medical descriptions of more than seven hundred drugs there is but one single medical incantation. But the fate of Egypt was already sealed when Cambyses conquered this ancient land. After the reign of Cleopatra, Egypt became a province of Rome.

MEDICAL THOUGHT IN GREECE

To be Greek in the era of classical Greece was not a matter of anthropometric measurements or of skin color; to be Greek was "to participate in a certain view of the world and in a certain activity in the world," in a word, to be initiated into the "Hellenic communion."

Greek culture had its origins in Crete and Mycenae, but its Oriental, Egyptian, and Indian influences cannot be denied. On bivouac, at the bazaar, in caravan camps, Greek mercenaries and merchants would discuss the enigmas of heaven and earth, and in their palaces Greek aristocrats would interrupt their dalliance with captive Oriental women to question them on the millenary wisdom of their ancestors.

Greek arithmetic and geometry were derived from Egypt, and Greek astronomy from Babylonia, but the Greek mind brought order to the wealth of knowledge accumulated pell-mell by the Orientals and established the trilogy of *philosophy* (the desire to know and understand the world); *history* (the investigation and study of the world); and *theory* (a coherent vision in the search for universal norms and laws).

In Greece, the sorcerer was replaced first by the priest and later by the philosopher, who began medical research and initiated the transition of medicine from an art of curing to an applied science. The priest practiced the cult of Apollo and Aesculapius, which lasted for centuries and which, in contrast to the Hippocratic cult of observation and naturalism, was a cult of psychotherapy and a ritual of suggestion. The Hippocratic system was ruled by the theory of the four humors, although both systems insisted on cleanliness, fresh air, exercise, pleasant surroundings, and few medicines, even if Hippocrates himself prescribed beef liver in the treatment of anemia.

Hippocrates unified medicine and surgery and separated magic and philosophy from medicine, accomplishing in this field what Socrates accomplished in philosophy.

In Greece, cradle of philosophy and scientific medicine, the latter passed from the hands of the priest to those of the philosopher—since many philosophers were also physicians—thus leaving the indelible influence of art on science.

Pythagoras defined philosophy as the love of wisdom and the study of the principles and causes of all things. The first Greek philosophers were physicians. Democritus introduced the subtle composition of the atom as the basis of existence when he asserted that all things are composed of infinitely small atoms; Alcmæon of Crotona (c. 500 B.C.) established the brain instead of the heart as the seat of intelligence; and Empedocles of Agrigentum (c. 490–430 B.C.) described the four elements, fire, air, water, and earth, and founded the doctrine of humors, which was to be the basis for medical practice for many centuries. But although the Ionic, atomistic, and Pythagorean philosophers studied the universe, they did so with excessive imagination and little discipline and experimentation; they were outstanding, however, in the arts that demand observation and description, such as astronomy and biology. We must not forget that political fluctuations also hindered investigation.

Socrates (c. 470–399 B.C.) made man—not the universe—a philosophic subject; Plato (428–347 B.C.) laid the foundations of psychosomatic medicine by pointing to the unity of body and soul; Aristotle (348–322 B.C.) initiated scientific biology; and Hippocrates endowed medicine with its own philosophy, partially completed by Galen, who used experimentation as a basis for medical doctrines.

The Greeks made three great contributions to medicine: first, they looked at disease objectively, regarding it as a natural phenomenon, a physicomental disharmony (they kept clinical records of cases, and established the unity of the organism and its functions thus showing that observation was the method for studying natural phenomena); second, faced by a waning Greek mythology even before the advent of Christianity, they created a moral code for medical practice, and this morality was reflected in the lives of such men as Socrates and in the philosophies of such men as Plato; and third, they established the physician as a factor indispensable to human society.

Greek medical philosophy appeared during an era of uncertainty and in a world under the sway of unconquerable gods, when epidemics came and went like waves on a wild sea. In that world and under the influence of Plato's philosophy, Aristotle systematically observed the surrounding world and, by dissecting animals, founded the study of comparative anatomy; by describing the heart as the seat of the emotions, he completed Plato's idea of the brain as the seat of the mind. In this way he was able to relate the Platonic idea of the soul to his philosophic idea of the body.

In Greece, investigation and science were synonymous with search and creation. The contemporaries of Plato and Aristotle did not have a precise word for "science." For them, history, investigation, and philosophy were synonymous with practice, research, and system. According to Ortega y Gasset, philosophy was born through realization of the difference between discovering that one knows and the discovery of knowledge.

The figure of Hippocrates (c. 460–377 B.C.) dominated Greek medical thought. He was revered more than he was known, inasmuch as Greek science was more empirical than we have heretofore believed. Hippocrates is an example of how dangerous it is when love of brevity leads one to a certain obscurity of thought. This is borne out in some of his aphorisms.

Of course, while ancient Oriental literature was concerned solely with cures by drugs and surgery or supernatural powers, the idea of spontaneous cures was established in the Hippocratic collection for the first time, a fact which separated theurgic-empirical medicine from scientific medicine. The school of Cos developed the theory of disease as an effort on the part of the body to restore its disturbed functions and to re-establish the natural processes. Hippocrates asserted that nature itself cures disease, the processes of which he had studied, particularly of acute fevers in which the corrupted humors are eliminated by secretion and excretion. At the same time, he admitted that the curative power of nature sometimes fails, recourse to medical aid being then necessary. For Hippocrates, the word "nature" embraced the whole human organism and the laws that govern it. Plato and Aristotle insisted on the lack of aim in that nature. Asclepiades (124–40 B.C.) later conceived of nature as the body and its movements, holding it to be dangerous in certain situations.

In the realm of ethics, our ideal is identical with the Hippocratic, not only from the point of view of morality, but intellectually as well. The Hippocratics insisted on the importance of studying the complete clinical picture and of treating not diseases but the diseased, whom they considered as members of one group. They overestimated the capabilities of the physician; but even so they employed the services of technicians, chemists, physicists, and anatomopathologists, who today enjoy equal status with the physician, but were at that time his servants. Even today the sick man in search of cure turns not to medical societies or associations but to the private physician. Hence, the ideal physician of the Hippocratics —individualistic, wise, humble, and humanitarian—remains the ideal physician today.

MEDICAL THOUGHT IN ROME

Rome represents in history a sudden explosion of military might and ambition to dominate the world. Her proud eagles spread their wings over all the known regions of the planet; but the extraordinary qualities of the Romans as soldiers, lawyers, and administrators contrasted with their meager creative powers as intellectuals. They borrowed their art, their science, and their medicine from the Greeks, only as an aid to practical living.

Honor was paid to such men as Cicero, Caesar, Seneca, and Varro, authors of seventy-four works in six hundred and twenty volumes, praised by Saint Augustine, Pliny the Elder, author of a gigantic natural history, and Lucretius, the poet of science, who discussed epidemiology in his work *De Rerum Natura.*

In the year 219 B.C., for the first time a Greek physician, Archagathus, established himself in Rome. In 46 B.C. Julius Caesar extended citizenship rights to all foreign physicians. About A.D. 30 in the reign of Tiberius, the elegant Celsus penned his famous *De Re Medicina.* About A.D. 130 Galen was born, and Aretæus composed his most important treatise, emphasizing the curative powers of the *physis* as the sum of the organic forces. Galen was appointed Imperial Physician in 168; he died around 200. And in 529 Justinian closed the doors of the Platonic Academy, thereby putting an end to scientific investigation.

Medicine as a profession was beneath the dignity of the Roman citizen, who cured himself by invoking the aid of the gods. There were no physicians in Rome until the arrival of the first Greek immigrants, although medical services were available to the rich. The first Greek physicians were slaves of Roman families, and prejudice against them lasted until the Christian era; they were the butt of jibes and criticism in the epigrams of Martial and other satirists.

Because the Romans, who dominated world civilization, treated their physicians as slaves, they were responsible for the stagnation of medicine for more than a thousand years, for medicine can flourish only in a free climate.

Various sects and cults controlled medical practice under Roman rule. The Hippocratic, dogmatic, empiric, formal, and pneumatic theories pervaded the air, electrifying it with philosophic subtleties. The Romans therefore eventually became eclectic in attitude.

Rome fell heir to the medical school of Alexandria, founded in the wake of Alexander the Great's amazing march of conquest through Greece, Asia Minor, Egypt, Persia, and India, which made Alexandria the spiritual and intellectual capital of the world. Here the first medical school had been founded—based on the Aristotelian natural philosophy—where Herophilus (335–280 B.C.) dissected the human body and Erasistratus (c. 310–250 B.C.) adopted the dialectic materialism of Democritus (c. 460–357 B.C.). The decline of the Alexandrian Empire and the rise of the Romans ushered in an era, extending from the death of Herophilus to the birth of Christ, in which, preceded by a procession of brilliant physicians such as Asclepiades, Celsus, and Dioscorides (first century B.C.), the figure of Galen emerged. After Galen's death (c. A.D. 201), there was a period of lethargy that lasted until the publication of Vesalius' *Fabrica* in 1543.

Galen was the dictator of medicine for more than twelve hundred years. His word was the supreme authority, and to dissent from his opinions was heresy. Galen arrived at the end of the classical period; he popularized Aristotelian ideas and held that the human body was simply a vehicle for the soul—an excellent basis for the monotheism of Arabs and Christians. He accepted the ideas of Erasistratus and Herophilus, believing with the former in the healing powers of nature and with the latter in the creative purpose of nature and God, a purpose that led toward a well-defined end. He was physician to gladiators and to the emperor. He traveled extensively, and in his span of seventy years he wrote more than five hundred medical treatises, dissected animals and human bodies, and through vivisection investigated the operation of the heart and the spinal cord. He based his medicine on the idea of the spirits that permeated the various parts of the body, and considered that the principle of life was a pneuma that man took from the universal spirit through respiration. His knowledge of other branches of medicine summed up everything that had been discovered up to his time. He asserted that matter was composed of four elements, and that the body was made up of solids, humors, and spirits that originated in the liver as natural spirits, and when they reached the heart united with air to become vital spirits, and when finally they reached the head through the arteries were transformed into animal spirits. He encouraged and himself created extraordinary combinations in polypharmacy, and classified the pulse into sixty separate varieties. He studied all of medicine, embellishing it with his knowledge and confusing it with his theories. He propounded that blood moves, but not that it circulates. He was obstinate and dynamic and was held infallible until defeated by Paracelsus' theories; his anatomic myths were destroyed by the illustrations of Vesalius and Ambroise Paré's principle of the physiologic cure of wounds.

Galen thought little of his compatriots, insulting them in his writings. He possessed a highly polished style and was exceptionally addicted to polemics, which redounded to the detriment of his authority. His advice was sometimes reasonable, but the grounds on which he based it were often trite. As a psychologist he stood above any Renaissance medical writer, since he realized that medical treatment of psychoneuroses required a psychologic understanding; but at the same time he revered authority and authoritarianism, ascribing his own opinions to his teacher Herophilus, as Saint Thomas Aquinas would refer his own to Aristotle.

Galen asserted that the body creates its own structures and functions in accordance with the end purpose of the supreme being; to provide justification for his research on animals, in his teleologic writings he attempted to demonstrate the superiority of the human organism. According to Galen, nature exerts on disease, through nutrition and life, the same forces as on the normal state. By accepting the Aristotelian concept of the relation between the body and soul, he prepared the world for the idea of individual responsibility and the Christian interpretation of human life, thus again reuniting medicine and philosophy, which had been separated by Hippocrates.

In Hellenic civilization, the Greek ideas of an abstract morality of instincts, of metaphysical gods, and of the survival of the human personality challenged the Hebrew idea of an agreement between man and a single, universal God. Because they were teleologic in content, Galenic ideas were pleasing to the new Christian faith, which preached the existence of the Holy Trinity, individual responsibility, original sin, and redemption by grace. Of course, by overestimating the power of the mind over the body, Galen retarded the progress of experimental medicine; thus, interest in the body and in medicine declined with the accession to power of the Church in the Western Empire after the death of Emperor Constantine.

Galen's authority was so lasting that as late as 1559 Dr. Heynes was summoned for trial before the College of Physicians in London for having cast doubt on Galen's infallibility. He was readmitted to the medical college only after he made a retraction in writing.

For the rest, although they mistrusted the theories of their predecessors, Roman physicians accepted the philosophy developed by the Alexandrian empiricists, and founded their own private schools, where within six months a student could become a physician using such universal panaceas as theriaca.

Viewed as a whole, the contribution of Rome to medicine was slight, since medical practice was almost entirely in the hands of the Greeks. On the other hand, they popularized the use of public baths and sunbathing for therapeutic purposes. Anthonius Musa cured Augustus with cold hydrotherapy.

The Roman water supply system has never been equaled in history. The swamps and marshes around Rome were drained, and magnificent aqueducts constructed to carry pure water over distances of many miles. At the height of her power, Rome was served by fourteen aqueducts providing more than 130 gallons of water per capita, an amount never again attained by any other city. The baths were furnished with gymnasia and swimming pools. The Romans established the first hospital, as the result of a plague on the island of San Bartholomeo, and several convalescent homes. However, the aqueducts and baths (eight hundred in Rome) were only for wealthy neighborhoods, and the poor lived in the utmost squalor in spite of the fact that Plutarch recommended prophylaxis as the first step in the fight against disease.

In contrast with the progress in the fields of architecture and sanitation engineering, medicine in Rome was based on the private physician, although up to a point army physicians performed the duties of public health inspectors in their capacity as wandering physicians (*periodeutes*) or as practitioners in the *iatreias* or clinics. A professional class consciousness began to grow, but public health was always in advance of medicine, as is proved by the admirable structures built for irrigation, sewage disposal, and ventilation.

In the year 162, the Roman physician would rise in the morning and immediately present himself in the large hall of the Temple of Peace, hear the master speak in exquisite Greek on medicine, literature, philosophy, and grammar, after which he would discuss these subjects with his colleagues. He would then return home and see his patients, on whom he would operate alone or with his assistants, and would visit other patients in their own homes. At consultations, physicians would often become so incensed that they would even stick their tongues out at one another. Fees gradually rose from sixty-five cents per visit one hundred years before Christ to the equivalent of twelve thousand dollars which Manilius Cornutus paid for a consultation with a dermatologist.

A physician was required to have a license to practice, and in the year 370 an imperial edict forbade medical students to visit bordellos.

Yet, medicine served the rich exclusively until the advent of Christianity. The pleasures of the table and the body ruled the life of the wealthy citizen, who ate his food covered with pepper sauce and caviar, drank mead and white wine, took a nap in his chamber, and performed gymnastics followed by a massage, while Rome marched on to her destruction.

The barbarian invasion, malaria, moral and political corruption, exorbitant taxes, and the decline of agriculture brought about the final collapse of Rome. From then on, that is, from the fifth to the tenth century, medicine was again linked to magic even more intimately than before. The end of the cycle of Roman culture ushered in the controversial period of medieval medicine.

MEDICAL THOUGHT IN THE MIDDLE AGES

The capitol shook, the buskins of the Northern barbarians trampled on bloody togas, and the Roman Empire fell helped by the exhaustion of the silver mines of Spain and Greece, which depreciated Roman currency and caused a catastrophic fall in prices, and by the havoc wrought by the malarial plague. Then began what we call the Middle Ages, a period not entirely sterile, since the seed was planted that would germinate in the Renaissance.

The Middle Ages, an era of bronze and iron which emerged enveloped in a historical cloud of dust, did not represent a complete retrogression in medical knowledge. True, the stars of astronomy became the flickering lights of astrologic symbolism, and the chemist's test tube was transmuted into the bubbling crucible of the alchemist searching for the philosopher's stone. But the cathedrals became temples of study where the essences of classical knowledge were translated and poured into occidental molds, and the Arabs advanced pharmacology, although they suppressed the knife in favor of cautery.

The medieval period had a thirst for knowledge. The people crowded into the market place to hear Abelard, Duns Scotus, William of Ockham, Albert the Great, Saint Thomas. It was a great and germinative age, comparable to scorched earth where vegetation again bursts through, bearing once more the seed of civilization. It was also the night before the dawn of surgery in the thirteenth and fourteenth centuries, an Oriental and Islamic night studded with stars, like Oribasius (325–403) and the monastic compilers and Avicenna (980–1037), the Arab Galen.

During the thousand years called the Middle Ages, from about 500 to 1500, man lived on the defensive, in continual struggle with his own body. Medieval man was tortured by thoughts of the hereafter and portrayed himself in cadaverous-looking figures in which the skeleton tried to break through prematurely, as if it were trying to rush death. It was an era of continual war, religious fanaticism, and contempt for the flesh. Entirely absorbed in the contemplation of the spirit, people dissembled their neglect of the body with strong perfumes and voluminous raiments, while they awaited the resurgence of their rejuvenated, purified souls. In medieval Europe, the only cities of more than one hundred thousand inhabitants were Rome, Florence, Venice, Barcelona, and, later on, Toulouse and Paris. These cities had water supplied from rivers, sewer systems, legislation regarding public and market places, leprosaria, municipal baths, and medical services; also some attention was given to social hygiene for moral purposes. The medical profession was confined to the clergy. Streets were dark and muddy; houses had small windows filled in by boards instead of transparent glass, and their interiors were indescribably filthy. People ate heavily and with their fingers. All therapy, explained in almanacs and medical calendars since the publication of the *Regimen Sanitatis Salernitanum,* centered on the expulsion of undesirable humors by purges, emetics, cupping glasses, or bleedings. This no doubt represented a cathartic process of mystical meaning, since disease was thought to be possession by a foreign body that had to be ejected.

Medieval man, ruled by fear of plagues and of God, was a strange conglomeration of faith, ferocity, sensuality, and respect for the authority of the classics, particularly of Galen. The revival of alchemy and astrology in turn revitalized belief in invisible zodiacal and magical bonds between men, the stars, and the world.

The practice of medicine began to be taken up by highly cultivated men who were accorded a degree of nobility parallel with or superior to that of senators and provincial governors. But it gradually passed into the hands of the Church, which began to combine prescriptions with sermons, medicines with relics.

Betwen 400 and 1200 the great Hippocratic-Galenic tradition disappeared and medical knowledge regressed. Anatomy was forgotten, prognosis became an affair of divination, therapy a list of fantastic drugs, medicine a collection of spells and litanies. Everywhere, except in Salerno and Monte Cassino, the return to magic and sorcery prevailed, and no real progress was made for more than a thousand years. Only a few drugs, such as belladonna, hyoscyamine, aconite, valerian, cinchona, and digitalis, were derived from medieval folklore and sorcery. But Byzantium, the monasteries, Moslem Spain, and the European universities provided the channels through which medicine, bridging the murky medieval ocean, arrived on the shores of the Renaissance.

With the collapse of the power of the Visigoths in the sixth century, the south of Italy became for centuries an international battleground and a mosaic of small states, usually under the power of Byzantium and the influence of several cultures. The northern invaders seldom reached the south, and Byzantium, from its vantagepoint on the Bosphorus, asserted its might against the local leaders and later on against the Saracens. Greek was the predominant language; it still colors certain dialects today. Unnoticed by the Byzantines, other languages filtered in, such as the Arabic *pabis* and Latin dialects. In addition, a vigorous Hebrew culture flourished. Art and literature were encouraged in Byzantium, where, in the ninth and tenth centuries, Greek manuscripts were collected.

The night of the Middle Ages is illumined by Byzantine medicine, which appeared before the fall of Rome. The collapse of the empire was delayed by Emperor Marcus Aurelius' (121–180) diplomacy and by Constantine's (274–337) removal of the capital from Rome to Byzantium. Here medicine survived from the death of Galen thanks to a series of historians among whom the most distinguished were Oribasius (c. 325–400)—physician to the emperor Julian the Apostate, the last ruler to oppose Christianity—Aëtios (396–454), Alexander of Tralles (525–605), and Paul of Aegina (625–690), the famous compilers who, although lacking originality, preserved classical medical thought in their writings. When Constantinople fell (1453), Hellenic knowledge emigrated to the West with the Byzantine savants, and Humanism (*humanitas*), the patrimony of man who is the measure of all things (*homo mensura*) according to Protagoras, began to stir.

MONASTIC MEDICINE

The medieval monasteries, stationed along the great travel routes in Europe, were a combination of religious temple, home, haven, and hospital for travelers, as well as journalistic centers where news from all over the world arrived by word of mouth and was disseminated by the resident friars in conversation with travelers. Gigantic nerve centers of medieval life, the monasteries acted as the world's loud-speakers, while in the silence of their cells monks, fleeing from earthly dangers, chose learning and classical literature as the road to heaven.

Salerno, the Greek colony that became later a Roman outpost, represented the last flicker of Hippocratic medicine, just as Monte Cassino represented the dawn of modern medicine. While Europe was steeped in medieval darkness, Greek dialects were still spoken in Salerno, and there were physicians in the area during the eighth and ninth centuries after the Saracen invasion of Italy. Toward the middle of the tenth century, Salerno became famous throughout the world as the first great European medical school in which the study of medicine was preceded by three years of preparation in logic.

Several cultural streams converged in Salerno, making it the meeting place for physicians of all races and creeds. It was the first school to award a diploma and the title of *Doctor*. In collaboration with Monte Cassino, many books were published there, among them the famous *Regimen Sanitatis Salernitanum,* a medical manual in verse, perhaps the most popular book on medicine for the home ever written, and in which "Doctors," "Rest," "Cheer," and "Diet" are recommended. It was compiled by many authors and the date of its publication is uncertain; it was dedicated to Robert, Duke of Normandy, the eldest son of William the Conqueror. With the invention of the printing press, it appeared in many editions, was the basis for subsequent treatises on hygiene, and was often imitated.

The name of Arnold of Villanova is now offered as the possible author of the Salernian epos. The school of Salerno is enveloped in a veil of romantic legends, among them that of its founding by four doctors—a Greek, a Roman, an Arab, and a Jew—symbolizing the blending of four cultures. The period of its greatness coincides with the time of the Norman invasion, when the old monks kept guard over the traditional Greek science and taught the value of gymnastics, diet, and hygiene. The first modern text on anatomy comes from Salerno, and in it human anatomy replaces the pig's.

Bologna and Padua replaced Salerno in the twelfth century. In 1224, Frederick II, the great enemy of the Popes, established a university in Naples, rival city to the papal Babylon. This dealt a mortal blow to the neighboring Salerno, where the university languished until it was closed by Napoleon in 1811. The pendulum of knowledge thus swung from Salerno, as the center of world knowledge, to Padua, Montpellier, Paris, and Leyden.

Monte Cassino, which carried on the Salerno heritage, was the cradle of modern western medicine. It lies slightly less than a hundred miles from Salerno as the crow flies. The light of the new Renaissance spirit shone from its vast monastery, a gigantic mass of stone set at the top of a hill, with a large cathedral and a series of beautiful cloisters of various periods. The trip from Salerno to Monte Cassino used to take a week. The monastery was founded in 529 by Saint Benedict of Nursia, and his tomb, as well as that of his sister, Saint Scholastica, can still be seen. Monte Cassino was sacked in 580 by the Lombards and was reconstructed in 720. It was once again destroyed by the Saracens in 884, was rebuilt in 950, and reached its zenith under Abbot Desiderius, who became Pope Victor III in 1086, the time of the Norman conquest.

Monte Cassino was the great occidental monastic center, reaching its golden age in the eleventh century, when the West was flattering the Orient by acknowledging the military supremacy, knowledge, and science of Islam, as well as its superiority in battle, industry, administration, and the arts. Oriental and Semitic words were adopted, such as *arsenal, admiral, tariff, algebra, almanac, theodolite, damask,* and others of pronounced Oriental flavor, including many anatomic terms (*basilica, cephalic, saphena*) and the nomenclature of certain drugs. Another great achievement of Monte Cassino was the work of Constantine the African (1020–1087), born to Jewish parents in Carthage or Sicily. An Arab orator and secretary in Oriental languages to the invader Robert the Norman who spent many years in Salerno, Constantine was converted to Christianity and became a Benedictine monk at Monte Cassino. During the last ten years of his life he translated into Latin, with the aid of a local scribe, the works of certain Jewish doctors from Kairouan. At the same time that the Archbishop of Salerno was translating Greek medical writings into Latin, Constantine brought to the West his translations of Arab learning, until then understood only by the Jews. Just as the Arab superstructure over Greek medicine affected all Islam, so did the Latin translations of Constantine affect the West. Among his most important translations are the treatises on fevers, diet, urine, and philosophy originally written by the Jew Isaac of Kairouan (845–940), and the works by the Persian, Abbas Haly (930–994), including a technical vocabulary.

But it is now time to discuss another phase of medieval medical thought: Arabic medicine.

ARABIC MEDICAL THOUGHT IN SPAIN

Arabic medicine was the result of prodigious historical juggling. The first personage to emerge in this great historical march was Nestorius, patriarch of Constantinople (from 428 to 431), who was born in Syria toward the end of the fourth century. An eloquent man and a subtle metaphysician, he broke with Orthodox Christianity by attributing two personalities and two natures to Jesus. At that time, when Christianity still glowed with the flame kindled by Paul of Tarsus, the prince of Christendom, it was easy to create a separate religious school based on a new interpretation of the dogma. The Nestorians claimed that Mary was not the mother of God but of Christ, and this slight dialectic difference brought Nestorius exile and death in an oasis in Libya, just as another theologic slip condemned Servetus to the stake under the regime of Calvin.

Exiled to the desert, with no one with whom to argue their theologic subtleties, the Nestorians dedicated themselves to healing the body, since healing the soul had cost them so dear. Disappointed with their times, they turned back to the lost glory of classical Greece. From the medicophilosophic waters of the Greco-Roman schools they filled their spiritual vessels. Generous with their science, they then poured the old Hellenic nectars into Syriac molds. And in Edessa and other Persian towns they founded schools of medicine and translated Greek writings into Syrian. Their purpose was to continue the brilliant Hippocratic-Latin medical tradition. When exiled to Persia, they founded on the banks of the Euphrates the medical school of Jundi Shapur, the point of departure for future Arabic medicine.

Up to that time the Arabs had been content to ride across the hot, yellow sands of Asia and Africa and to sip their aromatic wines and discourse on their ancient philosophies. But, a young and ardent people, inspired by the new doctrines of Mohammed (570–632), they suddenly launched into a fabulous historic cavalcade that took them across to India and from Samarkand through the Caucasus to Sicily. And when Tarik leaped from Africa to *Gebel-Tarik* (the mount of Tarik or Gibraltar) (711) their swords were to carve in Spain a slice of that Saracen civilization which was born with Mohammed in the seventh century and died with the sack of Baghdad by the Tartars and with the expulsion of the Arabs by the Spaniards in the West and by the Turks in the East.

This whirlwind of conquest gave them sway over Persia and possession, not only of men and towns, but of all the medicophilosophic treasure derived from the Greeks recorded in the ancient Nestorian parchments. That is why Arab medicine is clearly Persian and indirectly Hellenic in origin. Arab physicians drew from these sources, but since theirs was too vast an empire—it stretched from Medina to Finisterre—to be fashioned of a uniform fabric—on the contrary, it was really a multicolored mosaic of races and nations joined by the power of the scimitars and the prestige of the Saracen crescent—Arabic medicine was a compound of many more elements. For that reason it has been said that Arabic medicine should be called Moslem or Islamic medicine. For it was not race, but the Arabic tongue that united them. Arabic medicine derived from those men who spoke and wrote in Arabic, whatever their race or even their religion.

The history of Arab Spain is the history of medieval Europe. The Eastern or Baghdad Caliphate, under the rule of the Abbassids, happily took the initiative in extracting, to its own advantage as well as that of science, all the wisdom enclosed in the old Nestorian medical schools and the younger schools to which they gave birth. The caliphs took pains to endow their country with a flourishing cultural organization. Libraries, institutes, and hospitals which were veritable centers of learning similar to those of Damascus, Cairo, and Baghdad, vied with one another in research and in disseminating medical science. Moslem Spain in 1200 boasted seventy libraries replete with medical books—the library in Cordova alone housed two hundred and twenty-five thousand volumes—and seventeen schools of higher learning, lodes of intellectual gold that were mined by all the medical men of the time. The Arabs introduced in Spain aromatic gums and spices such as myrrh, cinnamon, and cassia. They also distinguished themselves in ceramics, in which activity the Persian influence can be detected. Their urns and jars were embellished with fruit and leaves after the Persian manner, and their tiles and majolica bear the same decorations as Persian rugs. The magnificence of their work is borne out by the fact that as a gift for Emperor Charlemagne (742–814), the Caliph Harun-al-Rashid (763–809) chose several jars which he had filled with unguents and precious trinkets.

The Arabs also introduced the palm tree, sugar cane, rice, cotton, and oranges, and they grew exotic medicinal plants in Andalusia with excellent results.

One certainly cannot accuse the Moslem Empire of intolerance. The Arabs, who adopted the science of Paul of Aegina, Oribasius, Hippocrates, and Alexander of Tralles without prejudice, allowed medical navigators of all denominations to sail on the vast Arab sea. Under the aegis of Islam, Jews, Spaniards, and Persians distilled their medical findings into a comprehensive bibliography which featured such medical treatises as the great *Pharmacopeia* of the Vizier Ibn Wafid al Lakhmi in Toledo.

At first the Arab physician carefully searched for threads of gold in the Hellenic strawpile, translating whatever Greek works fell into his hands into Aramaic and Syrian and then into Arabic. This frenzied resurrection of ancient learning lasted until well into the ninth century. The caliphs became the Maecenases of studious investigators; and in the Moslem court the melodious twang of stringed instruments alternated with grave voices discussing medicine. In every palace, next to the mysterious seraglio could be found the library, where hour upon hour men of solemn mien scrutinized yellowed parchments. During the period of the Omayyad caliphs, whose empire extended from Spain to Samarkand, the luxury, the lavishness of the Damascus court—inexistent in the times of al-Chiliyat and the nomad shepherds; later, during the lifetime of Mohammed, established in Medina—was extended to medicine, which reached its golden age in the eighth century and lasted until the twelfth century, when it began to decline.

It is a flagrant injustice to say that the Arabs were no more than compilers of Greco-Latin science. The Arabs did more than decant the Greek waters from spring to vessel. They added to them their intuition, their humanism, and their romantic spirit. Proof of their historic labors were the four hundred thousand volumes bound in leather and gold in the library of al Hakim II, books that recorded their great knowledge in a language rich, nervous, agile, virile, as adequate an instrument for exalting medicine as Vergil's was for agriculture. In their castles, redolent with the scent of sandalwood and humming with the melody of the rebec, they plaited the strands of a solid medical culture. They evolved their medicine on a logical basis, translating the works from Greek to Arabic and adding their own commentaries. They particularly studied epidemic fevers and eye diseases, both prevalent among them, and greatly contributed to pharmacology and pharmacy by introducing many drugs and new words in their terminology, and by their skill in the processes of chemistry, which they called alchemy. And their history boasts such physicians as Hunain (809–873), Avenzoar (1113–1162), Rhazes (850–925), and, above all, Avicenna (900–1037), the Arabic Galen, physician and philosopher, whose *Canon* has been the most famous medical book in the world, and who sought to harmonize Galen with Aristotle. The Arabs hated the surgical knife, preferring cautery, to which topic a book was devoted by the great surgeon Albucasis of Cordova. His fame was overshadowed only by that of Maimonides (1135–1204), who symbolized the fusion of Arabic, Hebrew, and Spanish cultures.

The thirteenth century marked the Hispano-Arabic-Sephardic union. In the narrow streets of Toledo, the grave accents of Sephardic Jews and Moors blended with the rich, sonorous Castilian. Three faiths worshiped in the mosques. In an intolerant Europe, Spain was a beacon of religious tolerance. Translators poured Arabic science into Latin molds, and then into Hebrew cruets. Talmudists, cabalists, philosophers, jurists, grammarians, and poets wove wreaths of Sephardic roses about the Spanish brow. Aristocratic philosophy went arm in arm with Catholic dogmas and the religions of Moors and Jews. The Strait of Gibraltar was spanned by a bridge of civilization supported by three racial arches. Toledo, Cordova, Barcelona, and Morocco were beads in the necklace of an erudite and tolerant medieval Spain. Like a towering colossus, Maimonides rose, a second Moses. One no longer had to dream of Jerusalem. The Arabs until their expulsion in the late fifteenth century and the Sephardic Jews until their expulsion in the early sixteenth were rooted in the generous soil of Spain. And like a rosebush, they often bloomed; and like a fig tree—the noble Biblical tree—they often eschewed the blossom to yield only fruit. For this reason the history of Arab Spain is the history of medieval Europe.

MEDIEVAL THOUGHT IN EUROPEAN UNIVERSITIES

European universities grew from the passionate desire for knowledge that characterized medieval thought. The center of learning moved then, as now, with political power: from Salerno to Bologna, Padua, and Montpellier.

In Bologna the unity of medicine and surgery was maintained, and such outstanding figures as Geronimo Cardano (1501–1576), a contemporary of Benvenuto Cellini, studied there. Cardano, a fascinating figure, whose *De Propria Vita,* with those of St. Augustine and Rousseau, is one of the three best autobiographies ever written, established the existence of what later was called "moral madness." In collaboration with the encyclopedist Konrad von Gesner (1516–1565), he later also developed astrology.

The School of Montpellier was founded by Arabs and Jews in 1208, and the faculty of medicine was created in 1220. It flourished during the thirteenth and fourteenth centuries, and again in the seventeenth and eighteenth centuries, producing such outstanding figures as the Spaniard, Arnold of Villanova (1240–1313), Henri de Mondeville (1260–1320), Guy de Chauliac (1300–1370) (whose text on surgery was the most outstanding in history and who pointed out the error of medieval medicine in separating itself from surgery), François Rabelais (1494–1553), Vieussens (1641–1715), de Bordeu (1722–1776), and Delpech (1775–1832).

The School of Paris flourished in the thirteenth century. It was a citadel of scholasticism and authoritarian and dialectic medicine as represented by Roger Bacon, Albertus Magnus, and Saint Thomas Aquinas. This university excluded books on surgery and obstetrics from its library and barber-surgeons from its benches.

Respect for dogmatic authority was combined in these universities with naturalistic observation; there was both research and teaching, and medicine was considered one of the so-called liberal arts. But students' textbooks were primarily the texts of Aristotle with commentaries by Averroës, Saint Thomas Aquinas, Ovid, Cicero, Plutarch, and other classics.

Oxford was founded in the twelfth century and Cambridge in the thirteenth. The former was classicist and conservative; the latter specialized in the exact and natural sciences and was furthermore of a much more liberal character. Chaucer described in his *Canterbury Tales* a dogmatic physician, a symbol of the time, and apparently used as his model John of Gaddesden, the author of the work *Rosa*

Anglica, so entitled because of its five parts which he compared to the petals of a rose. In the fifteenth century, the number of universities in Italy rose to sixteen, and in 1518 Thomas Linacre, a humanist comparable to Erasmus (1460–1574) and Francis Bacon, founded the Royal College of Physicians under Henry VIII, although Linacre was an authoritarian who aspired to re-create old classic culture as orthodox dogma for the medicine of his age. His image is tinted by the first dawn of Renaissance thought.

MEDICAL THOUGHT IN THE RENAISSANCE

The Renaissance, which began in Italy around the end of the fourteenth century and reached its apogee two centuries later all over Europe, was not only a revival of classic culture but a change in philosophic attitude toward life as well. With freedom of thought, Platonic humanism was reborn and supplanted medieval scholasticism. Medicine was separated from philosophy and combined with dialectic materialism. The Renaissance was a resurrection, a *re-birth,* which is more important than birth itself.

The printing press and gunpowder were invented; America was discovered; the heliocentric revolution of Copernicus (1473–1543) superseded Ptolemy's geocentric conception; the anatomic revolution of Vesalius (1514–1564) nullified Galen; navigation was facilitated by the mariner's compass; the earth was accepted as having a spherical shape; and the gold and silver of Mexico and Peru produced a certain degree of inflation that stimulated industry and commerce. All these factors contributed to swell the irresistible torrent of the Renaissance.

Taste for classical Latin was restored by the works of Petrarch; the "humanities" opposed the "divinities"; and the fall of Constantinople to the Turks forced many teachers to come to Europe, bringing with them their manuscripts. The unique multifaceted genius of Leonardo da Vinci (1452–1519) influenced all the arts and sciences, especially anatomy and physiology. The Vatican was transformed into a dynamic center of classic culture, and the Protestant Reformation re-established ecclesiastical discipline. Simple, primitive religious ardor returned, complemented by the humanism of men like Erasmus and the Spaniard Juan Luis Vives (1492–1540), teacher of kings, self-exiled in Bruges, who reasserted the equilibrium between God and man. Copernicus restored the universe's ancient plan and structure. Paracelsus (1493–1541) refuted the dogmas of Galen and Avicenna. Vesalius dissected the corpses of executed criminals, studied boiled, polished human bones, and published his *Fabrica* with splendid anatomic illustrations by Titian's pupil, Calcar, giving the world (1543) the first great scientific work in the history of mankind, and freeing anatomy from the dogmatism of the old masters. Michael Servetus, burned for heresy by Calvin, discovered the pulmonary blood circulation; and a realistic English army physician, William Harvey (1578–1657), taught King Charles I how the embryo of the chick develops in the egg. Later, on an April afternoon in 1614, alone in his study, Harvey added to the notes he was preparing for a lecture before the College of Physicians in London the statement that "blood circulates." He considered blood circulation as a problem of mechanics, based it on the ideas of Galileo, and carried out in his work the greatest advances in embryology since Aristotle, initiating modern scientific research. Malpighi (1628–1694) discovered the capillary system. Botanical gardens were revived in Padua, Pisa, Leyden, and in other European cities as the expression of an Aristotelian love of nature. Interest in medicinal herbs was reborn and zoologic gardens were created in Lisbon and other cities, while advances were made in work on magnetism and electricity, especially by William Gilbert (1540–1603). And, while ancient magic was paradoxically reborn in the form of enchantments and witchcraft, the philosophy of Bacon and Descartes (1596–1640) created a mechanical conception of the universe and of the human body.

The Renaissance therefore represented the birth of the physiobiologic sciences in the work of Leonardo da Vinci; of the biologic sciences in the studies of Vesalius, Harvey, and Malpighi; and of chemotherapy in those of Paracelsus. Renaissance medical thought, particularly that of Harvey, whose discovery of the circulation of the blood was literarily "anticipated" by Shakespeare in his *Coriolanus,* notably influenced the literature of the time toward the naturalistic, just as Claude Bernard (1813–1878) and Trousseau (1801–1867) were to influence the school of Zola in nineteenth-century literary France. The body was looked upon as a machine subject to definite laws, and, although the Church reacted against this depredation of the soul, the phrase of Leonardo da Vinci, "All knowledge (consciousness) comes from the senses," became the slogan for investigation. The soul was forgotten and medicine lost its philosophy.

Descartes, father of modern philosophy, described the body as a machine, although he conceded man a soul located in the pineal gland. The scholastic Aristotelian conception, overthrown by Galileo, Bacon, and Descartes, gave way to a mechanistic conception in which the cosmos and the human body were considered as machines composed of imperceptible parts, it being believed that with each movement the invisible atoms rearranged themselves according to a geometric law.

MEDICAL THOUGHT IN THE SEVENTEENTH AND EIGHTEENTH CENTURIES

With the passing of the iatrochemical and iatrophysical rage of Thomas Willis (1621–1675) and Pitcairne (1652–1713), there emerged the figure of Thomas Sydenham, the English Hippocrates. Thomas Sydenham (1624–1689), a stout fighter in the parliamentarian ranks of Cromwell, established diseases as clinical entities, just as later the Dutch Hippocrates, Hermann Boerhaave (1668–1738), restored the human aspect of medicine. Sydenham asserted the healing power of nature, claiming that it watches over us day and night and looks after our welfare. He was a good, simple, practical physician who sat by the patient's bedside instead of at an experimental work table like Harvey. He was not interested in the *why* of disease as Harvey was, but in *how* to cure. He studied patients, not biologic phenomena as Harvey did. He closed his books and opened his eyes, and revived the Hippocratic spirit in medicine.

Sydenham's shining example is eclipsed only by John Hunter's, the Scotch Titan (1728–1793) who demonstrated the value of pathologic and comparative anatomy in medical research. It is to him we owe the famous phrase—included in a letter to his friend Edward Jenner (1749–1823), the discoverer of vaccine—"Why think? Why not try the experiment?" Hunter anticipated modern scientific thought by uniting medicine and biology on his dissecting table.

Nevertheless, treatment by provoking salivation, emetics, purges, and bloodlettings continued into the eighteenth century. But the stage was being set for the great philosophic change in therapy.

MEDICAL THOUGHT IN THE NINETEENTH CENTURY

In the nineteenth century the true nature of scientific investigation was completely revealed when the curtain was raised on Claude Bernard. The father of modern physiology, he set down the steps of all scientific investigation: observation, hypothesis, and experimental proof. His philosophy, expressed in his *Introduction to the Study of Experimental Medicine,* is a classic study which since 1865 has oriented the modern research worker.

In that century therapy was based on pathologic anatomy, which led to therapeutic nihilism. But the introduction of hypodermic medication by Sir Thomas Clifford Allbutt (1836–1925) was already a considerable advance. Hospitals grew like mushrooms in a forest, among them the famous Hôtel Dieu, the Berlin General Hospital, and those in Oxford and Minnesota.

The 1890's saw the first endocrine medication (the precursors of which were Celsus and Galen, who administered extracts from organs, and the physicians who, in the Middle Ages, administered powdered heart), a thyroid extract prescribed by Murray (1891) to a cretin, the first antitoxin, and roentgen rays.

In the same century pathologic anatomy was born with Morgagni (1682–1771). Schwann (1810–1887) and Schleiden (1804–1881) established the cellular unit, on which Virchow (1821–1902) based his pathology. In 1859 Pasteur proved the bacteriologic origin of infectious disease, and Darwin published *The Origin of the Species.* From 1900 on the science of genetics and inheritance developed. The philosophic pendulum swung back to materialism and determinism in biology, and science came once more into conflict with the Church. Later, in the dawn of the twentieth century, brilliant new ideas started to burst like rockets.

MEDICAL THOUGHT IN THE TWENTIETH CENTURY:
THE NEW SYSTEM OF IDEAS

Modern medicine, as we see it today, is not pure art, since it rejects the sovereignty of intuition, nor is it mathematics, since it places experiment before statistics. Its ultimate purpose is that of modern civilization: to prolong life and improve health by eliminating the causes of disease and death and thus facilitate the integral triumph of the human being over environment.

Medicine as a science is now also *erudition*—facts, principles, theories, methods and rules—and *action;* that is, theory and practice. It tends to acquire new knowledge and methods through study and observation, transmits them by teaching, and applies those methods to the creation of an art of healthy living. *Research, teaching,* and *clinical practice* are therefore the three royal rungs on the ladder of medicine. The practicing physician, depositary of the art of healing, applies it like an artist to the improvement of the health of men and of peoples. The medical teacher's objective is to bequeath his erudition to the student. The researcher works on animals and chemical substances in his laboratory, on patients in clinics and hospitals, and on populations in social statistics. Hippocrates and Sydenham are symbols of the practicing physician, devotees of medicine as art, *ars medendi;* likewise, Haller and Osler are the incarnation of the teacher who makes of medicine a pedagogic discipline of the university; and Harvey and Finlay personify the research worker who makes of medicine a pure science. These three fight side by side against the three eternal enemies of humanity: pain, age, and death.

Philosophically, energy and matter are thought of today as aspects of one and the same reality, described by mathematicians as *quanta* in a four-dimensional space-time continuum. A given organized structure is established as the basis for life. The viruses are looked upon as complex molecules and are likened to genes. It is accepted that life creates form and structure and tends to maintain these immutable, resisting the maximum entropy which is death.

The concept of disease, which for the Greeks was functional disharmony between mind and body and for the Renaissance an accident in the human machine, is today something quite different. The mind is held to be the passage of impulses through the nervous system, just as the cardiac beat is the contraction of muscular fibers in the myocardium. The mind begins as reflex and later becomes consciousness. On a higher plane, the mind acts on voluntary life, and in the subconscious it acts through the autonomic system on involuntary life. The life span depends on the original genetic equipment, on the way we live, and on environment in the same way as the durability of a tire depends on the car, the driver, and the road. Disease is looked upon today as a deviation from anatomicophysiologic normality, and medicine is a more complicated affair than Sydenham imagined. Diseases are not items that can be classified like birds or flowers, but complex interactions in individual genetic structure, free will, and environment. Pathology gradually gains ascendancy over ecology, which means that we interfere with the equilibrium of nature when we treat disease.

Modern therapy has developed into several fields: immunobiology (vaccines, sera, and biologic agents); opotherapy; vitaminology; chemotherapy (arsenicals, sulfonamides, antibiotics); psychiatry and psychotherapy (psychiatric shock, leukotomy, psychosomatic medicine, psychoanalysis and psychosynthesis, narcoanalysis, hematosonography); surgery, and other fields of lesser importance.

On the other hand, individual, university, national, and industrial research has achieved extraordinary importance, distinguished by the fact that it seeks the dynamic interrelationships among things and by its pragmatic attitude. Public health is today a governmental responsibility, has a profound social and political significance and a universalist basis, as in quarantines, international health laws, antimalarial campaigns; it is military and civil in nature, both a weapon of war and a weapon of progress in peace. In synthesis, therapy represents the present stage of Hippocratic-Sydenham-Boerhaavian naturalistic thought; research is the application of the Harveian spirit of medicine as science (and therapy as art); public health is the modern channeling of Roman thought and work in sanitation.

NEW ORIENTATIONS IN BIOLOGIC THERAPY

Up to the last century there was no therapy in the strict sense of the word, the effects of several substances being known only empirically: most of these substances were vegetable, like digitalis, belladonna, quinine, and others. Up to the last century interest was centered primarily on diagnosis. Today therapy is drawing as much or more attention than diagnosis—a sign of a Hippocratic revival, of greater concern for the health of the individual, and of the growing need for community health. The beginning of the nineteenth century found therapy exactly as it was fifteen hundred years previously. Prehistoric ideas that disease was something foreign that had penetrated into the body still prevailed, and therapy centered almost exclusively on elimination by means of enemas, purgatives, diuretics, emetics, and bloodletting.

With a new concept of disease, there was a change in the approach to therapy, based on the comparison of physical signs observed in life with lesions observed in death; in other words, therapeutic nihilism. In the last decade of the nineteenth century appear the first biologic ideas on therapy as reflected in immunobiology and endocrinology.

ORGANIC, NATURAL, AND ACQUIRED DEFENSES AND IMMUNOLOGY

A new therapy was born with the discovery that the body and its functions could be influenced by chemical means, which sometimes, as with endocrine products, were a simple therapy of substitution to aid the chemical defenses of the body.

In 1894 it was found that the body could acquire new defenses against microbial attacks, through, for instance, antitoxins, the first of which to be used was the diphtheria antitoxin.

From then on, contagious disease was regarded as a contest between the capacity of bacteria to reproduce and that of the body to destroy them. The body possesses two mechanisms for the destruction of these infecting agents: (a) antibacterial substances contained in serum; (b) leukocytes which phagocytize bacteria. The antibodies are produced by specialized cells in response to the presence of infecting agents and are proteins capable of adsorbing the surface of microbes, rendering them susceptible to phagocytosis. Each antibody is specifically effective against a particular type of infecting agent. Chemotherapeutics may be bactericidal, killing germs, or bacteriostatic, inhibiting their growth and development. Therefore, in order to combat an infection, either chemotherapeutic agents may be used directly against microbes, or the organic defenses may be increased through the administration of sera rich in antibodies.

The discovery of the diphtheria antitoxin revolutionized cathartic therapy by showing that it is better to provide the organism with the necessary instruments to aid its natural defenses, whether phagocytosis or humoral principles. It was more effective to determine passive immunization by means of sera or active by means of vaccines—introduced by Sir Almroth Edward Wright toward the end of the past century—than to attack microbes by other means. The science of immunobiology was developed by taking importance away from the germ and giving it to its toxins. The conclusion was also drawn that there must be as many antitoxins as there are infectious diseases.

Consequently, active immunization was practiced against typhoid fever and tetanus, stimulating natural protective reactions in anticipation of a possible subsequent infection. Serotherapy reinforces these defenses after the infection. In diphtheria it was discovered that the bacilli are concentrated in the throat, but the toxins enter the blood stream, requiring treatment by antitoxin prefabricated in large doses; the presence of bacilli in the throat then ceases to be of importance, except as regards possible contagion.

We observe here a relationship between the concept of disease and the method of combatting it. As long as it was believed that disease was subject to malign external influence, magic methods were employed in treatment. When disease came to be thought of as a series of organic reactions to changes in the external environment, therapy was oriented toward utilization of an aid to the natural organic defenses. Between these two great phases a slow transition occurred during which magical properties were attributed to herbs and alkaloids were extracted from their juices and saps, thus marking the beginning of scientific chemistry.

Ancient pharmacopeias consisted mainly of remedies extracted from plants, the so-called Galenic preparations. In the sixteenth century Paracelsus turned his back on nature and introduced certain metals into the pharmacopeia, such as mercury, lead, iron, arsenic, and copper. From Galenic medicaments we have arrived at antibiotics and from non-Galenic remedies we derive modern chemotherapy, which began with the studies of Ehrlich in 1900 and was furthered by Domagk in 1932. The latter introduced TB-1, the antitubercular sulfonamide, precursor of modern isoniazid derivatives, which represent the greatest step forward in the therapy of tuberculosis.

MODERN CHEMOTHERAPY

"We must learn to make magic bullets which, like those of the ancient fable, cannot miss their mark, and will destroy only the pathogenic agents against which they are aimed." Thus spoke Paul Ehrlich (1854–1915), marking the beginning of modern chemotherapy, just as the rebel genius of Paracelsus founded classical chemotherapy in the Renaissance. The basic theory was the discovery of a chemical substance with an affinity for the syphilis spirochete that would be nontoxic to the human body. In his book-filled laboratory, Ehrlich led for some years the life of a recluse, a hermit of science, finally discovering a new staining agent for the trypanosome: trypan red. In 1905 he studied the effect of atoxyl on sleeping sickness, discarding it as excessively toxic. In 1907 he discovered a new formula, the six hundred and sixth in a series of previous tests. 606 proved to be the "magic bullet" against trypanosomes and spirochetes in chickens.

Present-day chemotherapy is based on Ehrlich's brilliant discovery: the treatment of parasitic diseases by chemical mastery over the infecting germ without marked toxic effects on the patient. Ehrlich's theory of lateral chains led him to consider the possibility of controlling toxins with a drug instead of with an antitoxin. Certain organic compounds could carry a strong poison on a lateral chain which upon detaching itself would neutralize or destroy a toxin or bacterium by attaching itself to it. 606 would destroy the protozoa in vitro only when the cells liberated the arsenic in pentavalent ionized form.

Ehrlich continued his work of creating a *Therapia Sterilisans Magna* and synthesized another new product, 914 or neoarsphenamine, the new "magic bullet for hunting microbes" which machineguns the parasites in the blood and leaves the organism unharmed. The German wizard started syphilotherapy as a chromotherapy, or treatment with dyes, and developed it into a true chemotherapy.

Chemotherapy was born therefore from Ehrlich's desire to find out why immunity is a real factor in many diseases produced by bacteria but not in diseases produced by protozoans, such as malaria. He knew that methylene blue dyed the parasites without harm to the human body. His scrutinizing eyes observed that the trypanosomes dyed by trypan red "swam gaily in a drop of blood" instead of dying, but were incapable of infecting rats into which they were inoculated. Reactions between the chemotherapeutic agents and the parasites, while not occurring in vitro, often took place in the human body, and, by releasing arsenic oxide inside the body slowly and in concentration sufficient to destroy the treponemas, proved lethal to the parasites which, rendered incapable of reproduction, were devoured by the phagocytes and destroyed by the defensive agents of the organism. Interference with bacterial reproduction had been finally achieved, as a result of coupling art and science in medicine.

The emergence of sulfonamides related the discoveries of Ehrlich with those of Domagk in 1935, who used stains that acted bacteriostatically on live tissue only. Ehrlich left the chemotherapy of spirochetal and protozoan infections well established, but only Domagk can be credited with having begun specific antibacterial chemotherapy. By taking the place of para-aminobenzoic acid and other nutritional factors essential to bacterial cells, sulfonamides act, so to speak, as a "wolf in sheep's clothing" toward the bacterium, since if, in the presence of pus or necrotic tissues, para-aminobenzoic acid in small quantities cancels out the bacteriostatic action of large quantities of sulfonamides, under favorable conditions sulfonamides biologically produce a real deficiency disease in bacteria. The sulfonamides therefore do not kill bacteria; they only stop their development. A sulfonamide is a kind of "bacterial hypnotic or anesthetic." If, however, the bacteria are not destroyed while "dormant" by the organic defenses, the infection bursts forth anew when they waken from their parasitic slumber.

The next step in chemotherapy was to compare the metabolism of bacteria with that of the human cell in order to select the agents least toxic to man and most toxic to bacteria; or to study—as in the work of Dubos—the specific complex sugars that form the armorlike capsule of certain pneumococci and that protect them against the organic defenses, and then to analyze farm soils in search of microbes capable of destroying this capsule with their digestive enzymes. In this manner it has been possible to attack type III pneumococcus and destroy its sugar carapace or shield.

The next step now is to study interference with microbial metabolic processes, to determine the chemical structures vital to bacterial life and to synthesize them in the laboratory, with a view to employing them as nutritional blocks against bacteria. This rational pharmacology involves hurling chemical compounds into the intramicrobial metabolism after the fashion of a monkey wrench thrown into the complex machinery of this metabolism, thus paralyzing its wheels, twisting its structures, and replacing the vital microbial metabolites by a veritable "fifth column" chemotherapeutic agent which, from within the bacterium, aids in its destruction. On this chemobiologic interference with the enzymic systems vital to the bacterium, the pharmacology of the future may be based.

So far, chemotherapy has achieved its greatest heights with the discovery of penicillin by Fleming in 1928 and of its clinical application by Florey in 1940. Between primitive antiseptics and modern antibiotics there is a long stretch that begins with Lister and culminates in Fleming. Antibiotics (penicillin, streptomycin, the three great broad-spectrum antibiotics—oxytetracycline, chlortetracycline, chloramphenicol—and others, such as neomycin, polymyxin, tyrothricin, erythromycin) have indeed achieved Ehrlich's ideal of maximum bacteriostatic effect with minimum toxicity; their power is extraordinary, since they selectively attack the disease-causing germ-lesioning organic tissues.

The era of antibiotics has started brilliantly. The antibiotics discovered to date are only the vanguard of a long series of antibiotics. Our therapeutic arsenal is being enriched every day with new antibiotics. Meantime, we are already successfully fighting syphilis, tuberculosis, and many tropical plagues.

NEW IDEAS ON ENDOCRINOLOGY

Modern medical thought toward endocrinology is very different from that which prevailed only twenty years ago, when endocrinology was considered an almost mathematical phase of medicine and its imponderable factors were overlooked. Endocrinology was very simple in its beginnings. Everything was reduced, first, to diagnosing excessive or deficient hormonal secretions in the patient and, second, to restraining excessive hormonal secretion through chemical or radiotherapeutic agents, or correcting deficient internal secretions through hormonotherapy.

With the discovery of the coexistence of endocrine hyper- and hypoactivity in many patients, the concept of endocrinology changed radically. It was also observed that there were patients with endocrine hyposecretion due to inability of their tissues to make use of internal secretions, although the endocrine glands were apparently normal; and, inversely, there were patients in whom normal internal secretion coexisted with a glandular hyperfunction syndrome produced by excessive utilization of the secreted hormones. All this revolutionized the old concept of glandular alterations; less importance was ascribed to hormones which we might call central, and more importance was given to peripheral hormones. In fact, no sooner have certain internal secretion glands, such as the adrenal medulla and the thyroid, secreted their particular hormones, than they disappear by oxidation into the blood stream and are no longer to be found from the moment they leave the glands until they reach their destinations, where they are reconstructed as peripheral hormones, which are the ones that really act on the tissues or organs. In brief, so as to facilitate the transportation of the extremely complex machinery of hormones through the blood, the organism disassembles and disintegrates them, recomposing them upon arrival at their destination.

Another new point of view is the establishment of the functional unity of the endocrine system, wherein the pituitary is considered its center, or, so to speak, the baton of the endocrine orchestra which, however, is wielded by the diencephalon, especially the hypothalamus which is so importantly related to the anterior pituitary. The hypothalamus, as small in anatomic size as it is important in functional activity, is the seat of our emotions and primitive instincts. The diencephalon is the brain of primitive life, wherein are located the centers of hunger, thirst, sleep, sexual activity, and other functions that were primordial in the life of primitive man; through the endocrine glands, it regulates these instincts, making them cyclical: daily for sleep, lunar for menstruation, and seasonal for the hibernation of certain mammals. All that mysterious life of the instincts compressed in the diencephalon represents the phylogenic subsoil, including pre-human existence, when the beings that preceded us had fur, feathers, or scales. Evolution and civilization placed over the diencephalon a curtain of restraints and inhibitions consisting of the higher cerebral structures. The resounding voice of primitive instincts continues to speak through the diencephalon, which in our anatomy and physiology is the equivalent of the unconscious in psychology, and its outlet for expression is the pituitary, through which it transmits its orders to the entire endocrine system. Hypothalamic disorders may destroy the normal expression of the emotions, a fact that has revived the old idea of the classic anatomists that it was a miniature brain, a functional mirror of its larger counterpart. Harvey Cushing (1869–1939) held it to be the base of elemental life—vegetative, emotional, and reproductive—over which man has superimposed a layer of inhibitions. Psychic stimuli in cows, for example, may create an impression of unpleasantness which is transmitted by the diencephalon to the pituitary, inhibiting the secretion of a particular hormone and thereby interrupting the lactic flow.

Modern endocrinology—which was born in 1891 with the treatment by Professor Murray of a myxedematous patient with extracts of calf's thyroid—proved that the excretory theory of endocrinology had to be abandoned and it established instead the hormonal theories, thereby ascribing more importance to hormones than to the internal secretion glands themselves. It is a fact that the hormone phylogenically precedes the endocrine gland, as has been observed in lampreys, in which adrenalin appears before the adrenal glands themselves. But it is known today that hormones are not the "chemical messengers" they were once held to be, since, in reality, they do *not* travel in the blood, but stimulate certain nerves which in turn determine the appearance of peripheral chemical intermediaries on the level of the corresponding nerve endings. Already in 1901 Langley pointed out that the stimulation of a sympathetic nerve ending not only could liberate adrenalin, but at times also acetylcholine; that is, all nerve impulses acted on tissues through peripheral chemical intermediaries.

The result of the study of these mechanisms and of the discovery of the processes of cholinergy and adrenergy at the nerve-ending level has revolutionized endocrine biology. In addition, new horizons have been opened in the study of organic interrelationships by the discovery of the clinical similarity existing between the hormones that regulate normal growth on the one hand and carcinogenic agents on the other, and by the establishment of the relationship among the chemical structures of certain vitamins very similar to those of some hormones.

Altogether, the new endocrinology is becoming each day more closely bound to neurology and psychiatry, as well as to allergy and vitaminology. The isolation by Kendall and Reichstein of cortisone (1940) and Hans Selye's new theories on the general adaptation syndrome and the diseases of adaptation open the door to a new era of the science that one day will be called neuroendocrinology.

SCIENTIFIC RESEARCH IN THE TWENTIETH CENTURY

In the current century, scientific research represents a new tool for the exploration of the universe. It is based on the reproducible experiment and is characterized by analytical thought, which passes from deduction to induction. It symbolizes the usefulness of knowledge and has that probing curiosity which, according to Flexner, is the most notable characteristic of modern scientific thought. It is a state of mind, an intellectual and social phenomenon, and it has a scientific and sociologic function and purpose. It is the desire to look at the world, observe it, and experiment with it, passing from the stage of logic and pure investigation to the subsequent one of application and methodology.

Research began with Adam, and slowly continued through thousands of years with the discovery of fire and of what heat could accomplish in separating iron and copper from ore. The curiosity that led prehistoric man to discover fire led him also to use a stick as a weapon and a tool, and to discover the lever, the wheel, ceramics, and the art of weaving. These secrets were then transmitted from family to family, and artisans and artificers came into being. Later, man went on to the observation of morphology before studying function.

Scientific investigation, as we know it today, was born in the Renaissance with the invention of the printing press, the discovery of America, and the onset of the Reformation. In its very beginning it rode on the shoulders of those two great iconoclasts, Paracelsus and Vesalius.

The Renaissance also saw the beginning of man's preoccupation with the nature of the world. Bacon introduced the inductive method and was the apostle of scientific societies. With experimental science were born in the seventeenth century the Accademia dei Lincei, the Royal Society, the Académie des Sciences, the Berlin Academy, and "The Invisible College." When the desire and the right of the mind to exert itself methodically toward no particular "practiced" aim were recognized, giants like Galileo, Newton, and Harvey made their ap-

pearance. Experimental science was transformed into a new philosophy. In the eighteenth century it underwent a subdivision, and such
men as Laplace, Lavoisier, Volta, Morgagni, Boerhaave, Haller, and
others, helped in the creation of the "systems." Observation was introduced, and importance was given to the dynamics of physiopathology
and to pathodynamics in medicine, delving into physiology, pathologic
anatomy, and therapy. "Ideas, given substance by facts, integrated
the science" of the last century, according to Claude Bernard. Comprehension and clarification of dynamic interrelationships were sought
after. To this end, basic data were gathered and dynamically inter-
related. To the structures and morphologies discovered by Vesalius,
Bichat, and Virchow were added the functionalism and dynamics
discovered by Claude Bernard, Helmholtz, Pasteur, and Ehrlich and
the morphologic and functional aspects of human beings indicated
by Hunter, Müller, Koch, and others.

While in the industrial field scientific research was being carried
out, resulting in such discoveries as the first Colt revolver, Fulton's
steamship, the sewing machine, the typewriter, and the mechanical
seeder, the research laboratories foreseen by Harvey, Lavoisier, and
Purkinje were being created.

Already in the eighteenth century Benjamin Franklin had founded
the American Philosophical Society and the American Academy of
Arts and Sciences which exist to this day; but in the nineteenth century there were as yet no American centers of investigation comparable to those of Europe, and the needs of life rendered professional
practice obligatory, leaving no time for pure research. Toward the
middle of that century, however, great scientific progress began. The
Wistar Institute of Anatomy and Biology was founded in 1808 at the
University of Pennsylvania; the Institute of Pathological Anatomy was
founded by William Henry Welch in 1886 at Johns Hopkins Hospital
in Baltimore, and the Smithsonian Institution in 1846 in Washington.

In 1901 the Rockefeller Institute for Medical Research was
founded, where Simon Flexner, among others, worked. This typically
American institution realized Bacon's dream of a House of Science.
Instead of centering around one man, it was created around its departments and institutions. Here biology was related to physics and
chemistry and antimeningitic serum was discovered; here Noguchi
did his research on syphilis, yellow fever, and Oroya fever, as well
as his study on infectious diseases and their epidemiology, the history
of which he traced by the observation of "mice cities"; here Carrel
worked on blood transfusion and tissue culture, and Loeb on par-
thenogenesis.

Next followed the McCormick Institute of Infectious Diseases in
1902 in Chicago; the Carnegie Institute in the same year in Washing-

ton; the Phipps Psychiatrical Clinic in 1913 in Baltimore; and 61 other scientific foundations. And finally industry joined research, making use of science in the solution of technologic problems.

The first laboratory for industrial research was built by Thomas Edison at Menlo Park, New Jersey, 1876, and the next one was erected by the General Electric Company in 1901. Today there are more than three thousand laboratories for industrial research in the United States with a total prewar expenditure of more than four hundred million dollars, of which only thirty-five million were spent by universities and schools.

Thus medicine came to the shores of America. The first medical school was founded in 1578 in Mexico; eight years before, the first book to appear on the continent had been published there. The heroic medicine of the first North American frontiers, when the physician was a pioneer with a gun in his hand, eventually produced many great figures.

Benjamin Rush was a pioneer in American psychiatry; Benjamin Franklin was the American Leonardo da Vinci; the first medical dispensary was established in Philadelphia; organized medical education entered the scene; Oliver Wendell Holmes tore the veil of secrecy from puerperal fever and blazed new paths in psychologic literature; the first studies on epidemics were made; medical botany became a precursor of modern studies on allergy; there was the figure of Daniel Drake and the genius of William Beaumont; the first studies were made in physiology; Wells, Morton, and Long discovered anesthesia; surgical gynecology was established by Ephraim Mc-Dowell; Physick became the father of American surgery; and all over the world great research laboratories sprang up: the Pasteur Institute in Paris, the Koch Institute and the Ehrlich Institute of Chemotherapy in Berlin, the Kitasato Institute in Tokyo, the Oswaldo Cruz Institute in Brazil, the Lister Institute in London, the Rockefeller Institute in New York, and the Biological Research Institute in Toronto.

Our century is a springboard from which medical research has dived bodily into a strictly scientific ocean.

But just as in the development of the nervous system progressive differentiation must be followed by progressive integration, so in present-day medicine, specialization must not undermine the integration of medicine as a whole. Being up-to-date in science must not interfere with medical education in the humanities. The world today is obsessed with the care of the body, while it neglects the soul. The more we know, the less we philosophize. Humanity is blindly crossing dangerous paths. The indifferent humanist regards penicillin as a curiosity until some day this magic drug saves his child. The scientist detaches himself from art and history until pain and suffering force him to return to them. Science, which seeks a definite answer to a general question, just as medicine requires a definite decision in a given case, must be reconciled with the humanities, if an intellectual equilibrium is to be established.

The excessive specialization that prevails in the field of medicine is compensated by a tendency to synthesize in the field of research. Specializations are regrouping themselves under new banners, although in some cases, as in the neuropsychiatric combination, they are new only because, faded by the sun of centuries, their original colors can no longer be distinguished. A cry for integration and universality fills the laboratories. The mind of the investigator is becoming a small firmament with a central sun of interest in one subject, but surrounded by many stars of diverse scientific interests. The research worker, having gone beyond the purely microchemical and analytic thought of the nineteenth century, once again becomes a philosopher. But his philosophy is that of an investigator whose mind is broad and free and whose purpose is to apply his discoveries to the art of healing. Fleming, a pure researcher, gave Florey, the experimental pathologist, a magic tool with which to write another page in medical art. The medical investigator who studies pathologic anatomy knows that, as William Osler recommended, the hospital and the medical faculty are centered around the humble marble of their dissecting table. Investigators can no longer ignore what is happening in other fields of modern science. A fine spirit of collaboration unites researchers from any area of medicine. From the merging of the work of physicists, bacteriologists, and electrotechnicians has risen the portentous electron microscope. The joint efforts of bacteriologists, biochemists, and clinicians led to the discovery of the new sulfonamides. Mycologists and veterinarians, chemists and pharmacologists, are wresting from the sphinx of nature the secret of antibiotics. The accumulated knowledge of entomologists, parasitologists, and biologists is yielding the new antimalarials.

To penicillin, blood banks, folic acid, blood globulins, new techniques in neurosurgery, antireticulo-endothelial serum, the new electronic physics of the laboratory—to all these are added other great discoveries. Gastric ulcers are treated with hydrolyzed amino acids; Rocky Mountain spotted fever is treated with para-amino-benzoic acid; the mechanism by which insulin liberates hexokinase from the anterior hypophysis is known; streptomycin is used against tuberculosis; cholera is satisfactorily treated with hematic plasma and trypanosomiasis with gamma-butyric acid; the whitish gelatin that befouls the piping in sugar mills is used in place of plasma in shock cases; hearts are transplanted in warm-blooded animals. And one of the most exciting discoveries in psychiatry, the hematosonography of A. M. Sackler, M. D. Sackler, R. R. Sackler, Co Tui, H. A. La Burt, and their collaborators, was born at the Creedmoor Institute and at the Van Ophuijsen Center in New York as a new tool in psychiatric research and a new diagnostic method in medicine.

Thus scientific research has arrived at this crucial time at a splendid stage of development. The investigator has written his own philosophy with his toil. Under his microscope and in his test tube, through his spectrophotometer and in his hematocrit, in his laboratory and his clinic, thirty centuries of historicomedical evolution shake hands with twenty allied sciences, from physics to agriculture. The medicine of the future will more and more be a *science* in its methods—pure and applied research—but it will also be an *art* in its moral end of serving mankind. The physician is each day more and more of an investigator, whether in his modest consulting office or among his books at the university. Fame will continue "sounding its long trumpets," but our admiration is reserved above all for those who work and disappear "without singing," as Wendell Holmes said, "but with music in their hearts." With the captains and generals of medicine and the foot soldiers of the white crusade, the world marches on, through "science and conscience" (Montaigne), to health and happiness.

L'ENVOI

When it crossed the seas and reached Latin America, medicine built shelters for itself in universities such as San Marcos in Lima, Guatemala, San José de Costa Rica, Santiago de Chile, Buenos Aires, Rio de Janeiro, Mexico, Havana, and others, and thus completed its historic course.

On another occasion we will trace the panorama of Latin American medicine and its contribution to universal medicine. We will evoke the procession led by the giants, Carlos Finlay, Hipolito Unanue, Cosme Bueno, Francisco Javier Espejo, Narciso Esparragosa, Carlos Chagas, Daniel Carrión, Oswaldo Cruz and the other standard bearers of Latin-American medicine. The memorable heritage of these architects of medical thought in Latin America is now in the hands of their present-day followers.

Had medicine taken still another leap, over the Pacific, and had it reestablished its throne on the Asiatic continent, the westward march of medical thought in history would have ended where it began—in the Far East. But the banner of medical science is securely hoisted in the soil of the Americas, already suffused with the light of a bright new dawn in the history of medicine.

SIGERIST AND SPAIN

I first met Henry Sigerist twenty-three years ago, in Spain, and then again five years later, many miles away, in Baltimore. The years rolled by. And then one golden day in September, 1954, in Rome, at the International Congress of the History of Medicine, I saw him again. Clothed in black, his broad-planed face looked pale as a candle, his wide brow and naked skull like a bare rock around which hovered the eagles of thought.

He graciously accepted my invitation to lunch at the Osteria dell'-Orso. We arrived at one-thirty. The streets of the Eternal City slumbered under the heat pouring down from glaring skies. Perspiration oozed from Sigerist's face as water from a jug left out in the sun. The Osteria was deserted. They say that there Dante wrote *The Divine Comedy*. If so, he improvised his picture of hell, for the Osteria is all heaven. To Sigerist it was a revelation. With his characteristic youthful enthusiasm he admired and praised the tapestries, panoplies, statuary, and paintings in this magnificent palazzo, built on the remains of a medieval rustic tavern of which there still stand the huge hearthstones, some ancient wooden benches, and the bricks blackened by age.

Sigerist's charm and graciousness had but increased with the years. Time had aged him as it ages the finest ivory. During the melon and *prosciutto* his delightful small talk was the spice that seasons a fine dinner; with the arrival of the *scampi a la griglia* and the golden wine from Verona, he led the conversation along deeper channels; by the

From *Journal of the History of Medicine and Allied Sciences 13*:244, 1958.

time the plump dark grapes bursting with all the sweetness and sunshine of the Italian autumn reached the table, his powerful intellect
was fully unfurled. He talked about many things, and about his work
plans for the future, and about Spain, a land most dear to his heart. I
sat quietly, listening intently to this man in whose brain, as in that of
Aristotle, was enclosed a vast empire without frontiers where, as on
that of Philip II, the sun never set. It was the last time I saw Sigerist.

FLASHBACK TO SPAIN

I had met him in Madrid, at the Tenth International Congress of
the History of Medicine, presided over by Dr. Gregorio Marañón. This
was indeed a memorable congress, perhaps the most memorable of
its kind ever celebrated. Over one thousand historians flocked to the
Spanish capital; and the great ones, too. Capparoni, Giordano, and
Castiglioni from Italy, Max Neuburger from Austria, Paul Diepgen
from Germany, Ralph Major from the United States, Suheyl Unver
from Turkey. And one *homo universalis*—Henry E. Sigerist. The
welcome accorded us was warm, the entertainment lavish. In Toledo,
at the Plaza Zocodover, hundreds of brilliantly colored kerchiefs,
waved in greeting by the beautiful Toledanas, fluttered in the air like
birds of paradise. At the Alcazar—later, in the Civil War, scene of
heart-rending tragedy—we were sumptuously feasted on the delicacies
of Spain: partridges from Toledo, hams from Estremadura, tomatoes
from Murcia, asparagus from Aranjuez, cheeses from La Mancha,
oranges from Valencia, cool white wines from Montilla, warm red
wines from Rioja, and the fiery cognac from Jerez de la Frontera.

I particularly remember one night during the congress. In the
velvety Castilian sky, thousands of stars, like eyes of celestial cats,
glowed with a bright amber light. Facing El Escorial, looming like
a giant ship of stone in the dark, Sigerist poured out to a few of us
surrounding him the love and devotion for Spain that filled his heart.
For Sigerist, who turned the history of medicine into the history of its
"great doctors" and ideas, a veritable sociology of medicine based on
the labors and achievements of man, Spain was an inexhaustible
spring of revelations. For Spain, as Somerset Maugham said in his
Don Fernando, owes her greatness to her men. Her grandeur and her
misery are built upon the virtues and defects of her people. A Spaniard
is a "Catholic Moor," intransigent yet tolerant, mystic yet realistic,
passionate yet scrupulous, enamored of Woman and women, a devout
believer in God and in the gods. Sigerist was fascinated by the contradictions of my native country, geographically the most Occidental in
Southern Europe, spiritually the most Oriental, where the European
garden becomes Moroccan desert and Africa really begins. Spain,
virgin and martyr, sensuous and mystic, voluptuous in Moorish Anda-

lusia, ascetic in Catholic Castile, which gave medieval Europe the greatest example of racial and religious tolerance when Moslems, Christians, and Jews coexisted in harmony in Toledo, held their religious rites in the same temple, and worked side by side at the College of Authors and Translators—Spain was a vast, intricate, colorful tapestry, and Sigerist yearned to examine not only all it portrayed on the right side, but above all the labyrinth of threads on the reverse that went into the making of the tapestry.

Many times I heard Sigerist comment on the politeness and dignity of the people of Castile. Nothing can better illustrate the impression this innate dignity makes upon the foreigner than the words of G. K. Chesterton. Traveling the dusty highroads of Castile in the company of the Minister of Education of the Republic, the late Don Fernando de los Rios, a kind humanist himself with the face of a Christ, Chesterton and his companion were invited by some peasants to share their repast of bread, cheese, and wine. Observing the delicate manner in which they handled the humble food, Chesterton exclaimed: "How civilized these illiterate Spaniards are!"

It was this inborn dignity of the Spanish people that captivated Sigerist's sensitive heart. Devoted as he was to the history, art, and culture of old Spain, he was deeply stirred in 1935 by the craving for culture that flourished under the Republic. He left the country wishing it, in impassioned words uttered to us, many years of greatness and fortune. But four years later, after three years of nightmarish bloodshed, Spain was cast back into the darkness of medieval times. Sigerist already anticipated the future tragedy of Spain when he wrote in a memorable article:*

The last such meeting took place in Madrid in September 1935. These glorious autumn days will remain unforgettable to all who were privileged in attending this gathering. The tragedy that was soon to befall the Spanish people was in the air already and could be perceived by whoever knows how to feel the pulse of a country. We were brilliantly received by high officials, archbishops and generals. We were entertained lavishly, but when we drove from Madrid to Toledo where the meeting was to be opened formally, we saw poor peasants tilling the soil with hand-plows and mills operated by blind-folded donkeys, while in Toledo, in the cathedral, we found buckets full of pearls and precious stones. Life was gay enough in daytime, but at night the streets assumed the aspect of a besieged city with large detachments of police, infantry and cavalry patrolling the streets. And in the hotel my elevator boy and waiter studied the works of Karl Marx. One year after we had been offered a magnificent banquet in the Alcazar of Toledo, the latter was blown up and the President of the Madrid Congress Gregorio Marañón is now living abroad while we are sending American physicians to help the Spanish people in their struggle for independence.

---

* From Yugoslavia and the XIth International Congress of the History of Medicine, *Bull. Hist. Med.* 7:99, 1939.

In 1939, at the end of the war in Spain, I visited Sigerist in Baltimore. In my nostrils there still lingered the smell of gunpowder and blood. The severe wounds inflicted upon my native land would take many years to heal. Sigerist received me with characteristic warmth. The fate of Spain had seared his heart. His greatest friends were in exile all over the world or dead. With the historian's keen perception, he perhaps realized that the epitaph for democratic Europe had just been written in Spain.

Sigerist tried to secure work for me near him, at the Welch Library in Baltimore, and generously signed on my behalf the affidavit required by the immigration authorities. Sigerist was not a politician; neither was I. Perhaps this is why he fully understood the tragic fate of the intellectual who for love of country and of democratic ideals winds up a victim of History, that same History which taught him for naught that intellectuals who meddle in politics wind up, like Plato, as slaves in the public marketplace.

Fate did not grant me the privilege of working close to Sigerist. From afar I followed his life and work as closely as possible. I corresponded with him regularly when he retired to Switzerland to engage in the titanic task of carving with his pen the colossal blocks for his monumental history. In his letters he spoke with affection of our past meetings and of Spain. To Sigerist, as to that great Spaniard, Miguel de Unamuno, "Spain was a great pain in his heart."

I remember you well [Sigerist wrote to me May 12, 1954], I remember you very well indeed, both our first meeting in Spain and your visit to my Institute in Baltimore. I shall never forget how tense the situation was in Spain just before the civil war broke out. You remember the banquet we had at the Alcazar, half a year later it was blown up. I still have not lost hope that Spain will be a democratic republic again, although the American support of Franco has certainly postponed the day of liberation.

Sigerist had often mentioned to me another great intellectual, the German poet, Ernst Toller, whom I had met in New York in 1938 and who committed suicide some years later, brokenhearted by the outcome of the Spanish tragedy. Toller had been affected far more by the Spanish civil war than by his years of incarceration in Germany in a cell where his only consolation was some swallows nesting on his window and to which he dedicated some of his finest poems. Despairing and disillusioned, Toller hanged himself in a gloomy hotel room in New York. The news chilled my heart, for I had seen him only two weeks before and I could clearly recall his thin pale face and his sad eyes when he said to me: "To look at Central Park from my window consoles me, but even there I still see the tragedy of Spain."

Sigerist reacted to the tragedy of Spain as did all true intellectuals throughout the world. Something precious and irretrievable had been flung over the precipice of History. Many times Sigerist spoke to everyone about Spain's misery and his Spanish friends, victims of the war. Great historians like Sigerist, who are gifted with the faculty to see the total perspective—in view of totality and eternity—and who live by their keen perception, can deduce from present events not only their historical roots but, what is even more important, their ramification into the future. The unfinished bridge across the river of Time, which ordinary mortals but barely perceive suspended midway in the mist, the Sigerists of this world can clearly trace with their prophetic vision to the very end on the shores of the future.

Perhaps that is why Sigerist wanted the United States and Russia to understand each other and particularly each other's history, for both countries made a late appearance in Western history, while Europe had already been through the Renaissance.

But men of small stature should not be expected to understand those whose heads are high amid the clouds. Sigerist was one of those. He was enamored with the history of Spanish medicine; he was a brother in spirit to the martyr Michael Servetus who, faithful to his ideal of man uncorrupted, died a slow death at a stake of green wood under the waxen skies of Geneva; he was a devout admirer of that kind artist and bard of science, Ramón y Cajal; he was a lover of the Spanish artists he knew so well, of El Greco in front of whose "Burial of the Count of Orgaz" in Toledo he stood rapt in ecstasy, and of Velázquez whose "Meninas" so entranced him in Madrid. Most of all, Sigerist loved *Don Quixote,* a copy of which was among the books kept by his bedside. Its pages must have afforded consolation to this wandering Quixote of History, forever in search of new kingdoms to offer to Science, his Dulcinea. Once, when I asked him to write for one of our journals an article on his favorite reading matter, he left out *Don Quixote,* and when asked why, he replied (July 2, 1954):

Very many thanks for your letter of the 25th June and cheque. I was delighted to hear that you liked my article. It was actually one that I had meant to write for a long time as reading and writing have been the essence of my life.

I do have *Don Quijote* among the 500 books and should have mentioned it but for the fact that I could not mention all of them. Please feel free to add it to my manuscript, the book really is one of the very great classics of world literature.

Thanks also for the reprint of your paper "The Artist as Physician" which I read with the greatest interest. One of the joys of living where I am now is that I am so close to Italy. The border is only one and a half miles away and whenever I have the chance I escape for a few days to Venice, Florence or Rome.

I liked what you said about Vesalius because I really think that the new anatomy was the foundation of the new medicine and I like your references to Jaspers. Long before he wrote his book I felt that it was extraordinary that Greece (Socrates), Persia (Zoroaster) and India (The Buddha) and China (Confucius), had a flowering of their culture at the same time. The same also happened around 800 A.D. when Europe was united under Charlemagne, the

Mohammedan East under Harun'Al-Raschid, and the T'ang Dynasty was ruling in China. It always seems to me that *Homo sapiens* needs a certain time to elaborate certain ideas.

I am looking forward to seeing you in Rome, and should you be in our region before I would be delighted to see you in Pura. John Fulton, Henry Schuman, Ilza Veith, Geneviève Miller, and a few other colleagues will be here before the meeting starts and we have a nice little hotel, Albergo Paladina in Pura, where you could all stay.

In the course of his life, Sigerist never shied from tilting at windmills, as if wishing to prove that, if there are people who, like the yokels in *Don Quixote,* mistake castles for inns, there are others who have the gift of turning an inn into a castle, a pigsty into a garden. If there are those who, afraid to attack giants, aver that they are but windmills, Sigerist attacked windmills merely to prove the falsity of the legend that they were giants. He often experienced the true meaning of the words uttered by Jacinto Benavente, Nobel Prize winner in Spanish literature: "It is a very sad thing in life when we are asked for gold and can only give copper, but it is far more sad when we give gold and are told, 'Copper would have been enough!' "

Sigerist greatly admired the tremendous achievements of the great Spaniards of the past, but had an equal eye for those of the present day, particularly Gregorio Marañón and Ortega y Gasset, the greatest and most clear-thinking philosophical mind of twentieth-century Europe. For Sigerist, Spain was a European Garden of Eden dotted with African cacti, a realm of the paradox and the unexpected, a barren land peopled by "giants" and Dulcineas, where he felt at home because his romantic soul found there a historical stage firmly grounded on age-old pillars and boundless inspiration for creation. He was as enchanted by the parched Castilian highlands, so beloved by Rilke and Cocteau, as by the Mediterranean, whose blue waters, so blue perhaps because they run with the blood of the Homeric gods, gently bathe the warm land where the flowering almond trees are like ivory goddesses. At heart, Sigerist was an Argonaut for whom, as for the ancient Greeks, "the main thing was not to live, but to sail" on all the oceans of life and of history.

All who knew him found in Sigerist some things that cannot be appreciated from mere reading of his works, great and warm though they are—a superbly human quality and a mind Aristotelian in its vastness, Leonardian in its creativeness, Quixotic in its undertakings, brilliant and powerful as the sun of Castile. Elsewhere I spoke of Sigerist's fame as a historian; here I have only wanted to bring together, in softly spoken words, as if we were standing before his tomb, two great loves in my life as a historian and as a man: Sigerist and Spain.

MEDICAL GEOGRAPHY AND HISTORY

man lives on a planet where he makes his dwelling and wherefrom he draws his sustenance. On earth he is born and to the earth he returns upon his death. The Earth-image, together with that of the star-studded firmament, is the most deep-rooted in the human mind. Despite the fact that modern astronomy and physics have shattered many important millenary-old beliefs about the earth's place in the cosmos, the emotional realization that the earth is the center of his very existence still has a stronger impact on man than the intellectual concept that the earth is just one more dynamic point in the mechanics of the heavens.

Though mentally man can travel through the whole of the universe and through time, physically he is anchored to one place at a time on the earth. Any change in man's relation to his "living space" profoundly affects his life roots. Hence he has sought to adapt himself to his environment by organizing his existence in time and space.

The earth is to man a symbol of stability, and so is the knowledge of his position at all times on earth. Maps show man his position on the planet, and plans his location in a city, just as the calendar and the clock show him his position in time. Visual orientation and intellectual recognition of his geographic position tell man where he is. And to know *where* he is, is virtually to know *why* he is there. To know his position on his planet is indispensable to man's peace of mind. Hence

---

Foreword to *The Ecology of Human Disease* by Jacques May, New York, MD Publications, Inc., 1958.

the tremendous psychologic impact of seasickness and other kinetoses, which by threatening man's spatial stability can destroy the roots of his psychic stability.

MAN'S TRAVELS

For thousands of years man lived a "bidimensional" life in a tridimensional world. From the very beginning, being the most restless of all living creatures, man roamed all over the earth, first on foot, later on horseback, and still later in power-driven vehicles. Until one day, having explored practically all of horizontal space, he set out to conquer vertical space. Technology, by abolishing distances, has launched man on vertiginous journeys through cosmic space far more exciting than any he ever made on the earth whence he came. But for his spatial restlessness man is paying a price. His mental and physical stability is being destroyed.

To live is beyond all else to travel. Life itself is a turbulent journey from the bright shores of birth to the dark portals of death. This conception of the meaning of life as an incessant journey was envisaged by the Greek Argonauts, who said: "The essential thing is not to live; the essential thing is to travel."

In prehistoric times man traveled forced by the elements, famine, or prehistoric monsters. Later, in the ancient world, civilized man traveled moved by a thirst for knowledge. Already classical Greece differentiated between sedentary physicians and *periodeutas,* or itinerant physicians. The medieval world witnessed large-scale migrations caused by wars and invasions, and the hazardous wandering life of the knight errant and the crusader contrasted sharply with the isolated life of the scholarly monks in their monasteries, veritable coffers of stone where, except for the sun, which stealing through the stained-glass windows spangled the floors with glittering colors, little from the outside world ever entered. The late Middle Ages marked the commencement of the great explorations, including Marco Polo's journey in quest of Kublai Khan, one of the most important historical gestures made by man in his search for what lay beyond the rim of the earth. Not until the Renaissance, however, were explorations conducted systematically, a sign of mankind's yearning to probe all the chambers of the planet he inhabited, of which he then knew only the anteroom.

This yearning crystallized into great expeditions in the past century. Voyages beyond the seas and into the hinterlands took man inch by inch across the whole face of the earth. So extensive and numerous were these explorations that with the arrival of the twentieth century very little remained to explore. Man, then, suddenly assailed by a fervent desire to explore his planet vertically, descended the abysmal depths of the ocean and ascended the dizzy heights of the stratosphere.

And, as G. K. Chesterton foretold, the modern world began to shrink with the airplane, just as it had expanded under the microscope. Simplification of travel, thanks above all to the airplane (which cast certain countries directly from the mule stage to the airplane stage), has drawn the world's continents so close together that they now virtually form one world, each of whose nodal points feels the repercussions of what happens in the others.

MEDICAL GEOGRAPHY IN HISTORY

From the moment man realized that his life was not only himself but also the world around him, he became interested in the medium wherein his life evolved and in the changing environment encountered in his travels. Thus the concept evolved that man is only one half of a reactive system whose other half is his environment, a concept perfectly summarized in the words of Ortega y Gasset: "I am myself and my circumstance."

Such "circumstance," compounded of a place in space and a moment in time as indispensable factors of human existence, is now the object of study of geography.

That geography has important medical aspects was obvious from the very beginning of this science. From remotest antiquity the most fearful epidemics—plague, cholera, smallpox—followed the great caravan routes. Death galloped at the heels of the endless processions of pilgrims and nomads, who, sandal-footed, slowly plodded across the burning deserts of Asia and Africa. Remedies from remote lands traveled the same routes as disease. The history of human communication is also the history of transmissible diseases and, often, of their remedies. The fabulous exploits of Columbus' vessels had a fearful climax when, together with their loads of gold and befeathered Indians, they imported to Barcelona and thence to the whole of Europe virulent strains of syphilis, which in the 1495 siege of Naples by Charles VIII of France unleashed the terrible pandemy of the execrable *mal d'amour.* The spread of Islam from Medina to Cordova, at the scimitar's point, introduced Arabian polypharmacy in the West; and the bloody adventure of the Crusades showered numerous Oriental ills upon Europe by way of Salerno.

As told by Leonard Olschki in his excellent work *Medical Matters in Marco Polo's Description of the World,* from the early Middle Ages onwards there was an abundance of travel books on Asia of medicogeographic interest, such as Gossouin's *Image du Monde*; Bartholomew the Englishman's *Liber de Proprietatibus Rerum* (1250) on the virtues of drugs and precious stones imported from Ethiopia, India, and the Far East; Brunetto Latini's *Tresor,* which revived the fabulous minerals and herbs described in ancient lapidaria and herbaria; and Francesco Balducci Pegolotti's *La Pratica della mercatura* (1340), listing spices, drugs, and other products from Asia. None of these accounts was as famous and spectacular as Marco Polo's *Il Miglione.* Before the Venetian adventurer, many others had traveled to strange, remote lands, among them Filippo, physician to Pope Alexander II, who in 1177 set out on a one-way journey in search of the legendary country of Prester John; the missionaries who went to the court of the Tartar Khans of Mongolia; the Franciscan Friar William of Rubrouck, who spent four months in the black sands of fabulous Karakorum, the first capital of the Mongolian Empire, and who, in 1254, half a century before Marco Polo set out, brought back rhubarb as a panacea. But it was the restless Venetian who confirmed to the physician Pietro d'Abano, the famous *conciliatore* of Padua and Dante's teacher, the habitability, denied by Aristotle, of the southern hemisphere, which Dante himself had called *mondo senza gente.*

All this, however, was not yet medical geography proper. Geography was for many centuries almost exclusively the province of a special type of man of science who appeared tardily among the Greek philosophers. The study of medical geography was already extremely important in ancient Greece, particularly to itinerant physicians, and so it was understood by the Wise Man of Cos, whose treatise, *Air, Water and Places,* describing the effect of topography and climate on man's health and character became, together with the medicogeographical notes in Books I and III of his *Epidemics,* the classical text of this specialty. Today physicians are not as conscious as our precursors were of the importance of climate and terrain in relation to disease, for we are not as much at the mercy of cosmic and telluric influence as they were. In Hippocrates' times the two most prevalent maladies, malaria and respiratory diseases, were manifestly connected with the geographic conditions of the environment. Of course, then as now climate was the basic factor in the treatment of certain forms of pulmonary tuberculosis as well as in the propagation of epidemics.

Later on, Paracelsus in his ceaseless wanderings through Europe and Asia preached, as part of his lay gospel of reform, the need for the physician to travel and be both geographer and cosmographer if he wished to understand the dynamic essence of disease. The Renaissance and the seventeenth-century world, consumed as they were on the one hand by the passion to explore the marvels of the human body and on the other by the passion to probe the mysteries beyond the seas, witnessed an avalanche of publications concerning medical geography and the marvelous things discovered overseas. Columbus' famous letter to the King's scribe recounting his first voyage to the Indies is perhaps the first account of medical anthropology and geography in the new world, besides which it throws a vivid and revealing light on the Great Admiral's own psychology.

But Columbus' epic and the years of "wooden ships and iron men" that followed brought new threats and perils to all who ploughed the seas. Besides infectious "fevers," traumas caused by accidents or boarding assaults, malnutrition as a result of a steady diet of ship's biscuit, hardtack, or bean soup, as in Philip II's galleys, and sailor's "vapors" or the mental disturbances that assailed the sailors during long sea crossings, confined as they were in a wooden hulk between two infinite walls of monotonous blue, the sky and the sea—besides all these there were so many other strange diseases that it became imperative to record the medical problems of remote regions.

Among the many treatises of this type we find, as mentioned by Sigerist, *De Medicina Indorum* (1642), a classical text on tropical medicine by a Dutch physician whose name is unknown and who resided in Indonesia; Daniel Drake's work on the medical topography of the Mississippi Valley (Cincinnati and Philadelphia, 1850–1854); a medical geography by a rural practitioner, Leonhardt Ludwig Finke (Leipzig, 1792–1795); the monumental treatise (1779–1819) of the great hygienist, Johann Peter Frank, father of modern public health; August Hirsch's *Handbuch der historisch-geographischen Pathologie* (1860–1864); and other more modern works.

Studies on medical geography were practically neglected when with the discovery of bacterial infection it was erroneously believed that to understand the epidemiology of an infection all that was needed was to know its causal germ, no importance being ascribed to the study of environment.

Revival of interest in medical geography had to await the convergence of two special factors. One was the First World War, which compelled the evacuation to new places of huge masses of people, both civilian and military, subjecting them to the threat of infections and subsequent epidemics. The geographic factor here was undeniable. Hindus from the Orient were decimated by tuberculosis in Europe, and Europeans were consumed by malaria in the Far East. Once again medical attention was forced to focus on the geographic theatre, where the drama of disease was played, rather than only on the leading actor, the causal microbe, and in 1929 the International Society of Geographical Pathology was founded.

The second factor was generated by the advances, after the First World War, in means of locomotion. Combustion engines contracted the world, and man traveled much faster and more often. But so did disease carriers. A mosquito stowed away in a French destroyer traveling from Africa to Brazil caused a wave of malaria that might have been cataclysmic for the latter country. A bus traveling from Mexico to New York transported, lodged in the body of an ailing passenger, the smallpox virus that unleashed an epidemic in Manhattan. Ticks, mice, flies, bugs, and other insects and rodents can propagate disease with the same speed with which they are transported by ship, airplane, or automobile. This again compelled a global view of the problems of infection and the intensification of interest in medical geography. To the epidemiologic problems were suddenly added psychiatric problems. In former times, slowness in travel afforded the traveler ample time to adjust himself physically and mentally to the place of destination. The airplane has radically changed this. A stagecoach traveler years ago arrived mentally at his destination days and even weeks before his poor battered body; today the body arrives at its destination long before the mind has had time to even anticipate, much less adjust itself to, the forthcoming changes in environment, people, food, habits, and perhaps even language, all of which may cause psychosomatic problems.

THE PHYSICIAN AND GEOGRAPHY

Thus it happened that the medical problems evoked by two world wars and numerous local wars, and by the progress in means of locomotion, demanded, every day more, the physician's active intervention in geographic problems in relation to disease and the health of men and nations.

Throughout history the physician has always been concerned with such geographic problems, partly because, tied to his patients like the galley slave to his oar, he cannot gratify his own wanderlust, and partly because he is interested in knowing the world in which we live, now that travel has ceased to be a matter of adventure or chance and has become instead a pleasure or a necessity. Ever since the travels of Democedes of Crotona (sixth century B.C.), the first physician-explorer whose travels united democratic classical Greece with the mysterious Asia of the tyrants, physicians have roamed with their science and their dreams throughout the length and breadth of the planet.

Among the many physicians who bear witness to the fascination travel has always exerted on physicians, we have the Portuguese García de Orta, who explored India in the sixteenth century; Mr. Monkhouse the surgeon, who defeated scurvy on Captain Cook's expedition to the South Seas (1769), on which expedition he was accompanied by Dr. Solander, a physician and naturalist from Upsala; Walter Russell, "Doctor of Physicke," who accompanied Captain John Smith in his explorations across the craggy Chesapeake region; the Scottish surgeon James Bruce (1730–1794), the first white explorer to discover the sources of the so-called Blue Nile; Mungo Park, another Scottish surgeon (1771–1806), who explored Senegal and Kaarta; Dr. Livingstone (1813–1873), discoverer of the Zambesi River and Victoria Falls; and the German physician Eduard Schnitzer (1840–1892), better known as Emin Pasha, the fabulous hero of the Sudan.

To naval surgeons also belongs part of the glory of having conquered the seas, men like James Lind, who finally vanquished the scurvy that had killed ten thousand men, as recorded in Admiral Hawkins' reports; Thomas Dover, of romantic memory, who on the island of Juan Fernandez, not far from the Chilean coast, rescued one Alexander Selkirk, later immortalized in Daniel Defoe's *Robinson Crusoe*; Eugène Sue, a novelist of immortal fame as well as a physician; Tobias Smollett, whose wreath of laurel is twined equally with medical and literary honors and who "discovered" the French Riviera; and countless other naval physicians who with their genius, bravery, and determination dispelled many of the fearful mysteries posed by the seas.

Having conquered land and sea, man, loath to remain chained to the earth, longed for wings to carry him higher than eagles fly. And in the conquest of the air, too, physicians were pioneers. The first human being to ascend in a balloon, on October 15, 1783, was one Jean Pilâtre de Rozier (1756–1785), a physician-apothecary from Metz. Subsequently, de Rozier became the first martyr to aeronautics when he perished in an attempt to emulate a Boston physician named Jeffries and the balloonist Pierre Blanchard, the first two men to cross the English Channel in a balloon. And it was Paul Bert, a pupil of Claude Bernard, who founded aeronautic medicine, today a vital part of modern medicine and the key to tomorrow's interplanetary navigation.

ON THE PREOCCUPATION AND OCCUPATION
OF A PHYSICIAN-GEOGRAPHER

"Anatomy is to medicine what geography is to history," said the great sixteenth-century French humanist-physician, Jean Fernel. With the passage of the centuries geography has increasingly become the dynamic anatomy of history, just as anatomy has become the dynamic geography of medicine.

To paleopathology, which studies disease in prehistoric times, have been added two main groups of studies, each of which has two different basic approaches.

The first group is called the *history and geography of disease,* or disease in time and space, and is the study of when and where a given disease was first observed, and what its incidence was, tracing it all over the world and examining the social, physical, and nonphysical factors responsible for it. When this group of studies concentrates on the disease itself, the approach is basically pathologic and the studies are then called *historical and geographic pathology;* when they concentrate on geographic factors, not on cholera or plague but on a geographic unit—the desert, the Arctic, Italy, India—the studies are then called *historical and pathologic geography.*

The second group of studies is called *history and geography of medicine,* or medicine in time and space, and deals not only with disease but also with medicine, that is, with health promotion and the prevention and cure of disease. Here again when the approach focuses on medicine itself, the studies are then called *historical and geographic medicine;* when the accent is on geography, that is, all the aspects of medicine, past and present, in a given country or geographic area, the studies are then called *historical and medical geography.*

Between these four aspects of medical geography, that is, of the ecology of disease, there are no discernible frontiers, as was so admirably pointed out by the greatest contemporary medical historian, Henry Sigerist, an ardent advocate of teaching medical geography and history of medicine as one single subject.

Outstanding among those who have labored unflaggingly to learn everything in this field that might be of help in health promotion, in world-wide prevention and curing of disease, and in making of geography not merely a geophysical delimitation of countries and oceans but a powerful instrument for research, is Dr. Jacques May, author of this book, whose title alone, *The Ecology of Human Disease,* indicates the wide philosophical perspective of his medical thought.

For many years now I have been honored with Dr. May's friendship and have received inspiration and enlightenment from his person and his work. There are men whose mere presence, word, and example are as pure a fountain of inspiration and stimulus as their thoughts and pen. European by birth and American by nationality, Dr. Jacques May is a true *homo universalis.* His devotion to his profession, his fervent sense of duty, and his acute awareness of his life mission place him among that illustrious minority of medical humanists who by their deeds and words exercise a transcendental guiding influence in the world. It suffices to listen to his quiet wise voice for one to realize that this man of the melancholy blue eyes and pensive pale brow is a shining example of greatness and simplicity, and of noble professional endeavor.

A man's original preoccupation is not only a clue to his future occupation but also to the carat content of his mind. Dr. May has always been interested in the problems of the geography and ecology of disease considered as a dynamic process in time and space, and has devoted his life to such problems, having published hundreds of scientific papers, several books, and a series of world maps of infectious and nutritional diseases, which are models of accuracy and priceless sources of valuable information. He has also done extensive work in the field of disturbances in human behavior, all of which has earned him world-wide acclaim and a rich harvest of honors.

Dr. May's philosophy on the ecology of disease has been developed in space by him as a geographer-anatomist of the earth; in time as a historian; and in thought as a humanist-philosopher who is animated by the noble urge to fight disease on a global scale. Being one of those "great doctors" of whom Sigerist spoke, Dr. May in his lectures and writings never fails to convey the lucidity and depth of his thinking. He is like a river carrying not only vessels but the seed that will render the land along its banks into fertile orchards and gardens. His books are the mirror of his mind, reflecting faithfully his ideas and ideals at the service of mankind's welfare and health.

THE CONCEPT OF "THE ECOLOGY OF HUMAN DISEASE"

This book is the fruit of many years of labor in medical ecology and geography. Dr. May begins by rejecting as inadequate the definition of disease given by dictionaries as mere impairment of health. In place thereof he gives a dynamic definition of disease as "that alteration of the living tissues that jeopardizes survival in their environment." By making disease synonymous with "maladjustment" and by stressing the importance of "organic survival" in a particular environment, Dr. May converts disease into an object of study for medical ecology, that is, into a study of the "seat" of disease.

The concept of medical ecology formulated by Dr. May conceives disease as a convergence in time and space within the person of the patient of environmental stimuli (organic, inorganic, or sociocultural). These stimuli are a challenge which induces a tissular response, that is, disease (communicable, degenerative, or behavioral), which in its turn eventually results in ecologic adaptation and survival or in total maladjustment and death.

Genotypic, or inherited, and phenotypic, or acquired, features control the individual's response to the stimuli, the response varying from the so-called "threshold" to the "ceiling" which is death. Adding to the study of these factors that of the individual's environment and that of races and populations, that is, of medical geography, Dr. May succeeds in charting the changing map of disease in time and space, in the world past and present. Knowledge of this map—which is a changing one either spontaneously or because of preventive and curative medicine— is for Dr. May the key to the study of the nature and prevention of disease.

One of the innovations in Dr. May's work is the study and integration of the cultural factors of disease, that is to say, of the concepts and techniques of which man avails himself in the different environments in order to survive the morbific impact of disease. Culture could influence disease by uniting or separating, whichever the case may be, the "challenges" of the environment, which would then change and so would the host population. For Dr. May the interrelation existing between culture and disease offers three possible approaches for the mastery of disease: to erect a protective wall between the human being and the pathogenic agent; to change the disease-producing environment in which man lives; or to change, intensifying and improving it, man's tissular response to the pathogenic stimulus.

The first part of this book, which expounds the author's philosophical concept of the ecology of disease, is perhaps the most lucid exposition made in our time on the problems of medical ecology. The book then proceeds to expound seriatim the ecology of the principal infectious, nutritional, and behavioral diseases. In each section, the author, with a geographer's culture, a historian's vision, and a clinician's eye, gives a vivid picture of disease of great interest and value as much to the physician as to the public health worker, the sociologist, the educator, and the traveling physician. In this book are indeed crystallized the author's many years of study and experience and the essence of his learning and Hippocratic philosophy.

GEOGRAPHY AND HISTORY

This book leaves us with a creative preoccupation regarding the connection, very important for medical historians, between geography and history, to which Hegel devoted some of his finest meditations.

The importance given by the author to the human element coincides with our own belief that geography must be supplemented by history in order to give a complete view of human ecology and the historical evolution of man.

Geography may not create history, but its importance to history is unquestionable. Geography by itself does not determine the history of a people, but it does influence it.

We must remember that, as Dilthey said, "Man is not only Nature; man is History." It has often happened that in the same corner of the earth the most diverse forms of history, that is, of being man, have taken place, for it is possible for one place on the earth to be inhabited at different historical periods by entirely different people. Hence it is essential to give man a basic position in this formation of history.

From the same geographico-anthropological background can rise the most diverse histories. Environment, more than the cause of our deeds, is an excitant, our deeds being free response and autonomous reaction. The influence of the earth on man must be studied by studying the influence of man on the earth. Geography may not propel history, but it does incite it.*

Every human race, however, just like every human being, carries within its primitive soul an image of the ideal environment, which it endeavors to fit within the surrounding geographic frame. Just as the woman of his choice is a clue to a man's character, so also is the environment accepted by a people a clue to their essential character. If the geographic topography is adverse to its psychology, a strong race will respond by emigrating to a more promising land. Of greater importance, then, than autochthony are the migrations of peoples. What matters most in history are migrating peoples who settle in one spot and thus create history. The important thing, then, is to understand *why* peoples migrate and appoint themselves to a new landscape that takes their fancy, just as a man surrounded by women is suddenly attracted by one and attaches himself to her.

All of which means that unquestionably there is an affinity between the soul of a people and the type of landscape they chose to inhabit, and between a nation and its territory. Peoples migrate in search of the environment they carry engraved in the depths of their souls. The "promised land" is really the environment craved for.

Hegel chose three basic types of landscape because of their capacity for making history: the high plateau, the valley, and the coast. From

---

* The essence of modern geography is the study of physical environment and of the adaptation of living creatures to it. Some years ago, K. Olbricht studied "bioclimatic" science, or the effect of climate and its changes upon the evolution and vital functions of living creatures, a science Huntington later expounded in detail in his *Climate and Civilization.*

Olbricht's concept was that the living creatures of the present day are *functions of space and time,* space determining the type of biologic organization (movement, coloration, form of the organs, metabolism) of each being, and time the biologic level. According to this, the science of environment (ecologic geography) and the science of the earth (geology) are two auxiliary sciences of extraordinary importance to biologists.

If such a concept is right, civilization, then, first developed in dry, subtropical zones, which compelled tribes coming from the north who were already versed in agriculture to devise canals, dikes, and reservoirs; thus creating an irrigation culture, which developed into a culture of states as the tribes spread into cities and finally into zones with steady favorable temperatures. This is what happened in Egypt, Mesopotamia, Mexico, and Peru, where the tribes first merged and then spread throughout regions with steady favorable temperatures, creating states out of the original settlements.

Prior to all this, the earth, according to Wegener, was at first one single block, which later split up into drifting fragments, forming finally our present continents. This theory could be proved, since the various coastlines could virtually be fitted together like the pieces in a jigsaw puzzle, and so could the mountain ranges and terrains and the fauna and flora. According to this theory, the Old and the New World are like a newspaper torn in two pieces which can be put together line by line.

this group he excluded those zones with extreme weather conditions, where man lives in a state of lethargy, overwhelmed or depressed by nature and unable to consummate that separation from her which is the prime requisite for spiritual culture. In his *Philosophy of Universal History,* Hegel pointed out that in such cases nature's violence renders man too weak and helpless to make his spiritual liberty avail against nature's might. Man cannot focus his attention on himself, he cannot dream and think, while fighting the threat of jungle and glacier. He cannot make history while he is unable, because it is a menace to him, to turn his back on nature and live within himself. Nature is antagonistic to the spirit and, in the form of steaming jungle, burning desert, or polar zone, can be a paralyzing prison from which man's spirit finds no escape. Extreme cold and heat preclude all blossoming of the spirit; the temperate zones on the contrary assist it.

According to Hegel, the dry impoverished tableland or high plateau historically induced nomadism, the urge to do things, to move here and there, nomadic pasturing of flocks, war, restlessness of spirit. The tableland terminates in slopes, which go straight into the ocean or are carved into valleys by rivers. Slopes are not propitious to fresh types of life. On the other hand, valleys are a new geohistorical principle, and mean fertile land and agriculture, property based on social classes and laws, regimentation of life according to the seasons, and coexistence. The valley binds man to the earth and generates fluvial civilizations which revolve upon themselves, confined as they are to a limited repertory of subjects and hieratic cultures, as was the case in Mesopotamia and Egypt. The coast liberates. The sea arouses bravery, it incites man to conquest and rapine, but also to profit and industry. Those who sail the seas are intent upon acquiring gain and upon satisfying their needs, but they also seek danger. The sea is the eternal spirit of unrest; it liberates from the limitations imposed by the earth.

TOWARDS A GEOGRAPHY OF HEALTH

Man throughout the centuries has fought against hunger, war, and disease, the three great threats that incessantly tend to change the map of humanity, just as medicine tends to shrink the empire of disease. Man's passionate craving for immortality has compelled him to fight incessantly against the forces that condemn him to the oblivion that is death.

In such struggle the best tools available today are perhaps a global approach to disease problems; integration in medicine of the human being with his environment (both used by Dr. May in this book); and protecting man by maintaining the "constancy of the internal milieu" (propounded by Claude Bernard) not only in his habitual environment, but also when he travels, by contriving for him artificial environments that duplicate those left behind. Protection against dangers proceeding from *within* (stress, anxiety, tension) and from *without* (infection, intoxication, malnutrition, trauma) must not be limited to civilized nations and great cities alone, but must be made available to the entire world. The only way to make our planet safe and habitable, as Dr. May states in this book, is to turn into adaptation the still frequent disadaptation between man and his environment, and into adequate the inadequate response of his tissues to environmental morbific stimuli.

This book is a blazing pennant announcing a new perspective in the study of disease ecology. With his philosophic concepts and his vast labor, Dr. May is the standard-bearer in that noble crusade for the conversion of the ecology of disease into a hopeful geography of health.

THE SPIRIT OF AMERICAN MEDICINE

MAN AS HISTORY

man is not only Nature; man is History," said the German philosopher Wilhelm Dilthey in his famous letter to the Duke of York. Nowadays historians as well as philosophers agree that the category of values represented by the "historical persona" of man is in a certain way superior even to his own biologic values. For though man's nature gives him his biologic being, his history, on the other hand, that is to say, his work, justifies him as a social entity. Hence the medical historian is increasingly concerned with the study of man as a problem in medical anthropology and with the study of medicine as a *social* science employing the methods of the natural sciences.

While man is eminently history, peoples are even more so. Every fragment of our planet, every one of those portions of the world we call nations, is a composite of land and people. The land is not, however, space alone but—what is even more important—time. Each land is at a different stage of culture or civilization in accordance with the cultural development of its inhabitants. It is not enough to speak of a country as an entity crystallized in its national characteristics; it is necessary to contemplate it as a moving force.

The dynamic concept of human life as movement and work, not only in space but also in time, must be applied to peoples also. Likewise, just as medicine today interprets disease as a pathologic accident

---

Foreword to the Symposium on the History of American Medicine, *International Record of Medicine 171:*317, 1958.

grafted onto the individual biography and studies it as a dynamic process indissolubly bound up with the life of the individual, so too must history interpret for us the reason for the rise or fall of a nation as a result of its course through time.

AMERICAN MEDICINE TODAY

American medicine today is indisputably leading in technological progress, development of some specialties, scientific research, and medical communication; in public health and social hygiene, it stands among the leaders; and when certain still existing gaps are filled, for instance, the lack of encyclopedism in professional training, it may also take a leading place in medical education.

Today the American physician has perhaps the best opportunities in the world for learning and for advancing in his profession. But in order to be able to fulfill his task with dignity and efficiency, he must know the history of medicine in his country. He must be acquainted with its social and psychologic trends, with its correlation with the great historical streams that nurtured the evolution of the United States, and with the struggles and achievements of the great figures in American medicine. He must, in short, be aware of everything concerning the turbulent, dynamic past of medicine in this country, if he wishes to comprehend its majestic present and its prospects for the future.

The American physician, often more familiar with the history of European medicine than with that of his own country, must learn to fit his knowledge and his work within the huge but simple frame of the historical evolution of American medicine. To do so would afford him a clear perspective in time and space and give his work and thought a double dimension of universality and eternity, which clinical work alone can never give him.

PLAN AND PURPOSE OF THIS SYMPOSIUM

It is now two years since we first began to organize this Symposium for the purpose of assembling the learning and thought of the outstanding figures in the field of American medical historiography. From the brilliant galaxy now gathered here, some distinguished historians are unfortunately missing through pressure of work, absence, illness, or death, as in the case of the beloved and irreplaceable master, Henry Sigerist; but those present here have unstintingly given of the knowledge and thoughts garnered in their lifetime regarding the basic themes of American medicine.

We have deliberately refrained from giving this Symposium a rigid textbook form with each subject strictly confined within its own chapter, preferring instead certain individual freedom in the selection and development of topics. Nor have we feared the repetition of concepts, data, and situations, since deliberate repetition lucidly made is the foundation of proper instruction. Perhaps when it appears in book form, we may enhance this Symposium with chronologies and appendices to make it a complete, instructive, and inspiring survey of the physicians and the medicine of this vast land, which so many have rightly called the Land of Promise.

The plan of the Symposium ranges over a series of works and writers the simple enumeration whereof has the electrifying effect of a clarion call to History. Let us now review briefly this list of fascinating subjects and of authors as distinguished as they are devoted to their chosen work:

"Guideposts in the History of American Medicine," by Dr. Benjamin Spector; "Medicine and Medical Practices among Aboriginal American Indians," by Dr. John Duffy; "Diseases and Medical Practice in Colonial America," by Dr. John B. Blake; "Medical Education and Medical Schools in Colonial America," by William Dosite Postell; "Medicine in the Era of the American Revolution," by Dr. William F. Norwood; "The Lessons of the War Between the States," by Professor Courtney R. Hall; "The Evolution of American Medical Literature," by Dr. Norman Shaftel; "The Evolution of Medical Research in the United States," by Morris C. Leikind; "A Brief Sketch of the Rise of American Medical Societies," by Dr. W. B. McDaniel, II; "The Nineteenth Century American Physician as a Research Scientist," by Mrs. Phyllis Allen Richmond; "Trends in American Public Health from the Colonial Period to the Present," by Dr. George Rosen; "American Medicine in the World Today: An Historical Perspective and Reappraisal," by Dr. Ralph H. Major.

It was not the purpose of this Symposium to make a synthesis of the multiple facets of American medicine, or to plait the many-colored threads of its separate components into a single braid. We preferred to let each writer open his window upon the vast impressive field of American medicine and reflect in the mirror of his own mind the men, facts, places, and things that have made it impressive. The reader will be able therefore to select his own favorite subjects or, after reading the whole Symposium, to effect his own mental synthesis, which after all is the best thing.

As a corollary to the present Symposium we may offer in a future volume the historical and philosophical perspectives of American medicine, what it was, is, and can become in scientific research, professional practice, medical education, and public health, and also its correlation with the sciences, arts, and economy of American society, and with international medicine. Such a task might help forge fresh bonds with other countries overseas, bonds that are indispensable if we wish medicine to add to its noble mission the function of ambassador of peace among peoples at present separated by distrust, but who could yet be united by a mutual endeavor to forge a healthier and more universal civilization.

ON THE BIRTH OF AMERICAN MEDICINE

American medicine was born on American soil; it is not as in Europe a continuation of previous autochthonous cultures. American medicine, like American culture and art, is of recent origin, for it is but a few centuries old. It was only in the sixteenth century that the first book on medicine in the Western hemisphere was printed and that was in Mexico by Spaniards. The importation into America of seventeenth-century European medical culture never succeeded in creating a medical "past" so solid as to bear upon the present with the force it still exerts in Europe. The result is that here it is easier to rebel and become emancipated from previous generations and their doctrines. Medicine in the United States has been optimistic from its beginning, perhaps because of its youth. Even some techniques to which the United States owes its spectacular progress were conceived in Europe largely during the eighteenth and nineteenth centuries, when this country was barely being born as a nation. In this great nation where everything is young, there has come about in medicine, as in everything else, a repristination or rejuvenation of ancient races, particularly of the European stock. There, in my opinion, we have the roots of one of the secrets of America's greatness—and also of one of its greater historical problems.

All human life is basically work and invention. We have to invent our own existence, and such invention cannot be a matter of caprice. If we apply here the basic concept of Ortega y Gasset's philosophy, we understand that life is work and that work in life must be directed toward what must be done and not just anything. Each particular person can possess only his own virtues, not those of his neighbor. The same happens with nations. Europe's virtue is its being old and enjoying therefore a long history and long memories. The United States, however, possesses the admirable simplicity of youth and still shows, in medicine as in technology, traces of its original "colonial" psychology.

THE "COLONIAL" SITUATION

How important this "colonial" character was, in time and space, in determining the future shape of the United States has not been stressed sufficiently. Colonial life—not modern "imperialist" colonialism but old-fashioned colonialism, a blending of exploration, pioneering, adventure, and technological conquest—has been lavish in historical harvests. The advent of philosophy on the earth was a colonial achievement. Medical as well as general philosophy, supreme achievements of the Greeks, did not blossom in Greece itself in the sixth century B.C.

but in Greece's Asian and Italian *colonies*. In those very colonies, not in the Greek peninsula, were born not only the first great Greek philosophers, but even the two greatest figures of Greco-Roman medicine: Hippocrates and Galen.

Colonial life was of supreme importance in forging the future shape of medicine in this country. A characteristic of colonial life is that it is not autochthonous, and the settler is not indigenous to the geographical space in which he lives.

As we said before, land is not only space but time, and each land is at a different stage of civilization in accordance with the cultural "time" of the people inhabiting it. Space and time are as inseparable in geography and history as they are in physics. In the United States there occurred in both medicine and history the inverse of what happened to the Nordic "barbarians" who invaded the old and overcivilized Roman Empire. The barbarians had little or no historical background; therefore, they had only benefits to reap. But the United States was a land historically young, while the people that flocked to it derived from old and highly advanced nations. These people were spiritually rejuvenated upon coming in contact with this land less civilized but younger than theirs. The first physicians, like the first explorers, traders, lawyers, statesmen, and soldiers, to travel the majestic, rolling, promise-filled spaces of America came face to face with races of an inferior culture, which filled them with superiority, but also with loneliness.

A century later other European, or European-educated, physicians arrived with concepts, techniques, and instruments numerous and efficient, only to find out that colonial America's problems were very simple. While colonial life is a bountiful life, historical life (from which these men or at least their professional education originated) was and is always precarious and subject to the dictates of destiny. The first physicians, surgeons, and clerics functioning as physicians had to face, then, problems easier, even primitive, but much more urgent than any they had encountered in Europe. The future United States was not yet a country but a historical *situation,* not a nation but a colonial state.

THE MAGNIFICENT HASTE

The American colonies proceeded with keen determination to face the two great situations posed by history: primitive colonial life; and the vertiginous growth of the country proportionate to the rapid progress in locomotion, industrial development, and the expansion westward by the pioneers. Thus they relived in a concentrated and vertiginous form, as in a motion picture, all the stages that had taken centuries in Europe. In medicine, they passed through the equivalent of medieval clerical medicine with Cotton Mather and the cleric-physicians; they employed magic, astrology, superstition, and folklore, as was done in the lower Middle Ages; in Virginia, young physicians were apprenticed to their elders who taught them and even boarded them in their own homes, as had been the custom in ancient Greece; they performed empirical heroic surgery during the Indian wars and the War of Independence, just as the barber-surgeons and the contemporaries of Ambroise Paré had done in the Renaissance; and in the Middle West they had "factories" that turned out physicians practically overnight, just as "Thessalus and his jackasses" had done in Imperial Rome.

The passage of the years led inevitably to greater historical maturity but did not diminish the craving to go full speed ahead, nor the magnificent pace of the new continent, nor the effort, like Proust's, "to make up for lost time," to cover by leaps and bounds in a few years what had taken many centuries in the old continent. The elements against which conquistadors and pilgrims had had to struggle were mastered; the virgin territories opened up by the pioneers were peacefully settled; the aboriginal races were completely subjugated; the Western frontier was thrust as far as the blue waters of the Pacific; the entire country was crossed by a network of railroads; independence was heroically wrested by force of arms from the British; political differences between the North and the South were washed out in a bloody civil war; industrial progress reached a zenith; huge cities sprang up everywhere—thus the United States marched forward, always at full speed, always in a hurry. The *festina lente,* the "make haste slowly" of the Romans, meant nothing in the young continent. Instead, to hasten haste, to accelerate acceleration, to run fast without fear of exhaustion, to do things quickly but well—such was the supreme goal of the American people.

THE PIONEERING SPIRIT

From the very beginning medicine played an active part in this welter of creative haste. Physicians flourished in private practice and teaching centers, in public health programs and research centers. Sacrificed on the altars of speed were values—not recovered yet—such as tradition, a stumbling block on the fast road to progress, and cultural encyclopedism, which, like a load of ballast, might impede the headlong flight of those who would rather jet straight up into the stratosphere than swing round sedately in less exciting but far more inspiring circles of culture.

The outcome of this effort is the dazzling panorama of present-day American medicine with its "typically American" triumphs, especially in the field of antibiotics, an American specialty despite its British origin; in psychosomatic medicine, again American in its rise but German in origin; in organ surgery, brought to the highest degree of perfection in the nervous system here; in the physiodynamic, metabolic, and organicistic approach to psychiatry, and in psychochemistry; in the application of nuclear and atomic physics to medicine; in the development of impressive physical instrumentation applied to medicine; and in public health and social rehabilitation programs.

If we put our ear to the chest of present-day American medicine, we still hear beneath its dazzling white jacket of technological progress the youthful heartbeat of the settler and pioneer, who knows that life is haste and that his problems admit no waiting and therefore theory must sometimes be sacrificed to practice. The spirit that moved the first medical pioneers to risk an ovariotomy without anesthetics in the Kentucky forests, to study gastric physiology experimentally beneath the open skies in the woods of Michilimackinac, to apply anesthetics without controls in operating rooms in Boston, to perform heroic operations in the Middle West because the patient could hardly wait for the benefit of experience and tradition—this spirit determined the two great traits of American medicine.

These two traits are the "colonial" spirit ("colonial" meaning exploring, adventurous, pioneering), that is to say, the yearning to reduce the complexity of medical problems to their most elementary lines and apply equally simple, bold, and speedy (that is, colonial, pioneering) solutions to them; and creative haste, the craving to do a great deal and do it quickly, to finish with it promptly so as to pass on to something else. This haste was the fruit of the spirit of a young pioneering nation, which learned how to speed up the construction of its buildings before the storm should strike; how to mind its cattle and harvest its crops before the wolves and frosts should come; how to forge new weapons before the enemy should attack; how to create a dynamic medicine so as not only to be on a par with but to excel the rest of the world, while at the same time attending to the constantly increasing problems indigenous to a young nation in full growth.

These are, I believe, the psychologic characteristics that explain the portentous rise and dynamic direction of American medicine. These are features of splendid and thrusting youth, today supplemented by the thought and deeds of many physicians, native and foreign, who have tinged American practice with the silver of maturity. This simple, vigorous, and impatient youth is what gives American medicine its finest characteristics. That dynamic historical youth of American medicine has brought to splendid achievement, now in the fullness of scientific maturity, the promise that throbbed in the great heroic and adventurous days so brilliantly narrated in this Symposium.

ON THE HISTORY OF PUBLIC HEALTH

edicine in our time is steadily approaching the concept
expressed more than one hundred years ago by Ru-
dolph Virchow: "Medicine is a social science . . . anthropology in its widest sense, whose greatest task is to build up society
on a physiological foundation. . . . Politics is nothing but medicine
on a large scale." For although medicine applies the scientific methods
of the natural sciences, its ultimate aim is eminently *social*.

A similar concept inspired the whole work of perhaps the greatest
contemporary historian of medicine, that wise, kind man, Henry
Sigerist—the concept of medicine, like art or sociology, is but one of
the many sides of the immense quarry of civilization.

And now this concept has inspired the creation of this series of
books, whose object is to depict with a modern approach and style the
vast mural of the history of medical specialties in relation to the history
of civilization.

Every day more and more we must accept the idea that there are
not sciences but one single all-embracing Science, that is, a "systematized positive knowledge," the only human activity that is truly cu-
mulative and progressive. Medicine is therefore an essential part of
science, culture, and civilization in every age. Medical history has true
meaning only when regarded as an efflorescence born of the evolution
of the human spirit, which like an underground stream has in every
age nourished the ground of History. This series of books will endeavor

Foreword to *A History of Public Health* by George Rosen, New York, MD
Publications, Inc., 1958.

to present each branch and specialty of Medicine in terms of its impact in time and space on human society.

The most important aspect of modern medicine is unquestionably that of Public Health, embracing as it does the four fundamental historical functions of the physician: to heal, to know, to predict, to organize. Even further, Medicine has been gradually changing from a personal relationship between physician and patient to a relationship between the physician as counselor and his community. From the *Techne Iatrike* of the Golden Age of Greece and the *Ars medendi* of Imperial Rome, Medicine has evolved into the Preventive Medicine—ultimate goal of Public Health—of today, which anticipates the Medicine of Tomorrow.

The history of Public Health is therefore the story of man's endeavors to protect himself and his community against disease. In this sense it is the story of the attitudes of society towards the sick throughout history. In primitive communities, down to the Middle Ages, society's defence against sickness, physical or mental, was to *isolate* or *destroy* the patient; later came the endeavor to *heal* the sick so as to prevent them from infecting or harming their fellow men or becoming a burden on society; and finally the establishment of positive *protection of the healthy* from the dangers of disease. Thus began the Era of Preventive Medicine with its rich arsenal of safeguards, such as quarantine, vaccination, sanitation measures, and other physical and mental health resources, which now take the place of those early rudimentary measures, the propitiatory spells of the shaman and the catharsis of the Greek.

In the philosophical sense the concept of the "individual" has been replaced by that of the "person," that is, the individual in relation to society, just as the concept of the "people" has been replaced by that of the "nation," which is the people in relation to the world. Person, society, nation, and mankind are the concentric circles wherein Preventive Medicine performs its Samaritan work.

The fascinating saga of Public Health is the subject of this book, which is the fruit of the thinking, learning, and doing of Dr. George Rosen. He is a man blessed with that modest simplicity that seems to be an inseparable companion to greatness. To this quality—frequently found in great historians as if it were the best lesson they learned from History—Dr. Rosen adds his brilliant perceptive thought, which has earned him a boundless harvest of achievements. To those in the field of Public Health, Dr. Rosen adds his achievements as a true teacher forever sharing his knowledge with others, as a vastly experienced editor of various distinguished medical journals, and as a world-famous medical historian. In the latter field, Dr. Rosen belongs to the modern school of medical historians who, instead of rendering history into a chronological succession of events, embroider the polychrome fabric of civilization with the figures and events of medical history.

Thus in this book his pen has skillfully traced the procession, sometimes noisy, even stormy, sometimes solemn and majestic, but always colorful and human, of the men, deeds, and facts that have played a vital part in the story of Public Health down the ages. As this historical parade, century after century, files before our eyes, we witness the perennial conflict between comfort and health, between the zest for life and the fear of death, between the satisfaction of physical cravings and whims at the risk of illness, and the sobriety in living and frugality in desires as ways to protect the health.

Reading this book sends flying through our minds a swift flock of thoughts about the correlation among the most diversified aspects of human existence. Progress in sanitary engineering had an important medical consequence—the reduction of typhoid cases. The poetry of an Elizabethan physician paved the way for the advent of the water closet. The burning desire at the heart of all religions to stand in the presence of God in a place of worship inspired the rules of dietary and physical hygiene adopted by all creeds to preserve the purity of the body, dwelling place of the soul. The philosophical individualism of the Greeks determined their highly personal hygiene, just as the political imperialism of the Romans dictated their unique public health system. The prevalence of "collective" enterprises in the Middle Ages was responsible for the fight against the Black Death and other "collective" diseases, just as Renaissance individualism was behind the concern with "individual" diseases, such as syphilis. Thus at every turn in this book, Public Health appears like a mirror reflecting the now anguished, now hopeful face of mankind in every period of history.

To the epic work in Public Health of the physician—sometimes aided by and sometimes in conflict with society—this book is a memorable tribute.

In this panorama of Public Health, painted with the assurance, richness, and perfection of a master, Dr. Rosen confirms the ever-increasing recognition of the *social* character of disease which is making the physician every day more a counselor, mentor, organizer, and, above all, a *preventer*.

ON THE HISTORY OF NEUROLOGY

*t*he history of neurology, far more than the history of any other branch of medicine, has been a gigantic conflict between dogmatic tradition and experimental observation. Only with the progress of modern scientific research in the last century did this conflict begin to subside.

In cardiology or dermatology, for instance, there being concord between philosophic tradition and the empiric observation of patients, medical thought progressed steadily. But in neurology, and consequently in psychiatry, progress was impeded by the notion, metaphysical in the conceptual sense and emotional in its personal connotations, that the organs that are studied in neurology, such as the brain and the nervous-system organs, regulate internally man's organism and externally his relationship with his environment, with God and Nature. This is the reason for the historical clash between the two principal attitudes governing neurological thought—the metaphysico-religious and the empirico-scientific. Although present-day neurology is oriented by scientific thought, one can still observe in primitive (or should we say "isolated?") peoples that curious dichotomy which so delayed progress in the knowledge of nervous-system physiology.

In this book, the second in our medico-historical series, a kindly and learned medical historian, Dr. Walther Riese, portrays the vast panorama of the history of neurologic thought, breaking it down into six panels, each one of which is a window through which he, with the luminous thought of the historian and philosopher, casts new

Foreword to *A History of Neurology* by Walther Riese, New York, MD Publications, Inc., 1958.

light upon the dark forbidding corners of the old somber mansion of neurology.

The author first considers the knowledge of the function of the nervous system, which in some respects preceded the knowledge of its anatomy; he then analyzes the history of the knowledge of the nervous impulse and of reflex action; he proceeds to present the historical evolution of the theory of cerebral localizations and of the rediscovery of the totality of the being; and lastly he examines the problem of pain in neurology. Like the panels of a hexatych, the sections of this book are beautifully integrated, conjuring a dramatic and colorful picture of man's search for knowledge of himself and of his basic medical problems by exploring the organs of the nervous system and its unfathomed functions.

Dr. Riese belongs to that school of modern historians for whom the history of medicine is also that of science, thus combining the study of events in time with that of inventions and discoveries in space, and the study of history-making ideas with that of their crystallization into technological achievements. Dr. Riese's internationally recognized works do great honor to this school. There cannot be many historians or neurologists with Dr. Riese's knowledge who have studied this subject, for his writings, as prolific as they are profound, include many studies on the history of neurology, on the philosophic aspects of modern medicine, and on the work of the great neurologists. History, regardless of what we may consider it—occupation, system, method, tool or lesson—must be philosophy if its delicate fabric is to have any meaning, and Dr. Riese has sailed across the high seas of history always guided by the compass of philosophy.

The history of neurology, considered as a medical specialty, did not begin with the simple anatomic description of nerve centers or of neurologic syndromes. It is one thing to observe something, and another to interpret it. The ancient Egyptians, as the Greeks before Hippocrates, observed many neurologic affections, meningitis and migraine, palsies and tremors, but failed to interpret them in terms of their relations with the nervous system, since the cranial cavity remained for many centuries an inner sanctum barred to the surgeon's scalpel.

The history of surgery may be summed up as the history of the surgeon's assault upon the three main cavities in the human body: the abdomen, the thorax, and the cranium, which were "invaded" in the order mentioned, perhaps because the abdomen was easily broached by both the enemy's knife and the surgeon's scalpel, while the thorax and the cranium, protected as they are by a wall of bone, were hard to reach by either one. The craniotomies practiced so frequently among aborigines were an attempt not so much to penetrate into the cranial box as to provide possessing demons with an outlet for escape. Parallel to the surgical fear in opening the great cavities of the body, there developed the idea—basic to Neurology and Psychiatry—of locating the seat of life in each one of them in turn. The first chosen, by the pre-Homerics, was the abdomen and its large viscera, particularly the liver, which, because of its size and the amount of blood it contained, was taken as the seat of the soul; later, in Homeric times, the heart was considered the seat of life and of the passions; and, finally, post-Homeric physicians deemed the brain to be animated with the magic breath that nurses the fire of life. There was therefore a certain concurrency among the empirical observation of the organic cavities, whether opened deliberately or by accident, the surgical invasion thereof, and the philosophic localization therein of the highest centers of life.

Neurology as a scientific specialty made its appearance comparatively late. The first professor of neurology was appointed only one generation ago. Neurology and psychiatry went hand in hand for many years, and their track can be traced, as we have done elsewhere,* merely by following the footsteps of organicistic philosophy in psychiatry and of the men and ideas responsible for its development.

It is possible to apply to neurology the conception the nineteenth century Spanish physician-philosopher, Leon Corral, had of medicine: a pyramid whose base is formed by the patients, its middle by the diseases, and its apex by the philosophic concept of disease. The base of the pyramid, therefore, is formed by the physician's experience, and the rest by his science.

The object of this monograph is to describe how physicians succeeded in developing this science. Quite correctly, Dr. Riese grants much importance at the beginning to the fact that orientation is inseparable from movement, and this from sensation. Of profound philosophic significance is his assertion, key to the whole outlook of his book, that all the qualities of the brain are spatial and only spatial phenomena occur within it, motion and sensation being the link between the soul and the brain. At the same time, he emphasizes that, since disease is a historic or biographic process, no structural diagram of the nervous system can accurately portray it. Only a film-track could properly follow its path.

Disease is a dynamic process and the human being is an entity, composed of soma and psyche, situated at an intersection of time and space, which keeps "making itself" throughout time. The history of neurology reveals how physicians passed from the study of the

* See page 433.

patient suffering from an ailment of the nervous system, which was considered with a semiological criterion, to the study of the disease itself considered with a nosological criterion, to the actual study of the disease considered with an etiological criterion and bearing in mind the total personality of the patient.

Today in healing the sick three criteria are applied: *objective,* whose purpose is to correct the symptoms of the patient; *subjective,* intended to make him *feel* better and to restore his social well-being; and *sociological,* intended to help the patient, by means of adequate rehabilitation, to become again a useful member of society. Let us not forget that semantically the word "*dis*-ease" is the opposite of health, which semantically is close to *holy* and *whole.*

There are two threads running through the story of neurology: the changes that have taken place in the anatomic concept of the nervous organs; and the notion of movement as an expression of the nervous functions in space.

The nervous system, and particularly the brain, was studied in three different ways down the ages: (1) as the operative principle, an instrument or organ expressive of the intrinsic function of the living being, a morphological "part" of and pure physical configuration in space; thus the ancients "saw" the brain up to the time of the Roman Empire; (2) as a static spatial or architectural arrangement, an allegorical representation, a mere piece of the whole anatomic figure built upon the religious idea of the microcosm as a reflection of the macrocosm; this idea prevailed in the Middle Ages; (3) as a process arising from a morphogenetic evolution in time.

An organ of expression, an allegorical representation, a morphogenetic process in time—these then are the successive views of the brain held by physicians at various stages in history. It would be illuminating to correlate the art and culture of any particular period with the particular view of the brain and nervous system in vogue at that time. Thus: the brain was a representative allegory in the symbolically minded Middle Ages; an architectonic structure in the sculpturally minded Renaissance; a mechanical movement in the dynamic Baroque; a physiological evolution in the biologically inclined nineteenth century; and so on down to the scientific synthesis of today.

The notion of movement, which, according to the author, is the rational principle upon which we evaluate the changes in Nature, a concept already recorded in the pre-Homeric *Panta rhei,* has kept pace with the ceaseless changes in the history of neurology. The nervous physiology of old was very dynamic, as shown by its eminently kinetic vocabulary (physis, kinesis, dynamis). Motion for post-Aristotelian philosophers was the step from potentiality to action, a qualitative variation in the being; while for the moderns motion came to mean merely displacement from one point in space to another. So also, while for the ancients Nature was in essence the cause of motion, for the moderns Nature is the law of motion. Form and function to the ancients was only function. But with the publication in Basel, by a brave Belgian anatomist, of the most famous anatomy work in history, which studied the "anatomy of the cadaver" and treated the body as a statue or fabric, "modern" science was born, opening the path for an Englishman in the seventeenth century to put anatomy in motion and make *anatomia animata* in space, today called physiology, and *anatomia animata* in time, today called embryology. Nervous physiology then ceased to be qualitative and intuitional and became mensurative and quantitative. From the new concept of *local* movement sprang the new trends in neurology described in this book.

In the last few years neurology has reached a transcendental stage of development, as is explained in so masterly a fashion in this volume. Though at first it adopted the methods, concepts and trends current in medicine, neurology today is of considerable help in the elucidation of medical problems in biochemistry, metabolism, organic integration, and particularly in psychosomatic and psychiatric nosology. The vast still unexplored areas of the human brain, and that *terra incognita,* the hypothalamus, which together with the pituitary, adrenal and thyroid glands may conceal the secret of so many endocrine, neurologic and psychiatric problems—all these promise to be the most important field of medical research in our century, as their padlocked doors yield one by one to the new keys, the ataraxics and the hallucinogenics.

On ancient Spanish maps, the unexplored zones of the Gobi desert were simply marked, "Here are lions," thus revealing the ignorance and superstition of the map-makers. Practically the same thing was done for many years with the areas of the encephalon, and only recently were functional explorations started which will in time dispel many age-old errors and shed light upon the truth.

Such is the panorama Dr. Riese has surveyed in the following pages. Reading them, one can readily appreciate how progress in clinical and in interpretative thinking have run parallel, though at different speeds, across the fields of history, as would a train and a river running parallel. The author has traced this panorama with science and art, which in medicine are one and the same. For art is but a part of science, and science derives from the Latin *scire,* meaning knowledge and learning, two ideals unattainable were the substance of science denied the esthetic form of art.

ON THE HISTORY OF OPHTHALMOLOGY

*t*he history of ophthalmology is a chapter apart from the rest of the history of medicine. The reason for this peculiarity of ophthalmology is the unique nature of the eye. While other sense organs were studied, at first empirically and later scientifically, by physicians through the centuries, the eye, the most vital of all senses to the human being, because of the importance of its functions and the mystery of its nature was closely associated in the human mind with superstitions, myths and legends. The eye thus became a *terra* not only *incognita* but also *mystica,* which man dared not explore for fear of offending the gods, of whose omniscience the ocular organ was itself a symbol. Hence, the history of ophthalmology is the history of a gigantic conflict between prejudice and necessity, a conflict that was settled late in history when the eye was explored scientifically. It is also the history of the attitudes of society toward not only the eye but also the visual function, attitudes so strong that they were reflected in the religions, art, and culture of each period and rendered knowledge of the visual organ difficult until the Renaissance, when the "visual" replaced the "auditive" attitude in medicine.

In this book Dr. George Arrington, as distinguished a historian as he is an ophthalmologist, with a vigorous pen vividly traces the story of ophthalmology from its beginnings in prehistoric times to its present-day scientific and technological achievements. Not only does Dr. Arrington tell us everything that can and should concern the ophthalmologist, the historian, and the physician regarding the prog-

---

Foreword to *A History of Ophthalmology* by George E. Arrington, Jr., New York, MD Publications, Inc., 1958.

ress of this medical specialty, but he does so using as a backdrop the vast multicolored tapestry of civilization, pointing out the great figures in art and science throughout history who themselves helped to weave the tapestry. Thus on one and the same distaff are interspun the threads of the story of ophthalmology with the threads of the story of culture and civilization, affording us the only way there is to understand them both properly. Only someone like Dr. Arrington could have performed such a difficult task so brilliantly, for he has been for many years passionately dedicated to the study of the delicate ocular structures in the anatomical specimen as well as in the patient, and has thus acquired the subtlety and patience indispensable to becoming a skillful architect of the history of his specialty.

This prologue is but a brief overture before the curtain rises, and I shall therefore only allude to a few points of interest in the philosophy of ophthalmological history, for instance, the symbolism of the eye in religions, which originated the conflict between the mystic respect for the eye, which impeded the academic study of this organ, and the need for attending empirically to its maladies. Another instance was the effect of the "visual" attitude on the progress not only of ophthalmology but also of medicine.

In primitive mythology the eye often represented the deity as a symbol of force and luminosity. As J. Eduardo Cirlot recently indicated in his excellent study on this subject, the eye was often employed in mythological iconography, in which its magic powers were stressed by three processes: *displacement,* or placing eyes in places other than the anatomically normal, for instance, heterotopic eyes in the wings of romanesque angels; *diminution,* or reducing the number of eyes, as in Cyclops; and *augmentation,* or increasing the number of eyes, as with the hundred-eyed Argus of Greek mythology.

To the aforementioned uses must be added the use of the eye as a magic protective talisman, such as the eyes painted on Greek galleys, Oriental eye-amulets, the eye painted on the faïence orbs used by Indochinese religious sects, and the eye symbolic of the Divine Providence stamped on ancient Christian Gnostic images. The eye was used as a symbol of the powers of darkness in some medieval allegories of satanism. The eye has also been considered a powerful magic symbol by artists, and in our own times it has been used in surrealist painting (Ernst, Magritte, Dali). Cirlot in his work contrasts the symbols of the three attitudes adopted by man when, facing the Infinite, he inquires about his fate: the symbol of the *wall,* for instance, the Wailing Wall of Jerusalem, which represents a feeling of impotence in face of the Infinite; the symbol of the *window,* for instance, the perforated jade disks of the Chinese, which represents a feeling of possible but restricted human activity; and the symbol of the eye-talisman, which is not impotency like the first symbol, nor an opening offering escape like the second symbol, but a *mirror* that provides an answer for man, for upon looking into the eye he finds in himself the answer to his anguished queries.

This intimate association of the eye with religious symbolism made the study of the eyes difficult for thousands of years. On the other hand, people living in areas, such as the Middle East, anvil of our civilization, exposed to unceasing sandstorms that caused ocular irritations, often followed by infection and blindness, were desperately in need of a solution to this pressing problem. That is why in ancient Egypt, as among the Arabs more than a thousand years later, there prevailed on one hand a servile submission to dogmatic Galenic ophthalmology, and on the other persistent attempts to develop ocular techniques and medications for eye diseases such as ophthalmia, cataract, and trachoma. Even so, the recurring mention of blind beggars in the legends of ancient Egypt and in *The Arabian Nights* bears witness to the frequency of blindness among Oriental peoples.

But the crucial change in the history of ophthalmology occurred in the Renaissance, with Leonardo da Vinci's *Eye Codex* and particularly with his new "visual" attitude, his unflagging determination to *saper vedere*—to know how to look at the world and at man with eyes freed of the medieval cobwebs, to observe, describe and portray things as they really were instead of distorted, as fear-ridden, prejudice-bound medieval man portrayed them in allegories and symbolism. It was this desire of the Renaissance artist to look at things closer and better that led to the study of the visual function and to a better knowledge of the organ involved in such function. Ophthalmology owes indeed a great debt to da Vinci and the Renaissance painters, not so much for their contribution to the anatomical study of the human eye, as for their having aroused a new and passionate interest in the act of seeing, in how to look at things, in the use of sight as man's most precious instrument for exploring the world around him.

Ever since then, the parallelism between certain mental attitudes, certain artistic periods, and scientific advances in ophthalmology has been continuous. It was in those periods of history when the yearning for Romantic "infinitism" was most acute that ophthalmology made the greatest progress, ophthalmology meaning the discipline devoted to investigating the mysteries of the human eye's visual "infinite." A beautiful example of such parallelism between investigators and artists, each impelled by a similar passion, is the fact that in the city of Delft, Holland, at the very same time that Leeuwenhoek, who enlarged the visible world with his polished lenses, was studying the function and structure of the retina, Vermeer, only a few blocks away from him, was painting those exquisite miniatures in which he depicted the most minute details of a Dutch interior with the same loving care that Leeuwenhoek devoted to the exploration of the minute world enclosed in the intraocular structure.

Similar parallelisms could be established in our own era, for instance, the attempt of impressionist painters at the end of the last century to capture light in their pictures (splitting it sometimes into tiny luminous dots, as in Seurat's *pointillisme*), which created new concepts about light and color that coincided with the advances realized in that field by contemporary ophthalmologists.

Such is the philosophical fabric of the fascinating story related in this book. For his many achievements the author has reaped an abundant harvest of laurels, but in my opinion what he deserves the greatest homage for is his humanistic point of view that the physician not only must once again look at the *whole* patient, but must himself be a *whole man,* who never allows himself to be dominated by technology but at all times applies a humane and Hippocratic criterion. This attitude of Dr. Arrington is all the more worthy of the highest praise for having emanated from a physician whose specialty is highly dependent upon physical instrumentation. Dr. Arrington thus proves that he is indeed an example of the humanist physician who places above his instruments his *saper vedere.*

III. the philosophy of medicine

THE BIOPHILOSOPHIC SIGNIFICANCE
OF ARTIFICIAL HIBERNATION

*t*hrough the gateway of his concept of artificial hibernation, Dr. Henry Laborit ushers us into that vast dark-roomed palace which is the physiopathology of the neurovegetative system. Ghostly shadows fill this area of neuroendocrine pathology, where proved scientific facts exist side by side with new theories. But Dr. Laborit walks ahead of us, opening windows and turning on the lights, banishing shadows and illuminating theories as new in their meaning as they are traditional in their empiricism. For artificial hibernation is not merely a new therapy but rather a widening of the horizon of modern medicine. It is based on a medical philosophy that promises to revolutionize classic concepts hitherto considered immutable. Let us reserve for the brilliant contributors to this symposium the task of explaining the techniques, applications, and possibilities of artificial hibernation. Our purpose here is to provide a blueprint for those unfamiliar with this therapeutic system.

Biology teaches us that man, like many animals, is a homeothermic being, capable of maintaining the stability of his inner milieu—intercellular fluids, vascular lymph, and blood—and the constancy of his body temperature through the functioning of thermoregulating physical and chemical mechanisms. Because of these mechanisms, man is a warm-blooded animal in contrast with the cold-blooded animals called poikilotherms, like the lizard, whose body temperature is on a par with that of their environment. As Claude Bernard demonstrated, the stability of the inner milieu permits us to enjoy an independent life, safe from environmental variations.

From *International Record of Medicine 167*:309, 1954.

The biologic instrument used by our body to guarantee the constancy of its temperature and the stability of our inner milieu is the neurovegetative system—and certain mysterious areas of the nervous system, like the thalamus and hypothalamus—whose vast network is integrated with the endocrine glands, thus forming a neurovegetative-endocrine system without which man could not enjoy biologic freedom and would be at the mercy of any change in external temperature. Because of this system, the body of an Eskimo in icy Lapland and that of a Zulu in the burning heart of Africa have the same temperature. Many years after Claude Bernard established this basic concept of modern physiology, Walter Cannon baptized it *homeostasis,* and from then on it has been considered the ineluctable condition of independent life and the most precious physiologic gift enjoyed by man.

Several years ago, in the wake of the new concepts introduced by Reilly and Selye, who established the consequences of that powerful, unspecific external aggression called *stress* upon the human being, it was observed that the reaction of the human body to external aggressions could be so violent that it could cause a state of shock frequently resulting in death. The mechanism of this biologic catastrophe is the overreaction of the organism to aggression from the environment; the body violently mobilizes a series of drastic defensive reactions whose purpose is to maintain the thermic autonomy of the organism, that is, its homeostasis. These reactions can be intense enough to exhaust the individual. Mobilization of the body's defenses against external aggression frequently produces a collapse of the organic fortress, as if the suddenness and magnitude of the defense measures were even more harmful to the fortress than the possible attack from without.

The neurovegetative system, the hypothalamus, and the endocrine glands are the factors in these reactions, which can consume the last bit of organic energy and produce a sudden drop in blood pressure, a reduction in the volume of circulating blood, shivering, and other symptoms characterizing shock. This occurs because our organism attempts to defend itself against an aggression that is greater than its means of defense. Shock is a typical example of the fact that—contrary to the claims of classical medicine—not all physiologic reactions are beneficial, and it also further confirms that pathology and physiology make up one area in which frontiers are arbitrarily defined.

Our neurovegetative system is capable of defending our lives under normal or moderately abnormal conditions, but when it is faced with aggressions that are exceptionally violent, it can exhaust and kill us. As the classic proverb has it: "The cure is worse than the disease." In such cases, the attempt of the neurovegetative system to maintain the stability of our inner milieu may be made at the price of our lives.

When Laborit began his search for a means of combating shock reactions, he was guided by the desire to solve a problem common to physicians of all times. In the course of his reading, he had come across old reports from physicians at the Val de Grâce Hospital who had taken care of soldiers wounded while fighting under the Napoleonic banner; these reports stated that the patients had survived tremendous ordeals under very low temperatures. Such claims dovetailed with others made a century before Napoleon by French explorers who had survived great privations and wounds in the frozen wastelands of Canada. Laborit also read more recent books on the subject and was drawn to the work of Finnish and American scientists on the production of experimental hypothermy in animals. The information he acquired led Laborit to suspect that blind acceptance of the principles of Claude Bernard might entail risks, and, after studying Reilly and Selye, he began to wonder whether the solution to the problem of shock should be based not so much on man's capacity to resist unusually intense external aggressions as on his ability to adapt himself to them, to yield to them temporarily without any struggle. If we may be permitted the use of a pugilistic term, in such cases it might be more useful to "roll with the punch," like the boxer who deadens his opponent's blow by allowing his body to be carried by the impact of the blow rather than meeting it full force.

The work of Laborit and his school had for a backdrop a very rich folklore and a vast treasure of empirical "know-how" among countryfolk. If human vitality could be temporarily reduced without causing any lesion, it might be feasible to let a physical agent play an important part in vegetable and animal biology. If nature teaches us that extreme cold is the mortal enemy of living beings, it also shows us that, paradoxically, extreme cold may also ensure survival. Horticulturists know that the best time to transplant plants and even trees is in midwinter, the colder the better, for then the plants and trees are not traumatized. Marmots and other hibernating animals live all winter *au ralenti,* and their organisms suffer no lesion.

Jentzer, of Geneva, found many trout imbedded in a frozen lake in Gothard. Observing that they were as stiff as wood, he traumatized them in various ways with sufficient intensity to kill a living trout several times over. Yet when he returned them to frozen water and warmed the water, the trout revived without showing any ill-effects from the traumatisms. This means that poikilothermal animals, like insects, lizards, and batrachians, instead of defending themselves against aggressions from without, especially cold, simply resist them by adapting their temperature to that of the environment. Such a phenomenon is possible, according to Jentzer, because such animals do not have a neurovegetative system. But the human being has a highly developed neurovegetative system, more so than that of any other species, which in response to any *external* (thermic, surgical, physical, etc.) or *internal* (chemical, medical, etc.) aggression sets in motion a series of reactions in the nature of a neuroendocrine defense of homeostasis. These reactions are usually beneficial, but in cases of unusual aggressions they may exhaust and even kill the organism. This "dragon" of excess threatening "the Saint George" of homeostasis—to use Cannon's picturesque image—was recently named *hyperexis* by Dickinson W. Richards. *Hyperexis* is a Greek word meaning a reactional excess and was first used two thousand years ago in the dialogue *Timaeus,* written by that great Athenian called Plato.

Refrigeration of the body as a means of lowering defense reactions is a revolutionary measure. For centuries the obsession of the physician has been "to increase organic defenses" as a means of preserving the constancy of the inner milieu and fortifying it against pathologic or traumatic aggressions. Therefore, the idea of refrigerating the body to enable it to adapt itself *passively* to an aggression instead of fighting it represents a reorganization of classic physiology from the ground up.

Hypothermy of the body reduces the organic requirements and the consumption of oxygen, lowers the metabolism, and, with the reduction of capillary circulation and loss of radiating heat, changes the bright flame of metabolism and cellular oxidation into a tiny flickering light. This obviously would be of great advantage in brain and heart surgery when the attempt is made to interrupt the flow of blood to vital organs. For some time now physicians have had recourse to *refrigeration* of a part of the body as well as of the *entire* body (hypothermy) with a lowering of its temperature to 77 F. or even lower (deep hypothermy). This method was employed by Bell as far back as 1812 to treat pain, and by Arnott one hundred and three years ago to treat carcinoma. The term "artificial hibernation" was originally employed by Simpson in 1905 and revived in 1951 by Laborit and Huguenard, who were the first to strengthen anesthesia by means of certain drugs and then to provoke a neurovegetative block accompanied by induced hypothermy. The term artificial hibernation therefore should not be applied to the method itself but to the state of autonomic block and reduction of body vitality to a minimum.

In order to block the neurovegetative system and prevent it from liberating chemical substances, which, like a clarion call, mobilize organic defensive reactions, Laborit experimented with substances that might provoke a "lysis" or interruption of the defensive mechanisms of the body, a *neuroplegia* or disconnection—on all possible levels—of the neurovegetative system and even of the central nervous system if possible. Laborit and Huguenard tested different neuroplegic or lytic drugs, mixing various ingredients of diverse effects and often of unknown total results, and they finally developed a mixture that produced a certain "intoxication" followed by a twilight state, which justifies the term *lytic cocktail,* or *liberation cocktail,* introduced in 1953 by Huguenard. In point of time, neuroplegia had been induced prior to the work of these two scientists: e.g., the medicophilosophic systems described in Hindu yogas, the anoxi-anesthesia of Crile, the deep anesthesia of Bigelow, the muscular relaxants of Krogh, procaine perfusions, high rachianesthesia with vagal cervical block, the sleep cures with local anesthesia of Vijnejkij, and the cortical blocks of Russian psychiatrists who were the forerunners in the use of neuroplegia in psychiatry as applied today in France by Delay and his collaborators.

What Laborit and his co-workers aimed at from the very beginning was to effect an artificially induced hibernation in man, similar to that of hibernating mammals and cold-blooded animals. This means that hibernation is more than just inducing a prolonged sleep. It entails calming the disorganized reactions of the neuroendocrine system at a given crucial moment, thus imitating the physiologic attitudes of certain animals that are not as highly developed as man but are, on the other hand, less fragile. As Laborit has said, it is a matter of "temporarily abandoning a metabolical luxury with which we can no longer maintain life and adopting a more modest type of life, in order to await a return to a regime of free interexchange and more favorable conditions of life in the environment." Artificial hibernation therefore is, particularly in cases of civil traumatisms or war wounds, more than a therapeutic technique; it is part of a treatment by which we can survive, as has been shown in surgery, psychiatry, and especially in military medicine, and which has saved innumerable lives.

The search for the royal road to artificial hibernation led to the search for chemical compounds that would strengthen the effect of refrigeration of the human body through iced sheets and other means that would not cause dangerous bronchopulmonary reactions when such compounds have deprived the body of the ability to react against cold. The combination of a *lytic cocktail* and refrigeration may revolutionize the treatment of shock. No longer are the defenses of the body stimulated as hitherto by heat, stimulants, or tonic medications, which sometimes increase organic reaction so out of proportion that the body, exhausted by its own natural reactions and those induced by stimulants, succumbs like a worn-out horse that is suddenly whipped violently. Instead, the organic functions are now reduced to a minimum bordering on the inertia of hibernating animals.

After several attempts, Laborit decided to use a drug with a phenothiazine base of strong lytic effect. Later a derivative—chlorpromazine—was obtained, which has one of the broadest known spectrums of activity on the nervous system, since it is sympatholytic, vagolytic, spasmolytic, and sedative. To this drug Laborit and Huguenard added two more (promethazine or Phernergan, and Demerol or Pethidine) whose effects are primarily sympatholytic, adrenolytic, and vagolytic, and secondarily hypnogenic (lobotomisant) and analgesic, the *cocktail* being administered by intravenous perfusion drop by drop.

Thus, the combination of induced neuroplegia and refrigeration of the patient produces the state of artificial hibernation characterized by hypometabolism, hypothermia, hypotension, hyposecretion, and biologic indifference of the organism to external aggressions. The neuroendocrine system is stabilized and the rhythm of life is slowed down by pharmacodynamic mechanisms while the lytic cocktail "sends the adrenal-pituitary couple on a vacation," as Laborit, with typical Gallic humor, put it.

When the organism is deprived of nutrition it draws on its own reserves of proteins and lipids, since the metabolism of the glucides is blocked. Laborit also used injections of pituitary somatotropic hormone (STH) to favor protein anabolism and catabolize lipids, in imitation of hibernating animals which during their winter sleep consume their fats but not their proteins or sugars, which they need when they awaken in the spring.

The cold of hibernation eliminates the antistress reaction (often very dangerous in states of shock) of the organism and protects it from the aggressor factor, at the same time that it lessens, by its narcobiotic action, microbe pullulation and toxic reabsorptions. And so, of the two factors necessary for the development of a disease— the pathologic aggressor factor (traumatism, microbe or toxin) and the reaction of the attacked organism to it—the second factor is eliminated and instead homeothermic life is protected at the cost of putting conscious life to sleep, thereby sheltering the organism from the threats of stress, whether it be traumatic, toxic, infectious, or even emotional and psychiatric in nature. And all this is due to the chemically induced "vacation" of the neurovegetative-endocrine-hypothalamic system.

From this we can see that artificial hibernation is as ancient as nature herself, since it imitates the method she has given trees, plants, fish, reptiles, and many other animals of defending themselves from bitter winters and the attendant lack of food. Prehistoric man must have possessed this quality to a certain degree but lost it as he learned to defend himself consciously from cold and hunger. Animals still sleep during the long months of cold and hunger. Their breathing, as well as their pulse, slows down, their temperature falls, their consumption of oxygen decreases to a minimum, organic elimination is interrupted, and the neurovegetative block and coma of certain sensorial areas of the brain eliminate external sensations, such as cold, which would make them wake up and consume energy. Instead they feed on small amounts of fat stored up in the organic pantry of their own body. These fats are consumed and burned up so slowly that they last until the animal awakens.

Man has done nothing more than imitate scientifically the mechanism of natural defense used by animals. Lecomte de Nouy (quoted by Jentzer) said: "The criterion of adaptation is usefulness, while the criterion of evolution is freedom." The error of early research and conclusions was to mistake evolutional features for vital phenomena. Instead of exalting means of defense—which often accelerate exhaustion of cells and precipitate death—the new artificial hibernation deprives us temporarily of our freedom through a neurovegetative block of harmful reactions, and gives the hibernating organism a period of repose and sleep during which to recover and save its life.

Laborit and his collaborators have led us into a vast mansion of mysterious shadows—artificial hibernation—and have opened some of its treasure rooms that they may be explored by investigators the world over. We stand on the threshold of a new era of research into vegetative and endocrine phenomena, perhaps also into new psychiatric methods, with the consequent widening of our knowledge of biology and human pathology. Artificial hibernation does not correct Claude Bernard. It broadens the horizon he described and provides a new theory and promising tools for the research biologist, so that he may constantly progress toward that ideal of happiness—unattainable in medicine—enjoyed by the man who knows the cause of things. For, as Vergil said, *Felix qui potuit rerum cognoscere causas.*

PHILOSOPHIC PERSPECTIVES
OF MOTION SICKNESS

for thousands of years man lived a "two-dimensional" life in a three-dimensional world. While man used his legs, the horse, or the carriage as his principal means of transportation, the physical displacement of his body involved a number of difficulties and discomforts which, however, rarely affected his mental and organic well-being. But when man abandoned *terra firma* and took to the water, when he furrowed rivers, lakes, and oceans in rafts, canoes, and boats, he had to pay the penalty exacted by nature: seasickness.

Nausea and vomiting were associated for thousands of years with seafaring, hardly ever with land journeys. Seasickness overtook Ulysses and his companions in the Homeric saga; it was a scourge to the Spanish *Conquistadores* when their proud boats sailed uncharted seas; it laid low the Portuguese heroes who first circumnavigated the globe; and it continues to vex those who, through necessity or pleasure, cross the seas in modern transatlantic liners.

Since literature and history record so few instances of motion sickness overtaking horsemen—no matter how distant, fast, or exhausting their travels—we cannot subscribe to the ancient theory that nausea is caused by mere visceral displacement. It is possible, however, that the men who rode on the backs of the lurching elephants responsible for Pyrrhus' victories suffered from motion sickness. The men who rode the camels—the ships of the desert—led by Colonel T. H. Lawrence during his famous rebellion in Arabia

From *International Record of Medicine* 167:621, 1954.

Deserta, told of the nausea that overtook them on the shifting hot sands so reminiscent of a vast gray sea.

At the beginning of our century, man, who had moved horizontally for several millenia, decided to attempt the conquest of vertical space. The great motility of airplanes added new violence to motion sickness and made this condition a tremendous problem particularly in countries—in some South American countries, for instance—where there has been a sudden transition from mule to plane. It was then that medical research workers began to investigate motion sickness, not as a vexatious if inevitable companion of the traveling mortal, but as a medical riddle whose physiopathology was a question mark and whose therapy had been compounded of folklore and crude empiricism.

The progress made by civil and military aviation has increased the importance of studying and preventing motion sickness produced not only by airplanes, but also by boats, automobiles, trolley cars, and other means of physical displacement. The immense progress made in the physiopathology and therapy of motion sickness is illustrated by this current symposium, which represents the first international monograph ever published on this subject.

The historical and literary references to *mal de mer* are as ancient as they are numerous. Cicero, the golden-tongued Roman statesman, said that he "would rather be killed than again suffer the tortures of *nausea maris.*" Before him, Hippocrates pointed out that when a hellebore draught was administered to a patient to provoke emesis, the patient "should move about and sleep and rest as little as possible." This advice was based on his concept that "sailing the seas shows that movement upsets the body."

Throughout the history of medicine we find frequent references to seasickness as well as attempts to interpret it medically. William Hyde Wollaston (1766–1827), the eminent ophthalmologist famous for his research on the physiologic mechanism of central vision, tried to show that seasickness was caused by "oscillatory alteration of the blood," especially in the brain, brought about by the movements of the ship.

The notion of seasickness suddenly widened with the expansion of the semantic cage in which the elusive problem was imprisoned. In 1881 J. A. Irwin used the term "motion sickness" for the first time; he felt that seasickness was a misnomer because this condition could "be induced by various other motions than that of turbulent waters." His term was universally accepted only at the beginning of the Second World War, when the unforgettable Sir Frederick Banting stated that the expression "motion sickness" could include a series of syndromes resembling seasickness but resulting from "frequently repeated oscillatory movements of the body." [1]

Finding a name for an illness is often tantamount to focusing light on possible treatment. This has occurred time and again in the history of medicine. We need only recall the therapeutic implications in the coining of the name "syphilis" by the great Renaissance physician and poet Fracastoro. At any rate, as the semantic concept of classic seasickness changed to "motion sickness," a conceptual revolution took place: the idea that the sea caused nausea was replaced by the theory that *movement* was responsible for such a disturbance, a concept pregnant with new therapeutic possibilities.

Next, the ideologic scope of the word "nausea" was extended. Since *nausea* was derived from *naus,* the Greek word for vessel, it at first meant only seasickness, but eventually came to mean an urge to vomit arising from other causes. In his recent novel *La Nausée,* Jean-Paul Sartre used the term existentially to signify the physiologic expression of a supreme philosophic disgust with life—an idea whose physiologic roots certainly bear a strange resemblance to the anxiety factor in motion sickness.

The study of motion sickness, or kinetosis, parallels that of certain reactions observed in the human being when he undergoes changes of position, e.g., the change from the supine to the erect position in the orthostatic, or orthotic, reaction. Among the different types of kinetosis, investigators began to include physiologic reactions provoked by oscillations passively imposed on the body, either in a swing or in a boat, by rhythmic or irregular movements, angular, linear, radial, circular, or seesaw accelerations.

Clinical facts accumulated quickly. It was observed that motion sickness ran the gamut of pallor, cold sweat, difficulty in breathing, weak pulse, nausea, vomiting, and physical and moral prostration. Certain sensory, visual, tactile, and olfactory excitations produced a similar picture, for instance, acute tobacco intoxication. The neurovegetative system actively participated in motion sickness, and there was a marked analogy between this syndrome and the phenomenon of vagal excitation produced by physostigmine. Paradoxically, visceral shaking-up was not enough to excite the nerve endings in the abdominal viscera, since ordinary shaking provoked by racing and jumping did not produce motion sickness. Notice was also taken of the absence of motion sickness in deaf-mutes and of the similarity between motion sickness and Menière's syndrome. Proof was adduced that odors, fear, and anxiety aggravated motion sickness, or provoked it in certain cases. Motion sickness of long duration, during extended sea voyages when the weather is constantly stormy, could cause arterial hypertension, loss of weight, dehydration, exhaustion with acidosis, and mental depression.

This avalanche of observations made in laboratories and clinics created a doctrinal corpus around motion sickness, but it was an amorphous corpus that needed a patient hand to transform the chaos into cosmos, to give organic structure to the huge pyramid of empirical facts, and to train a clear light from the experimental apex of that pyramid to its wide clinical base.

The most revolutionary step taken in the study of the factors causing motion sickness was to study motion sickness independently of its most obvious organic localization, the stomach; it was decided to seek its genesis in the recondite areas of the organs governing equilibrium. Today it seems logical that motion sickness should be studied in connection with the organs responsible for equilibrium. But years ago it did not seem so, because the predominant tendency in the historical evolution of medicine was always to begin the study of an illness in the area of its principal symptom. Only in our time has medicine begun to evolve philosophically from outside in, from the symptom to the etiology, from the dramatic picture of the manifestations of an illness to a subtle grasp of its causes.

In this brief introduction, which is like the diffuse tuning-up preceding the start of a concert, we are concerned solely with pointing out some of the philosophic aspects of the research into the causes, prevention, and treatment of motion sickness. Such work is of the utmost importance if we bear in mind that more than twenty-five million people travel by plane every year, and that plans for interplanetary navigation are taking more concrete shape all the time.

The philosophic concept of motion sickness can be summed up by saying that this condition is caused by changes in the spatial stability of the environment in which the human being lives. Man is bound to the earth by a number of factors. He is born on the earth; he lives from the earth; and to the earth he returns upon death. Psychoanalysis—especially the Jungian school—has shown how deeply the archetype of Mother Earth is imbedded in man's unconscious mind. It is of little consequence that the new physics and modern astronomy have taught man that the earth is not his true cosmic center. Psychologically, the earth has been man's focus from the time he first appeared on it, and the emotional realization that the earth is the center, axis, and basis of his existence is more important to man than the intellectual concept that the earth is not the center of the universe. The earth is as much a symbol of stability to the human being as his knowing where he is at each moment. Maps break down his location on the planet: the country, the city, where in the city. This visual and intellectual recognition of his geographical placement tells man *where* he is. And to know *where* one is is, to a certain degree, to know *why* one is there. To know one's location on earth at all times is an indispensable requisite for peace of mind.

Man mentally is everywhere in the universe, but physically he is bound only to one spot on earth at a time. All changes in the relation of man to space affect the very roots of his life. Man has adapted himself to his environment and has arranged his life basing it on distance and space. Ironically, technology has abolished distances and thrown man into the vertiginous whirlpool of an age in which, in order to conquer space, he has destroyed his own philosophic and physical stability. Motion sickness is a penalty for man's spatial restlessness.

The sensation of man's position on earth is physiologically located in three sensory organs: the vestibular apparatus, the sight organs, and the proprioceptive system. Orientation, coordination, and regulation of all these organs are indispensable in the maintenance of equilibrium. As De Wit has stated,[2] the sense of equilibrium is connected with the inertial system of the earth. The principal function of the vestibular apparatus is to register at all times the position of the body on the earth. Equilibrium in the human being is maintained by collaboration between the vestibular organ, the proprioceptive system, and the muscular system.

Any number of examples would bear out these basic principles. A person without labyrinths would drown if thrown into water. Skaters gliding through a thick mist on a frozen lake would trace circles indefinitely if they lost their spatial orientation. A dove without labyrinths cannot fly; and if its eyes are bandaged, it will return to earth.

Motion sickness occurs when there are disturbances of the vestibular function along with kinesthetic and psychologic alterations. Irritation of the vestibular apparatus produces nausea and vomiting, and destruction of this apparatus causes total immunity against swing sickness. Such disorders are also caused by disturbances in visual orientation, for instance, when the horizon seems to move as a result of the movements of a plane or a ship. The common denominator of all motion sickness is the exposure of the human being to angular, linear, or radial accelerations.

According to Christopher Shaw, the dynamic cause of motion sickness is the same on earth as on water or in the air, it being the sum of linear accelerations and decelerations according to longitudinal, lateral, and vertical axes and around them, especially so-called linear accelerations of pitch, roll, and heave and, to a lesser extent, of yaw, surge, and sway.

Apparently, all the higher species of animals suffer from nausea under the same conditions that produce nausea in human beings, as De Wit has observed in monkeys, dogs, seals, and parrots. On the other hand, persons with altered vestibular function brought about, for example, by an extended streptomycin treatment, with the consequent auditive nerve lesions, are immune to motion sickness.

The initial psychologic symptom of motion sickness is disorientation about one's spatial position on earth. Optical illusions, such as the feeling that things around are moving or that the horizon is shifting, contribute to an increase of motion sickness. Psychologic disorientation creates a state of psychic discomfort followed by a sensation of uncertainty. The proprioceptive system then sends an avalanche of abnormal alarm stimuli to the brain to warn it that the body is occupying an abnormal position in space. These alarm stimuli—flash signals warning us of impending danger—cause a dis-inhibition of the mesencephalic center and bring about symptoms of alarm, thereby aggravating motion sickness. Then when we become conscious of sick people around us, the exogenous psychic factor—psychologic contamination—may intervene. The victim of motion sickness, threatened by the disturbances of his equilibrium, becomes aware of a cosmic threat to the stability of his ego. This important aspect of the motion sickness threat, which reaches into the depths of one's psychologic structure, is one of the philosophic roots of motion sickness still to be explored.

The therapeutic and prophylactic revolution in motion sickness began with one of those "lucky" accidents so frequent in medical history. In 1947 Gay and Carliner used dimenhydrinate at the Johns Hopkins Hospital to treat a female patient suffering from hives, and accidentally cured her of automobile and trolley car sickness, which had plagued her all her life. Every time the patient took dimenhydrinate for her hives, she could travel by automobile or trolley without difficulty. Later, on November 27, 1948, on board the thirteen-thousand-ton ship "General Ballou," sailing from New York to Bremerhaven with thirteen hundred soldiers, "Operation Nausea" took place. Dimenhydrinate was then successfully used during a violent storm, the test being made with controls. Since then this drug has become part of the therapeutic arsenal against seasickness, to which have been added several other drugs. Anti-motion-sickness agents, such as meclizine hydrochloride, are successfully used today against pernicious vomiting during pregnancy (the "disease" that killed Charlotte Brontë!),[3] as well as against vomiting caused by radiation therapy, Menière's syndrome, fenestration, and cerebral arteriosclerosis.

The history of motion sickness is as ancient as man, for it was born with him and has always followed him, first in his horizontal wanderings on earth, and later in his vertical ascent through endless space. Yet until quite recently no work had been done on it. But a new horizon in physiology, pharmacology, and prophylaxis is open to research workers. The symbolic centaur, Chiron, still gallops through the plains of medical history. And only the future years shall tell what new and promising therapeutic results research workers will derive from their present investigation of *nausea maris*. Their success will enable man, already master of the seas, to proceed with the conquest of outer space.

THE SEARCH FOR THE NATURE OF DISEASE

*t*he noblest preoccupation of the physician throughout history has been to establish a unified concept of the nature of disease. From Hippocrates to Sydenham, the task of the physician was to *describe* what he observed in his daily practice. *Experimentation,* that supreme instrument of the clinical research worker, began very late in history. It started with Roger Bacon in thirteenth century England, was later introduced by Galileo into the field of natural sciences, and ultimately was raised to a philosophic category by Francis Bacon. Ever since then visual observation in the Goethean sense has been closely linked to that sovereign questioning of nature that is experimentation. Man has been pressing nature to answer basic questions concerning its most secret biopathologic motives.

Pre-Hippocratic medical thought was motivated by a terror of the unknown. The nature of disease was thought to be demoniac by the Chaldeo-Assyrian civilizations. Hippocrates introduced the first naturalistic concept of disease by analyzing each patient as a natural phenomenon subject to the laws of space and time that govern all life. His humoral theory of disease had been preceded by Empedocles' concept of disease as an imbalance among the four basic elements (fire, air, water, and earth) of life and was followed by the theory of Asclepiades of Prusa, who considered disease as a disturbance in the mechanics of our atoms.

Two centuries after Christ, Galen made of the *pneuma* the essential principle that maintained organic equilibrium. Later, in the Renais-

From *International Record of Medicine* 167:179, 1954.

sance, Paracelsus considered man a microcosm, a constellation subject to the influence of cosmic forces. Vesalius and Harvey were the heralds of a new anatomy and pathology based on genuine observation and experimentation. The avalanche of theories and systems that marked the seventeenth century—Galileo in physics, Van Helmont in chemistry, and Descartes and Bacon in philosophy—was followed by a revival of the Hippocratic spirit with Sydenham, who established the first natural history of diseases considered as natural processes. From then on there have been numerous attempts to unify the theories about the nature of disease. Stahl re-created animism; Boerhaave started true clinical observation; Morgagni emphasized postmortem anatomy; Haller described the sensibility and irritability of nerve structures; Bichat made organic lesions the basis of pathology; Laënnec created organopathology; Virchow established local organic lesions as the cause of disease; Claude Bernard created physiopathology; and, under the aegis of Corvisart and Auenbrugger, clinical pathology was born.

Toward the end of the nineteenth century, Pasteur and Koch contributed their concept of bacteriologic causality and Kretschmer his constitutionalist theory. We must also remember Bergmann's functional pathology, Brown-Séquard's hormonal pathology, Fredrick Kraus's neurovegetative pathology, Speransky's theory of neurodystrophy, Siebeck and von Weizsäcker's biographico-personal pathology, and the modern psychosomatic and anthropologic concepts of disease.

The physician of today, heir to a rich historical tradition, regards the problem of disease not so much as a study of syndromes and lesions but as an etiologic question. He is interested not so much in the pathogenesis of a disease as in its etiology, which is the principal basis of a truly scientific therapy. Disease has become a historical problem integrating time and environmental circumstances, and an anthropologic question involving a philosophicoscientific concept of human life. The sovereign individuality of that pathographic story we call "clinical history" merges today with the universality of scientific knowledge, of which the clinical history is the true basis.

Today we know that disease does not exist outside the patient but is located *within* the patient, who is influenced by the confluence of his genetic constellation, his environment, and the interrelationship—whether voluntary (free will) or accidental (ecologic influences)—between his being and its environment. Every disease is an evolutive process, a way of life, not a parasitic life grafted upon normal existence. Gregorio Marañón has said: "The brief paragraph devoted to the study of the *course* of diseases in the treatises contains for the most part the key to the concept of those diseases."

The greatest ambition of the modern clinician is to unify his ideas within a concept that will embrace all the etiopathogenic essences of disease considered as a form of life, as the way a being reacts to the *endogenous* influences (the cenesthesic reflections of his own body) and the *exogenous* influences (the pathogenetic interrelationships between the precipitating situation of the surrounding world and the individual organism) that act on him. The human being appears to the physician of our day as an entity situated in time and space—between *nature,* which is his own organism plus the reality of the outside world, and *history,* which is the chronologic evolution of his individual life and his historical reality.

Through his senses—the windows through which the outside world penetrates and acts on him—each being screens a fragment of the world from the cosmos. From the moment of birth, each being creates for himself a world of his own in which he lives; from the sum of the stimuli he receives, he forms his environment. In this sense, health and disease are modalities of the same physiologic functions. All disease involves a vital teleologic impulse toward cure. That is why modern biology, starting with von Uexküll, tends to reject the Darwinian concepts and creates not mere biologic mechanics but authentic biology. Modern biology tends to study not so much *organized* life, the use of organs, which is secondary life, as *organizing* life, which is basic primary life. Modern biology does not study the struggle for life, which is such an important factor in Darwinism; instead, it investigates those main factors of life which are the "strugglers" themselves. It studies that original *unorganized* life that creates organization. The human being thus becomes a system involving a series of reactional possibilities and capable of responding adequately to a series of *new* situations and variable—internal or external—tensions.

The philosophic objective of the modern physician is to learn how to read the secret of the nature and history of disease in the patient. He must therefore avail himself of a concept of the nature of disease. Half a century ago the Spanish pathologist León Corral said that disease is *"an abnormal way of life* in which the organism reacts against some harm." For, paradoxically, the essence of physiology is really pathology, just as the most typical features of our face are those that can be exaggerated in caricature.

And in answer to this deep-rooted desire of the medical research worker throughout history to integrate his knowledge within the framework of a philosophic doctrine, Hans Selye, creator of the theories of *stress* and the *general adaptation syndrome,* which have so radically changed the picture of endocrinology, has outlined a theory to unify medicine. This theory in a way binds together all the doctrines and concepts cited in this introduction, theories that represent the effort of human thought to arrive at an understanding of the nature, causes, and course of disease as the best way of knowing how to cure it. We reserve evaluation of this theory for another article. Here we only wish to set the theory within the framework of earlier medical philosophies.

There are still people who look upon theories with a contempt born of the excess pragmatism so prevalent in modern medicine. But we must respect theories, for they have provided the bases for the most important practical discoveries. Leonardo da Vinci understood that when he said: *"La teoria è il capitano, la prattica sono i soldati."* (Theory is the captain; practice, the soldiers.) In the case of Hans Selye, however, both the concept of *stress* and his theory unifying medicine represent a harmonious flight of philosophic thought made on the reliable wings of experimental research and clinical observation.

A FOOTNOTE TO MEDICAL HISTORY

DISEASE AND HISTORY

One of the most important and least known facets of disease, philosophically considered as a nosologic entity, is the role it plays in heralding historic situations. Because of its impact on man as a living being and on society as a community of men, disease can change the face of history. Malaria contributed to the disintegration of the Roman Empire, and the bubonic plague dug the grave in which the Middle Ages were buried. Sometimes, however, instead of changing a historic situation, disease announces its coming. Syphilis, then a "new" disease, announced the imminent arrival of the Renaissance, while psychoneurosis, raised almost to a poetic level by Freud, was a sort of medical prelude to our century. Stress, a concept first formulated by Hans Selye in 1936, is perhaps the most typical exponent not only of new directions in medicine, but of the gravest social and psychologic problems of our civilization.

Human beings can no more invent disease than disease alone can create history, even though it may change it. Very often diseases incarnate historical crises. The medieval plague marked a crisis in public health or hygiene, which had been raised to a high level by the Greeks and Romans but had decayed with the advent of Christian philosophy. Syphilis foreshadowed the Renaissance crisis, a crisis motivated by other factors—the discovery of gunpowder, the crossing of the Atlantic, the end of feudalism, the return to classic philosophies —but which was translated into a "new" disease that was to obsess

---

From *International Record of Medicine 168*:288, 1955.

man until Ehrlich's day. Neuroses, as Freud explained them to a timorous society embarrassed by an excess of taboos, revealed the crisis that existed between the individual's innermost life governed by the pleasure principle and his outer life governed by the moral conventions of society.

When Selye formulated his stress theory, he crystallized a new historical current and anticipated the newest tendencies in medicine which were just then being adumbrated.

THE "DEFENSIVE" STAGE OF ENDOCRINOLOGY

Modern endocrinology is scarcely sixty years old, if we establish its birth on the day G. R. Murray treated a cretin with thyroid extract. For the first ten years, the new science was inspired by the concept that the endocrine glands possessed a predominantly *antitoxic* function and that their secretions neutralized circulating blood poisons.

The next ten years saw the birth and progress of the idea that the function of the endocrine glands was *metabolic*, an idea that still prevails in medicine today, for we have proved that the endocrine glands govern the finest and most subtle enzymatic processes on which the functioning of the entire organism depends.

Less than twenty years ago Selye formulated the idea of the *defensive* function of the endocrine glands. That function was not defensive in any specific sense against given poisons, as it was believed in the antitoxic stage, but rather *defensive* in a generic way against all infections, intoxications, tensions, shock, excesses of all kinds, and stress, which both body and mind may suffer.

The stress theory propounded by Selye, who in spite of being essentially a research man has always had a subtle clinical insight, is a revolutionary reaction against the etiologic tyranny of specificity, which dictated over medicine ever since the beginning of the great bacteriologic discoveries at the end of the last century. Contrary to the etiologic concepts that from Pasteur's time on directed the course of diagnostic and therapeutic studies in medicine, Selye's work, with clear perspective, has restored the importance of the terrain as against the germ, of the body as against its toxic or microbial aggressors. Thus the current "new" ideas of organic functional unity and psychosomatic medicine have been harmoniously integrated into the concept of stress, which so typically represents the historicultural spirit of medicine in our times.

THREE BASIC PRINCIPLES OF THE STRESS CONCEPT

Hans Selye's article, "Stress and Disease," ratifies the growing conviction that the concept of stress has introduced into modern medicine several principles of enormous practical value:

First, that the *whole* organism, especially the neuroendocrine, humoral, and enzymic systems of functional correlation, responds to the most heterogeneous and least specific aggressions. This concept has been important in pointing out new directions for the treatment of the *entire* patient, integrating, for example, antibiotics with vitamins in the treatment of infections, thus combining in one single medication highly specific therapies with therapies that represent the acme of therapeutic unspecificity.

Second, that the general adaptation syndrome reveals more and more in the clinic how disproportionate the organic reaction is with regard to the stimulus or aggression. The organism responds to nonspecific or specific aggressions with an excess of circulating corticoid hormones and vascular reactions, excesses that may lead a patient of "slight endocrine reserve" to adrenocortical exhaustion. The alarm signal of the pituitary-adrenal axis (why doesn't Selye add the thyroid to his "stress axis"?) excites an emergency—and excessive—response of the organism to the danger that threatens it at the moment of stress.

And finally, that in all organic reactions, specific and nonspecific, to aggression, the organism responds in such a way as to denote a return to a *less differentiated biologic phase*. Our physiology and psychology are organized to respond to "normal" situations, but in an emergency, the civilized physiopsychologic rigging collapses and we return—even biologically—to a "prehistoric" epoch of undifferentiation; in other words, when there is danger, the glands, the organs, the different organic systems, return to a phase of undifferentiation or at least of less differentiation. Under these conditions, the organism responds with excessive inflammatory (in the *local* reaction to stress), humoral, and psychic reactions to the stress situation that threatens its organofunctional unity.

The human being possesses several "defense planes," the most superficial being Cannon's classic sympathicoadrenal "emergency system," and the deepest Selye's diencephalic-pituitary-adrenal axis. On these "planes," a delicate chain of endocrine correlations enables the organism to defend itself against the stress that threatens the constancy of the "inner milieu," described by Claude Bernard, and the continuity of human life. Paradoxically, although the human being can live without his "system of acute alarm" and yet face emergency situations, he cannot survive without his "system of chronic alarm," which responds to that "chronic situation of alarm" that is human life itself.

STRESS AND MODERN MEDICINE

Selye did not usher in what some call the "Adrenal Age" of medicine; but when he focused universal attention on stress as the bio-pathologic crossroads of modern medicine, he contributed to the harmonious integration of psychiatry, neurology, endocrinology, and nutrition, the normal and the abnormal, in a syndrome that is of enormous importance not only clinically as a research tool, but from the historicocultural point of view.

It is understandable, then, that stress has become one of the main fields of study in modern medicine in our Atomic Age, which, with its tremendous international tensions, its constant threats of nuclear holocausts, and its apocalyptic visions of a future of destruction, has replaced the peaceful "Aspirin Age," as Ortega y Gasset called the last century, when people assuaged their small ailments with mild drugs bearing musical names.

A historic situation frequently crystallizes into a discovery. This is what happened with chloroform, which ushered in the era of anesthesia; carbolic acid, which ushered in the antiseptic era; the smallpox vaccine, which initiated modern immunology; and penicillin, which started the antibiotic era. The response is to a pressing medical need, and clinical interest in a problem that suddenly becomes very important to society announces the fact that such a problem contains one of the keys to the philosophic currents prevalent at that particular moment of history.

The universal interest centered on the concept of stress nowadays is the harbinger of what the next objective of medicine will be: concentration on disease coming from *within* (psychotic, metabolic, and degenerative diseases) as progress is made in eradicating diseases coming from *without* (infections, shock, and exogenous intoxications). The human being today is preoccupied with stress because stress is the biopsychopathologic subsoil of his organism, as well as of society and of the present historical moment.

We might use von Weizsäcker's classification and say that, as we have overcome *bioses* or the reversible modifications of cellular structures caused by infections, toxins, or shock and manifested in the entire human body, there has been an increase of *neuroses,* or diseases caused by pure functional alteration of the rhythm and proportion of the biologic phenomena of absorption, secretion, and chemism, and of *scleroses,* or irreversible structural modifications located in only one part of the body. From the chronologic point of view, *scleroses* represent what is historicobiographic and permanent in disease as against what is temporary in *bioses,* and as against what is achronologic, or not situated in time, in *neuroses.* The stress theory is a common denominator for the three aforementioned disease categories of von Weizsäcker.

The stress concept is revised and brought up to date every year, thanks to the zeal and application of its originator. Hans Selye does not allow his theory to petrify in time and to become—as has happened with so many other theories—a fossil of thought; he keeps it alive, growing, changing like a living being, reappearing with new colors and additions every season.

"Death goes wherever the body goes," says an old Spanish proverb. Stress goes everywhere hand in hand with the healthy or diseased human body and represents as important a perspective to the clinician, who is interested in the human body and tries to ascertain the reason for its reactions so that he may complete and correct them, as to the medical philosopher, who is interested in diseases as exponents of the historicocultural climate of each period.

The stress theory represents furthermore a sober therapeutic lesson. The body in its "autopharmacological efforts"—to use Selye's expression—is excessively generous in its reactions and may injure itself in its adaptation efforts. The best physician is the one who in his therapy soberly supplements these efforts of the organism and *nothing more*. He applies to therapeutics the classic advice on what every knight should do with his sword: "Never unsheathe it without reason, and never put it back without honor."

*W*e have now come to the end of the journey through time and space on which this First International Symposium on Health and Travel set out. The philosophic principle that guides medicine as applied to travel is that the constancy of the inner milieu of the traveler must be maintained, a principle already conceived in the nineteenth century by Claude Bernard.

Two main techniques are used today to translate this principle into reality: first, to protect the traveler by means of drugs and physical agents against the dangers originating *within* his person, such as motion sensitivity, stress, psychosomatic reactions, and the aggravation of already existing organic diseases. Second, to protect the traveler against the dangers originating *without* his person by helping him take with him as much as possible of his habitual environment, as if he were a Robinson Crusoe carrying with him his own private little island. Among these external measures are pressurized cabins with uniform temperatures, mechanical devices to reduce excessive motion in ships and planes, special diets, and the administration of antibiotics for protection against or to fight infection.

The main problems studied in this symposium can be grouped into the following five categories.

THE PROBLEM OF MOTION SENSITIVITY

The moment that man moves in any kind of vehicle—car, train, ship, or plane—he is exposed to motion sensitivity, which may affect

From *International Record of Medicine 168*:583, 1955.

even the most experienced sailor or the most daring air pilot, regardless of his physical strength or moral fortitude.

Motion sensitivity is probably the greatest menace to the health, comfort, and pleasure of the traveler; it may disturb him both physically and mentally, making his trip one of agony instead of pleasure.

Motion sensitivity develops with such common early symptoms as general apathy, disinterest in the environment, pallor, respiratory anguish, mental depression, cold sweat, chills, headache, subnormal pulse and temperature, hypersalivation, and, when motion sensitivity finally becomes motion sickness, nausea and vomiting. The chain reaction of physiologic events that leads to motion sensitivity is set off by the motion of the traveling vehicle; it includes labyrinthic, extra-labyrinthic, and psychogenic factors as well as pure hypersensitivity or idiosyncrasy, which in some individuals becomes a true allergy to motion. Motion sensitivity can be successfully prevented or treated with the new anti–motion-sickness drugs, such as meclizine and similar compounds.

THE PROBLEM OF STRESS

Stress, that physiopathologic taxation of civilization, is one of the main etiologic factors of disease in the traveler. The usual causes of stress are nonspecific factors such as excessive fatigue, mental exhaustion, overexposure to sun, air, water, heat, cold, and motion, as well as an excess of visual impressions. We may also add the mental tension created by the necessity to cope with new horizons, faces, and foods and strange languages, all of which are encountered on every journey no matter how pleasant it may be. Furthermore, there is also a biologico-philosophic factor of the utmost importance in the cause of stress in travel—*change*.

Man lives consciously through his brain and emotionally through his hypothalamus, and he establishes liaison with the outer world through his endocrine system. Between stress-causing factors and man's organism, which may react to stress with a series of psychosomatic and even organic conditions, stands only the defensive curtain of his adrenal cortex. All that protects the human being against the nonspecific aggression of stress is a tiny gland, the adrenal. In the strength of the adrenal cortex lies the key to the successful resistance of the traveler to the burdens of stress.

Human tissues are vulnerable to the menace of the stimuli unleashed by any change of environment. Although not specifically noxious, these stimuli however can, by merely altering the normal interrelationship between the human being and his environment, threaten the constancy of the inner milieu. Whether the traveler returns to his original environment in good health depends on the capacity of the adrenal cortex to adapt to the continuous *changes* entailed in a journey.

To fight stress, aeromedicine, naval medicine, and the technical industries connected with travel have created artificial environments that mimic all the conditions of the traveler's familiar environment. They protect him against sudden external changes by making available to him vehicles with uniform temperatures, adequate lighting, proper atmospheric pressures, noise-reducing devices, and choice of proper diet. Adequate mental and psychosomatic hygiene will further help the traveler to bear these external circumstances and avoid the increase of stress, that unavoidable price we pay for being human.

THE PROBLEM OF INFECTION

Throughout history infection has been the greatest threat to the traveler. Today it is perhaps the easiest one to fight. In the past the fight against infection was *passive,* being limited to isolation of the sick traveler by the classical quarantine in order to protect the other travelers. Today the fight against infection is *active.* Infection is considered the result of the interaction of two factors: the etiologic infectious agent and the human organism host to the infection. To fight the etiologic agent we now use antibiotics, especially the broad-spectrum antibiotics, either as prophylactic or therapeutic agents. We also use new pesticides and disinfectants to make habitable and safe huge areas of the earth that centuries ago were colossal caldrons in which malaria, cholera, and other dreaded germ broths brewed perennially. The fight against epizootics has contributed to this global hygienization, although there is still much to be done to render all human dwellings on this planet healthy. To strengthen the traveler's organic defenses, other biologic immunizations—vaccines, toxoids, and serums—are enforced. Hygienic measures are also taken, and special regimens with vitamin supplementation are used to reinforce his organic strength. But, above all, it is through the therapeutic use of the antibiotics that we can today prevent infections among travelers, restore the sick traveler's health, and protect his traveling companions from the risk of contagion.

THE PROBLEM OF NUTRITION

Food is one of the most important indexes of the culture and economic progress of a nation. Adequate nutrition, provided nowadays in planes, ships, trains, and hotels the world over, protects the traveler against diseases caused by toxic food in former times.

If we eat to live and not live to eat, then we must learn what to eat so that we may travel like air pilots and not like Brillat-Savarin, who traveled only to eat.

Disease, nutritional or otherwise, develops at different levels, of which the one most recently studied is the tissue level, to which may soon be added a subtissue level comprising the physiochemical and bioelectric changes in cell activity. The best way to enable the tissues to resist trauma, infection, or stress is to nourish them adequately. The healthy nutritional diets available today while traveling permit the traveler to face the stress of travel with a good probability of overcoming it.

THE GEOGRAPHIC PROBLEM OF DISEASE

The ever-growing knowledge of the geography of disease—the geography of infections, nutritional deficiencies, parasitic infestation —is priceless in planning the fight against disease and in safeguarding the traveler.

If disease is caused by maladaptation of the traveler to his environment and the inadequate response of his living tissues to environmental stimuli, the only way to make our planet safe and comfortable is to know thoroughly the geography of diseases in order to protect ourselves against them. Protection against disease, then, is conditioned by transporting *together with the traveler* the basic factors— food, clothes, artificial climate—of his familiar environment and by the use of antibiotics, anti-motion-sickness and other drugs which help him fight from *within* his body, from the tissue level, the specific menace—trauma, microbes, toxic agents—or the nonspecific menace—stress—originating in the new environment to which his travels take him. The new global philosophy in the fight against disease, by extending to the entire planet those prophylactic and curative measures and drugs which in the past were limited to the great capitals only, must inevitably change the geography of disease into the geography of health. We should then be able to use this geography of health as a blueprint of happiness that shows us how to make the best use of health factors—sunshine, fresh air, pure water, wholesome food—wherever available in our travels around the world.

L'ENVOI

When, according to Greek mythology, beautiful, inquisitive Pandora opened the box given her by Jupiter and let fly all the miseries and evils that afflicted man, only Hope was left. On this planet of ours, where land and sea have already been conquered, Hope is represented by Medicine, which will make possible space travel—man's new goal—and the conquest of health and peace on the shoreless ocean of Time.

IV. on medical communication

ON A NEW CONCEPT OF MEDICAL JOURNALISM

B efore the first truly scientific journals were born, medical progress was communicated orally. The physician discussed his work verbally with his colleagues and his disciples. Only upon his death did he bequeath to future generations the harvest of his knowledge and experience collected in monumental works, which, like the *Canon* or the *De Re Medica,* became fossils of thought with medical ideas petrified within their covers and blindly repeated from generation to generation, thus standing in the way of scientific progress. The creation of scientific academies represented a considerable advance in the dissemination of medical knowledge. But there remained the overwhelming difficulty of circulating the papers submitted to them beyond these restricted circles. When the manuscripts finally found their way into printed form, the original interest had already abated, and they were ultimately relegated to the dusty shelves of some medical library, where they slept for many a year until such time as they were awakened by the hand of a restless reader.

Our age has witnessed the launching of thousands of medical journals that are intended to be vehicles for the prompt and wide diffusion of medical thought. Just the same, *communication* is still one of the greatest problems in the medical world.

Despite the great number of medical journals in existence today, there are not yet enough of them to guarantee prompt publication of the incessant flow of papers pouring daily from clinics and labora-

---

From *International Record of Medicine* 167:243, 1954.

tories. This situation makes it difficult for the physician to impart promptly to a medical audience the findings he has made in the calm of his laboratory or the hustle-bustle of his hospital. Also, the justified reluctance felt by research workers to make public anything that is not aged by time delays not only the diffusion of their work but their research itself. If reliable findings were made public in advance reports, instead of being withheld until the entire project has not only been completed but has multiple corroborating reports, then investigators doing parallel research and many a patient would benefit. Finally, the physician today, overwhelmed by daily tasks, finds it impossible to carry out that vain dream of "keeping abreast" of all phases of medicine.

The confluence of these factors makes the communication of medical progress a vital problem still far from solution.

Because we believe that the studies on the clinical use of xanthine derivatives, which are reported in this issue of the *International Record of Medicine*, are of general interest, we are making this journal available for this new type of medical reporting. The findings of authoritative investigators must, of course, pass the tests of time and general clinical verification. We would welcome comments from our readers on this project of devoting a symposium to a new therapeutic agent as soon as sufficient clinical reports by competent investigators become available.

The success of our past symposia on Atomic Medicine, Endocrinology and Psychiatry, Premenstrual Tension, Cardiovascular Diseases, Blood Diseases in Children, and Chemotherapy, among others, has encouraged us to tread this new path, which combines medical journalism and advance clinical investigation.

It is not enough that laboratories are constantly launching new drugs; it is also necessary that we know how to use these drugs so that optimum clinical effect with maximum safety is obtained. For such a purpose, it is indispensable to conduct controlled experiments in both the laboratory and the clinic. Some of the papers published in this issue represent a branch of research of great interest to the medical practitioner, which we could call *clinical pharmacology,* that is, the therapeutic testing of new drugs on patients to enable the physician to establish the exact nosology and define clearly the therapeutic spectrum of such drugs.

In publishing this symposium, we are attempting to advance a new philosophy of medical journalism. Instead of waiting years for a complete authoritative monographic article or for the appearance of many papers at varying times in different journals, we shall from time to time publish a symposium of advance papers, each one of which will be a spotlight trained on a particular fragment of an important medical topic. The articles will combine to form the same vast mural of pathology that otherwise would have been denied us until the scattered results of research had been laboriously collated.

These advance reports of the progress of a research project will not only help other investigators interested in the same problem, but, because of their concision, will also be of help to the overworked physician who cannot keep abreast of medical progress. In the daily experiments he makes at his patients' bedsides, he can promptly put to practical test the latest developments in the field of therapeutics.

This symposium again confirms that modern medicine is trying to understand clinical phenomena from a physiologic point of view. Someone may point out that these observations are based on the treatment of pathology. But there is nothing more physiologic than the correction of medical pathology. Medical pathology is not something foreign tacked on to physiology; pathology is the reverse side of the physiologic tapestry. Those pathologic accidents called diseases are only accelerated phases of the most physiologic process of life, which is the relentless progress toward death.

These articles also reconfirm the belief that scientific language must be simple, clear, and euphonic if it is to be easily understood— an ideal achieved by Vergil when he described the diseases of cows and pigs with the precision of a scientist and the sensibility of a poet. These papers are also brief, for as Baltasar Gracián, Jesuit philosopher of seventeenth century Spain, said, "A good thing, when brief, is twice as good."

WORDS AND RESEARCH

or the fifth time in as many years, physicians, investigators, and clinicians of many nationalities are gathered here to cement further the bonds of friendship, to assess the year's harvest in antibiotics, and to gaze at the new day rising above the historical horizon.

MAN AND HIS PROBLEMS

The object of this Symposium is easy to define. Like that other famous symposium recorded by Plato and presided over by the physician Eryximachus amidst the quiet silver-green shades of the Greek countryside, we have gathered here to discuss problems of mutual interest. That we *have* problems indicates that, more than scientists, we are human beings, for only man has problems. It is the very fact of his problems, wherefrom spring all his misery and all his greatness, that makes man human.

The dictionary defines the word "problem" as a "question proposed for solution." Etymologically the word derives from the Greek *pro* and *vallo,* meaning something thrown before our eyes. Any difficulty one may encounter—physical, economic, intellectual, or, as in our case, scientific—is therefore a problem.[1]

Our problem is to develop fresh weapons for combating diseases in general and infectious diseases in particular. This is a scientific problem. We must also forge these weapons into instruments that will

---

An address presented at the Fifth Annual Symposium on Antibiotics, Washington, D. C., October 2, 1957; published in *Antibiotic Medicine and Clinical Therapy* 4:740, 1957.

help us understand the natural history of a disease and the biological cycle of its causal germs. This is a historical problem, for it affects the knowledge and advances of our time.

To each one of us individually, scientific research involves at least one of the two afore-mentioned problems. Were this not so we would not be here at this meeting. Whatever our particular interest may be— clinical, experimental, biochemical, industrial, agricultural, veterinarian, or, as in my case, historical—research to all of us philosophically represents something vital. This is so much so that we have traveled here only to tell one another what we have thought and done and what we contemplate doing further in the antibiotic field. Reporting our thoughts and our past or future work is, in short, the intrinsic purpose of this Symposium.

WORDS AND MEDICINE

Were we to ask a historian living at the turn of our present millennium exactly what did, say, eight hundred people, which is our number here today, do year after year at symposiums, I am sure he would answer, "Talk." But to talk is to use words to communicate. Nothing, then, is more fitting than to spend a few minutes together speaking about words as a means of communication.

Words, whether spoken or written, are the most powerful means of communication between human beings. From the time when the last Neolithic men developed a speech system until the invention several centuries later of tablet writing in Assyria and papyrus writing in Egypt, speech was the sole means of communicating and transmitting knowledge. Until the printing press was invented in the fifteenth century, the spoken word was the paramount vehicle for medical instruction, and ours indeed was the most *vocal* of all professions. Then, when human knowledge began to be transmitted in print, there came a reversion of medical pathology to its original *visual* form.

Nowadays the written word, after a transient period of domination over the spoken word, has to wage incessant battle against our modern radio, television, and electronic methods of transmitting voices and sounds, which now seem to be the predominant and most powerful means of communication between men. For all that, the written word may yet come out the winner. In the antibiotic field, the volume of scientific information published in the last fifteen years is far greater than that in any other field of contemporary medicine.

WORDS AND TECHNOLOGY

Some of you may possibly be asking yourselves why we are devoting so much attention to words in a Symposium whose foremost objective is medical technology—that is, the practical application of scientific knowledge to the solution of problems of direct practical importance. The answer is that words form the most important facet of human personality and particularly of the scientist's personality, for science is based on the transmission and assimilation of knowledge.

Anatomists and philosophers have not, even yet, agreed on a definition of what Man is. However, we do know—as Singer[2] has pointed out—that all men possess one characteristic in common that distinguishes them from all other creatures—man makes things. But then, so do certain animals. Man fashions tools and instruments out of various objects, but so do a few animals. But only man can make tools with which to make still other tools! The most characteristic and constructive—and sometimes the most destructive—of all the instruments fashioned by man are *words*.

Animals use actions and sounds as *signals;* only man learned to use them as *symbols*. This was the simplest form of technological advance. Man became proficient as a toolmaker and tool-user simply because he was a *maker* and *user* of words. Only after making considerable progress in constructing language, that is, in the technology of creating symbols, did he acquire the ability to improve his tools. Ever since then, for half a million years now, man has been making words and tools.*

WORDS AND MEDICAL PATHOLOGY

I am a physician and a historian speaking to persons with a vested interest in the diseased. Hence, I am in a position to maintain that medical progress throughout the ages has always been founded upon fresh methods of "looking at" the morbid reality that is the patient. Hippocrates looked at the patient as a sufferer; Galen viewed him as a function not only of his humors but also of his diseased organs, much as we ourselves do these days; Morgagni related the patient's symptoms to determinate internal organs, which in turn inspired Laënnec's work; Addison with his investigations of the suprarenal

---

* It took man hundreds of thousands of years before he ceased to rely on his hands alone in collecting food, and became a hunter and fisherman with arrowheads and spears made of flint and stone, bone and wood. Two facts in this pageant of history are worthy of note: first, that for a million years mankind made little or no progress in using his hands, then reached the highest skill in the days of ancient Egypt and Babylon; and second, that technological proficiency in the Far East was always far ahead of anything in Western Europe. While Greek thinkers were weaving philosophies more tenuous than the finest gossamer, the Chinese had already invented gunpowder, block printing, projectiles, ceramics, cosmetics and plastic surgery, anesthesia, and even the pocket handkerchief, while Plato and Aristotle were still wiping their honorable and learned noses on the inside of their togas.

cortex showed that endocrine lesions were possibly the core of certain diseases; Claude Bernard—that mighty figure who was not a physiologist but Physiology itself in human form—taught us to think physiologically, to base our opinions not only on experimental data and statistics but also on the normalities and abnormalities of the body processes; Virchow brought this notion down to the level of the cell; Pasteur initiated the "tyranny" of the microbe, which was to last so many years; and Ehrlich and Fleming contributed not only fresh forms of therapy but also fresh approaches to the problem of disease, fresh vantage points from which to track down the sources of disease. But all these men, with the exception of Galen, had one factor in common: They were able *lucidly* and *accurately* to report their observations of the sick human being.

An example of how lucidity in reporting may affect the results thereof is provided by the interesting fact, revealed by Arthur Jores, Professor of Medical Pathology at Hamburg, and commented on by Rof Carballo,[3] that of the two thousand human diseases recorded in textbooks the etiology of not more than eight hundred is known. Of many of the rest—asthma, gastric ulcer, hypertension, for instance—we know in detail many of their pathogenic peculiarities, but we know little about their true etiology.

These diseases, whose pathogenesis is known and whose etiology remains unknown, are diseases specific to mankind; they are not observed in identical fashion among animals. On the other hand, those diseases against which we have efficient etiological countermeasures are the ones man has in common with the higher mammals. Present-day pathology is "prosthetic," not etiological, for it only makes temporary prosthetic replacements; it is etiological only in so far as it relates to the pathology of the higher mammals.*

Progress has been greater in those fields—such as the naturalistic description of human and mammal pathology—in which reporting has been clearer and more precise and hence less theoretic or interpretative.

Infectious diseases are an excellent example of how accuracy and excellence of description, from Hippocrates to our own days, can smooth the path of research. On the other hand, in schizophrenia, atherosclerosis, asthma, and cancer, multiplicity of interpretation and semantic confusion have greatly hindered diagnosis and therapy. The better we learn how to describe the etiology, symptoms, and course of a disease, the easier it will be to hit upon the proper treatment.

---

* Thomas Sydenham already stated that acute diseases were *biological* or *animal* (or, as we say today, epidemiological) and that chronic diseases were *biographical* or *human* (or, in our language, psychosomatic or degenerative).

Clear, detailed, and prompt reporting is therefore an active, vital part of the solution to medical problems.

WORDS, SEARCH, AND RESEARCH

Two prior steps are involved before an investigator undertakes the task of making a report in actual words. In the first place, he must have *thought* about a particular problem, that is, it must have preoccupied him; second, he must have *done* something about it, that is, he must have occupied himself in investigating that problem. Only after such meditative and cognitive acts will he perform the conative act of communicating his thoughts and experiments in the form of a scientific paper.

Inquiring thought, probably the oldest thinking in medicine, began when man began to explore the world and discovered how to use fire, metals, the ax, wheel, and lever, and how to make pottery. During succeeding ages it bloomed into the analytical thinking of the Greek philosophers and the introduction of the first experiments capable of reproduction. In this path of progress, alongside the work of the Italian scientific academies and the Invisible College in London, which replaced the medieval universities, men like Galileo, Harvey, Newton, and Haller stand out brilliantly. Their curiosity and self-abnegation gave new life to the noble Aristotelian tradition of wanting to know the reason for things and to understand Nature scientifically.

In every investigation the *search* for elementary data, often of a morphological character, preceded the search for the dynamic interrelationships among objects, i.e., *research* properly so-called. The flame has always preceded the light. So also the thirst for learning is born with human life. Aren't children always asking the how, what, and why of things? The eyes of the researcher light up with the same curiosity as a child's eyes, which look at everything in astonishment and wonder.

The scientific investigator who, as Cicero counseled, "strives to render himself strange to the familiar," converts such curiosity into a guide in his work. In finding his way through the jungle of fact, the investigator must be guided by his imagination as a navigator is guided by the distant stars. Imagination can be a torch to illuminate his path, but he must always be ready to recognize that, as Huxley said, "the tragedy of all inquiry is that a beautiful hypothesis may be slain by an ugly fact." He must realize that not every experiment ends in achievement, and he must appreciate the value of negative data. If, besides, he admits that his research is founded upon the work of his predecessors and feels himself at one with them in time and space, his investigation will then become the mission, direction, and glory of his life.

The inquiring mind has altered little in its basic directives throughout human history. Hildebrand[4] brilliantly describes how Merezhkovski wrote in *The Romance of Leonardo da Vinci* of a "duel of learning" that took place in the court of Duke Ludovico il Moro in Milan in the year 1498. There were gathered "sundry doctors, deans, and magisters of the University of Pavia, in quadrangular red caps, in scarlet silk capes, lined with ermine, in gloves of violet chamois, with gold-embroidered pouches at their belts. The ladies of the court were in gorgeous ball apparel.

"Soon the Countess Cecilia proposed to the Duke that he ask Leonardo to take part in the tourney. His topic was sea shells.

"His exposition was received with hostility. An old doctor of scholastics maintained that 'the disputation was being carried on improperly,' because 'either the problem . . . belonged to the lower, "mechanical" knowledge, foreign to metaphysics, in which case there was nothing to be said of it, inasmuch as they had not convened here to contend over subjects not related to philosophy, or else the problem was related to the true, higher knowledge—to dialectics; in such case, it must even be discussed in accordance with the laws of dialectics, raising the subjects to pure mental contemplation.'

" 'There is no higher or lower knowledge,' Leonardo replied, 'but one only, flowing out of experimentation. . . . For, in considering subjects not open to proof, men cannot come to any agreement. Where there are no sensible deductions, their place is taken by shouts. But he that knoweth hath no need of shouting.' "

Upon this, bedlam broke loose, but Leonardo was silent. "He perceived his isolation among these people, . . . saw the uncrossable abyss that separated them from him."

But that thought of Leonardo's still inspires science and the methodology of research today.*

INDUSTRY AND RESEARCH

Research methodology has been put to its best use by industry, which these days is giving tremendous aid to the researcher, particularly in the antibiotic field. Research itself has become an industry

---

* This methodology might be summarized in four stages: (1) fortuitous or deliberate observation of an incident; (2) immediate provisional hypothesis; (3) search for significant data to confirm or refute the original hypothesis; (4) new hypothesis, tested by observation and experimentation.

Such methodology is founded on the force of ideas, since, as Claude Bernard taught, "the idea is the seed, the method the soil in which it flourishes. Since only what is sown will grow, nothing will develop by the experimental method except *the ideas* submitted to it."

in its own right, for by creating new products and opening up fresh markets it has added a dynamic strength to world economy. Industries no longer compete in markets but in the creation of new necessities, so as to determine what discoveries need to be made and then make them. Industry has found that it is possible to harness science and invention with production, to systematize the search for knowledge, and, by having huge research teams working simultaneously on the same project, to achieve in a few months what otherwise would take years or even decades.

ART, MEDICINE, AND SCIENCES

Equally important in understanding the language of science are the interrelationships between art, medicine, and other sciences.

In what we today call "modern" art, despite the fact that Gauguin, van Gogh, and Cezanne all painted their pictures before the turn of the century, the influence of scientific progress has been enormous—as Melicow[5] has pointed out—not because the artists themselves were well versed in science, but because the cultural atmosphere of their day was so permeated with it that it could not but influence their minds and, consequently, their work. Thus, the discovery of the refraction of white light through a prism into the colors of the spectrum had its artistic reflex in Seurat's *pointillisme,* the splitting of light into an infinite number of separate, luminous dots of color on canvas; the new notions on physics and on form and light illuminated *impressionism,* or rendering with the brush subjective impressions of outer reality, as in the paintings of Manet, Monet, and Pissarro; the explorations into the unconscious were related to *expressionism,* or the projection of the painter's mind and feelings onto his work, as in the case of van Gogh; fragmentation of the human frame and penetration into its inmost tissues and recesses consequent to the discovery of roentgen rays and the progress of radiology influenced the original *cubism* of Braque and Picasso; atom-splitting physics with its threat of universal disintegration was reflected in the works of abstract painters and in Dali's atomic fragmentation; the modern concept of the unity of time and space forming a single space-time continuum is evident in Picasso's later work, which depicts one and the same person, both full-face and profile, at various stages on the same canvas, together with views of his body seen from different angles, thus introducing a new *time* dimension into painting—a hitherto purely *spatial* art. Lastly, the advances since Freud in psychiatry and psychology illuminated Kandinsky's *non-objective* art and the *surrealism* of Miró, Tanguy, Klee, and de Chirico.

In present-day scientific research, such integration of thought has ousted the fragmentation of scientific findings. Thus, the electrical industry has provided us with new chemical substances; modern mathematics has aided neurologists in charting of brain maps; the hydraulic pumps of the automobile industry have been modified and used in hospitals to pump liquefied foods into the stomachs of patients just operated upon, thereby sometimes eliminating the need for intravenous feeding; and another improvement in the same industry, a sensitive apparatus for testing car parts, has been employed in the development of an electronic stethoscope.

THE DUTY OF BEING LUCID

The harvest of the investigation that constitutes the second step in research is finally put into words. These words must be transparently clear. Lucidity of expression is synonymous with quality of thought. The more of a naturalist a scientist is, that is, the more he observes natural phenomena and the less he theorizes, the clearer his thinking becomes.

The lack of progress in psychiatry during the past 50 years, barring Freud's contributions to medical anthropology, may well be attributed to the fact that, although psychiatry deals with the obstacles that reduce man's ability to communicate with his fellow men, it has failed to express itself clearly. For half a century psychiatry has employed a strange language ever more and more confusing and obscure. Fortunately, it is now pulling itself out of this mire, thanks to the success of physiodynamic and organicist psychiatry, which speaks the plain, clear language of biology. Thanks to this, numerous successes have been achieved during the last five years in the psychochemotherapeutic field, and many more will no doubt follow these, until one day the sphinx of mental disease will finally surrender its secret.

This goal demands that psychiatrists cease to be mystics and theoreticians and become biologists and physicians in their explorations into the tenebrous world of mental disease.

THE WORD, CREATOR OF KNOWLEDGE

Antibiotic medicine, on the other hand, has progressed considerably in a few years because it has used a clear, definite, biological language. In chemistry, biochemistry, pharmacology, and clinical medicine, only one vocabulary is possible, that of biological science. In biology each term has a unique meaning. Lack of lucidity occurs mostly when we formulate new concepts. Now, without new concepts to integrate the results of research, no progress can be made. Hence it is indispensable that the scientist convey his thoughts with lucidity, clothing them as tights clothe the circus acrobat, without hiding their form.

It is also essential for the researcher to learn that, whatever his field, he must complement the study of things in *space* (which is the function of *science*) with the study of events in *time* (which is the mission of *history*) and with the study of the basic concepts of life in its biologic, social, universal, and human aspects (which is *philosophy*).

A lucid philosophy of science has led to our present advances. That is why the fabric of the scientist's words, if these are to become his basic instrument in expressing his thoughts, must be woven from his combined knowledge of science, history, and philosophy. That does not mean that he must become a bookworm and forsake his scientific chores for the theoretical study of these other subjects. It does mean, however, that at all times he ought to know how to keep a total perspective, seeing things, as Spinoza said, *sub specie aeternitatis* (in view of eternity) and *sub specie totius* (in view of totality).*

To live perceptively in this manner—as an investigator, as a man with a sense of history, who bears in mind that our present work is the result of the heritage handed us by our forebears and itself the heritage of the future, and as a philosopher at heart who loves wisdom although he never attains it, just as sailors never reach the stars they follow on their path across the ocean—to live thus is to be a complete man. He who is able to do this will always speak with the clear, simple, friendly tongue of the biologist and the naturalist.

THE WORD, CREATOR OF HUMANITY

Words, however, have another mission besides imparting knowledge —a most important mission in a symposium such as this, where old friends meet year after year and where they become acquainted with new friends as well. That mission is for us to approach each other and, by talking among ourselves, to turn our cosmic loneliness into companionship. It is, perhaps, the noblest work that words can do— to act as carriers of sincere friendship among men. For the simple act of two people meeting and stirring the air with the sound of words of greeting establishes the human basis of history with all its glory and grandeur.

---

* The investigator must do that with the same *tenacity, humility,* and *passion* that Pavlov recommended as the three greatest attributes of the inquiring mind. He must not seek to possess the truth but to become a philosopher in the true original meaning of the word, namely, a "lover of wisdom," a lover fated—as in Keats' "Ode on a Grecian Urn"—never to possess but always to desire and adore, for it is far more rewarding to wish than to possess.

V. the mirror of psychiatry

THE HISTORICAL AND PHILOSOPHIC
BACKGROUND OF PSYCHOBIOLOGY

THE HORIZON OF PSYCHOBIOLOGY IN 1956

*W*hat three great contributions can psychobiology make in our time? First, the philosophic integration of psyche and soma not only in psychosomatic medicine but also in clinical psychiatry, and in both cases in etiologic research and diagnosis. Second, inclusion in the clinical history of the element of time, the *biographic* component, basic in anamnesis and of vital importance in prognosis. Third, the introduction of biochemical and chemotherapeutic agents in solving etiologic, diagnostic, and therapeutic problems in psychiatry.

Psychobiology, as a new trend in psychiatric investigation and as a happy union of three factors in psychiatry—biographic, biologic, and pharmacologic—has challenged the philosophic dictatorship that existed in psychiatry and is investing it with the full dignity and stature of a science.

Psychobiology has also made it possible for psychiatric congresses such as this one to be more purely scientific, practical, and universal than ever before, for it has opened their doors to an enthusiastic and energetic legion of physiologists, chemists, biologists, physicists,

A paper presented at the Round Table Dinner Meeting of *Journal of Clinical and Experimental Psychopathology and Quarterly Review of Psychiatry and Neurology,* American Psychiatric Association, Chicago, Ill., May, 1956; published in *Journal of Clinical and Experimental Psychopathology and Quarterly Review of Psychiatry and Neurology 17*:360, 1956.

and even mathematicians, who can bring enlightenment to psychiatry with their wisdom.

Above all, psychobiology has accomplished an important scientific vindication. It has made it possible for the psychiatrists of state mental hospitals—those forgotten back-bench workers, in fact, the infantry of psychiatry, whose clinical material, the "small change" of psychiatry, has enormous practical and statistical value—to retrieve the place of honor they so richly deserve.

Psychobiology, furthermore, has made it possible for etiology to add to its psychiatric roots metabolic, endocrine, and biologic roots, just as it has made it possible to add the biographic and anthropologic aspects to the nosologic phases of the clinical study of a disease.

All this has made psychiatric diagnosis wider and deeper, although in becoming multidimensional it has also become more ambiguous, since we still lack objective criteria to evaluate its components. Prognosis has also gained a social and chronologic dimension, although it still is not given the importance it deserves, probably because of its uncertainty.

Finally, therapy is also moving toward new methods that, although slower, are more lasting than the shock therapies to which the patient's physical integrity is still subjected in the haste to cure, a haste that has made both the patient and the psychiatrist stop trying to help nature effect a spontaneous recovery. This haste also explains why we are no longer interested in the metaphysical problems of death that so fascinated psychiatrists in the past century. If today we lack time for living, how can we possibly find time for worrying about death and the hereafter?

Psychobiology has also opened new biologic roads for psychiatric research into the organic changes in schizophrenia: the effects of mescaline and LSD in normal subjects and in mental patients in order to produce "pocket-size" psychosis; the decomposition products of epinephrine in the organism of the schizophrenic; hormonal balance; the alteration of the tricarboxylic cycle in cerebral metabolism; adrenal changes; brain lipoproteins; cerebral circulation and oxygen consumption; and the nervous tissue and its possible hormones. These "classic" brain hormones—the "nervous juice" that already intrigued Spanish physicians, such as Sabuco, in the Spain of Don Quixote—are perhaps the secret of the activity of the pituitary-hypothalamus-adrenal block, that *terra incognita* where the mystery of psychoses may be hidden.

THE SEARCH FOR MENTAL PEACE

What underlies the obsession of twentieth-century man to know and to cure mental disease? Down through history each century has had a basic preoccupation that served as a guide to man's activities in that period. In the sixteenth century, man searched for the ideal form in art, just as in the seventeenth century he searched for a philosophy in science. In our century, man searches for mental health and peace of mind.

Half a century ago, the great philosopher Ortega y Gasset, one of the most luminous minds of our time, called ours the "Aspirin Age" because, instead of looking actively for happiness, modern man was satisfied with the modest happiness afforded by a handful of drugs with melancholy names. Ataraxia, peace of mind, has become an obsession with modern man, whose mind is unceasingly being shaken as never before in history by wars, revolutions, and the juggernauts of technical progress.

We have succeeded in reducing the incidence of *accidental* diseases of *external* origin (traumas, infections, intoxications), but, on the other hand, we have witnessed the increase of *personal* diseases of *internal* origin, such as mental, sclerotic, and degenerative diseases. Faced with this new powerful menace, we looked for quick solutions. It therefore became more important to cure than to *know*, which would be acceptable if we could cure without knowing. We accepted therapies of a highly aggressive and even brutal nature, but we neglected the search for the root of things. We created a quick but not a *deep* science.

Fortunately, the pendulum is swinging back again. The necessity to cure led to the yearning to know; this in turn led back to the desire to cure but in a more rational way, for, in science, as in life, the shortest way may be that pointed out by the poet who said that the shortest way between two points is the one that crosses the path of the stars.

THE PHILOSOPHIC ROOTS OF PSYCHOBIOLOGY

What are the philosophic roots of current psychobiologic trends in psychiatry? The history of psychiatry may be summed up by saying that it was five thousand years of demonology and one thousand years of painful groping in the dark for a scientific principle. For over one thousand years it accepted the Hippocratic endeavor to establish a physical cause for mental disease, mania, and melancholia as effects, and the elimination of *materia peccans* as its therapy.

In that historic cycle the therapy and management of mental patients proceeded from the phase of *isolation* of the patient to an *institutional* phase, to the *management* phase induced by Pinel, to the *seismotherapeutic* phase of *shock therapies,* and finally to the phase of the *physiodynamic therapies.*

During the historicophilosophic evolution of psychiatry, the three great goals were: elimination of the symptoms—hallucinations, agitation, and negativism—that made the mental patient "different" from other patients and made his therapy and management difficult; establishment of communication with the patient, isolated as if on a deserted island by the invisible walls of his disease; organization and management of the patient on the same basis as any other disease, that is to say, maintaining the patient's contact with the outer world and hospitalizing him only during the phase of acute paroxysm or extreme chronicity of his disease. To these therapeutic and management objectives has been added the desire *to know,* not by waving subtle philosophic patterns but by ventilating psychiatry with the clean fresh breeze of a biologic criterion and new technical resources.

As a result of Virchow's theories, up to the end of the past century when scientific psychiatry really began, the microbe reigned as supreme dictator in medicine. Then suddenly something of tremendous historic importance happened: the biologic essence of the patient's life was rediscovered. From a mere thing, the patient became a living *being.* The organic totality and the neurophysiologic and humoral unity of the living body were also rediscovered. In a way, it was a renaissance of the old constitutional pathology—the classic *idiosynkrasia* and *temperies*—and the symptom began to be considered as a response to a biologic situation created in the organism by the disease.

Totality, constitution, and responsiveness became the three new points of view of the psychiatrist, together with the principle that the patient's personality is situated in a certain *environment* at a certain moment of time; that is to say, that man is a *social* person but he is also a *historical* person. The psychiatrist, and later the physician, was suddenly faced with a new unknown land to explore: the *total person* of the patient.

From the old Galenic concept of disease as a passive affliction, the psychiatrist passed to the Sydenhamian concept of disease as an active effect of nature intended to cure man. Disease became then an abnormal and painful way of life, but still *a way of life.*

THE GIANTS OF PSYCHOBIOLOGY

Cajal, Pavlov, Sherrington, Kraepelin, Bleuler, Freud, and Meyer —these men laid the foundations of the psychobiologic revolution in the concept not only of mental disease but of disease in general. By a striking coincidence, they were all born within a period of seventeen years (1849–1866), the most outstanding in the history of psychiatry for the number of geniuses it produced. In this same period Adler, Jung, and others were also born.

Cajal established the anatomic basis and Pavlov the physiologic basis of psychiatry; Sherrington introduced the concept of integration, supplementing the classic concept of evolution and dissolution of J. Hughlings Jackson; and, later, Freud introduced the concept of regression, and Bleuler, autism and introversion. All of these concepts were of the greatest neuropsychiatric importance. Kraepelin converted into a cosmos the nosologic chaos of psychiatry. Under his commanding voice, psychiatric symptoms and syndromes aligned themselves like well-disciplined soldiers into his rigid imperial Prussian army of nosologic entities. Thanks to Kraepelin, systematization in psychiatric methodology and nosology was achieved.

FREUD AND ANAMNESIS

Chronologically, Freud was a contemporary of Kraepelin. Conceptually, Freud belonged to a new generation that was not to be satisfied with merely classifying mental diseases as the entomologist pins down butterflies in his specimen box.

Freud's centennial is now being commemorated not only by psychiatrists but also by other men of science the world over, for Freudian psychoanalysts do not have a monopoly on the man who today would probably be less "Freudian" than they are.

Freud converted pathography into biography, incorporated the disease of man into medical pathology, and considered the sick man as a *man,* thus starting the trend in psychiatry toward a biologic anthropology.

In the line of mankind that goes from the ameba to God, the mission of genius is to unveil a new fragment of the universe and to formulate objective truths. Freud created a psychologic image of man, and as a result man's image will never again be what it was before Freud, just as the images of the universe and the living being will never again be what they were before Galileo and Darwin.

Freud was above all a biologist, and as such he studied mental diseases using biologic methods. His work culminated in the creation of a biologic psychiatry.

The Freudian concept of anamnesis actually resurrected the ancient Assyrian ritual of studying not only the disease but also the biography of the patient. In contrast to the etiologic and pathophysiologic concept of the neuroses prevalent in his time, the great physician of the Berggasse demonstrated the extreme need for the dialogue with the patient. He thus transformed mental pathology from a visual science, as it was with Charcot, to an auditive science. Charcot *saw* neuroses; Freud *heard* them. Charcot dramatized neuroses; Freud practiced "auscultation" of the patient's monologues with the same loving interest with which Laënnec auscultated the chests of his patients for râles.

Freud was an "auditive" type. Even when he wrote he was actually speaking, and when we read him today we are listening to his voice. For Freud each word was an iridescent bubble charged with intimate meanings, a delicate mold imprisoning an emotion.

It was given to Freud to establish the value of the instinctive component in human life, to demonstrate the different modes of consciousness and the influence of the psyche upon the body, as well as the comprehensive, orderly integration into the biography of the patient of the event of disease. Freud began by studying man from the point of view of the natural sciences and pure biology and finished by having the patient accepted as a person and psychiatry as an anthropologic science.

To explore the dark region of the patient's instincts, Freud used that subtle instrument, the dialogue, a new version of the old anamnesis. The difference was that the traditional anamnesic dialogue was purely descriptive. The patient spoke as a witness or as a spectator of himself and his environment, whereas Freud invited the patient to be an *interpreter* of himself. Afterward he taught psychiatrists to interpret the interpretation.

All this was not completely new. In his *Charmides* Plato mentioned cathartic rituals of a verbal nature. However, since Freud's discovery of the priceless tool of anamnesic dialogue, the psychiatrist has been able to explore the complex etiologic, semiologic, and configurational interrelationship between the body and the mind of the patient, between his intimate nature and his environmental reality.

In spite of all the opposition, Freud illuminated psychiatry with his concepts. As Cajal once said, "Geniuses, like abyssal creatures, move on illuminated by their own inner light."

MEYER AND PSYCHOBIOLOGY

The work of Freud coincided chronologically, although somewhat preceding it, with that of Adolf Meyer, the originator of the term psychobiology, that incandescent word whose glow illuminates this round table.

Although Meyer was Swiss, he was responsible for the definitive split between American and European psychiatry. In spite of his being a foreigner, he was ultimately incorporated into the life of this nation, just as the Greek El Greco was incorporated into the Spain of Philip II.

When Meyer came to this country two principles prevailed in European psychiatry: *nosologism,* which considered mental diseases as mere nosologic entities no different than any other disease; and *somaticism,* which accepted the concept that mental diseases had organic bases, specifically encephalic, according to the dominant thesis of Griesinger.

Meyer rebelled against the patterning of psychiatry after medicine and the idolatrous cult of diagnosis. The fact that Meyer resided in this country saved him from being overwhelmed by the weight of historical tradition. In this country the past does not weigh on the present as heavily as in Europe, which makes it easier to become emancipated from it, since one is not so grateful to it.

Meyer created a psychiatry of common sense which he called *psychobiology* and converted mental disease from an abstract nosologic entity to the flesh and blood reality of the mental patient.

Meyer created a mental pathology based on individualistic principles and resurrected the Hippocratic concept of treating *patients* rather than diseases, thus replacing the nosologic by the personal. Disease for him was a chapter in the biographic-psychobiologic evolution of the individual. By accepting the common root of pathology and physiology in human life, he eliminated the distance then existing between the "normal" man and the mental patient. He rejected the point of view that the brain rather than the personality is more interesting in the mental patient, and he demonstrated that in the normal or in the sick person this personality must be understood in its constant interaction with the environment.

At the time that Freud was invited by Clark University to deliver a series of lectures (1909), Meyer's ideas had already developed in the United States. The Freudian concept of symptom and disease as defensive manifestations of the individual against the pressures of life helped to shape the concepts of Meyer. And when Meyer's wife began to visit patients' homes with the purpose of investigating their sociobiologic environment, there was started what later became the profession of psychiatric social work.

Meyer created new objectives for psychiatry by concentrating not on the disease but on the patient. First he enlisted neurotics, and then normal persons, in the movement of mental hygiene founded by Clifford Beers. By using psychiatry to teach civilized man how to live, he completed the "Americanization" of psychiatry and gave new impetus to the cultural anthropology originated by Freud.

American psychiatry was then transformed not only by the psychiatrists but also by the patients themselves and by public opinion. Meyer converted psychiatry into one of man's basic sciences by stimulating mental hygiene and psychiatric social work and by enlarging the scope of clinical psychology and psychosomatic medicine. He even tried to study the prevention of war by analyzing the psychologic factors responsible for human aggression.

Meyer was fascinated above all by psychoses, as Freud had been by neuroses. His concept of the personality that pantingly hides in the entangled bushes of a psychosis permeates all modern psychopathology, just as his other ideas have replaced Kraepelinian psychiatry.

When Meyer died in 1950, he left a glittering heritage: his concept of the *whole man*. Instead of looking with a magnifying glass at each facet of man, Meyer examined his image as if through a reducing glass, which produces a sharper, clearer image. He attempted to integrate psychology and biology and he studied the behavior of the whole man as a reaction against environmental stresses, representing in his diagrams the chronologic and the clinical history of the patient's disease. If Kraepelin went from general concepts to individual facts, Meyer reversed this process by replacing the nosologic with the personal.

Meyer's main contributions to psychobiology may be summed up thus: (1) the concept of disease as a simple chapter in the biographic integral evolution—psychobiologic—of the individual; (2) the integration of the environment and its influences in the study of mental disease, a concept that inspired present-day psychiatric social work; (3) the extension of the province of psychiatry to a study of the "normal" individual, thus stimulating the movement of mental hygiene; and (4) the study of the total personality of the patient and not merely the nosology of the disease.

PSYCHOSOMATIC ROOTS

Let us now consider another current of thought, that of psychosomatic medicine, a term that up to 1948 was still written in italics, indicating that it was not accepted "officially."

Psychosomatic medicine was the inevitable historical reaction to the situation that prevailed half a century ago, when the ideas of Johannes Müller and Claude Bernard were still dominant. The prevalent concept then was that medical pathology was but changed physiology. This confined psychiatry to the laboratory, or at best to the hospital, and prevented the recognition of the *extrasomatic* components—social, historical, and psychologic—of the individual biography until the advent with Freud of the new anthropologic concept.

The progress of psychosomatic medicine was the result of three main factors: the ever-growing pressure of the clinical problems posed by the increase of neuroses and chronic diseases; the study by Cannon and James of the somatic expression of the emotions; and the advances in the psychology of behavior.

All this made possible the scientific study of emotion and the restoration of its true meaning, which had faded just as the image on a coin finally fades from constant use.

An avalanche of contributions in the field of psychosomatic medicine finally chiseled out of the mountain of psychiatry the new profile of psychobiology. We need only remember the work of Groddeck (1908), considered by some as the father of psychosomatic medicine, the psychogenesis and psychotherapy of organic symptoms formulated by Schwarz in Vienna, the work of Ludwig Krehl in medical anthropology, the studies of Siebeck and von Weizsäcker in Heidelberg creating a biographic medicine—a *graphos* of the human *bios*—and the work of Karl Jaspers differentiating diseases predominantly *biologic* from diseases essentially *biographic*.

After that, psychosomatic medicine flourished in this country, where it represents an important current of contemporary American medical thought—the triumph of the philosophy of psychobiologic unity over Cartesian dichotomy.

HALLUCINOGENIC DRUGS

The newest and most revolutionary method of research and therapy in psychobiology is the use of hallucinogenic compounds.

The use of drugs in psychiatry dates back almost to the dawn of history. Greek physicians used hellebore to treat "lunatics," and the literature of medieval times is prodigal in examples of brews and concoctions that could induce insanity and in some cases "cure" it.

Drugs were used in psychiatry always with the idea of soothing, calming, or drowsing the mental patient by affecting his conscious mind. Ninety-nine years ago bromides were discovered and, later, barbital. In 1934 seismotherapy was introduced with the shock therapies.

None of these agents, however, served to reach the three great goals of psychiatric management already mentioned: to consider the mental patient as a *patient,* to reduce his agitation, and to improve communication between him and the psychiatrist.

In 1943 there occurred one of those happy accidents that have often contributed to the progress of science. Hoffman of Basel, Switzerland, accidentally induced in himself a pocket-size psychosis by swallowing some lysergic acid diethylamide. This was followed by a splendid study by Stoll, demonstrating that this and similar substances afforded psychiatry chemical keys that would open doors and project some light into the dark world of psychoses.

These hallucinogenic drugs, called in the past "phantastica" by the Germans, were used for many centuries by primitive people to provoke religious ecstasies (among them was the cohoba used by the

American Indians in the times of the Spanish *Conquistadores*). They were also amply used in medieval brews. In the second half of the nineteenth century some of these drugs, for instance, hashish, were consumed by the so-called decadent French poets to stimulate mental imagery, such as embellishes the poems of Rimbaud and Baudelaire.

A new way of communicating with the mental patient was through the use of agents like mescaline, bufotenin, and others which act as chemical keys that open and close at will some of the locked doors that lead to the mental imagery and perhaps to the pathogenetic mechanisms of mental disease. The replacement of shock therapies, in some cases by a more humane psychochemotherapy, has started a revolution in the management of the mental patient and in psychiatric research.

RESERPINE AND CHLORPROMAZINE

While this work was in progress, Dr. Rustom Jal Vakil, of King Edward Hospital in Bombay, India, had been, since 1940, using a centuries-old Indian root called *Rauwolfia serpentina,* an *ajurvedic* medication of mythologic lineage. Vakil treated with *Rauwolfia*—today called reserpine—thousands of patients suffering from hypertension and published the results in 1949 in the *British Heart Journal.* This paper eventually reached Dr. Robert A. Wilkin, of the Massachusetts Memorial Hospital, who obtained and used samples of *Rauwolfia,* describing in 1952 its sedative effect at a meeting of the New England Cardiovascular Society.

In 1953 Dr. Raymond Harris, of the Albany Medical College, confirmed the tranquilizing effect of *Rauwolfia* on mental patients, and in 1954 he was followed by Dr. Nathan S. Kline, Director of Research at Rockland State Hospital in New York. The mythical *ajurvedic* drug of the Orient, whose tranquilizing effect was known several centuries ago in India, was at long last confirmed by the modern science of the Occident.

Meantime, in Paris an investigation of antihistamines had been started, with the purpose of finding one that would not produce excessive drowsiness. This research eventually led to the discovery of 4560 R.P. (chlorpromazine) at the Rhône-Poulenc Laboratories. With this compound, Madame Courvoisier in 1951 "cured" the anxiety experimentally produced in rats and Laborit, in 1952, the anxiety suffered by human patients including pregnant women. In the same year, Jean Delay and Pierre Deniker used it successfully in mental patients; in Canada, Lehmann, and, in the United States, Winkelman and others introduced it in different clinical fields of psychiatry.

Thus it became possible to use a group of drugs that since then has increased to more than twenty-five tranquilizing agents now under investigation. Some are endowed with the property of interrupting experimentally induced psychoses and tranquilizing mental patients.

Supporting a suggestion from the professor of classical languages Alister Cameron, Dr. Howard Fabing of Cincinnati gave the name "ataraxics" to these drugs. Under this name is included a variety of drugs pertaining to the groups of indoles, piperidines, and phenothiazines. Their effect is said to produce ataraxia, that is to say, they leave the patient *ataraktos*—without confusion, with peace of mind—this being a beloved word of the classic epicurean philosophers because it represented their most cherished philosophic goal.

A PAUSE BEFORE THE MYSTERY

We still do not know the mode of action of the ataraxics, the most powerful weapon of psychobiology. Maybe they act on the hypothalamus—that tiny islet of nervous tissue, refuge of whatever instincts remain from our hairy prehistoric ancestor who lurked in the dark primeval forests. Maybe the ataraxics act also on the neurovegetative system. They especially seem to act upon the reticular formation of the cerebral cortex, the archaic paleocortical-hypothalamic-mesencephalic system that regulates the primitive urges of hunger and sex and the interrelationship with other living beings; they also act upon the mesocortical-reticular-endothalamic system, which adapts the human being to the temporal-spatial circumstances of the outer world and contains a condensed representation of the peripheral structures.

It is also possible that the ataraxics, to paraphrase Selye's concept, in their action "imitate and if necessary correct and complement the body's own auto-pharmacologic efforts to combat the stress factor in disease."

The possibilities that these compounds offer for research in psychochemotherapy are unlimited. For example, the mental imagery observed in patients treated with these drugs coincides with the imagery in the literature produced by great poets and mystics, such as Baudelaire, Coleridge, Poe, De Quincey, St. Theresa, and St. John of the Cross. Conversely, the artistic productions of persons treated with the hallucinogenic drugs have a striking resemblance to the early works of Picasso, Braque, and some of the surrealist painters. We welcome in this direction the work in progress of

Werner Wolff, who is trying to determine the relationship between drugs and poetry.

Considering the similarity between the mental imagery of geniuses and that of persons under the effects of these drugs, one is bound to think that perhaps the organic production of certain substances—a gigantic chemical mistake of the human body—may in some cases originate schizophrenia. In milder instances, when these substances are produced under the stimulation of fast, self-hypnosis, or toxic drugs, they may determine literary and artistic imagery. Perhaps some day we may discover part of the secret of genius through the study of body chemistry. The horizon is unlimited. This is only the beginning, the dawn of a new day.

THE PHILOSOPHY
OF ORGANICISM IN PSYCHIATRY

THE CONCEPT OF THE MIND IN CLASSICAL GREECE

O*iscipulus est priori posterior dies*—each day is the scholar of yesterday. To understand better the transcendental importance in modern medicine of the new psychiatric somatotherapies, one must study the evolution of the philosophic thought that led from the mystic shadows, which for so many millennia obscured the concept of mental illness, to the radiant dawn of modern psychiatric therapy. Although application of these therapeutic methods began less than a quarter of a century ago, philosophically they represent the crystallization of a thought with a history of more than twenty-six centuries.

Let us, therefore, first of all, outline the evolution of the organicistic concept of the human mind, the historical trajectory of the idea—which today seems elementary, yet for so many centuries was considered revolutionary—that the brain is the core of the mind. Following this, we shall trace the historical roots of the forms of therapy based on the somatic treatment of mental diseases. Historically and philosophically, one concept presupposes the other. For once the brain was recognized as the core of the mind, it became logical to treat mental disturbances by therapies intended to correct alterations in the cerebral tissues.

Some five hundred years before Christ, the figure of Alcmæon of

From *Journal of Clinical and Experimental Psychopathology & Quarterly Review of Psychiatry and Neurology* 15:179, 1954 (with Raymond R. Sackler, Arthur M. Sackler, and Mortimer D. Sackler).

Croton, pupil of Pythagoras, emerged on the horizon of history. His work entitled *Concerning Nature* was the basic textbook on medicine prior to Hippocrates. Alcmæon of Croton declared that the brain, not the heart, was the organ of the mind, and that through it, sensorial impressions reached our consciousness. A physiologist of stature, he carried out experimental studies on the functional alterations caused by brain lesions. But his viewpoint, an isolated beacon in an age clouded by the fog of mysticism, was not shared by his contemporaries or by the majority of the Greek philosophers who followed him. Their favorite pastime was to discuss endlessly the nature and core of the consciousness and the mind, ascribing intelligence, passions, and sensibility to such organs as the heart, liver, and lungs.

The true founder of anatomiconeurologic thought in psychiatry, however, was Hippocrates (c. 460–355 B.C.), who held the view that psychic functions had a cerebral substratum, a concept accepted by Aristotle (384–322 B.C.) and Herophilus and Erasistratus (c. 310–250 B.C.). Hippocratic thought, which was naturalistic in outlook, was based on observation and experimentation at the patient's bedside.[A] It challenged the mysticism of the Asclepiades by insisting that mental disturbances resided in the brain, thus opposing the prevailing belief in demonism with its natural-physical doctrine of psychopathologic alteration.

In *The Sacred Disease,* Hippocrates states: "Men ought to know that from the brain and from the brain only arise our pleasures, joys, laughter, and jests as well as our sorrows, pains, griefs and tears. . . . It is the same thing which makes us mad or delirious, inspires us with dread and fear, whether by night or by day, brings sleeplessness, inopportune mistakes, aimless anxieties, absent-mindedness and acts that are contrary to habit. . . . Madness comes from moistness. When the brain is abnormally moist, of necessity it moves, and when it moves neither sight nor hearing are still but we see or hear now one thing and now another, and the tongue speaks in accordance with what has been seen and heard on any occasion. . . ."

Hippocrates declared that intelligence reached the brain borne by the air that circulated through the veins—for such was the accepted explanation of circulation at that time—and that when the veins were obstructed by cold phlegm, the patient lost consciousness, and an epileptic seizure ensued. In attributing the latter to irritation of the brain by acid or sour substances, Hippocrates established the first indication recorded in history of the localization in the brain of certain pathologic processes of the mind. He also described mania, "phrenitis" melancholia, puerperal psychosis, and hysterical phenomena. To treat mental diseases he used physical and chemical medications, such as rest, baths, a bland diet, purgatives and emetics, and extracts of plants, such as black hellebore and mandrake, for their cardiotonic, narcotic and gastrointestinal effects.

The doctrines of Hippocrates and the earlier ideas of Alcmæon of Croton subsequently influenced Plato (427–347 B.C.), the portentous Athenian who emblazoned the Golden Age of Greece. Plato also believed that the core of intelligence—and of its disturbed form, insanity—was the brain. He attributed epilepsy to the obstruction of circulation of air in the head by a mixture of white phlegm and black bile. Commenting on Aristotle's concept that the sole function of the brain was to cool and purify the air or vapors carried by the blood through the veins to the brain, Plato, in his *Phaedo,* has Socrates say: "It is the brain which creates the sensations of hearing, sight and smell, from which arise, in turn, memory and reasoning; and from these sensations, once they are established, knowledge is born. . . . There is no cure for the body apart from the mind. First, then, and above all, the mind must be treated if the body is ever to be made whole. . . . Just here the mistake is made in regard to man: the attempt to treat the body independently of the mind." In these words Plato condensed the Greek credo that all the illnesses of man were psychosomatic in nature, a thesis which is accepted today by a number of schools of psychiatry.

Asclepiades of Prusa (c. 124 B.C.) classified insanity into acute and chronic; while Aretæus of Cappadocia (c. early second century A.D.) recorded clinical descriptions of cerebral palsy and in his lifetime spread the views of Hippocrates concerning the brain. The elegant Celsus (first century A.D.), the Cicero of medicine and possibly the greatest medical mind in classical Italy, studied hallucinations and deliriums and described the neurovegetative functions in the insane.

FROM GALEN TO STENSEN

This gigantic wave of naturalistic doctrines concerning the brain, the mind, and mental disturbances, was confirmed and supported by Galen (A.D. 138–201), who maintained that the brain was the organ of the mind and of all sensation and movement. This concept of the Roman Dictator of Medicine persisted through the centuries that followed,[B] despite the fact that during this era (with the exception of the concept of cerebral localizations worked out by Constantine the African (1015–1087) and a few sporadic references by Arab authors[C] to the cerebral localization of mental disturbances) organicist thought in psychiatry lapsed into the lethargy of the long medieval night and was lulled by the chants of religious fanaticism and demonism.[D]

Since the Church regarded suspiciously any opinions that did not agree with its notions of witchcraft and demons as the only explanation for mental diseases, physicians had to fumble along as best they could. For many centuries, observation and experiment were replaced by the dogmatic authority of the classic writers. As Sir Thomas Browne was later to say in his *Religio Medici,* authority has always been "a powerful enemy unto knowledge."

In his *De Humani Corporis Fabrica,* prelude to modern science, Vesalius (1514–1564) reaffirmed the possibility of the cerebral localization of mental diseases. A contemporary of Vesalius, Johann Weyer, is considered by some authors as the father of modern psychiatry. In his book entitled *De Proestigis Doemonum,* Weyer assailed the welter of belief in devils and witchcraft that prevailed in his day. Along with his precise clinical descriptions of mental patients, he launched a crusade against the Inquisition for treating the insane as creatures possessed of the devil, thereby introducing humanitarianism in the cure of the mentally sick.[E]

At the time when the Renaissance[F] was radiating its beams of clarity to the farthest reaches of Europe, the French philosopher René Descartes (1596–1650) dedicated his years of voluntary exile in Amsterdam and Sweden (from 1628 until his death) to solving the problems of biology and medicine by mathematical methods supported by anatomical observations. To this very day, medicine is influenced by his philosophic system, which is known as Cartesianism and is directly linked with the ideas of Giordano Bruno (1548–1600). Descartes liked to wander along the sleepy, melancholy streets of old Amsterdam, collecting anatomical specimens from butcher shops, which he would take to his room to dissect. In a treatise on physiology, *De Homine,* forerunner of the philosophies of iatrochemistry and iatrophysics, he localized the soul in the pineal body.

At about this same time, Niels Steno (Stensen) (1638–1686), discoverer of the parotid and lacrimal ducts, in a discourse delivered in 1665 in Paris at the home of Melchisédech Thévenot, patron of the sciences, declared: ". . . Those who seek for solid knowledge will find nothing to satisfy in all that has been written about the Brain, but it is, quite certainly, the principal organ of the soul and the Instrument which works very wonderful effects."

This prevailing ideology subsequently had a brilliant supporter in Georg Stahl (1660–1734), founder of animism and one of the precursors of biological medicine. Stahl distinguished between delirium due to physical causes and that due to emotional causes. He fought to achieve recognition of the integral unity of man as against the concept of dualism between mind and body, which in his day reigned supreme.

Towering astride two centuries, the figure of Giovanni Battista Morgagni (1682–1771), who laid the anatomicopathologic basis of modern medicine, stands forth as a revolutionary in the field of medical concepts. In his magnum opus entitled *De Sedibus et Causis Morborum per Anatomen Indagatis* (1761), a monument of clinico-pathologic descriptions, he enunciated the concept of insanity as an organic disease. He introduced in medicine what Virchow later called "the anatomical concept in the study of disease."

Morgagni's views on anatomy were carried on by the French alienist Joseph Daquin (1733–1815). In his *Philosophie de la Folie* (1791), Daquin recommended humanitarian treatment of the insane. He also warned against the excesses of anatomical interpretation of mental illnesses, which were already beginning to be observed, stating: "A good many of the lesions found in the brains of the insane were, to all appearances and in all probability, not formed until the latter years of [the patient's] life and represent the effects rather than the cause of the disease."

Other authors who supported the anatomical concept of mental disturbances were Sementini (1743–1814) and the humanitarian Vincenzo Chiarugi (1759–1820). The latter wrote *Della pazzia in genere e in specie,* which is devoted to the diagnosis, prognosis, and pathologic anatomy of mental diseases. They were followed by F. J. Gall (1758–1828), whose views on anatomy were to be confirmed a century later by Nissl and Ramón y Cajal.

Although he offered no proof for his statements, C. W. M. Jacobi (1775–1858) was the first German psychiatrist to present systematically in his writings mental disturbances as symptoms of disturbances in the functions of the brain, indicating that mental disease was a misnomer for what should be called brain disease.

The standard-bearer of vitalism, the anatomist J. C. Reil (1759–1813), described the structures of the cerebellum and the insula ("island of Reil"). He recorded a study of a process similar to the present-day concept of a psychoneurosis. During this same period, J. Haslam (1764–1826) described the syphilitic nature of dementia paralytica. Meanwhile, Philippe Pinel (1745–1826), glorious liberator of the mental patient and initiator of a new era in humanitarian assistance, declared in his *Traité Médico-Philosophique sur l'Aliénation Mentale* (1801) that mental diseases were based on pathological alterations of the brain.

THE NINETEENTH CENTURY

In the nineteenth century, psychiatry acquired the category of an autonomous medical discipline. "From Hippocrates to Boerhaave," wrote Heinroth in 1818, "bile was the sole cause, melancholy and mania the sole effect, and elimination of the *materia peccans* the sole remedy in mental disease."

Three German clinicians—Griesinger, Meynert, and Wernicke— started the parade of great scientific figures in the nineteenth century, —a century destined to see psychiatry established on firmer organic foundations. They studied and reported the anatomicopathologic alterations that take place in the brain of mentally sick patients.

Wilhelm Griesinger (1817–1868), author of the first textbook on psychiatry (1845), sought to demonstrate that every psychosis is determined by specific cerebral lesions. Thus, he identified the activity of the psychiatrist with that of the physician treating diseases of the body and advocated common methods of investigation in the natural sciences.*

Theodor Meynert (1833–1892), a pupil of the great pathologist Rokitansky, studied the structures of the brain and the physiopathology of the nervous system in man and animals. He established the functional antagonism existing between the cerebral cortex and the deep cerebral nuclei and emphasized the importance of cerebral circulatory disturbances in the genesis of mental disturbances. He is regarded by some authorities as the forerunner of modern investigators of cerebral cytoarchitecture and also of those who treat mental ailments with agents that modify the circulation and nutrition of the cerebral tissues.

Karl Wernicke (1848–1905) presented "focalist" concepts, many of which he supported with anatomicopathologic evidence, and also published an excellent atlas of the brain.

Around the middle of the nineteenth century, German and French contributions reinforcing the organic concept of psychiatry began to spring up in greater number. Even as its influence was ebbing, the Romantic school of psychiatry in Germany was recreating the medicine of Paracelsus in the works of Neinroth and Gross. Some psychiatrists, such as Morel and Magnan, became partisan to the criteria of genetics and attributed mental disease to heredity in the sense of a degeneration or a polyvalent hereditary disposition, while others, like Krafft-Ebing, saw it as a pure encephalic lesion.

The French psychiatry of the first half of the nineteenth century, as represented by Pinel, Esquirol (1722–1840), Georget and Fodéré, is rather equivalent in its nosology to the anatomical chapters into which works on pathology were divided prior to Sydenham.

In the latter part of the century, Liébeault (1825–1893), Charcot

---

* Griesinger's pupil, Karl Westphal (1833–1890), specialized in the study of histopathologic psychiatry.

(1825–1893), and Bernheim (1840–1919) established the scientific bases of the use of hypnosis in psychiatry and medicine, giving stimulus to a psychologic orientation in psychiatry. Paradoxically, the great neurologists, such as Charcot and Janet (1859–1947), encouraged the development of a psychologic psychiatry! It was in this atmosphere of neuropsychiatrists obsessed by the desire to discover what the *species morbosae* of psychiatry was that the future psychogenic concepts of mental disease first began to germinate.

The historical delimitation of separate clinical entities within psychiatry was firmly underway at the turn of the century. This was necessary for the individualization of psychiatric therapy and for the establishment of therapy on a rational basis of the etiology and pathogenesis of each mental disease. Thus, the separation of dementia paralytica patients from the great mass of hospitalized psychotics was arrived at. Falret and others laid the foundations of clinical diagnostic criteria. It remained for Richard von Krafft-Ebing (1840–1902) to demonstrate the correlation existing between a syphilitic infection previously existent in a patient and subsequent dementia paralytica as established by the patient's immunologic response to inoculation with *Treponema*. Subsequently, Aloys Alzheimer (1864–1915) described the histopathologic alterations in cerebral syphilis, while Emil Kraepelin (1856–1926) established that a previous syphilitic infection is an indispensable condition for the development of dementia paralytica. Treponema was discovered in the brain of paretic patients by Noguchi and Moore. In 1910 Paul Ehrlich introduced salvarsan (arsphenamine) in the treatment of syphilis. Ehrlich's "magic bullet" was followed by malariotherapy, introduced in 1917 by J. Wagner von Jauregg.*

Toward the end of the nineteenth century began the era of almost explosive progress in somatological psychiatry, starting with the monumental work of Emil Kraepelin. After elucidating the historically common elements in groups of psychotic patients, Kraepelin proposed a scientific nosology of the two main psychoses. As early as 1896, he began to develop the organophysiologic concentration in psychiatry, systematizing it as a science. He gave it a pseudoclassical perfection by setting up, together with Kahlbaum, the "descriptive types" which are still basic in our present-day psychiatric classifications. In the later editions of his splendid textbook, Kraepelin, by

---

* In this way, following delineation of etiological and pathogenetic mechanisms, a considerable part of the mentally ill population was afforded relief, later arrest of pathology, and in more recent days specific therapy and control. Of even greater importance, late cerebral manifestations have been practically eliminated by proper prophylaxis and therapy with antibiotics.

integrating the somatologic and psychologic approaches, foreshadowed a metabolic trend, and thereby laid a biologic basis for psychiatry.

As a corollary to this avalanche of somatologic contributions to psychiatry stands the statement made by Professor Benedict before the International Congress of Psychiatry held in Paris in 1899. After the great Korsakow (1854–1900) had finished reading his historic paper on "A Form of Mental Disease Combined with Degenerative Neuritis," Professor Benedict rose to remark: "We thank Dr. Korsakow for his interesting study. He has confirmed to the maximum the theory that all psychopathology can be reduced to lesions of the brain and the nervous tissues."

In 1890 Sigmund Freud (1856–1939) began his monumental contributions to the study of psychiatry. With Freud, psychologic psychiatry gained pre-eminence and made a number of revolutionary contributions to medicine. Among these are:

(1) the description and definition of the unconscious and the important role of such psychic material in motivation of behavior; the formulation of the existence of various levels of psychologic consciousness, namely, unconscious, preconscious, and conscious;

(2) the concept of a "structural" stratification of the psyche with id, ego, and superego;

(3) the psychosexual development through oral, anal, and phallic stages in the achievement of adult genital sexuality as well as the concept of regression to earlier stages;

(4) the use of dialogue and free association—an outgrowth from Freud's work with hypnosis in hysteria—as a therapeutic tool; the relationship of resistance and dreams to this procedure; the role of transference in the psychoanalytic process and its use by the therapist;

(5) the controversial concept of instinctual forces, including the libido, and their psychodynamic significance and therapeutic applicability.

Before Freud, hysteria, in the Charcot manner, was *ex visu;* since Freud, it has developed greater depth: *hysteria ex audita*. Pathology, before Freud, was observed as exclusively visual and tactile. Since Freud, the study of psychopathology gained an *auditive* dimension (symptom complexes are defined *ex audita*). Attention was directed to the zones of being and human life susceptible to verbal audition, comprehension, and interpretation, but not to eidetic intuition. Freud's later years were marked by an orientation—also adopted later by Eugen Bleuler (1857–1939)—toward the integration of the somatologic aspects within psychiatry and an ever more biologic emphasis on psychologic phenomena.

In the history of organicist ideas, psychiatry finds itself, in the twentieth century, beneath the brilliant constellation formed by the work of Freud; the transcendental achievements of Santiago Ramón y Cajal (1852–1934) in the histopathology of the nervous system, which were later to constitute a source of inspiration for the whole newer somatologic approach to psychiatry; the work of I. P. Pavlov (1849–1936) on the physiology and physiopathology of the nervous system, with his studies of higher nervous functions through the use of his method of conditioned reflexes; and the accomplishments of Charles S. Sherrington (1861–1952) demonstrating the complex integration of the nervous centers and their functions. These four names alone constitute one of the most electrifying pages in the history of scientific progress. The genius of these investigators had as its common denominator the acceptance—even by Freud—of the premise that the substratum of nervous diseases not due to structural alteration is a functional disturbance of the nervous tissues invisible to the microscope, but which may be revealed through biochemical analysis.

THE PHILOSOPHIC BASIS OF PHYSIODYNAMIC THERAPY

This concept of mental diseases having a physiopathologic, organic, sometimes histologic and always endocrinologic and biochemical substratum served as a philosophic basis for the development of somatotherapies in psychiatry. In these newer treatments we cannot help but see the immense impact of the latest discoveries in histology, physiopathology, biochemistry, and physics upon psychiatric thinking.

The therapies embrace the modes of treatment that concentrate on the somatic substratum of the phenomenon of consciousness. Though the methods are empirical, they may help uncover physiopathologic data and lead to greater specificity in the treatment of mental disease by physical means as well as biochemotherapeutically. These methods, which today are fundamental, particularly in the treatment of the more malignant disturbances, can be classified into three major groups, viz., physicotherapeutic, biochemotherapeutic, and psychosurgical.

The treatment of insanity by means of agents that profoundly agitate the organism has been used in an infinite variety of empirical forms in all ages. Hippocrates, Galen, and Boerhaave, in fact, mentioned cases of mental illnesses cured as a result of febrile diseases contracted at the same time as the mental process.

We cannot consider the trepanations so profusely recorded in prehistory—like the Peruvian *huacos*—as a forerunner of present-day somatotherapy, except indirectly, for in primitive times disease was regarded not as a natural phenomenon, but as a religious and magical punishment. Trepanation was practiced to relieve those "possessed"—tormented by terrible headaches or by epilepsy—by opening a hole in the skull with a trepan or punch made of bone or sharp stone in order to allow the evil spirits possessing the patient to escape *from his head,* not from his brain, inasmuch as the latter organ was not recognized as the core of consciousness but only of the soul and of the spirits that possessed the soul.

Somatotherapies in psychiatry did not really begin until it was understood that just as disease cannot exist without a patient, so mental disease or the mind cannot exist without a brain. The human mind, in relation to a somatic structure, and its ailments affect the human being in his totality, the whole person, and not just his psyche. It is precisely because the psyche and the soma are simultaneously affected, however, that it was thought that even as physical disturbances could be corrected by treatment of the psyche, so probably could mental disturbances be corrected by the application of certain therapies to the brain and the body in general.

THE HISTORICAL ANTECEDENTS OF SOMATOTHERAPY

The most ancient report in existence of the use of electroshock *before* the discovery of electricity was recounted by none other than the discoverer of electroshock, Ugo Cerletti (b. 1877 in Italy). At the First International Congress of Psychiatry in Paris (1950), Cerletti reported that Scribonius Largus, physician to the Roman Emperor Claudius, wrote in his *Compositiones Medicamentorum* the following: "A chronic and intolerable headache which insistently manifests itself can be eliminated at once if treated by applying a live torpedo fish (electric eel), black in color, to the site of the pain and leaving it there until the pain stops and the part is swollen (*obstupescat*). As soon as this occurs, the remedy should be removed, in order not to abolish sensibility in the region affected. It is necessary to prepare a certain number of these torpedo fish; for the benefit of the cure, or reactivation—which is the index of the utility of the effect obtained—is often only achieved after two or three applications."

The therapeutic nihilism that prevailed in psychiatry until well into the eighteenth century was interrupted only occasionally by some spark of light that anticipated the somatotherapies of the future. In 1804 Joseph Mason Cox, the English physician, in his booklet entitled *Practical Observations on Insanity,* stated: "It is evident that any considerable excitement, some new and violent action provoked in the course of the manic disease, often has the effect of considerably alleviating the mental disorder or of permanently improving it." Cox recommended the inoculation of smallpox or scabies and irritation of the skin with emetic tartar, vesicants, or setons to produce suppuration.

Spasmo spasmus solvitur. . . . This same principle was reflected in the discovery—though not in the development—by G. Burrows of London, of convulsive shock therapy in 1828, more than a century before its rediscovery in our times. In his *Commentaries on the Causes, Forms, Symptoms and Treatment, Moral or Medical, of Insanity,* he notes: "In a case of insanity in which two scruples [of camphorated oil] were applied, a convulsive seizure was produced, and a complete cure followed."

As early as 1845, Griesinger employed ether, chloroform, and opium in the treatment of psychotics. In 1870, Britsch and Hitzig, followed by Batelli, Viale, Chiauzzi, and others, studied the electrical stimulation of the cerebral cortex and the production of convulsive crises in man. A. S. Loevenhart studied the use of carbon dioxide to stimulate cerebral circulation in mental patients in 1918, twenty years before the rediscovery of the same treatment! Leduc, in 1902, succeeded in producing the inhibition of the cerebral hemispheres in mental patients, causing sleep and general anesthesia during the application of electric current to the cranium of his patients. Zimmerman and Dinier, in 1903, applied Leduc's method to produce epileptic coma experimentally by electricity years before the definitive contribution of electroshock therapy by Cerletti.

In its turn, the discovery by Klaesi (b. 1877 in Switzerland) in 1920 of *Dauernarkose,* or therapy by prolonged sleep, with the use of somnifene and dial, was preceded by the use of trional by Wolf in 1901 for the same purpose.

Insulin coma therapy, discovered by Sakel (1900–1957), was historically preceded by G. Klemperer's (1865–1946) discovery that insulin improved the general state of mental patients by producing hypoglycemia, as well as by the doctrines of Pascal and Davesne concerning colloidoclastic shock.

Convulsive shock therapy with cardiazol, discovered by Meduna (b. 1896 in Hungary), had as a precedent, besides the curious experiments of Auenbrugger—mentioned by Meduna himself—the observations in 1929 by Nyro and Jablonski concerning the effectiveness of antiepileptic medication when epilepsy is associated with schizophrenia. G. Mueller reported (1930) two cases of catatonic schizophrenia that were cured upon development of epileptic convulsive crises. Glaidus (1931) cited eight cases of epilepsy associated with schizophrenia in which there was an eruption of the schizophrenic symptoms when the epileptic ones disappeared. Comparable historical precedents could be listed in connection with the use of hormones in psychiatry.

The fact that a tree has deep roots does not detract from the importance of its fruits; if anything, it enhances it. To Cerletti, Klaesi, Meduna, Egas Moniz (b. 1874 in Portugal), and Sakel must go the glory of having introduced in modern psychiatry a series of somatotherapies that today make it possible to treat with greater success the two most important endogenous psychoses, schizophrenia and manic-depressive psychoses, as well as some neuroses.

In 1934 Manfred Sakel of Vienna published his method of treating psychoses by producing a state of coma by means of insulin injections. That same year, Laszlo Joseph Meduna of Budapest reported his method of producing convulsive attacks through the injection of cardiazol. In 1935 Egas Moniz of Lisbon described his first leukotomy (prefrontal lobotomy), thereby introducing surgery into the psychiatric field and creating the new specialization of psychosurgery. And in 1938, Ugo Cerletti and L. Bini of Rome demonstrated their electroshock technique.

Without going into the always delicate matter of historical priorities, the account of how these discoveries were arrived at and their re-evaluation a score of years later, in the light of present-day developments, is of great historical and practical importance. We were privileged to present such an appraisal by the discoverers themselves in the book, *The Great Physiodynamic Therapies in Psychiatry*.

To the achievements described should be added those that have been realized in the field of biochemical and endocrine therapy by Hoskins and several current groups of investigators, who are reviving the naturalist tradition in psychiatry with their attempts to conquer mental diseases with organic methods. These investigators are using clinical and physiologic data as their point of departure, with a view to discovering and developing new physiologic and pharmacologic agents.

Accomplishments in the field of somatotherapy in psychiatry may be likened to a majestic bridge having as its first pillar the historical therapies described; as its central pillar, the convulsive shock therapies and psychosurgery; and as its pillars still in the process of construction, the biochemical therapies (thyroid, testosterone, adrenal hormones, histamine, and acetylcholine) and, most recent of all, pharmacologic therapies (chlorpromazine and *Rauwolfia serpentina*). It is not yet possible to see the completed bridge which will carry us to the shore of the future. But following with a visionary eye the sweeping curve of the unfinished bridge, it is possible to project it toward the future and to see that some day the remaining pillars will be completed. It will then be possible for Psychiatry to cross by the bridge of somatotherapy over the conquered waters of the restless river of mental disease.

NOTES

A. Hippocrates localized the residence of the soul in the brain: *"Cerebrum illo organium est, ex quo insania originem ducit . . . Insanit homo ob humiditatem cerebri, in quo animi sunt officia"* (The brain is the organ where madness is born . . . Man becomes insane due to moistness of the brain, where functions of the soul are located). *"Cerebrum insanimus et deliramus. . . . Insania enim contingit, si cerebrum nimis humidum est."* (The brain makes us become mad and delirious. . . . Madness ensues if the brain is excessively moist).

B. Caelius Aurelianus (203–249) strongly advised against the use of violence, chains, and starvation on the insane, the three universal "remedies" used in his times. His suggestion of using "irritant injections in the ear" as a way to reach the meninges with medications when treating mental patients is most interesting.

C. The psychiatric conceptions of the great Avicenna (980–1037), the Persian "Prince of Physicians," could be summed up as follows: mental disturbances are originated by morbid changes in the proportion and composition of the brain and are divided in alterations of the imagination and memory, and true psychoses (melancholia, mania, imbecility, and dementia). Anomalies of the anterior brain cause alterations in the faculty of perception, anomalies of the midbrain produce imbecility, anomalies of the fourth ventricle and its surroundings cause disturbances of the memory. He recommended cold aspersions, diet, derivatives, and bloodletting as therapy for mania, and derivatives and emetics as therapy for melancholia. Avenzoar (1113–1162) was the first to recommend cauterization of the head as somatotherapy for manic patients.

D. Arnold of Villanova (1235–1311?), the great medieval Spanish physician of kings and popes, established in his incunabulum *Practica Medicinae Arnoldi de Villanova,* the relations between manic and melancholic states and menstrual disorders.

E. According to a great many historians, the first mental hospital created in History, was the Hospital de Nuestra Doña Santa María de los Inocentes or *Casa de Orates* in Valencia, Spain. Established in 1409 as a result of the preachings of Brother Juan Gilaberto Jofré in the time of King Martin I, it was converted into a general hospital in 1484. In this *Casa de Orates* the humanitarian principles of treatment of the insane were applied for the first time, anticipating Pinel by a few hundred years.

F. The Spanish philosopher Juan Luis Vives (1492–1540), teacher at Oxford and Louvain and self-exiled liberal in Bruges, accepted by some authors as the Father of Modern Psychology, represents the liberation of philosophic thought from the dogmatism of authority and the introduction of sound experimental criteria, as in his book the *Anima et Vita,* first of the great biologic psychologies. He also defended the scientific and social functions of psychiatry in his *Tratado del Socorro de los pobres* (1525). Vives, because of his splendid study of the passions, has been considered by many as the precursor of Freud.

THE GREAT
PHYSIODYNAMIC THERAPIES IN PSYCHIATRY

THE EVOLUTION OF THE MANAGEMENT OF MENTAL PATIENTS

In the panorama of man the place of the mentally ill was for centuries determined primarily by the traditional prejudices of society toward the misunderstood sufferings of those it termed "insane." Psychiatric therapy, its history, and its present status also reflect society's attitude toward the psychiatric patient. And now as psychiatry evolves toward a more mature biologic science, it is seen more clearly to follow the historical course of its sister sciences.

In man's earlier days the mentally ill were deemed possessed and, in some later societies, even criminals. The disorder was often held to be either possession by devils or a divine punishment. The predominance of therapeutic nihilism was therefore inevitable. Since there was no recognition of illness, there was no attempt to cure it. Confronted with the incomprehensible behavior of the mentally sick, society reacted by adopting self-protective measures.

The institutional period was the first phase of society's approach to management of the mentally sick. The "insane" member, after an attempt at exorcism or punishment for his "crime" by chastisement, was confined. Unhappily, the vast walled communities and mammoth window-barred buildings of this our "enlightened" age are vestiges

---

Foreword to *The Great Physiodynamic Therapies in Psychiatry* by Arthur M. Sackler, Mortimer D. Sackler, Raymond R. Sackler, and Félix Martí-Ibáñez, with the personal contributions of Ugo Cerletti, Roy G. Hoskins, Laszlo Joseph Meduna, Egas Moniz, and Manfred Sakel, New York, Paul B. Hoeber, Inc., 1956.

of the first phase—the removal of the mentally deranged from the society of their fellow men.

Incipit vita nova. Then, like the dawn of a new era in Dante's poem, came the day when the mentally ill were recognized as sick, and the concept of guilt and of antisocial danger began to be rejected and the stigma of "insanity" to recede. Confinement as a therapeutic measure gained a new aim—to protect the patient from himself, to isolate him from some of the emotional stimuli believed responsible for his disorder and from situations with which he could not cope. The beginnings of modern drug therapy wrought further changes by adding to the primitive physical methods, first, pharmacologically induced isolation by sedation and, later, physiodynamically active modalities—insulin, electroconvulsive therapy, metrazol, hormones, and histamine.

More recently, pharmacotherapy has come to the fore with narcobiotic drugs developed through German and Swiss research in artificial hibernation. In France, Laborit combined the use of refrigeration and drugs and opened the way for clinical attempts to reduce the reaction of the neurovegetative system to the effects of homeostatic-disruptive forces. The internal environment was "chemically isolated" from the external environment and, in fact, from the possible aggression of other endogenous psychogenic or metabolic elements.

Historically, *isolation,* accomplished by sedation through physical means and drugs, was followed by the *seismotherapeutic* stage or treatment by means of shock techniques, firstly empirical *pyretotherapy* by *chemical methods, malariotherapy,* and the use of the various agents that provoke convulsions and coma.

Philosophically, shock therapy can be viewed as an attempt to stimulate active defense of the organism to resist disorganizing forces, while the recent use of ataractic drugs attempts to foster passive "defense through submission."

The seismotherapeutic approach (the shock therapy era that bridged the early and the recent pharmacotherapies) can be viewed as being based on "defense through physiologic reorganization" of the organism's metabolism. Although the physiodynamic techniques evolved empirically, we hold that they are destined to lead us to the fundamental etiology and pathogenesis of mental disorders, to a "new" science of psychiatry based on a metabolic understanding of chemical dysequilibrations.

The physiodynamic therapies, as well as the more recent pharmacotherapies, should in turn lead to studies of neuroendocrine and other metabolic alterations produced by these procedures. We may thus advance from empiric therapeutic benefit to a clearer understanding of the metabolic processes that mediate them and to the ultimate biochemical deviations out of which the disease process arises.

THE SEARCH FOR THE AITIA

Psychiatry in the twentieth century started with Kraepelin's interest in the disease entity—in the psychiatric *nosos*. This was followed by the post-Kraepelinian curiosity as to the *semeios* or symptoms as exemplified by Freud's already classic concepts in the psychodynamics of symptom formation. The current trend of psychiatric investigation is to search for the *aitia*—for out of understanding the cause will come not only more basic psychiatric nosology but the most definitive measures for the control of mental illness.

The search for the *aitia* will be hastened by a physiodynamic philosophy and perspective. Mental disease cannot exist without an organic structure whose function is disrupted, and this dysfunction derives from metabolic alterations (psychogenic or pathophysiologic in origin) which can affect not only structure but also function. The mind itself has no possible existence other than as an *expression* of the activity of the brain. Physiodynamic psychiatry must accept the fact that psychoses and other mental disorders cannot exist except as they are related to metabolic disturbances operating within organic structures regardless of the origin of the disturbing forces.

In this day of psychosis-inducing chemicals and of drugs capable of "curing" such artificially induced syndromes, it is difficult to conceive of the struggle during the past decade, particularly in the United States, to strengthen and forward a biologic orientation. Kraepelin's clinical intuitions and the isolated but lucid comments of Bleuler and Freud on the biologic roots of psychiatry were for decades overwhelmed and submerged by a wave of "scientific" quasi mysticism. This then led to distortion of the originally brilliant concepts of the dynamics of symptom formation into etiologic forces. Talk superseded basic research, and unsupported hypotheses were propounded as dogma. The defects of nineteenth century psychiatry, in which the systematizing philosophy was based on the work of alienists in mental asylums whose observation material was largely restricted to severe psychoses in the later stages, were replaced by the weaknesses of early twentieth century psychiatry. Then, too many ideas were predicated on the subtle theoretical disquisition of psychotherapists whose experience for the most part was limited to non-hospitalized "neurotics."

The somatotherapies brought a healthy naturalistic trend. Studies began to bridge the gap between hospitalized and nonhospitalized patients. Fundamental criteria for diagnosis, therapy, and signs of improvement began to make their appearance. The challenging chasm between the results attained with the somatotherapies and our lack of knowledge as to how these came about led some investigators to intensify biologic research in psychiatry. Weakness was turned into an advantage, just as the carpenter in the old fable converted his proud sword into a useful saw when its edge had become jagged.

Present-day search for the cause of disease or *aitia* will integrate Kraepelin's interest in the idea of the disease or psychiatric *nosos* and post-Kraepelinian curiosity as to the *semeios* or psychiatric symptoms. Such transition from the nosologic criterium to the symptomatologic and, finally, to the etiologic criterion, repeats once more in psychiatry that inevitable historic evolution that has occurred in all branches of scientific medicine.

THE PROBLEM OF HISTORICAL PRIORITIES

It is of significance, of course, to know who is the father of any important discovery, but in the spirit of strict justice it is of equal interest to know who is the mother and who is the obstetrician who assisted in bringing it forth into the world.

It happens with scientific discoveries, as with literary works, that once the umbilical cord joining them with the mind of their creator is cut, they cease to belong to one person, and they take on a life of their own, ready to grow and change. The original and true features can then be appreciated only if we look at their reflection in the mirror of their creator's own mind.

How instructive it would be, for instance, if the great figures of the past in psychiatry could tell us what they think of their own discoveries re-evaluated in the light of our present-day knowledge! What a lesson in humility and tolerance it would be for many "Freudian" dogmatists if Freud himself were to give us a new estimation of his psychoanalytic theories in the light of the new biologic signposts in psychiatry!

Such is the experiment, unprecedented in the annals of the history of medicine, undertaken by the organizers and editors of this Symposium. The great somatotherapies in psychiatry were selected: insulin shock therapy, metrazol shock, electroshock, prolonged sleep therapy,* psychosurgery, and hormonal therapy; and their chief

---

* Unfortunately, ill health prevented Klaesi from submitting his reappraisal of the prolonged sleep therapy, the historical roots of which go back as far as the sixth century when Alexander of Tralles recommended the sleep cure as a remedy against insanity. We have every hope that the absence of so valuable a paper will be remedied in some future edition, since no review of the somatotherapies would be complete without a survey of this important technique, so much in use nowadays in several countries, which is credited with a vast wealth of successful statistics.

protagonists* were asked to tell simply the circumstances leading to discovery or orientation, and to examine the latter in the light of present-day psychiatric knowledge so as to give it a current evaluation.

Each one of the contributors was invited to relate the historical development of the method associated with his work, its evolution, and the opinion that he himself has of it at the present time, some years after its introduction. Their answers will be found in the ensuing pages, in which is assembled a quarter of a century's labor in tracing distinctive features on the vast mural of contemporary psychiatric knowledge.

These reappraisals take us back to the original fountainhead whence these discoveries sprang, for the somatotherapies nowadays are like transparent glass vessels that take on the color of the liquid contained in them. In the hands of certain psychiatrists these techniques were a prelude to psychotherapy; for others they represented the best physical means of breaking down the vicious circle of certain psychoses; while for the remainder they constituted the best clinical means of treating psychoses.

The physiodynamic therapies are now a basic element in the therapeutic arsenal of the psychiatrist. But, though he may be thoroughly acquainted with the correct ways of using such techniques, it is a rare psychiatrist who has had the time and opportunity to study their origin, development, and comparative value, and to integrate them philosophically into the present psychiatric panorama as a whole in order to evaluate correctly their future possibilities in psychiatry.

Only by listening to the words of the original protagonists of these methods can we trace their true historical roots and learn exactly what the original worker was after. To drive home the drama of such a historical lesson, it is necessary to confront the author with his work, the discoverer with his discovery, and thus have an opportunity of evaluating afresh in the light of present-day knowledge what these methods may stand for in the psychiatry of the future.

The men assembled between the covers of this volume do not breathe in an atmosphere of Olympian detachment and infallibility. The reader will observe discrepancies and contradictions here and there among them. We have no qualms in this respect.

The good of humanity has been forwarded by each one of them; a common eagerness for research made them orient their thought navigation into uncharted seas of scientific investigation, and a common success has crowned their endeavors. Each and every one

---

* Ugo Cerletti, Roy G. Hoskins, L. J. Meduna, Egas Moniz, and Manfred Sakel.

of them submits himself to the historical test of confronting his own work in retrospect, which is a prophylaxis against the danger of dogmatism, that ever-present insidious enemy and campfollower of science. If we all learned, as Osler suggested, how to die each night in order to be resurrected the next morning, to make a daily reappraisal of the merits and value of our thoughts and work, modern psychiatry would be liberated from the perilous burden of dogmatism that still clogs its progress.

From the contrast between what the physiodynamic therapies actually are in the crucible of daily psychiatric practice and what they are in the ideal image that exists in the mind of their discoverers, the present symposium derives its striking and tellingly personal values. In addition to enlightenment on the historical facts of the past, it provides a hopeful prospection for the future.

TO KNOW AND TO CURE

It is essential *to know* if we are *to cure*. In the past, empiric therapy predominated over diagnostic classification. Today, we acknowledge that every medical or psychiatric action entails a feat of cognition as well as of conation. Therefore, in the personality of the psychiatrist, clinical intuition must coexist with both naturalism and criticism. These facets must be combined into that "attitude of scientific expectancy" in the presence of facts that Pavlov, the physiologist and one of the great founders of modern psychiatry, with Kraepelin, the nosologist, Cajal, the anatomist, and Freud, the psychodynamicist, professed and demanded.

The psychiatrist, like the general practitioner, must be, first of all, a naturalist capable of observing with the eyes of a true investigator the signs that nature places before him in the form of the suffering of the sick person. He must learn to observe before trying to experiment, for it is in the careful observation of nature and in the correct interpretation of what nature offers that he will find the most fertile source of scientific progress.

The psychiatrist, however, much more than any other physician, must admit the importance of doubt and of constructive criticism as effective tools with which to carve out new concepts in his field and to smooth the rough edges of the structure he seeks to create. He must not accept a semblance of pathologic fact at its face value; he must learn how to penetrate its façade, which may be deceptive; he must reach the true, deep causes of what he observes on the surface.

Since the best way to appreciate a picture properly is to place it in its proper setting, it was deemed helpful to begin this Symposium with an historical introduction relating the evolution of the organicist philosophy that through the somatotherapy techniques culminates in physiodynamic psychiatry, and to end it with a chapter tracing the future course of modern psychiatric trends, integrating these somato-techniques into the endless scientific progress of psychiatry. To reminiscence we have added prospection.

Fame has crowned the writers we have collected here for their effort, their tenacity, and their achievements. As to determining the niceties of historical priorities, that is the mission of the historian, who must not allow an obsession with chronologic sequence to blind him to the fact that in medicine, as in all aspects of life, "no man is an island," and that no discovery exists that is not bound in both time and space to the toils and achievements of many who have gone before, often in other times and other lands.

To the merely chronologic fame of a discoverer must be added the truly historical glory of being the first to gather together in his hands the many threads of medical knowledge with which to weave the unique pattern of his contribution. Such renown is not merely a reinvigoration of the past but a dynamic prelude to the future, and that is what true fame is: A fame whose green laurels are represented by the gratitude of the mentally sick to the men who devote their lives and genius to their treatment. To all such men this volume renders the best possible homage—it is a living pedestal to their collective work.

Claude Bernard once said: *"L'art c'est moi; la science c'est nous."* To that *we,* the stuff of which science is made, this book is respectfully dedicated.

THE QUEST FOR FREUD

ON FREUD'S GREATNESS

One hundred years have gone by, but the quest still continues. The passage of time has intensified the effort to understand fully Freud's influence on many fields of human thought—history, art, pedagogy, and religion, as well as medicine—an influence that has spread like ever widening ripples in a disturbed pool.

A measure of the social importance of any human activity is the number of new words it bequeaths to the common language of all nations. Modern language is studded with scientific neologisms. The medical ones are evidence of the generous contribution made by medicine to popular wisdom and the progress of civilization. Perhaps no other branch of medicine, not even the field of antibiotics, has added to the vocabulary of the writer, sociologist, and common man as much as Freud and psychoanalysis. Not only in literature but also in everyday language a discerning ear can easily detect the familiar ring of psychoanalytic terminology.

Another key to a man's effect on the world about him is the gap separating the literature published in his particular field of action before and after his influence was asserted. The breach between a book on psychiatry written prior to 1900, when Freud announced some of his most important discoveries, and a book on psychiatry

From *Journal of Clinical and Experimental Psychopathology & Quarterly Review of Psychiatry and Neurology* 17:117, 1956 (with Arthur M. Sackler, Mortimer D. Sackler, and Raymond R. Sackler).

today is indeed astounding. The progress in psychiatry in this last half century due to Kraepelin, Cajal, Pavlov, Sherrington, Bleuler, and Freud is so enormous that the gap is wider than that between any two books on psychiatry written in the prior two thousand years.

Today, all over the world, men of culture, as well as men of medicine, are commemorating the centennial of the birth of the man who conjured up a new method of psychologic research, who gave mental hygiene so much of its modern form, and who wielded so great an influence on art, sociology, religion, and anthropology.

An anniversary is often merely an occasion for a man's admirers to flick off the dust that has collected on their hero's bust. With Freud, however, his thought and work are so dynamic and disturbing that his birthday should be a time for reappraisal of his contributions to science. It is also a moment for orthodox psychoanalysts—many of whom are more Freudian than Freud himself—to do more than place another crown of laurel on the pale forehead of the great Viennese thinker. They should join, not fight against, the efforts to integrate his contributions into the whole body of scientific medicine with the objectivity that has brought all science to its present high level.

Was Freud a genius?

Genius is made up of intuition, efficacy, and effort and is the happy compounding of three contingencies: intellectual aptitude, a suitable ground for such aptitude to flourish (for genius can be good only if it finds a favorable environment), and the right historical moment. If these three factors—aptitude, place, and time—do not concur together, genius can wither away unheard, unhonored, and unsung. These three essential factors did coincide in Freud's case.

Freud was a great man, and greatness is often combined with genius. During his lifetime, Freud possessed the insight of the great. His personal conviction was reflected in his reply to Princess Marie Bonaparte when she graciously reminded him that he was a great man: "I am not a great man; I merely made a great discovery."

Despite this apparent modesty, Freud nursed a vision of greatness throughout his life. It is said that the midwife attending his birth foretold his future triumph and that her augury stayed with him and gave him inspiration all the years of his life. His own words after having made his mark indicate the influence he attributed to the opinion of those dear to him: "A man who has been the unquestioned favorite of his mother retains through his whole life the feeling that everything must yield to him, thus engendering that confidence in success which is frequently the determinant of success itself." Freud's career made a reality of the fireside prophecies of his genius. Today there are few who begrudge him the recognition that he coveted so deeply.

Freud always considered himself a child of destiny. The man who "knows" he has a mission in life is filled with a supreme impatience to fulfill it. Freud was anxious to reap his destiny while he was still alive. "I want no posthumous glory," he said on one occasion. That is the why of his creative haste. At the root of his genius also lay the power of his will. His concentration on his desire to create was one of the secrets of his whole existence.

"History," said Emerson, "is the biography of Greatness," because "man just waits, but genius acts." Thus true greatness is man's forestalling of immortality. To be great is to live in perpetual defiance of what is close by and in everlasting search of what is eternal and universal in man.

Looked at in this light, history is not a journey through darkness but an exploration for the torch of creation in the primeval jungle of the human mind. The ordinary man feels himself restricted spatially by his biology and chronologically by the shortness of his life. The genius, however, knows that his dreams are sufficiently powerful to become reality propelled by his creative *élan,* which draws its energy and motive power from that infinite reservoir of the mind that every human being possesses. For, as Cajal remarked, "Geniuses, like abyssal creatures, move on illuminated by their own inner light."

No one can possibly object to the attribution of genius to Einstein. His was the genius that knew how to discover and reveal a new fragment of the universe, how to formulate a lineage of *objective* problems and then point the way to their accurate solution. Such discovery of universal facts and objective truths was the work of a Newton or a Max Planck. But when the creation is the fruit of a *subjective* act, as was the case with Freud, should not the palm of genius be awarded in this instance also?

Perhaps we can get at the answer if we consider the case of Descartes, whose philosophical thinking is still the cornerstone of the modern scientific world. His was an eminently subjective creation, but its fundamental validity was ultimately revealed as a universal objective truth. It may be the same with Freud. We trust that his original ideas were more than a subjective imagining, that they did more than burgeon out of some mystic enlightenment. Were they not the fruit of his naturalistic observation of man as he saw him wending his way along the cold corridors of the Salpêtrière or in his modest office in the Berggasse?

Is great fertility a characteristic of genius? There is one group of geniuses whose immortality rests on more than a single scientific discovery, a single literary masterpiece, or a lone immortal symphony

—Leonardo da Vinci, Goethe, Balzac, and Rembrandt. O. those who are remembered for only one particular discovery, invention, or masterpiece such as Fleming for penicillin, Cervantes for *Don Quixote,* Helmholtz for optics, we soon realize when we examine the setting of their "one" great accomplishment that it was of such outstanding brilliance as to outshine all their other work. Their other discoveries, being less brilliant, are overlooked, despite their value or the continuity and directed effort they gave to a creative life.

Thus Freud's interpretation of dreams should not obscure his other psychologic formulations, just as his concept of psychoanalysis should not blind us to his broader understandings or confine to limbo his labors in the pharmacologic and neurologic fields that filled out the confines of his life.

At the end of the nineteenth century Freud's concepts burst upon a stodgy Victorian world with its cult of individualism and of will power, the "I am the master of my fate; I am the captain of my soul" philosophy of W. E. Henley.

Freud's ideas on the unconscious motivation of our thoughts and deeds excited much irritation in his time—a time when middle-class society lived a commonplace, genteel public life (apparently in harmony with middle-class conventions), with a private life ruled by the principle of pleasure.

Freud set himself up against all that this represented. His interpretation of neuroses was in reality a condemnation of the historical backsliding of middle-class society in Victorian Europe. The general reaction was unanimous, and Freud's doctrines were "officially" proscribed.

Some men attain glory by discovering a single drug. Freud contributed new *principles*. These principles afford us a key to Freud's greatness, to his contribution not only to psychiatry but also to modern medicine in general.

FREUD'S SCIENTIFIC ENVIRONMENT: CHARCOT AND KRAEPELIN

A proper understanding of Freud's work cannot be achieved without knowing the surrounding circumstances in which it was developed.

The latter half of the nineteenth century was of tremendous importance to the whole world of science. The great events—discoveries or confirmations of discoveries—that occurred in that period fill a stirring page in the history of science: the physical theory of the conservation of energy; the theory of evolution; the cell doctrine; the glycogenic function of the liver; the neuronal theory; conditional reflexes; the chemistry of metabolism; chemotherapy and biochemistry; the microbial origin of infection; immunity; the quantum theory; the structure of the atom; the rediscovery of Mendelian heredity; and the integration of the nervous system. As this epochal half century of discovery was coming to its close, Freud brought forth his interpretation of dreams and laid the beginnings of psychoanalytic concepts.

Psychiatry in the nineteenth century was in the process of becoming an autonomous discipline. The "natural" Hippocratic theory on psychopathologic alteration had held sway for two thousand years. As late as 1765, Anne-Charles Lorry still held, as did Hippocrates, that alterations in the bile (to which Lorry added the elasticity of the organic "fibers") were responsible for insanity. Then, in the first half of the nineteenth century, French psychiatry (Pinel, Esquirol, Georget) became established on a structure somewhat like that of medical pathology. Mental diseases were classified in a manner reminiscent of the chapters of medical pathology prior to Sydenham. Only much later was the idea of the evolutionary process—disease in the time dimension—added to the concept of the morbid species —disease in space.

On this stage stepped Charcot, a fine observer of clinical pictures— in his own words, a "visual." In his time, hysteria was the condition that most expressed the "personal state" of the patient. The future psychosomatic approach had roots in his study of hysteria and of other neuroses. Charcot devoted ten years of his life (1883 to 1893) to the grouping of hysteria symptoms. He studied them nosographically as a morbid species, and also pathogenetically, and concluded by classifying hysteria—until then considered a functional disease of the brain—as a psychoneurosis, in other words, as a functional disturbance psychically induced. It was at this point that Freud entered on the scene.

Charcot "saw" the motion of hysterical symptoms in time, "anatomy in motion"; Freud was interested in their *nature*. The cause of neuroses appeared to Freud as "a repressed affection," and "vital instinct," as libido. Future historians have the task of ascertaining how much influence the repressed, puritan, middle-class society of Vienna in Freud's time had in setting ablaze the spark of his revolutionary theories. Even if Freud's postulate of the origin of neuroses appears like a sudden flash of inspiration, since every human idea is born from previous ideas, we must render due tribute to Charcot and recall his favorite phrase, which Freud heard so many many times while at the Salpêtrière: *"Mais, dans ces pareils c'est toujours la chose génitale, toujours, toujours, toujours."* ("But in these and similar cases, it is always a genital [sexual] matter, always, always, always.")

But if Charcot restricted his thinking to the dramatic theater of the hysterical cases at the Salpêtrière, Freud's thinking started off with the enunciation of an empiric theory on neuroses to which he added further postulates until he even encompassed a speculative theory of religion and culture. Perhaps Freud was driven by the idea he had of himself—based on a phrase borrowed from Hebbel—of having "disturbed the sleep of the world."

Furthermore, we must not forget the effect of German as well as French ideas on psychiatry in the early years of Freud's work.

The psychobiologic trend of the fifteenth to nineteenth centuries was pushed back by the wave of histopathology aroused by Virchow. The dictatorship of the microbe ruled in medicine. Certain voices were being raised: Darwin (1873) in describing emotional reactions as an important biologic phenomenon; Cannon in his two basic works (1911, 1915) on the study of the physiology of the emotion; Oliver Wendell Holmes in his "Medicated Novels" (1859–1885); and others who dared to set up the role of suggestion and bodily emotions in contraposition to the all-powerful etiologic empire of the microbe.

Kraepelin's nosographic work, chronologically contemporary with Freud's, historically came before Freud's. He sought to convert the then existing psychiatric chaos into an ordered, even though arbitrary, cosmos. Though his ideas were ridiculed by some as an "imperial German psychiatry" because of their didactic rigidity, through him psychiatry advanced its evolution from a philosophic discipline toward a natural physical science to become more intrinsically part of the science of medicine. Thanks to Kraepelin the working methods of the psychiatrist began to acquire an organization along lines similar to the methods practiced in clinical medicine.

Although they were contemporaries, Freud took a different path than Kraepelin. Psychologically, they were antipodes, for Kraepelin sought objective systematization, while Freud probed subjectively and his psychoanalysis is the "literary" aspect of psychiatry. Freud was a romantic,* despite the fact that he was trained by some of the greatest purely scientific teachers of his time—Billroth, Arlt, Claus, Brücke, Meynert, Nothnagel—and that he was an associate of Wagner-Jauregg, the first psychiatrist to win a Nobel prize. Freud's romanticism is reflected by the fact that while for Charcot an *idea* could originate psychosomatic symptoms, for Freud the cause of such symptoms was an *emotion* or feeling.

Among the main factors that went into the formation of new theories in neuropsychiatry, it is important to note three new con-

---

* As literary precursors for his work, Freud had the great Greek and Shakespearian tragedies, Zola's naturalism, Mallarmé's romantic symbolism, and Nietzsche's philosophy.

cepts formulated during that time: John Hughlings Jackson's "evolution and dissolution," Sherrington's "integration," and Freud's "repression."

THE CONTRIBUTIONS OF FREUD TO MEDICINE

The historical chronology of psychoanalysis is well known. In May, 1896, Freud explained, based on his previous work with Breuer, his interpretation of dreams and used the word *psychoanalysis* for the first time to denote a method of inquiry, a doctrinal corpus, and a special therapeutic technique.

Until 1902 Freud worked alone, investigating the psychology of the unconscious, reporting many of his observations in his strange and fascinating correspondence with Wilhelm Fliess. During 1902 he formed his first group of followers, among them Adler, Rank, and Jung. In 1908 Freud met with his followers in Salzburg, and in 1910 the International Association of Psychoanalysis was founded. From then until 1930, when interest in psychoanalysis began to decline somewhat, Freud saw his principles grow and develop and extend to other fields of medicine.

Freud was interested in etiology, pathogenesis, nosography, and mental therapy. He divided etiopathology into *conditional* (hereditary), *concurrent* (emotions, stress, traumas), and *specific*. Ignoring the existing nosographic descriptions, he passed from nosologic to personal diagnosis. As basic therapy he accepted catharsis and transference. Integrating psychologic study with psychiatric clinics, he focused attention on the world of the unconscious, sought to evaluate psychogenic factors, built theories of psychodynamics, and added new values to the clinical case history.

Prior to Freud, diseases were considered morbid cysts in the external life history of the person. After Freud, psychopathography became an integral part of the patient's biography, for Freud included the patient's inner life in anamnesis, making of the patient a *person*. Thus he began his most important contribution to medicine, which was to help link more closely psychiatry with anthropology.

With Freud, the technique of association became a basic method of investigation; the Hippocratic interrogation was broadened by a dynamic interview in which both the patient and the physician, instead of only the latter, are active participants. This serves to delve more deeply into the intimate, inner life of the patient, who ceases thereby to be a mere witness and becomes also an *interpreter* of himself. Pathography thus becomes *biography*, combining not only the environmental factor and the pathophysiologic facts but also the patient's unconscious instincts.

Psychoanalysis advanced the clinical case history because it stressed associative speech as an instrument of exploration and therapy. Freud was an "auscultator" of dialogues.

"Behavior is a mirror in which everybody reflects his image," said Goethe. For Freud the truest mirror of the mind was the spoken word. Mental pathology with him ceased to be visual and became *auditive*. Before Freud anamnestic dialogue was merely declaratory; the patient related things of which he was a passive witness. Freud turned anamnesis into an *interpretative* art; the patient interpreted his life and the physician interpreted the patient's own interpretation. Freud therefore turned the spoken word not merely into a research instrument but also into a therapeutic agent.

Freud's word turned into metaphor, and metaphor is the enemy of dogma. Such metaphor was for him expressive of an instinctive, eminently erotic existence. Man was for Freud *homo sexualis*, for whom the word could become a cathartic agent, just as it was, in the religious and medical sense, in the classical Greek *katharsis*.

Elsewhere we have mentioned the contributions made by psychoanalysis to modern medicine, to wit: firstly, engaging in dialogue with the patient in order to integrate the event of disease in his biography; secondly, the therapeutic and diagnostic evaluation of the instinctive factor in human life as an intermediate link between the body and the ego (perhaps foreshadowed in Sydenham's *inner man*) and the influence that mental life exerts on the mechanics of the body; thirdly, the discovery and interpretation of the various levels of psychologic consciousness and the influence of the subconscious and the unconscious on a person's life.

Freud began as a biologist and a scientist; thus, though he used an "old" tool, the word, for exploring his special domain, his interpretations tended toward the mechanistic, and even his own vocabulary belonged more to physics than to psychology. His concept of "the instincts" was that they were *qualitatively* equivalent while their disturbances depended on *quantitative* variations. His phraseology— "condensation," "displacement," "repression,"—seems to have been borrowed from the semantic arsenal of physics.

WAS FREUD A SCIENTIST?

The basic formative years of Freud's career were spent in a scientific atmosphere, steeped in pathology and pharmacology. Freud's first scientific task was in zoology, dissecting four hundred eels to confirm, at the behest of his instructor Claus, whether the small lobulate organ discovered by the Pole Syrski (1874) was the until then unheard of testes of the eel.

Did Freud prefer to be a medical practitioner or a scientific investigator? He stated: "After 41 years of medical activity, my knowledge of myself tells me that I have never really been a doctor in the true sense of the word. I became a doctor because circumstances compelled me to diverge from my original intention. I do not recall whether in my childhood I ever had the least desire to aid humanity. . . ." These rather ruthless words belie the great service to mankind of a man who gave so intensely in his search for knowledge. On another occasion Freud stated: "I am not really a man of science, not an observer, not an experimenter and not a thinker. I am nothing but by temperament a Conquistador—an adventurer if you want to translate the word—with the curiosity, the boldness and the tenacity that belongs to that type of being."

We know that Freud labored greatly on problems of pathology and pharmacology during his more youthful years. He investigated the medulla oblongata of the lamprey with Brücke, the nuclei of gray matter and fibers of the human spinal bulk with Meynert, and the properties of cocaine with Fliess.

As an investigator without a laboratory, Freud turned his office into his laboratory and each patient into an object of study. By the application of naturalistic observation, his clinical interrogations became psychologic studies.

Freud's fundamental scientific honesty is expressed in his counsel that the best attitude to take in psychoanalysis is one of "benevolent skepticism." The force of his personality, however, was such that it unfortunately made of many of his followers not pupils but proselytes who turned doctrine into dogma. Freud gave new directions to clinical medicine and to psychiatry, whereas the dogmatism of his fanatic followers has hindered the progress of a truly scientific psychiatry.

Freud hoped for the day when psychology, endocrinology, and neurophysiology would be integrated, as when he asserted, "All our provisional ideas on psychology will some day be based on an organic substructure . . . This brings up the possibility that special substances and special chemical processes may control the mechanics of sex, allowing the continuity of individual existence within the species."

Freud loved science. Though science today is becoming a discipline of organization and teamwork, in the time of Freud scientists still worked alone and had to be endowed not only with genius, but also with courage, determination, self-discipline, and a spirit of self-sacrifice to be able to set out on the long, lonely, uncertain road of investigation. Freud possessed all these qualities in the highest degree.

Freud was also a true teacher. A true teacher knows above all how to inspire and to give. Freud, who had been accused of being merely a divulgator, a "transmitter" in the Oslerian sense, was a true teacher. Unamuno said, "To divulgate is also to create." Freud did more than create, he propagated and communicated.

FREUD'S CONTRIBUTION TO THE KNOWLEDGE OF MAN

Freud's revival of the ancient Assyrian method of questioning directed at the patient's memory and inmost thoughts did more than vindicate the "personalism" of the ancient Semitic medicine. It made psychiatry, and then medicine in general, concentrate upon another aspect of the patient. Thanks to Freud, the patient became more of a multidimensional organism in the eyes of the physician.

The clinician for centuries had been treating his patients, sometimes with considerable success, as a biologic mechanism. Sydenham, Trousseau, and Osler did that. The medical pathologist looked upon his patient as a physical object or as a disturbed biologic entity. Freud was among the first to compel medicine to examine the patient more as a historical and sociobiologic organism.

As against the concept of *homo aeternus* or *homo coelestis,* Freud was interested in *homo natura* and wished to define his psychology, introducing anthropologic and "auditory" attitudes in the study of mental diseases.

Freud's conceptions of man as a biologic and historical organism inspired his hypotheses that sought to explain psychologic phenomena. In this task Freud was interested more in *why* his patients were suffering than in *what* they were suffering from, in the forces responsible for their complaints, stresses, and changes in the mysterious mechanics of his theoretic entities—libido, eros, and aggressive and death instincts. His concepts have done much to mold the image that the Western man of today has of himself and have deeply influenced modern literature, just as Claude Bernard's work influenced Zola and much of the literature of his time.

Rebelling against the Hegelian interpretation that identified the rational with the real, Freud adopted an arrogant Dionysian pose, asserting the will to love and have power in a Nietzschian manner and formulating such concepts as his "geological" view of the mind and his "deep psychology," rooted in the psychology of Nietzsche.

Whereas Nietzsche and Kierkegaard conceived of a psychology that was isolated at topmost spiritual heights, Freud originated a psychology that is universal in its acceptance.

Before the first World War, medical thought followed the lines set down by Johannes Müller and Claude Bernard to the effect that "pathology is nothing but disturbed physiology" and gave the laboratory pride of place over the hospital. The *extrasomatic* factors— social, historical, and psychologic—of the individual had yet to become prime subjects for study. The newer biographic and anthropologic concept of illness is today of the greatest importance in clinical medicine. Freud's contribution to this development may be among his most significant and may successfully integrate Claude Bernard's basic principles into the spatial and temporal components of man's life.

L'ENVOI

These thoughts, hovering around the figure and the work of Freud, are our tribute on his birth centennial.

Today psychiatry stands on the threshold of a new era. Biochemistry, metabolic research, endocrinology, neurophysiology, pharmacology, and nuclear physics—all may help to open wide the doors and let in the light that will dispel the shadows in which our knowledge of mental disease has dwelled for so many centuries. It is therefore now more important than ever to recall the true stature of Freud, which transcends the narrow limits of psychoanalysis.

To keep pace with scientific progress, to renounce the fanaticism of dogma and sect, to rectify when beliefs are exposed as mistakes, and to regard properly the complex wonder of health and sickness, the psyche and the soma, not with the limited instrument of a single theory or a single technique, even though it may be remarkable as psychoanalysis was, but with every available scientific tool—these afford the best way to honor the memory of Sigmund Freud. The adoption of such an integrated attitude in psychiatry may bring the best success in the quest for the greatness of Freud.

THE CHALLENGE OF BIO-
AND CHEMOTHERAPY IN PSYCHIATRY

*t*he purpose of Chemistry," said Paracelsus, "is not to produce gold, but to study the basic sciences and use them against disease."

The new narcobiotic, chlorpromazine, represents a crystallization of Paracelsus' dream, which has come true as modern medicine keeps adding synthetically produced drugs to the psychiatric arsenal.

For almost two thousand years the physician has been steadily progressing in the field of clinical diagnosis and enlarging his etiologic knowledge of disease. But therapy has been the slowest wheel on the wagon of medical progress. Perhaps as a result of the Galenic concept of the treatment of disease, which often confused symptoms with causes, at the end of the last century therapy was in some respects as symptomatic and empirical as it was in the days of the school of Salerno, for it drew heavily from herbs and plants.

Our century has provided medicine with a springboard of new biologic, endocrinologic, and antibiotic therapies. The researcher has thrown himself into laboratory work to discover chemical substances endowed with therapeutic powers—Paracelsus' ancient dream was finally fulfilled in Ehrlich's laboratory.

Ever since the first salicylates were synthesized in the last century, medicine has steadily grown richer in chemotherapeutic substances. As the physician has learned to aim his weapons at the etiologic cause

From *Journal of Clinical and Experimental Psychopathology & Quarterly Review of Psychiatry and Neurology* 17:15, 1956 (with Arthur M. Sackler, Mortimer D. Sackler, and Raymond R. Sackler).

of disease, the quest for specific chemotherapeutic agents has become keener.

For the last ten years the pharmacologic laboratory and the pharmaceutical industry have inverted the historical order in the quest for therapeutic agents.

At the beginning of the bio-chemotherapeutic era most drugs were born out of the practicing physician's need for a concrete answer to abstract problems of disease. Today drugs are born of the slow, methodical quest carried out by the chemist for compounds that are then cast by the clinician into the living crucible of a hospital to determine their range of action.

No longer do drugs arise directly from the pressing needs and daily frustrations imposed by medical practice on the physician, who in the past had little with which to treat his patient. Today they arise from the ceaseless search of the laboratory investigator for chemical substances whose clinical usefulness can only be determined by the physician at the patient's bedside.

Chlorpromazine—one of the greatest pharmacologic aids to modern psychiatry—is the result of research at the Rhône-Poulenc Laboratories (Paris) into the pharmacologic properties of phenothiazine derivatives, which were considered effective against trypanosomiasis and malaria.

One of these derivatives, promethazine, was shown to possess low toxicity and antihistaminic properties, and it, therefore, was used at first in the treatment of allergies. However, it was discovered that one of its secondary effects was sedative and hypnotic; Moindrot showed this to be true in fifty-eight per cent of all cases, while Halpern and Briot demonstrated that its action was located in the diencephalon. These facts led to the search for further derivatives. Diethazine, isothiazine, and thiazinamium (3554 R.P.), with their notable anticholinergic properties, were isolated. The tireless search then continued.

In December 1950, Charpentier (Research Department of Rhône-Poulenc) synthesized 10-(3'-dimethylaminopropyl)-2-chlorophenothiazine, whose pharmacodynamics were studied under the laboratory number 4560 R.P. by Courvoisier, Kolsky, Fournel, Ducrot, and Koetschet. This preparation was introduced to the medical profession in Europe in November, 1952, as Largactil.

Chlorpromazine, as it came to be called, was found to exercise its effects on the central and peripheral nervous systems and was also established as having a thermoplegic, anticonvulsive, ganglioplegic, and sympathicoplegic action. This drug was later described as a narcobiotic by some and as a neuroleptic or an ataraxic by others.

The semantics of these drugs are truly fascinating. As Decourt has stressed, we must differentiate between the *pharmacodynamic action* of a drug as shown in the laboratory and its *therapeutic* technique—the use, alone or in combination, of pharmacodynamic resources having a common therapeutic goal.

We must also differentiate among *neuroplegia* (deep, controlled, and temporary inhibition of the neurovegetative and central nervous systems in order to provoke a healthy hypometabolism), *artificial hibernation* (neuroplegia plus refrigeration), *potentiated anesthesia* (total effect of two or more combined medications that is greater than that obtained by merely doubling or multiplying their dosage), and *narcobiotic action* (a drug-induced inhibition of certain basic metabolic activities of the living cell, total or partial, reversible or irreversible).

Chlorpromazine was the result of twenty years of research directed toward the discovery of a drug that would prevent or correct the effects of the phenomena of Reilly—the hemorrhage, vascular and lymphatic lesions of the alimentary tract, and necrosis of the adrenal glands that occur subsequent to the irritaton of the sympathetic nerves.

The trial of antihistaminic drugs led to the isolation of phenothiazine derivatives; promethazine proved to be a "potentiator" of certain anesthetics (Laborit, 1950). Chlorpromazine protected seventy per cent of guinea pigs (Reilly et al, 1935) against splanchnic irritation and prevented the response of the pituitary-adrenal axis to nonspecific aggression through its central depressant action on the reticular formations of the brain.

Laborit and Huguenard used chlorpromazine as part of their "lytic cocktail" (in combination with Phenergan and Dolosal) to block the neurovegetative nervous system to induce "artificial hibernation." Thus, they sought to combat shock, facilitate surgery, potentiate anesthesia, and intensify the effect of barbiturates and narcotics. This was of immense importance in treating patients with inoperable cancers who were condemned to a life sentence of narcotics to relieve the tyranny of pain.

Artificial hibernation, and its modification as prolonged narcosis, had been under fairly intensive investigation abroad, especially since Klaesi's basic psychiatric work in the second decade of this century. However, while many investigators—among them the eminent clinician and psychoanalyst Johan H. W. van Ophuijsen—were encouraged by the therapeutic benefit afforded by this procedure, the mortality rate led to a reaction against its use. The revival of interest in this approach came during the first years of the current decade—with the advent of antibiotics—and more recently, when Henri Laborit (France) reported the marked effects of chlorpromazine on the autonomic nervous system, including the temperature-regulating mechanism.

The use of chlorpromazine in psychiatric disorders soon followed. It was first reported in France by Hamon; Paraire and Velluz; Deschamps; and Delay, Deniker, and Harl. In the report of the last group (Delay et al), the relationship to artificial hibernation as well as its sympathicolytic central action was noted.

Following upon research work overseas, Lehmann and Hanrahan (February, 1954) and Winkelman (May, 1954) introduced this new pharmacodynamic agent in Canada and the United States, respectively.

The clinical spectrum of chlorpromazine increases every day, and reports relate to its use in acute and chronic alcoholism, manic-depressive psychoses, control of agitation in schizophrenic patients, symptomatic control of confusions of a toxic origin, alleviation of tension in psychoneurotics, acute toxic delirium, and epileptic confusion.

The most promising field for chlorpromazine appears to be psychiatry. It is postulated that by depressing the autonomous nervous system and interfering with the synaptic transference of excessive psychomotive excitation between the cortical areas and the diencephalon, chlorpromazine tranquilizes without producing narcosis, coma, or amnesia. Inhibition of anxiety increases the patient's capacity to respond to psychotherapy.

From the vast range of clinical investigations under way today, it seems that chlorpromazine helps control hyperactivity and anxiety as well as improves communication with the patient, thus permitting the utilization of psychotherapy.

It is our hope that further investigation of the mechanism of action of this and other pharmacodynamic agents, together with continuing studies of the earlier physiodynamic therapies (insulin, thyroid histamine, testosterone, and electroconvulsive therapies), will bring to light new clues to aid the search for etiologic and pathogenetic mechanisms at the root of the most distressing psychiatric disorders. The so-called "functional pyschoses" will be seen more clearly as psychoses due to dysfunction, and the basis of the dysfunction will be more readily comprehended. And, with increased insight into etiology and pathogenesis added to the present store of knowledge of symptomatology (as established by Kraepelin and Bleuler) and psychodynamic symptom formation (as described by Freud), we believe the development and growth of a mature scientific psychiatry is heralded. With this, the fundamental fusion of psychology and biology—the most comprehensive concept of psychobiology—will be exposed to analysis and synthesis.

If we hold the sixteenth century to be the century of anatomy, the seventeenth that of the birth of modern physiology, the eighteenth that of medical philosophy, and the nineteenth that of histopathology and clinical etiology, the twentieth century is the century of biochemotherapy—and thus the new key to the future of psychiatry as well as medicine.

VI. through the psychological glass

ON CHRISTMAS AND NEUROSES

THE HOLY DAY AND THE HOLIDAY

*t*he bells are ringing. The King is here. Once again the miracle unfolds. Rosy flesh trembles on the golden straw in the humble manger misted over by the breath of mule and ox. But for most people this festival, which began as a *holy day,* is now merely a *holiday.*

Christmas cards, depicting snowclad hamlets beneath blue velvet skies sprinkled with glittering stardust, fleeting sleighs with tinkling bells, tables groaning under the weight of brown roasts, golden loaves of bread, casks of cider and brandy, steaming Christmas puddings, and spiced punch, recall memories of the season as immortalized by Charles Dickens, that gay benevolent dictator of all the Christmases in history. ("They arrived [Mr. Pickwick and his friends] high and dry, hale and hearty, safe and sound . . . they sat down by the huge fire of blazing logs to a substantial supper, and a mighty bowl of wassail . . . in which the hot apples were hissing and bubbling with a rich look and a jolly sound. . . .")

Washington Irving's *Sketch Book* (". . . the Yule log and the Christmas candle were regularly burnt, and the mistletoe, with its white berries, hung up, to the imminent peril of all the pretty housemaids") anticipated "Dickens' Christmas" by seventeen years, and in turn was anticipated by Addison's *Notebooks of Sir Roger de Coverley* (1772), which mentions that that worthy knight had eight huge

From *International Record of Medicine 168*:812, 1955.

boars slaughtered for Christmas, added "a double quantity of malt to my small beer," and set "a cold beef and a mince pie upon the table" for the delectation of his poorer tenants.

And so, Christmas combines, in the words of Chesterton, "a trinity of eating, drinking and praying";[2] but there is one aspect of Christmas, unknown to most people, of considerable interest to physicians.

DEATH STALKS AT CHRISTMAS

The December, 1953, issue of the journal *Pastoral Psychology* was devoted entirely to "Christmas and Suicide." The title alone indicates that not only neuroses, but also Death, stalk at Christmastime. It is not to be wondered at, therefore, that we have chosen a subject that from time immemorial has beset man at Christmastide. Because at Christmas the thought of death suddenly pervades the mind of some people whose personal conflicts are intensified during this season and become involved in their unconscious mind with great religious mysteries whose origin fades away in the mists of history.

But the extraordinary thing is not that *some* people commit suicide during the Christmas season, but that *more* people do not. Mortality from "natural" causes is higher during the dark cold months of the year than in the bright warm summer months, being, in general, in inverse proportion to the light and warmth of the environment. On the other hand, the highest death rate from suicide is recorded during the summer months; the lowest, in winter. It is almost as if the sharp contrast between the smiling summer world and the despairing state of mind of the individual were one of the chief factors in pressing the trigger of the suicide's gun.

In winter there is no contrast between the dismal cold world and a mind equally desolate and beclouded, and this seems to reduce the temptation to put an end to one's own internal tragedies by suicide. In fact, one of the highest suicide rates in the world is recorded for certain South Sea islands where life is gentle and easygoing under turquoise skies. Perhaps because life in a paradise is unchanging from day to day, the only thing left to bring variety in such heavenly monotony is to take the great leap into the Land of Shadows.

There is great wisdom in celebrating the birth of Christ in the most dismal month of the year. It is like frightening away the deepest gloom with the brightest torch, like setting a glowing beacon of hope in the midst of the winter shadows. We must remember that the King of Kings was born amidst straw in a stable, as though to establish for all time that we must regard the facets of a gem, not the setting.

Let us also remember that, long before psychiatrists, poets already knew about neuroses related to certain hours of the day, days of the week, months, and seasons. Because the human mind, like a mighty ocean, is subject to the ebb and flow of tides governed by the course of the hours, days, months, and seasons.

SUNSET NEUROSIS, SUNDAY NEUROSIS, AND SPRING NEUROSIS

There is, for example, that vague disquieting "five o'clock" feeling, the "sunset neurosis" sung by the poets, which invades many secretaries when, the occupations of the day over, they go out in the nostalgic twilight, their souls hungry for companionship or amusement that perhaps is not available.

Then there is the "Sunday neurosis" or the "week-end neurosis." How many people on Friday evenings are overtaken by an undefined dread as they hear the office doors close behind them! Those long, empty, restless, soul-consuming week ends when, free from weekday responsibilities, they are alone with themselves! Can they face for two whole interminable days the specter of their true personality, which during the week was kept submerged under the pressure of work and stress?

Ferenczi has investigated "Sunday neurosis" and the cyclic recurrence of cephalea and gastritis as evidence of the fact that for certain neurotics Sunday is a holiday from all taboos, internal or external. These symptoms develop when all impulses and instincts are released by these neurotics in their daydreams about what they imagine they can do during the week end. Cattel has described a "holiday" syndrome, lasting from Thanksgiving Day to New Year's Day, distinguished by anxiety, depression, irritability, and "wishes for the magical resolution of problems," which reaches its peak at Christmas and occurs in patients with broken homes who find it difficult to establish any emotional relationships and feel isolated, lonely, and bored.

There are also "spring neuroses," linked historically with the old seed-sowing festivals and their explosive accompaniment of wine, women, and song, and the springtide intensification of manic-depressive psychoses. Similarly, we might consider "autumnal neuroses." Autumn is the great sunset of the year, just as evening is the little autumn of the day.

CHRISTMAS NEUROSES

Dr. L. Bryce Boyer, in a splendid scholarly study of Christmas neuroses, analyzed four cases of neuroses, intensified at Christmastime, which had as a common denominator an unresolved rivalry for the love of the deceased father, each of the patients identifying himself with the father's favorite child. "In them the birth of Christ, a fantasied competitor against whom they were unable to contest successfully, reawakened memories of unsuccessful rivalry with siblings, real or fantasied, in their pasts." [1] Some of these patients identified themselves with Christ, and regarded the psychiatrist as their lost God-Father. Christmas served them as a stage on which they acted out the birth of new hopes, with the whole of humanity as audience and history as the spotlight.

All those authors—reviewed by Dr. Bryce Boyer[1]—who have studied Christmas neuroses agree that it is a period when unconscious birth fantasies and unresolved conflicts come to life, and that people seek to resolve them by means of the family Christmas reunion (Jones), thus eliminating the two great traumas of infancy: oral deprivation and sibling rivalry, to which is added (Jekels) the identification with Christ as a means of equating the son with the father and so resolving the eternal conflict between domination and subjection. Even for the "normal" individual, Christmas is a period of intensification of many conflicts: dread of solitude, financial, social, and emotional insecurity —in a word, fear of life.

MYTH, PAGANISM, AND THE HISTORICAL ORIGIN OF CHRISTMAS

The Christmas we celebrate today originated sixteen hundred years ago in Rome, but the true Christmas started some four thousand years ago in Mesopotamia, today Iraq, the ancient Biblical country situated between two legendary rivers, the Tigris and the Euphrates. The white-robed Mesopotamian priests, who from the rocky summit of the hills spied the resplendent cavalcade of the stars, held that the god Marduk created the Earth out of chaos and darkness. When autumn descended upon the land, presaging death for all plants, Marduk returned to defeat the monsters from Chaos, so that the planet might not perish. When each year ended, the Mesopotamians sought to purify themselves by means of a scapegoat to which their sins were magically transferred. At *Zagmuk,* their New Year festival, they burnt in effigy Marduk's enemy, holding masquerades and feasts by the light of bonfires.

Later on, the emperor Aurelianus (A.D. 270) set a fixed date for the celebration of Christ's birth, coinciding with that of the *Dies Natalis Invicti,* the day on which Baal, the Syrian sun god, was worshiped.

From the middle of December until Christmas Day was the period of the Saturnalia, during which feasting, singing, and love-making prevailed, ending with the sacrifice of an effigy of the god Saturn. Almost immediately the *Kalends* followed, with pagan celebrations lasting until Ash Wednesday. During these festivals license ran free. With masked faces and dressed in wild animal skins, the people surrendered themselves to all kinds of Bacchic and love excesses. On the last night, everyone sallied forth into the streets with lighted torches, concealing their anxiety under the mask of celebration.

The Christian Church endeavored to combat paganism by the subtle adoption of those rituals. In the year 601, Pope Gregory the Great ordained that the pagan rituals be adapted to Christianity and that eating, dancing, and love-making take place outside the churches in honor of God, instead of within the temples in praise of the Devil.

Christmas therefore does not figure among the most ancient festivals of the Church. Prior to the fifth century, there was no general decision as to when this feast should appear in the calendar. A passage from Theophilus of Antioch (c. 180) shows that the birth of Christ was to be celebrated on the twenty-fifth of December, which ruling was confirmed in the calendar of Philocalus (354), who also transferred the date of Christ's birth from January 6 to December 25. At that time this was a Mithraic date, and this was sufficient for the Romans to be accused of paganism by the Syrians and Armenians, who kept the sixth of January, today's Epiphany, for the Christian anniversary.

December 25 was originally a sun feast, motivated by the fear of the inhabitants of the earth, whose life depended on the sun, that the latter would not return from his yearly journey into the heavens. To ingratiate themselves with him, pagan offerings were made at the winter solstice to the solar god. In the icy northern lands, the winter solstice was the moment for lighting huge bonfires to lend strength to the winter sun and bring it back to life. The idea of the winter solstice—the return of light—was crystallized in the symbol of the birth of Christ, Light of mankind.

In the year 440, the Fathers of the Church chose the winter solstice as the best date to celebrate the birth of Christ, thus uniting it symbolically with a date of tremendous pagan importance. Christmas then gathered rituals and symbols from the whole world: the Christmas tree from Germany, which replaced the Odin oaks, the wreaths from the Roman Saturnalia, the Druid mistletoe, and the Saxon holly, all of which recur to this day in the Christmas cribs, the Spanish *belenes,* the Italian *preseppio,* and the Mexican *posadas.*

During the old *Kalends,* the Christmas banquets were loaded with ritual offerings to the dead, including the Fates. From that time on, Christmas became a season of fairy tales about goblins, ghosts, and witches. Robert Louis Stevenson wrote his fearsome story "The Body Snatcher" as a Christmas tale, and Dickens wrote his most hair-raising ghost stories for publication at this time of the year. Christ himself was born at midnight, the witches' hour, and since then it has been said that at dawn on Christmas Day the cocks crow louder "to frighten away the ghosts."

Winter solstice festivals, such as Christmas, were man's tribute to the sun for giving him successful harvests. Afraid that, because of his sins, the sun might not reappear, man expiated his sins by invoking the rebirth of the sun.

CHRISTMAS AND NEUROTIC RITUALS

Four thousand years after the Mesopotamian rituals, modern man is still trying to expiate his sins, to be reborn and forgiven by transferring those sins to a scapegoat. Certain neurotics[1] relive at Christmas the ritual of sin, punishment, rebirth, and salvation, passing through a phase of intense depression succeeded by the hypomaniac excitement of the New Year.

In Christianity, Christ is the scapegoat who dies so that the faithful may survive. At Christmas we still witness the pagan combination of feast and orgy of a totemic cult. The excessive gorging indulged in during these festivities compensates for the loss of loved ones, who in this manner become assimilated in our own person, thus making them immortal. In this way a type of communion is achieved similar to the ritual participation in the Host.[1]

RELIGION AND PSYCHOLOGY

On this subject P. W. Martin has written:[3] "Individuation, wholeness, how in fear and trembling a man may come to work out his own salvation, has always been the central theme of religion.

". . . Jung's experience on this score has been widely quoted: 'Among all my patients in the second half of life—that is to say, over thirty-five—there has not been one whose problem in the last resort was not that of finding a religious outlook on life.'

"T. S. Eliot, referring to Christianity, sees psychology as an 'indispensable handmaid': 'Psychology has very great utility in two ways. It can revive, and has already to some extent revived, truths long since known to Christianity, but mostly forgotten and ignored, and it can put them in a form and a language understandable by modern people to whom the language of Christianity is not only dead but undecipherable. . . . Psychology is an indispensable handmaid to theology; but I think a very poor housekeeper.'

"Toynbee, from the standpoint of universal history, likewise sees religion as primal; often mistaken, often twisted to meet man's desires, inevitably adapted to the exigencies of the age, but in itself the vision of 'a Kingdom of God which is not in Time at all but is in a different spiritual dimension . . . able to penetrate our mundane life and to transfigure it.'

"From these widely different angles of approach substantially the same conclusion emerges. Religion, rightly understood, has nothing to fear from psychology. On the contrary, psychology, properly so called, is in a position to serve religion."

THE CHRISTMAS "SPIRIT"

Christmas is not only Dickens' gay season, but also the magic night when the wolves in the icy wastes raise snow-crusted muzzles to a moon of silver and break into lugubrious howls. And it is the night when ghosts press icy nostrils against the frosty windowpanes to peer at the glowing logs crackling in the fireplaces and at the tables sparkling with fine damask and cut glass, loaded with smoking dishes and hot punch, surrounded by fair ladies more resplendent than a morning in May and their escorts as gallant as the knights at King Arthur's Round Table.

But Christmas also holds hours full of ominous shadows, and physicians must look with open eyes and an alert mind for the neuroses and conflicts that afflict their patients at such hours. And they must do this with simplicity and kindness, with the same humility and humanity that ensure that the true greatness of Christmas rests on its being the birthday not so much of the King of Kings as of the Christ Child who, like any other infant, preferred the humble gifts brought by the Magi to the splendored trappings of kingship.

This is also a time to help both patients and "normal" individuals who fall under the shadow of the "Christmas neurosis" to realize that insecurity in living may be a noble spur to progress.

Life is of itself a thing of uncertainty and risk. But the dangers and snares of life are preferable to absolute peace and absence of danger, which are attributes of death, for to fear life is to be already halfway dead. Let us ourselves learn, and teach everyone else, not to fear life but to accept its ups and downs as precious offerings in the same cheerful spirit as the gay heroes of Dickens accepted their Christmas gifts.

ON THE PSYCHOLOGY
OF SYMBOLISM IN ORIENTAL RUGS

THE LANGUAGE OF SYMBOLS

In the beginning was the symbol. . . ." The symbol was the very first means devised by man to express himself. Symbolism heralded all human languages. The language of symbols is the most universal in space and is the one that has best survived through time. A symbol is a veritable fossil of human thought.

Man began creating symbols as soon as his brain awakened to the realities of the world about him. Scorched by prehistoric suns, shivering with cold in his cave during the endless nights of the Ice Age, primitive man lived in panic over two fears that he had continuously to face: loneliness and death. At the bottom of his fear of loneliness lay his reproduction instinct, which demanded companionship; underlying his fear of death was his instinct of self-preservation, which warned him that only through health and strength could he conquer death.

To fight these terrors, man evolved an animistic interpretation of the universe and peopled it with intelligent forces. Thus animistic religions began, and the first myths, projections of man's hopes and fears, were born. In the course of time, myths were succeeded by legends—expressions of history distorted by the imagination. Myths were collective hallucinations; legends were the delusions of peoples. The first were perceptions without object; the latter, with object. Both still are the most archaic and spontaneous form of expression of all peoples.

From *International Record of Medicine 169*:651, 1956.

A symbol has been defined as "something that represents and hides something else." The word "symbol" stems from the Greek *symballein,* meaning to throw together, to join. A symbol is something whose outer appearance conceals a much broader inner meaning. It is a nodal point from which different rays of meaning emerge. It has a *conventional* meaning: the relationship existing between any object and the word that designates it; it has an *accidental* meaning: an object may affect a happy or a sad connotation depending on a person's experience with that object; and it has a *universal* meaning, the most important of all, for symbols are similar in all ages and among all peoples.

Symbolic language is not only the most ancient but also the most universal of all languages. It was used by primitive man at the dawn of history; it is still used by modern man in his dreams, by the child in his fancies, by the neurotic in his rituals, and by the artist in his creations. The common denominator of all people who resort to the language of symbols is a creative compulsion to extract from the subconscious a wide variety of images with which to disguise realities bearing a deep universal meaning. By analyzing these symbolic images, it is possible to dig into the unconscious of peoples, where their mental archetypes are buried in darkness and, like precious stones exposed to the light, can be made to sparkle only when exposed to a quick flash of consciousness.

Graphology was born before writing, with the simplest of human gestures—a motion of the hand, which is the first gesture made by the newborn babe as if greeting the world, and the last made by the dying as if bidding the world good-by. The finger of primitive man scratching on the sand of his cave—on the sands of time as it were —gave rise to subsequent graphism, just as his dreams, fancies, fears, and hopes gave rise to myths, legends, and fables.

Later, in his daydreams and night dreams, in his neurotic rituals and his artistic creations, man individually continued to use the same symbols that occurred in the collective language of peoples. Symbolic language is invaluable for studying the psychology of peoples as well as of man individually. Man's dreams today, whether in New York or in the African jungle, are the same as man's dreams in the times of the Egyptian Pharaohs or the Roman Caesars.

Time never stops in its endless march, but man, as Goethe observed, remains the same. This immutability of the human being, modified only by such biologic differences as are imposed by ecology and evolution, is also characteristic of symbolism, to which man has always resorted to hide those subconscious desires and terrors that are the quintessence of his being.

Man has always used symbolism in his thinking, in his writing, in all his creative endeavors. Symbolism was the basis of the so-called primitive magic thought that governed the mind of ancient man. It was the basis of the ideographic writing of many Oriental peoples, which has so amazingly survived to our day, as it was also the basis, subtly distorted and disguised but rediscovered by modern graphology, of Western writing. Even punctuation marks can reveal something of the collective soul. For instance, the Spanish language is perhaps the only one in the world with two question marks (¿?) and two exclamation marks (¡!), placed respectively at the beginning and at the end of a question or an exclamatory sentence, as if to translate the tremendous emotional capacity of the Spanish people when curious or surprised.

Symbolism is the basis of most modern art, and it has also exercised a great influence on the ornamentation of many objects of daily use.

The "lost language" of symbols has represented throughout history the way of all peoples of expressing their repressed fears and desires. Harold Bayley, in his book *A New Light on the Renaissance* (1909), formulated the theory that from 1282 (when they were introduced) to the second half of the eighteenth century watermarks represented an uninterrupted coherent chain of emblematic symbols. Such symbols were, so to speak, fossilized or crystallized thoughts; they preserved in the sanctuary of a cryptogram the aspirations and traditions of many of the mystical and puritanical sects that abounded in Europe in the Middle Ages. They are indubitably historicopsychologic documents of great importance.

Through the symbolism in watermarks we know that the art of papermaking was introduced in Europe by Protestant sects—the Albigenses and Vaudois in France and the Cathari or Patarini in Italy—antedating the Reformation. These sects continued to exist secretly for several centuries after they were excommunicated and outlawed by the Pope. An identical origin may be ascribed to the symbolic decorations used by printers in the Middle Ages. Printers, papermakers, and other such artisans were the precursors of the Renaissance, the period when symbolism became more manifest in art.

The same may be said about symbolism in Oriental rugs. Like the fossil that imprisons within its bed of stone the skeleton of a fish or the petals of a prehistoric flower, the symbols in rugs preserve many a dream and fear of the ancient peoples who fashioned them.

Onto the objects he creates, man always projects a varied collection of symbols representing the psychologic harvest of many centuries. All art handed down to us, however crude or humble, is encrusted with symbols in which the great fears and preoccupations of many generations palpitate. This is particularly true of Oriental art, for symbols have played a more vital part in the Oriental than in the Western mind, and they have been used with bounteous hands in Oriental art, and particularly in rugs, of which Sargent and Holmes have said: "There is more art in a great Oriental rug than in any picture of any period."

ON THE HISTORY AND PHILOSOPHY OF RUGS

If the value and importance of an object are based on the multiplicity of its uses and its historical tradition, then the rug indubitably outshines any other object used by man for utilitarian or ornamental purposes. For no other object has as many uses or has as faithfully kept man company in his cavalcade through history as the rug.

The origin of rugs is lost in prehistoric mists. Felt rugs (the Pasyrik rugs of the Altai Mountains) have been found that are thirty thousand years old and belong to the Paleolithic Age. But no one has thoroughly investigated the origin of rugs.

We can imagine how rugs came into being when prehistoric man, crouching on the muddy floor of the cave he shared with the snake and the frog, felt the necessity of protecting his body from dirt, cold, and dampness. Perhaps he began by covering the ground with leaves and branches, and then tried braiding roots into a mat to keep out the cold and humidity. Later, during the interminable prehistoric nights, women wove thick mats of vegetable fiber. Thus, perhaps, the first rugs were born. The vegetable rug was undoubtedly cleaner and more practical than animal skins, which attracted insects and vermin.

Slowly the rug became a vital necessity for man. Wherever he went, on his own back or on the back of his horse, buffalo, camel, or elephant, he carried his rug with him, so that he might always cover the ground on which he lay. On the backs of men, horses, buffaloes, camels, or elephants, the rug became a vital part of the baggage of the hunter and the primitive nomad. And when in crucial centuries—which the psychiatrist and philosopher Karl Jaspers called "time-axis," designating thereby those periods in the evolution of nations when modern humanism and culture began to flower—Asiatic cultures invaded Europe, they brought with them on the backs of their horses the rare gift of rugs.

The rug thus attained a sovereign position among the domestic articles used by man. Originally the rug was used to cover cold damp floors; later it became a curtain over windows and walls or a hanging to conceal the entrance to a room. Used as tapestries, rugs were indeed a blessing to feudal lords, who bedecked themselves like playing-card kings and queens and drank from solid gold goblets, yet shivered with fever and chills caused by the dripping walls of their castles. The rug was pillow and mantle and even a mattress for people who had nothing else to sleep on. Piled one on top of the other, rugs were bed or sofa in the luxurious dwellings of Oriental satraps. When a man, rich or poor, died, the rug he used during his lifetime became his shroud or covered his coffin. Cut in strips, rugs lined the floors of long corridors, and cut in small foldable rectangles, they protected the knees of the believer when he said his prayers. Orientals used them as money, and in many countries they were the most precious gift that could be offered. The nomad hunter used the rug as his tent, and rugs covered the flanks of the restless mounts that bore the hordes of Genghis Khan across the Asiatic steppes. Folded and tied with cord, rugs were used as satchels by pilgrims. In palaces and churches, the rug as an ornament was often unsurpassed in sumptuousness. Along with jewels, silks, spices, and lovely female slaves, Oriental potentates offered gifts of priceless rugs woven by deft hands. Rolled up, the rug was used as a hiding place for fugitives and as a weapon to asphyxiate an enemy. Cleopatra, rolled up in a rug, gained access to Julius Caesar, and in the same fashion the last Caliph of Baghdad escaped from the besieged city. Multicolored rugs formed a polychrome frame for Scheherazade while she bewitched her Caliph for one thousand and one nights.

A history of mankind might be written by studying the evolution of rugs and the historical role they played in the drama of nations, just as Bachofen wrote a history of the ancient Greeks by studying the bas-reliefs on their tombs.

The rug is a powerful symbol of home. When an Arab street vendor rolls out a rug on the pavement he magically turns the spot into a home. That little square of many-hued fabric spread out on the sidewalk can counteract man's subconscious fear when he passes from the security of his home to the insecurity of the street. It is as if the Arab had cut out a piece of the earth and transfigured it into a home, with the sky for a roof and the stars for lamps. No wonder the Arab street vendor and the streetwalker have for generations plied their trade in the open air!

An object so intimately tied up with his life as the rug naturally impelled man to enhance its value by adding lovely ornamentation to its practical ends. Man embellished rugs with patterns and figures almost from the beginning, and onto these he projected those symbols of greatest importance to him, to his race, his country, or his times. As time passed, the rug became a magic cloth on which skillful fingers wove signs that imprisoned as in a magic cage the restless birds of symbols. To decipher the symbolism in Oriental rugs is to peer into a fabulous cryptographic world harboring the psychologic secrets of the peoples of the ancient Orient.

MAN'S CREATION AND ITS MEANING: ON AN AUTHOR AND HIS UNIQUE WORK

Surely there is nothing more important in life than understanding the meaning of one's work. At least once in his lifetime every man should ask himself two questions: What meaning is there to what I do? What does my work mean to me and to others?

Human labor may be classified into the practical and the theoretical. The first is related to man's immediate reality; it embraces all utilitarian and some scientific occupations. These occupations— mason, geologist, physician, carpenter, physicist, astronomer, farmer —refer to man's present and try to consolidate or improve it. The second group of noble occupations may focus on the past instead of the present. These are of a theoretical type and concentrate on tasks that at first sight may seem to be foreign to man's urgent needs. Among these are the research scientist, who is concerned with abstract questions (just as the physician is concerned with concrete questions), the historian, the sociologist, the mathematician, and the collector and preserver of rugs.

To be interested in rugs and to make of them one's lifework, one has to be a romantic. Only a man whose soul is open to the lyrical breezes of the universe can dedicate his existence to what is for so many simply an ornament or a utilitarian object. Every occupation is preceded by a *pre*occupation. Hence I was intrigued some time ago with *The Hidden Language of Oriental Rugs* by Harry Raphaelian, a man whose preoccupation and occupation have happily blended. For this book I had the pleasure of writing a short introduction on the subject of symbolism in modern psychology, and ever since then I have been interested in the symbols in Oriental rugs.

Harry Raphaelian has lived almost half a century among rugs, collecting them, exchanging them, preserving them, studying them, and finally—this was the purpose of his unique book—glorifying them. Not satisfied with pointing out to the world the beauty of rugs, he imparted dignity to them by showing their psychologic value and their usefulness as instruments of historical research. He changed the rug from a merely decorative object to a scholarly book containing fragments of the soul of the peoples who wove the polychrome fabrics.

His book introduces us to a strange, dreamlike world. The horizon of Oriental history opens like a fan before us. The geographicohistorical belt whence came the loveliest Oriental rugs includes Turkey, Asia Minor, the Caucasus, Persia, the old Ottoman Empire, China,

Turkestan, Indian, and Tibet. (It would be interesting to study why this "rug culture" concentrated around the waist of the planet. Such study would no doubt supply the key to the psychologic motivations behind the desire of these people to immortalize themselves in the art of rugs.)

The history of rugs has lent itself too much to the anecdotal and the adjectival and too little to the basically substantive.

It is possible to understand the gigantic leap from rustic rugs fashioned from Mesopotamian straw to the "Spring of Chosroes," 1051 square meters large, that decorated the Royal Palace of Ctesiphon in Khusraw near Baghdad. This rug, made of silk, gold, silver, and precious stones, symbolized might and power to the visitor, and ostentation and relaxation to the monarch. Not only its fabulous value —which today would be over two hundred million dollars—but also its exquisite beauty inspired Persian art in the centuries that followed. It is possible to understand the sharp contrast between the magnificence typical of Oriental rugs and the simplicity and sobriety of the sixteenth-century Spanish woolen rugs from Alpujarras, and to understand why in periods of abundance and prosperity the opulent rug was preferred to the austere rug of lean years. But to this day no one has delved into the meaning of the symbols depicted in rugs. To descend into the rich mine of the symbolism of Oriental rugs and to bring the treasures of meaning out into the sun of our modern knowledge is the purpose of Harry Raphaelian's book.

To read through the pages of that book is to enter a palace with huge chambers representing the countries of the world, chambers reached through the long dark corridors of time. Fortunately, the author walks in front of us on this expedition through the night of centuries, opening windows and turning on lights. Under the spell of his word and the light of his torch, the figures on tapestries and rugs come to life, whisper to the reader, and open up a psychologic chest until now sealed. The author reveals by word and image—his word is simple and instructive, his image, brilliant and evocative—an exotic world palpitating with enigma and promise. He reveals the principal groups of symbols which century after century have preoccupied man. The author—born in Sivas, Anatolia, the fabulous land mentioned by Marco Polo in his *Travels*—presents enough material to write a history of the Orient based on the study of its textile symbols.

THE PSYCHOLOGIC ORIGIN OF SYMBOLS

A symbol is not a rigid immutable entity, but something flexible that changes according to time and place, although preserving its basic emotional charge.

However important the individual analysis of a symbol may be, it is even more important to study it in correlation with other symbols and with the same symbol in other places and times.

Primitive man, who suffered from cosmic loneliness and confused the laws of his thought with those of nature, created a means of communication and a technique to try to dominate demons and show his submission to the gods of the universe.

In his ignorance, primitive man ascribed the laws of nature to superior beings—demons and gods. Fearful of these invisible powers, he devised means to fight them and to appease them. Thus man passed from the creation of myths to the rituals of magic. Especially impressed by the sun, the moon, and the stars, man's most primitive myths and symbols and even religions are of solar essence. The biography of every great Oriental religious reformer recounts the birth, apogee, and death of the prophet-god, apostle, or Messiah, that is to say, the dawn, high noon, and setting of the sun on its course from east to west. The sun is symbolized by the inner light and the mystic halo of the great religious reformers.

Everything related to the sun represents what is conscious and above the surface, and everything connected with the moon and stars represents what is submerged in the unconscious. The ancient symbols of tree, cross, and snake were at first identical with the symbol of the sun saving humanity after the Flood, since they represented the same images of death, salvation, and resurrection. The snake and the tree come to life in the spring and take on new skin and leaves, respectively. Paradise contained the tree of life, later symbolized by Christ on the cross; that is, the ideas of death and salvation, since the original sin was committed in the Garden of Eden. The deluge was meant to punish man, but the sun shone over the waters and saved him, just as Christ rose from the dead to save man.

With each myth there was born the magic rite capable of establishing ritual communication with gods and demons. That similarity of all primitive myths stems from the fact that their symbolism is born from the secret or latent experiences of man. One might draw up a map of primitive symbolism throughout the world, and its psychologic cartography would reveal that the conception of the world entertained by all peoples was identical.

With the passage of time, people forgot the meanings of their mystic symbols, but their individual associations of ideas and dreams still maintained their correspondence with the collective symbols and myths of mankind. That is why the study of symbols is so valuable to the psychiatrist and the historian. Through symbols we can delve into the deepest strata of the human soul, depths to which we would otherwise have no access.

An original if simplistic interpretation of some of the symbolic images observed in ancient art, especially in tapestries and rugs, is that offered by the anthropologist Edmund Dacque, who said that giants, hippogriffs, fairies, and fantastic animals really existed, and that primitive man was terrorized for thousands of years by the strange world about him. When those fabulous creatures disappeared, the psychic trauma, the scar left on man's mind, was so deep that in order to liberate himself man created symbolic images—the dragon, the giant, witches—representative of those very same past terrors. If plumed serpents, winged bulls, hippogriffs and dragons, gnomes and fairies existed, the influence of alcohol or of a psychosis would be enough for modern man to establish contact again—in his delirium, hallucinations, or dreams—with those evil legions, which took refuge in his unconscious when they disappeared from the face of the earth.

But this fantastic photographic interpretation by Dacque of primitive symbolism cannot compare with the study of symbolism as it stemmed from primitive magic and religions, in which men wished to dominate demoniac powers through magic rituals or invocation, or to submit to beneficent deities through religious rituals and the cajoling influence of prayer. Magic was a way of conquering; prayer was a way of submitting. Magic was aggressive; religion was defensive.

Gradually man created religions of fertility to overcome his fear of loneliness and religions of mystery to overcome his fear of death. Thus he abandoned his earlier worship of demons. The fertility religions overcame loneliness by glorifying the idea of reproduction as symbolized by harvest festivals and the worship of Mother Earth. The mystery religions provided spiritual refuge for man, who craved immortality, and produced the rituals celebrated in the Eleusinian temples.

THE PSYCHOLOGY OF ANIMALS THAT NEVER WERE

Later, magic evolved and became the individual ritual of the neurotic, while religion changed into collective neurosis. But there still remained some of the individual fears, and these were projected as animal symbols.

The bird became a phallic symbol, just as the peacock became the symbol of death. The horse, which found its maximum symbolic expression in the Greek centaur—as savage as Eurythion or as beneficent as Chiron—was the archetype of sexual power. It originated in Thessaly, where the idea of the hunter of bulls who loved his horse and the idea of the horse itself were fused into one symbol. Bulls, goats, and insects symbolized the primitive passions in Egyptian mythology. In the cult of Ishtar, Siva rode on a bull and symbolized death; Indra rode an elephant and symbolized rain and thunder. The fish was the symbol of the Saviour (his Greek name was an acrostic of the words designating "Jesus Christ Son of the God Saviour"); the boat was the symbol of the Church on the sea of life. The lion also was the symbol of Christ, "Lion of the tribe of Judah" (Revelations 5).

These fabulous animals, which never existed except in people's imaginations, make up one of the most interesting groups of symbols in Oriental rugs. Many of these animals belong to the beginning of mankind, and in many instances were created in an attempt to explain the inexplicable in the universe. Later, the Assyrian priests, who from the peak of lofty hills scrutinized the stars, projected into the heavenly constellations the figures of the animals—goats, fishes, scorpions—that inhabited their fancies.

Fantastic animals do not appear only on rugs. Greek plates of the Corinthian period (600 B.C.) show terrible creatures with three heads —in front they are lions, in back, serpents, and in the middle, goats. These were the enemies against which Greek heroes pitted their strength. We have already mentioned the centaur, half man, half horse, which six centuries before Christ symbolized for the Greeks the savage aspect of man. Two thousand years before Christ there existed sphinxes—the ancient Egyptian symbol of royal power—with a human head, usually resembling some Pharaoh, and with the body of a lion to indicate the strength of royalty. When they reached Greece almost fifteen centuries later, these sphinxes were no longer royal symbols. Winged horses, which nine centuries before our era stood watch over the doors of the ancient Assyrian palaces to prevent the entrance of evil spirits, gave rise to Pegasus, the winged horse that the Greek hero Bellerophon broke in with a magic bridle. These effigies were immortalized in the Greek vases of Campania in the fourteenth century A.D., and later in the winged lion of Venice, the symbol of Saint Mark, patron saint of that romantic city. In the Middle Ages the griffin appeared in church architecture with the head and wings of an eagle, to indicate the power of the Church in heaven, and a lion's body, to denote its strength on earth. Fantastic birds like the Chinese *fêng-huang,* which appeared only in times of peace and prosperity, still seem to beat their wings on the polychrome woodcuts of the Ming dynasty. Another fabulous animal was the *chi-lin* of Chinese bronzes. It has a stag's body, horse's hoofs, and the tail of an ox, and it treads delicately to avoid crushing the grass and insects. In Japan, this animal was called *lirin,* and alongside it were placed sea serpents, hydras, griffins, and especially unicorns and dragons.

The unicorn was a graceful beast with the body of a horse, the hoofs of a stag, the tail of a lion, and a single horn protruding from its forehead like a petrified sprout. During the Middle Ages, it was the symbol of purity and tenderness. Bronze unicorns pouring forth holy water may still be seen in old churches. Flemish tapestries of the fifteenth century depicted the hunt with hounds of the unicorn, "that austere and noble animal" of blond mane, but only the pure hands of a virgin could overcome it. Later, medieval folklore changed the unicorn into the symbol of Christ, the virgin-huntress became an emblem of the Virgin Mary, while the chase became the allegory of Christ's passion. The legend of the unicorn, mentioned as far back as Pliny, was born in the Orient, where it was considered the spirit of the earth, just as the dragon was the spirit of the air and the phoenix the spirit of fire. The pointed, polished horn of the unicorn was a universal panacea. Only four centuries ago it still brought a high price in Dresden, although it was probably only a piece of ivory endowed with curative powers by the faith of the times. The power of the unicorn's horn against poisons derived from its being the symbol of Christianity, the emblem of mystical purity, capable of disintoxicating souls and specific poisons. At the same time, its prolific magic powers (it was the symbol of the Earth, the Mother of all living things) conciliated the attributes of virginity and fertility.

Even before the unicorn, the dragon, another favorite symbol in Oriental rugs, appeared in folklore. Of this, G. K. Chesterton said, "The dragon is certainly the most cosmopolitan of all impossibilities." Many years later, still fascinated by fantastic animals, Chesterton, out in the country, drew with colored chalk the soul of a cow: ". . . and the soul was all purple and silver and had seven horns and the mystery which all beasts carry in them."

In China, dragons were considered friendly animals; in other places, they were symbols of Satan. Some inhabited the sky and ruled the winds and the rain. In all mythologies the flying dragon, the earth-dragon, and the fire-dragon were the basic elements of myths, fables, and legends. Today, in children's fancies as well as in the nightmares of adults and the deliriums of psychotics, the dragon still is the symbol of man's greatest fears. In weaving dragons into rugs, man perhaps tried to come to terms with them by offering them artistic tribute as well as shelter in his home, and perhaps subconsciously he also allowed himself the pleasure of stepping on the effigy of the much feared animal.

Primitive animism and Oriental rugs are full of these theriomorphic symbols, which can be explained psychologically by the fact that man at once loved, hated, and feared the animals with which he lived, and in order to express his emotional ambivalence with regard to these animals, he projected into symbols this complex of contradictory emotions.

Behind every symbol there is a real fact disguised or hidden. Symbols are closely allied to myths, and it is well known that myths are born historically at moments of national peril, when the imagination of men is fired. Excavations in Crete, Mycenae, and Troy have revealed that Greek myths symbolized the struggles that took place three thousand years ago between the old Minoan civilization of the South and the invaders from the North. The myths, such as the minotaur, adorning many Oriental rugs in the form of symbols were developed in a similar manner. The bull was Crete's national symbol, and the palace of Cnossus—in which the image of the bull was everywhere—was its labyrinth. The Athenians represented the bull symbolically as a cruel monster which every seven years demanded a tribute of fine young men and beautiful maidens. In truth, the bull was the symbolic projection of the fact that for many years the Cretans demanded tribute from the Athenians. The myth of the Argonauts represented symbolically the effort of the invaders from the North to colonize the area up to the Black Sea, after the destruction of the Mycenaean civilization of Troy.

Dreams today are the myths of the individual, just as myths were the dreams of peoples. The human being is essentially a creator of images. Most animals proceed by instinct, and action follows perception automatically. But in man, perception is not immediately transformed into reaction. With man some time intervenes during which selection is made, and at such time our images, ideas, and symbols take shape. Our frustrated desires, our unfulfilled dreams, what we love and what we hate, everything that is of importance in our mind we project in the form of symbols that eventually find their way into works of art and decorative objects, especially objects that play, as rugs do, an important part in the history of mankind.

By integrating the symbols, one could explain why the favorite motif on Persian rugs is the garden; why birds, peacocks, human figures, and bright colors are omnipresent on Turkish rugs; why the Tartars loved browns and purples; why the Chinese preferred blues and yellows, the Persians, red-browns and dark blues. One could correlate these symbols with historical periods and trace the geographic profile of each country, and interpret them not only in the light of the psychology of a specific nation and its time, but in relation to similar symbols at other times, keeping in mind the different meanings of the same symbols in different countries. The result would be a history of nations in the light of their symbols, a history in which the rug would play a unique role in revealing the deepest strata of the popular soul.

After all, the fingers that wove every rug were propelled by a brain bathed by the historicultural currents of a given period and a specific country. The symbol that the artisan's hands wove into the rug was the projection not only of his subconscious motives, but also of those of his people and of his time. The rug thus became a blackboard on which a people wrote its secret dream life in the cabalistic language of symbols.

If all the rugs produced by any one country throughout its entire history were put together, they would make up the multicolored pages of a fabulous book containing the unwritten story of its fears, loves, hates, ideals, frustrations, and ambitions. All together the rugs produced in the entire world at a given period would, like magic stained-glass windows, reveal the differences and affinities between their symbols, and would trace a polychrome map of the human unconscious as projected on the screen of history.

SYMBOLS AND LIFE

For the second time, led by the hand of a learned and dedicated man, we venture into a vast and mysterious palace, seemingly boundless in time and space. It is fortunate that the author of this book, an expert and confident guide, precedes us, opening windows and turning on lights, illuminating the dark corners of the world of symbolism.

In my opinion, this exploration of the symbolism of Oriental rugs, because of its wider horizon and greater depth, is even more important than the one the same author conducted a few years ago. Like the second part of Beethoven's *Third Symphony,* the second part of *Don Quixote,* and Mark Twain's *Huckleberry Finn,* this sequel is far superior to the first work. With his mind in inspired flight, with the treasure chest of his scholarship, the author attains a splendid cultural maturity in this fascinating book.

Since symbols have become one of the most important components of our civilization, anything that may help to understand them better will also help to a better understanding among men. The language of fanatic dogma is based on rigid terms; the language of science, on metaphors. And the metaphor is basically a symbol, the expression of something ineffable. For this reason the language of science needs the vividness of similes and images. The ever-increasing progress of atomic physics, psychiatry, and all the natural sciences is based on the bold and prodigal use of metaphors and symbols.

Foreword to *Signs of Life* by Harry Raphaelian, New York, Anatol Sivas Publication, 1957; published in *International Record of Medicine 171*:116, 1958.

Our modern life as a whole is influenced by symbols that sometimes stimulate world harmony and progress and sometimes, unfortunately, incite hatred, destruction, and war. Man has always been, as Goethe said, "outwardly limited but inwardly limitless."

Man first appeared on our planet as a pitifully frail and helpless living being. But in the bony box of his skull a treasure was hidden. The spark of intelligence harbored in his brain compelled him to defy and eventually to master Nature.

One momentous day he learned how to increase the strength and the length of his arm by carving the first eoliths or stone axes, which he used first as weapons, later as tools, and finally as chisels. With this new tool, man was able to engrave upon a fragment of Nature a psychic form that existed only in his mind. On the day he began drawing on the moist stone walls of caves—first for *magic* purposes and later for *aesthetic* reasons—man created *art* and *science,* his two future supreme activities.

Sometimes he drew representations of the *natural* forms he saw around him—women, hunters, beasts, and bees; from these baroque biologic forms, the surrealistic art of our time developed. At other times, he enjoyed producing purely *geometric* forms—which Plato would later consider the most authentic expression of pure beauty and from which the cubist and abstract art of our time developed.

Art, therefore, preceded writing. Since it is the transmission of thought by means of graphic or plastic signs, writing in the beginning was ideographic and pictographic. Images were used before man learned to represent sounds in phonetic writing. The representation of objects and persons was the first means of communicating thought. This was followed by symbolic and hieroglyphic writing. When language and writing were developed to what they are today, there were buried in the spoken and written word countless images, emotions, and concepts that could not be adequately expressed in words and therefore became symbols.

These limitations in the expression of thought had two consequences: human communication became more and more difficult and even dangerous, originating semantic misunderstanding among individuals and peoples that resulted in quarrels and wars; it also repressed at the bottom levels of art and human thought fragments of ideas, concepts, and emotions that took refuge in the symbolic art of primitive, archaic, and classical peoples and in the art of the individual artist in all eras. Like sleeping fossils of the mind, these fragments have been waiting for centuries for the loving hand that would awaken them and expose them to the light that would reveal their true color and meaning.

Such has been the patient labor of love accomplished by the author of this book. As a psychiatrist, I applaud his achievement. Today the new organicistic approach to psychiatry confirms the existence of a metabolic and biochemical substratum of psychoses. But if we are able to understand the psychologic content of neuroses by interpreting the data of personal biography, the psychologic content of psychoses *cannot* be interpreted on a personalistic basis. If we want to understand the meaning of the broken mirror of delusions, of hallucinations and dreams of the psychotic, we must study the images existing in the *collective* stratum of the unconscious mind. These images are the same as those found in the myths, legends, and lore of primitive peoples as well as in hieroglyphic and symbolic art. This explains why the study of symbols is so valuable as a means to understanding the significance of the psychotic material found in schizophrenia and other mental diseases.

Symbols are also invaluable in understanding ourselves and our fellow men, in the appreciation of art, and in facilitating human relations and communication. Human gestures are also living symbols, and gestures are made with the hands—the first thing to move when a human being is born and the last to move when he dies.

If the tongue as a vehicle of intelligence represents the brain, the hands have always symbolized the heart. Classic authors believed that special veins linked the hands with the heart, particularly the finger on which the wedding ring is placed, a gesture symbolic of the surrender of the heart.

The hand that created symbols, whether with the polished stone tools of prehistoric man or with the brush and chisel of the Renaissance artist, was the supreme vehicle of human impulses charged with emotion. The knowledge and understanding of such symbols, as presented in this book, may one day lead us universally to that most noble of all symbols representing peace and love—hands clasped in brotherhood.

ON THE PSYCHOLOGY OF CHESS

The King immediately fell flat on his back, and lay perfectly still.
Through the Looking Glass (Lewis Carroll)

C hess, a harmless-looking game, is one of man's bloodiest and most erotic battlegrounds.

Through the ages, over the little carved pieces of ivory, gold, bone, wood, and even clay have shone the sunlight through stained-glass windows in convents, the candlelight from silver candelabras in castles, the flickering blue flame of oil lamps in roadside inns, and the silvery moonlight through prison windows. The enigmatic little pieces have always captured man's soul and have made men like Charlemagne and Napoleon, John Huss, the philosopher, and Alphonse X, the Wise King of Spain, spend impassioned hours at the magic board.

At the chessboard have sat sultans, kings and caliphs, knights, monks, artisans and peasants. And almost always they have been men. For women seldom play chess. Women, who have attained greatness in art, science, and sports, have never displayed much interest or talent in chess. Women here and there have played chess but have never become outstanding players. Sinclair Lewis, with the mysterious intuition of the artist, wrote in *Cass Timberlane:* "He was worried. When she [Jinny Marshland] just loved chess, a game which has been truly mastered by no woman since Queen Elizabeth, she was hiding things." This seems strange, more so when one considers that the most active and aggressive piece in chess is a woman—the daring Amazon of the chessboard—the Queen.

But the answer to this riddle is simple. Women do not play chess because psychologically they *do not need* to play chess. And because men *need* to play chess, the great chess players of the world have been men.

The history of chess has been told many times and always in different ways. Its invention has been attributed to Greeks, Romans, Babylonians, Egyptians, Hebrews, Persians, Indians, Arabs, and Spaniards.

Chess was probably born in India about 5000 years ago. The poets of India referred to it frequently by its Sanskrit name, *chaturanga,* meaning the four elements of an army: elephants, horses, chariots, and men. In the sixth century the game spread to Persia. The Mohammedans, together with their swords and their sweeping empire, carried it west. The Caliphs after the seventh dynasty brought it to Europe. Around chess legend spins its multicolored wheel, and the names of the fabulous Harun-al-Rashid, the Caliph of *The Thousand and One Nights,* and Charlemagne glitter in the history of chess.

Spain, France, Scandinavia, and England learned to play chess, and the Crusaders already knew the game when ragged but victorious they reached the Holy Land.

Lasker, the great chess player, for 26 years champion of the world, wrote in his book *Lasker's Chess Primer:* "Chess originated from warfare. In olden times two armies opposed to each other took up their positions in nearly straight lines, separated by a nearly level plane. A general, to make his plans clear to his officers, sketched the position and indicated movements of bodies of men. In this way military games such as chess were generated. Possibly Hannibal before the battle of Cannae drew lines and placed stones on a board to explain his intended strategy for that battle. For the purpose of teaching strategy, the battlefield was represented by the chessboard. It was given the shape of a square, divided into 64 squares, usually coloured White and Black alternately."

To understand the psychologic meaning of chess, we must know first the psychoanalytic equivalence of the symbols in the subconscious mind: *God-King-Father,* the triad representing in its respective cosmic, hierarchical, and family spheres the supreme power over man; and *Virgin-Queen-Mother,* the protective triad where man always found refuge, whether as a believer, a subject, or a son.

Man, in the prehistoric period, had a holy terror of gods, particularly of the gods of vengeance of primitive mythology, the unknown supreme cosmic power he believed was responsible for everything that happened to him. This terror he later transferred to the king, or the chief of his tribe, who ruled over him, and ultimately to his father or the head of his clan or family, who continued to rule his actions and life. Unconsciously man has harbored a hidden desire of revenge against this unceasing power over him throughout his entire evolution, and has nursed the desire to destroy such power— *God-King-Father*—and become his own master. This deicide-regicidepatricide desire has flourished in man's subconscious mind since the beginning of mankind.

In contrast, the *Virgin-Queen-Mother* triad, always kind and prolific, was a life-giving, benevolent, and protective symbol that man could and did use against the hated and feared *God-King-Father,* as exemplified in Greek mythology by the struggles of the goddesses against the gods, in Roman history by the intrigues of the empresses against the emperors, and in daily life by the frequent domestic alliance between mother and son against the power of the father.

According to the psychoanalytic concept of a child's emotional problems, every child in his unconscious mind relives the history of our primitive past and inherits the feelings of hate, fear, and passion ascribed to our prehistoric ancestors. The child between five and seven years of age goes through a stage—the Oedipus complex (from the Greek legend of Oedipus who killed his father Laius and married his mother Jocasta)—where he wishes to kill his father, whom he unconsciously hates and fears, with the help of his mother, whose love he wants only for himself, just as his prehistoric ancestors wanted to kill the head of their tribe and marry his wives.

History and literature offer countless examples of the Oedipus complex: Henri Beyle (Stendhal), reminiscing about his childhood, once said: "I was in love with my mother. I was seven when I lost her. I always wanted to kiss her. I hated my father when he interrupted our kisses. . . ." The philosopher Diderot remembered his savage impulses as a child "to wring his father's neck and marry his mother." Baudelaire, the violent French poet, before he was seven "secretly and passionately loved his mother and fiercely hated his stepfather Aupick," in whom he sensed a rival.

When a child grows up, he overcomes the incestuous phase of the Oedipus complex, but he never rids himself of it entirely. His unconscious retains it and will respond to any call that symbolically may satisfy his patricidal yearnings.

Chess offers a unique way to accomplish this unconscious desire to kill the father with the help of the mother. For what is the purpose of chess? Coriat, the psychiatrist, answered this question by quoting Lewis Carroll: "The King immediately fell flat on his back and lay perfectly still." The object of the chess player is to *checkmate* the opponent's King. The word *checkmate* is of Persian origin: Check means Shah, monarch, and mate signifies death. To capture the King and destroy him is the goal and end of a chess game.

There are different ways to destroy a man. Man has always considered his masculine virility his supreme attribute of power and domination. The Mad Monk, Rasputin, referred to his sexual organ as "the real scepter of Russia." To destroy such power by castration, thus condemning him permanently to the tragic sexual incapacity of the eunuch, is the surest, most absolute, and cruelest way to destroy man. In prehistoric times parricide meant not only to kill the chief of the tribe, but also to castrate him and then, in a cannibalistic ritual, to devour the symbol of his masculine vigor, thus not only depriving him of the source of all his power, but also absorbing that power and becoming one with him. Savage tribes still practice this symbolic ritual. And patricide by castration is the psychologic interpretation of the *checkmate* in chess.

As in Lewis Carroll's *Through the Looking Glass,* the King and Queen in chess are subconsciously identified by the players with their parents. One's Queen is one's mother and the opponent's King becomes one's father. Oriental chess pieces have the shape of human figures. But even modern pieces have a phallic symbolism which has been pointed out by psychoanalysts. We must remember that the Castle or Rook originally was an elephant, which psychoanalytically is a phallic symbol. The Bishop also has been described as a phallic symbol. The erotic symbolism of the horse (Knight)—direct descendant of the centaur and the satyr—is also obvious.

A chess game becomes a sublimation of the unconscious desire to commit patricide, latent in all men, and dramatizes on the board the internal conflict and the horrible doubts of a Hamlet. It gratifies the aggressive instinct of a son toward his father, and it has the antagonistic as well as the homosexual character that the struggles between father and son have. To *checkmate* the opponent's King in chess is equivalent to castrating and devouring him, becoming one with him in a ritual of symbolic homosexualism and cannibalistic communion, thus responding to the remnants of the infantile Oedipus complex.

Kreymborg called chess "a war in the most mysterious jungles of the human soul," and Oliver Wendell Holmes qualified it as "brutal."

Psychoneurotic persons find in chess a unique way to free their repressed tendencies. For such players every game is a chance to become the aggressor (subconsciously renewing infantile activities such as playing with toy soldiers) and to dramatize their pattern of life and sadist-masochist tendencies. Chess magically eliminates their anxiety by erasing the frontiers between reality and phantasy. It has a therapeutic value because it shelters, protects, and liberates them at the same time.

Psychoanalytically the personality of chess players can be divided roughly into two groups: the romantic chess players, who *want to win* and use the attack and combination technique, and the classical chess players, who *do not want to lose* and play a static war of nerves game. Extroverts play an aggressive game with the white pieces, while introverts prefer a defensive game with the black pieces.

Even chess moves have a profound psychoanalytic meaning. Some players constantly protect their Queen-Mother in order to attain greater power over the King-Father. To crown Pawns and to exchange them for Queens is to reinforce the attack against the King, by converting Pawns—weak little men, psychoanalytically interpreted as castrated—into strong Amazon-like women with a tremendous sex and war drive.

Some players are afraid to lose the Queen and play that piece with great caution because subconsciously they associate it with their mother whom they were afraid to lose when they were children. For the same reason, the capture of the opponent's Queen reinforces the mother fixation by separating the mother from the father. The opposite type is the player with a complex of maternal omnipotence, who risks his Queen time and again because of his blind faith in the strength and invincibility of his mother. Still other players are pathologically afraid to lose a Bishop or to knock down a Pawn—which subconsciously they identify with phallic symbols—because it means castration to them.

Thus have psychoanalysts attempted to interpret the impetuous tactics of Morphy; the closed games of permanent positions of Steinitz; the unorthodox games of Tartakower; the imaginative strategy of Alekhine; the war of nerves games of Lasker; the splendid finales of Capablanca; the optimistic intuition of Bogoljubow, and the tactics of the rest of the masters of the chessboard.

But we must not be carried away by the extreme enthusiasm of such investigators. The genius of the great masters of chess cannot be interpreted only on the psychoanalytic profiles of their tactics. No, the demon in the genius is too powerful an eagle to be caged by psychoanalysis.

Psychoanalysis, however, has helped to lift the veil from the mystery of Paul Morphy, the greatest of all American chess masters. He was born in New Orleans, June 22, 1837, of a Spanish father and a French mother. His father taught him to play chess at the age of ten. Two years later he could beat all his relatives at the game, including an uncle who was then champion of the city. At the age of twelve he beat the French champion, Rousseau, and the Hungarian champion, Lowenthal. During the next eight years he studied law. At twenty he won the International Chess Tournament in New York. The following year he went to London and Paris, where he beat the best chess players of Europe blindfolded and playing several games at the same time. The entire Chess Club of Versailles played against him in a body and lost. In Paris' Café de la Régence, the mecca of chess players and scene of the past glories of the great Phillidor, Morphy played against eight men at the same time with his eyes blindfolded. After seven hours he beat the first one and three hours later all the others. While the game was in progress he did not eat or even drink water. After the game he escaped to his hotel with a delirious and cheering public at his heels. After a few hours of sleep, he dictated from memory all the moves in the games he had just won, as well as hundreds of variations of each one.

His chess prowess made him famous almost overnight. Duchesses and princesses fought over him in Paris. At a banquet in his honor he was presented with a bust of himself crowned with laurel leaves. When he returned to New York there were more banquets. He was given a chessboard made of mother of pearl and ebony with pieces of gold and silver. He was also given a watch with chess figures in place of numerals. At another banquet in his honor in Boston, Oliver Wendell Holmes, Longfellow, and Quincey were among the guests who paid him homage. He received a eulogy unparalleled in history: "Morphy is greater than Caesar, for he came and, *without seeing,* he conquered."

Morphy returned to New Orleans, where he issued a challenge to one and all. He offered his opponents the advantage of a Pawn and the right to start the game. No one accepted and his meteoric career of barely eighteen months came to an end.

The rest of Morphy's history is shrouded in mystery. Seized by a sudden hatred for chess, he decided to give it up and to start life anew. But he could not shut out the past. People saw in Morphy only an ex-champion of chess. He failed as a lawyer and he failed in love. After aimlessly wandering through Cuba and France, already affected by paranoia, he died of apoplexy at the age of forty-seven.

Ernest Jones made an excellent study of Morphy. His theory is that Morphy was destroyed by a success that he could not resist. Already as a child he wanted to defeat his father, who had been his first chess teacher. Later he transferred the father-image to all his opponents; subconsciously he continued to see his father in each and every one of them and wanted to defeat them, or, psychoanalytically, to castrate them.

Morphy's genius at chess was an effort to sublimate the neurosis that threatened him, hiding like a scorpion in the innermost recesses of his spirit. As he won one game after another, Morphy's uninterrupted success in defeating-castrating all his opponents-fathers began to weigh on his mind. This Raskolnikow of chess finally felt the full impact of his crime and was overwhelmed by subconscious guilt. The paternal image, castrated in each game, would reappear again and again with each new player, and Morphy had to keep on destroying it in an effort to liberate himself from the invincible ghost.

When he finally reached the pinnacle of his glory, Morphy discovered that the pedestal of his genius had become a wall that fenced him in. Chess, which at first had liberated him of his complexes, had finally set him apart from the world of reality.

Perhaps Morphy, short, frail, childish-looking, kind, and unassuming, unable any longer to fully satisfy on the chessboard his erotic fantasies of aggressive and homosexual encounters with his father, completely surrendered himself to his neurosis and finally became a paranoiac. For some happy months he had been able to relieve and overcome his neurotic conflict in chess. When he gave up chess, he could not return to reality and was lost. He never loved a woman, and he never succeeded in any other way in the world of men. When chess, which had become a sickness, was eliminated from his life, the last flicker of genius in his spirit also died. Nietzsche said that "there are sick people who would die if cured of their illness, because it is the only thing they have in life."

Thus we see that men play chess for a psychologic reason. And for the same reason women rarely care for chess. Over the chessboard men come to grips with the Oedipus complex latent in all of them and satisfy their patricidal impulses. Women go through the Electra complex, which is love for the father and hate for the mother. Therefore, they have no need to play chess. When they do so, there is a psychiatric reason, as in the following case.

Years ago I had a patient in Valencia, Spain, who had married at the age of fifteen. She was sickly and frail and had frequent undiagnosed pains and body ailments. Her husband, a young man as mentally immature as she was, came from a very religious and conservative family. Consequently, his wife was subjected to all sorts of social and religious restrictions imposed on her by her husband and his family. My patient tried to convince herself that she was happy. She lacked the courage to free herself and was being slowly choked by her surroundings.

And then her husband and her father-in-law taught her chess. Soon after, she could beat all her relatives. She had identified the opponent's King with her husband. That little carved wooden piece was for her the symbol of the husband she loved and hated in the same breath. To defeat him in the final checkmate was to fulfill her most cherished subconscious dreams of revenge and freedom. The Queen was a symbol of the woman she herself wanted to be, an all-powerful and fearless Amazon who on the chessboard could do everything she herself wanted to do in real life. Every time she "castrated" (checkmated) her opponent's King-husband, she attained her much-desired liberty.

This charming lady is still playing chess and has become a sort of local champion. Should she ever become strong enough to regain her freedom, she will stop playing chess and will even hate the game, which today for her is just a stage where she is fighting and winning her marital battle.

And this is perhaps the secret of that sphinx called chess, which, like most sphinxes—aren't most sphinxes women?—yields her secret only to men: Chess is a magic board of dreams where man fights one of the most transcendental battles for his peace of mind.

VII. the artist's world

THE PSYCHOLOGIC IMPACT OF
ATOMIC SCIENCE ON MODERN ART

THE PHILOSOPHIC BACKGROUND OF THE NEW ATOMIC SCIENCE

The new scientific ideology of the twentieth century.

*t*he year 1900 is a decisive date in the history of human thought. In that year there began to appear on the intellectual horizon of the new century a series of new ideas that differed radically from those that formed the philosophic and scientific subsoil of the nineteenth century. Now, half a century later, these new concepts have already become integrated into an ideology peculiar to our time.

Man today is demonstrating the great creative value of ideas. Backed by new theories of physics, he is succeeding in harnessing even the remotest stars in equations formulated by a human brain in the solitude of a laboratory. Just as the Copernican theory was the educating principle of the modern age, so the ideas of a four-dimensional universe, curvilinear space, and finite spheres, joined to the present-day autonomy of each scientific discipline, mark the historic countenance of our century. Just as the sun sheds different colors on the countryside as it rises, so the new ideology of the twentieth century is coloring all human activities, from scientific thought and artistic accomplishment to the humblest routine tasks.

The year 1900 also marks the beginning of a historical crisis in the evolution of scientific thought. It is a date comparable to the

A paper presented at the Thirteenth International Congress of Psychology, Stockholm, Sweden, July, 1951; published in *Journal of Clinical and Experimental Psychopathology 13*:40, 1952.

year 1300—Dante's hour—when a new conception of the world was born that was to prevail for many generations. One system of scientific convictions has succeeded another, not by continuity but in jumps, which makes the transition even more dramatic.

The crisis in scientific thought, which brought in its wake a crisis in artistic thought, left modern man without a solid universe by upsetting his convictions, by isolating him in a vacuum, and by shattering the ideas that underlay the world of the nineteenth century. But thought, like nature, abhors a vacuum, and tends to fill it immediately with culture patterns, just as the body fills with conjunctive tissue any hollow that occurs in it.

In modern life, science acquires the character of a supreme organ that pumps animating strength into other artistic or philosophic organs, which are more adipose or conjunctive and less vital than scientific thought. To sketch the lines of modern scientific thought is to trace the framework within which the other forms of contemporary life, especially that plastic creativity we call modern art, can be interpreted.

At the turn of the century it was thought that everything had already been invented: since 1880 people had been using internal combustion engines, which later made possible the development of automobiles and airplanes; electromagnetic waves had been discovered by Hertz in 1887; the first radiogram had been sent from the Isle of Wight in 1898; the first public telephone had been inaugurated in New Haven, Connecticut, in 1879; the germ theory had been in circulation since 1860. Yet if a man who had been in a state of suspended animation for the last half century were to wake up today and look about him, how dumbfounded he would be by the changes that have occurred in the world around him!

Has the universe changed, then? No, the universe has not changed throughout the course of history; what has changed is only our mental attitude toward the universe. Life has existed for twelve hundred million years; man has existed for about a million years; he has made use of his brain for his own progress for fifty thousand years; he has been able to record his thoughts for about six thousand years; but he has been using science as an educational factor for only about three hundred years. In the last three centuries, the mission of science has been to draw up for man an inventory of the universe, to reveal to him all available possibilities and how to use these possibilities for his own betterment, and sometimes for his own destruction.

Perhaps no other science has influenced human thought as profoundly as physics. Starting from that historical crisis that we call the Renaissance, physics has tried to discover the laws governing material objects in time and space. Only a century ago physics was still subject to the laws of causality that ruled the universe with an iron hand. But the development of mathematics—genius' chosen field—has revolutionized the physics of the twentieth century, thus marking a critical moment in the history of civilization. The new physics has brought forth manifold geniuses, just as the Florentine art of the *qauttrocento* produced a plethora of artists.

The change in our mental attitude toward the universe has signified notable progress for man. This progress is due less to scientific discovery than to the conception of new relationships among various ideas; it is due more to man's ability to see old physical and mental phenomena through new eyes, following the rule set down by the German mathematician of the last century, Karl Jacobi: *Man muss immer umkehren* (One must always turn things around).

This new spirit of scientific research has caused the basic concepts underlying the universe up to 1900, such as space and time, inertia, energy, and symmetry, to be upset by a demon that has shaken physics, shattered the Aristotelian notion of natural motion and converted these classic ideas into theories like space-time intervals, the curvature of the universe, and atomic vortices.

HISTORICOPHILOSOPHIC ROOTS OF THE NEW ATOMIC SCIENCE

By "atomic science" we understand the new physicomathematical thought initiated at the beginning of the century, which has supported the most revolutionary changes in the history of human thought.

In the mind of the layman atomic science is usually associated with the spectacular explosions that marked a supreme advance in the science of killing. But in our study we shall not speak of the atom bomb, which is only a "practical" aspect (what was Dante's *Inferno,* after all, in comparison?) of the physicomathematical thought that has governed the development of atomic energy.

What we shall do here is to sketch the philosophic profile of the principal advances in physical and mathematical thought in the last 50 years, and to study its repercussions in other intellectual activities of man in our time.

Man needed so many years to develop his ideas about the atomic structure of matter because the conceptions of the atom were from the very beginning in apparent contradiction with the testimony of his own senses. Sight and touch tell us always that our body, and everything that surrounds us, is solid and continuous matter. The idea that matter is neither solid nor continuous is as fantastic to certain people in 1952 as it was, even to the most enlightened, in the fifth century B.C., when the Greek philosophers expressed for the first time the theory of the atomic structure of matter. So fantastic was it considered that when a wandering philosopher called Democritus of Abdera said, in 420 B.C., that things were made up of an infinite number of invisible atoms separated by large spaces and in constant motion, educated men thought he was mad, and advised him to take treatment from a physician called Hippocrates. Democritus, a legendary figure, adopted the atomic theory of his master Leucippus—the true creator of that theory, according to some—who established that the "essence" of the matter that forms water, or, in other words, the immutable particles that change only with reference to their spatial relationships, does not vary when the water changes to ice and then changes back to water.[A] Democritus, one day at the beach, picked up in one hand some sand and in the other a little sea water and explained to his disciples that matter, like sand, was formed of minute grains which he called "atoms" (that is, indivisibles) and that the structure of matter was not continuous as the water he had in his hand seemed to be. We are also indebted to Democritus for the idea that the light emitted by the Milky Way proceeded from innumerable stars invisible to ordinary sight, a hypothesis that Galileo confirmed two thousand years later as he looked through his telescope at the stars in the skies of Venice.

A century later, Epicurus of Samos continued this theory, establishing the existence of atoms endowed with "internal liberty, or free will" allowing them to break away from their directions, which, according to Democritus, were predetermined.

But eighteen hundred years had to pass before chemistry would become a scientific discipline and atomism could be confirmed, thereby establishing atomic structure as the only explanation for the laws governing chemical reaction. Dalton, in 1808, and Avogadro, in 1811–1817, confirmed the molecular atomic structure of matter; Lavoisier in the eighteenth century discovered the law of the conservation of matter; and Mayer and Helmholtz discovered the law of conservation of energy. These contributions clinched the doctrine of atomism, full confirmation of which came in our time when it became possible to count atoms. In biology, atomic structure was also confirmed when it was established that the transformation of one type of molecule into another in the metabolic processes of organic matter came about through the liberation or absorption of energy, as happens in the physical reactions that take place in inanimate matter. With the advent of these doctrines, the world keeps on being a machine, but a machine made up of much tinier parts than before.

The seventeenth and eighteenth centuries are dominated by mechanistic thought, making of the inanimate world a self-perpetuating system in which all changes take place in accordance with natural laws. Copernican thought scientifically replaces the old ideas symbolized by Dante's concept that the earth is the center of the universe and is encircled by ten spheres.

Nevertheless, even in an age as scientifically important as the age of Newton, science attempts to prove that God is the creator of the law of gravity and of the other physical laws of the universe. The role of man in the universe is both elevated and lowered in this supreme attempt to conciliate science and faith. In that eternal conflict between tradition and observation, the history of human thought can be summarized.

For the physicists of the nineteenth century, the universe was built on the scaffold of Newtonian laws of motion. They took no account of the idea of force, only of material changes. Matter was thought to be immutable. The most they accepted was the idea that combustion liberated energy, although they did not believe that matter was transformed into energy. The chemical elements were considered indestructible and it was not thought that one atom could be transformed into another, as in the romantic dreams of ancient alchemists. Only the impossibility of explaining phenomena such as atomic stability, roentgen rays, and radioactivity indicated that classic, mechanical, and deterministic physics were incapable of interpreting all the phenomena of the universe.[B]

The quantum theory: milestone in atomic physics.

In 1900, Max Planck, in Berlin, was convinced that the spectrum of radiation of dark bodies could not be explained by the principles of classic mechanics. Instead, he thought that irradiated energy was not emitted continuously but rather in quanta or finite quantities, proportionate in each case to the frequency of the radiations, expressed in a figure that was later called Planck's constant.[C]

This theory was received with great skepticism; it seemed strange to abandon the wave theory and return to the old corpuscular concept of light, but Einstein proved this theory by applying it to the emission of electrons by metals and to the thermic properties of crystals.

The inspired intuition of Max Planck inclined him to the hypothesis that the emission of light by radiant bodies came about through tiny indivisible explosions, an idea that struck people as fantastic as that of a bullet reaching its mark by short leaps.[D] This hypothesis was expressed with the modesty characteristic of genius, and remained submerged in the stormy ocean of speculative theories raging at the beginning of the century. But it meant that atoms, too vast to be considered the cornerstones of the universe, were being replaced by something infinitely tinier: the *quanta* or leaps of energy.

The quantum was thus born: the smallest possible action at play in a physical phenomenon. It was a bold concept that later would grow gigantically and become a veritable quantic revolution, forcing the dethronement of the rigid laws of ancient physics by laws of probability. Planck had demonstrated, at first only to a select elite of physicists and mathematicians, and as the years rolled by to the whole world, that the philosophic concept of continuity in the universe was only statistically apparent. The classic theories were the confirmation of the imperfection of our senses which created the idea of continuity in a universe where everything was discontinuous and spasmodic.

Planck's theory represents the cornerstone of the entire atomic science of our century, and its formulation was perhaps the most crucial act in the history of science. The layman is still not fully aware of its importance. The man responsible for it has not yet received his due. Laurels do not always crown the heads of true victors in the Marathons of science.

The quantum theory proved that not only matter was discontinuous, but also energy.[E] This theory contained the germ of the theory of relativity. The atomism of energy also implied the atomism of time, since the new vision of the universe could not be static, but dynamic. In a way, it was a pity that the quantum theory was formulated five years before Einstein published his theory of relativity, because had it been the reverse, it would not have been difficult to conceive that if matter and energy were simply different facets of the same reality, and if matter was discontinuous, then energy had to be also. The veil that hid this elementary truth could not be lifted for research men because in 1900 relativity was unknown and the ideas of Planck were considered by many as simply the expression of an empiric thought. Planck had to wait more than a quarter of a century to see the blossoming of his concept, which would entirely transform the structure of the universe in the mind of the present-day scientist.[F]

The quantum theory reduced matter, until then considered solid, to "waves of probability," an idea from which would be born, forty-five years later, the atom bomb. At first the public did not perceive the importance of the theory, perhaps because it is still so difficult for the popular mind to grasp anything expressed in terms of pure, higher mathematics without symbolic, graphic dramatization. But the scientific revolution was already on the march. Physics had been shaken to its very foundations.

The philosophic meaning of Einstein's theory of relativity.

The next stage in the development of the new physics began with the revelation of Einstein's theories which reduced to naught the old concepts of space and time. It was claimed that the concept of absolutely simultaneous events in different places had no physical meaning because the speed of the most rapid signals (light) is the same for all observers.[G]

Einstein's contribution to modern "atomistic" thought is that he revolutionized ideas about space and time, just as the quantum theory revolutionized ideas about matter and energy. The physics of the last century was materialistic and mechanistic. Today, matter is no longer considered solid, but rather a hollow in space and time, a tangle of electricity, a wave of probability undulating in a void.

Einstein has changed the twentieth century as well as mathematics. Instead of level Euclidian space, he has created curved space, the curvature of which varies from one point to another, and the intensity of which at one point measures the intensity of the field of gravitation at the same point. But the fundamental philosophic significance of Einstein's ideas lies in the creation of a theory incorrectly called "of relativity" (since the relativity refers only to the values of reality—space, time, matter, energy—which were until then considered absolutes), in contrast with the absolute, which is human awareness of the aforesaid values minus the classic notion of the infinite. What this theory does is to make the universe in which we live a finite sphere, subject therefore to laws which can be investigated by man.

The fundamental metaphysical concepts of space and time, matter and motion, cause and effect, have therefore been replaced by new ideas and have suffered a holocaust under the impact of the new science.[H]

Philosophic topography of the new atomic science.

Recently a voice (E. M. Forster) was raised making the "implacable offensive of science" responsible for the present chaos. But the civilization of the twentieth century, like a bicycle in motion, cannot stop short, because the only thing that supports it is its own motion directing it to new frontiers of energy. Just the same, the impact has been terrible. Scientific tradition, with other traditions, has suffered a tremendous shock. Once again science has collided with tradition—made up of the ideas of the past, according to Freud's concept of the superego—which plays a very important role in human life.

As a result of these portentous years, the complex structural edifice of classical science has crumbled. Modern science speaks a language totally different from that of former times. The practical difference between the Newtonian theory of gravity and Einstein's is probably small, but the theoretical difference is tremendous. When we speak, for example, of space-time instead of space and time as separate entities, we are simplifying scientific language, just as a physician by the name of Copernicus did in his own doctrine many centuries ago. When we describe the universe as a four-dimensional sphere of finite diameter, we are simplifying the concept of this universe. When we refer to curved instead of straight lines in the theory of relativity, we are witnessing a semantic change alongside a scientific one. Ideas have changed and with them, language.

If we examine this gigantic revolution in the spheres of physics and mathematics, we see that it has resulted in the disintegration of the old ideas prevailing up to 1900, conceiving the universe as a solid and immutable stage on which our life is acted out.

This picture has been converted into one of a fluid world where nothing is constant, fixed, or immutable, and in which waves of energy, laws of probability, discontinuity, change by leaps, relativity of space, and the unity of space and time have replaced the former rigid notions.[I]

To sum up, the characteristics of physical atomism that have left an indelible mark on the face of our times are the following: (a) a new science has been established—atomic physics—idealistic in its conceptions and so hypothetical that one of its basic factors, the concept of the electron, is purely imaginative; (b) as against observation and experimentation as bases of the biologist's work, and as against the physicist's measurements, the new mathematics accepts reason as superior to experiment for arriving at an integral comprehension of the universe; (c) the discontinuity of matter is accepted; (d) matter and energy have been accepted to be identical; (e) it has been admitted that space is finite; (f) the relativity of time has been accepted; (g) the continuity of time and space has been indicated; (h) it has been accepted that the universe is curved and four-dimensional; (i) it has been indicated that matter moves by leaps of energy, and the latter has been accepted as the basis of modern physics; (j) the substratum of mental life has been reduced to molecules and irreversible processes subject to physical determinism.[J, K]

These principles summarize the new scientific philosophy elaborated from 1900 onward. The psychologic impact of such philosophy on the mind of the artist has determined the features of modern art.

THE PSYCHODYNAMICS OF MODERN ART

Interrelations of scientific and artistic thought.

One of the characteristics of modern psychology is the broadening of its field of action so that it can be applied practically to a better understanding of human experience and conduct. In the ninety-odd years that have transpired since its birth as the stepdaughter of philosophy and physiology, psychology has become wide enough to embrace problems as varied as the neurohumoral mechanism for transmission of the nervous impulse and the determining factors of man's desire to understand the universe.[L]

Like the new physics, modern psychology is a science of relationships. For that reason, we consider as worthy of study the interrelation between atomic science and modern art, both genuinely representative manifestations of the spirit of our age.

All through history scientific truth has influenced artistic thought and vice versa. The artist does not deliberately reflect scientific truth in his art, but if the climate of an age is saturated with new ideas, the artist—the most sensitive barometer there is—reflects those ideas in his work. Here we cannot help recalling Zola's wise dictum: *"L'Art c'est la Nature vue par un tempérament."* This temperament of the artist is subject to the influence of anything that happens on the horizon of his time. To evoke the scientific revolution of our century and its psychologic impact on the artist is to point out unperceived facts that may impart new significance to ideologic tendencies influencing the artist's future activity.

In attempting to establish the impact of atomic science on modern art, we are anticipating to a certain extent the interpretations of the historians of the future, when the perspective of our time will be more serene.

Just as physics and mathematics in the seventeenth and eighteenth centuries helped to discover the circulation of the blood and respiratory physiochemistry, so scientific progress in the nineteenth century has had widespread cultural repercussions.

In 1865, Claude Bernard in his *Introduction a l'Étude de la Médecine Expérimentale* formulated the principles of a new medical science, which was considered a positive science based on reason and the experimental method. His lectures and experiments at the Collège de France attracted physiologists, chemists like Berthelot, philosophers like Janet, and historians like Renan. At the same time, Trousseau's clinical lectures and later those of Charcot at La Salpêtrière, were attracting numerous writers, philosophers, historians, and artists.

The repercussions were disconcerting. Renan asserted that history was a science like chemistry; Taine affirmed that vice and virtue were chemical products like vitriol and sugar, and, inspired by Claude Bernard, formulated his deterministic theory of heredity and environment; Victor Hugo declared in 1859 that the mission of the poet and the philosopher was to treat social problems as the naturalist treated zoologic problems; Flaubert affirmed that the novel should be scientific. These influences gave rise to novels that were real clinical histories, like those of the Goncourt brothers and Émile Zola, just as later on Freud and psychoanalysis were responsible for the psychologic novel, which is still the most widely read literature of our day.

The artist and his times.

For the artist, to live is to accomplish the bidimensional task of experiencing life from without and giving free play to his own spontaneity. The artist is above all a man subject to a double series of biologic stimuli, proceeding both from his milieu and his own individuality.

Ortega y Gasset has spoken of man's double dimension: his historical dimension (his heredity) and his ambition for the future. History and destiny: both factors are the determinants of the equation of life, the unfolding of which may be at times as clear-cut as the demonstration of a mathematical theorem.

The artist, who is first a man and next a professional, determines his organic adjustment through his sensory organs, and his being is made up of himself and his "circumstance," as Von Uexküll has shown.

The artist of the last half century has been subjected to the historical climate of our time, in which the most prominent influence has been the scientific revolution. In past ages the artist used to translate the ideas of the governing class, using as his raw material the landscapes, figures, and backgrounds of his time. In the atomic age, which started at the beginning of this century, the artist has been governed by the force of the new ideas forming the ideologic organism of the new century.

More artisan than bohemian, the modern artist is both a businessman in his transactions and a scientist in his techniques. That is the principal difference between the artist of today, who puts everything into the profound study of his theme and puts his technique to the service of an idea, and the classic artist of yesteryear for whom inspiration and improvisation were supremely important.

Let us not forget that behind every stroke of the brush there is a hand directed by a man whose brain is permeated by the ideas of the century in which he lives. It *is* important to him that he lives in a century shaken by political movements and world wars, a century also of tremendous scientific advances that are being applied in fabulous technologic projects and apocalyptic orgies of destruction.

The brain of the modern artist, like a small cosmos, has been illuminated by the sun of new ideas, and his hand is moved by the new scientific techniques just as surely as the hand of the technician in his laboratory.

Psychohistorical profile of modern art.

In the first part of this paper we selected the date 1900, the year in which Planck formulated his quantum theory, as marking the beginning of the new atomic science.[M]

We select the year 1907, when with his "Les Demoiselles d'Avignon" Picasso gave the world his cubist manifesto, as marking the beginning of nonobjective abstract art. The connection between this new art and atomic science is the subject of the second part of this study.

Let us review briefly the historical development of modern art, its general characteristics, and the psychologic impact of atomic science on the abstract art of our time.

Up to the eighteenth century, the artist depended almost exclusively on the patronage of the Church and the royal court. After the French Revolution, it was the merchant who supported the artist with his commissions of pictures on peaceful bourgeois themes. The artist was forced to choose subjects "that would be understood." But some painters, like Courbet, Manet, Pissarro, and Seurat, rebelled, and in their rebellion were moved to use a semiscientific objective method to register light, consisting in employing pure colors that would blend in the eye of the spectator instead of on the palette of the painter, thus abstracting the form of things. Light, which so fascinated these impressionists, subconsciously undermined their interest in the form of things and in landscape as pictorial subjects.

As a reaction, and to restore the architectural structure of a theme, Cézanne later used geometry, making of "the cylinder, the cone, and the sphere" the essence of all things; and "pointillist" Seurat employed vertical, diagonal, and horizontal lines to achieve the denaturalization of persons and objects. In this way, both artists limited and denatured Nature, making of it a *continuum* of space-time, as the physicists and mathematicians would later do in the exact sciences.

Cézanne equalized the value of still life and human form as themes. As the years went by, intellectual rebels projected into the twentieth century their unorthodox impulse to analyze in abstract art the practical forms found in still life, while those rebels opposed to the supremacy of reason emphasized the dynamic space of landscape in their surrealistic compositions. Such were the psychologic determinants of the two great trends in modern art.

Cubist painting was born at the beginning of this century, under the tutelage of Braque and Picasso, out of the cult of the exotic, the ballet, the study of African masks, the interest in Negro folklore and primitivism, as well as from the hunger for knowledge sharpened by the new science.

The objective of cubism was not to achieve visual pleasure but rather to make of art a scientific-philosophic instrument of investigation, to bring into relief new concepts of the reality of the visible world. This was a revolt, analogous to the scientific revolt, against classicism. Doubting the efficacy of the senses as vehicles of knowledge, cubism fell back on the logical and plastic mind, rejecting architectural and schematic concepts of classic order.

Cubist art is incoherent because it adopts musical liberties and utilizes new combinations of known forms; in doing so, it breaks objects up, putting them together again in a new order. Its purpose is the organic development of nonsymbolic pure forms in an imaginary bidimensional space; the idea is not to paint themes, but pictures.

The planes of cubism are those of synthetic vision, which approaches the observer and does not withdraw in deceptive space, as happens in classic paintings. The frame of the picture is not a window looking out upon distance, but a limit of space. The picture is monochromatic and bidimensional, so that it may come closer to the spectator. This is a cloistered art of still life, of static interrelations and immobility.

Cubism represents the final stage of the cycle initiated by the classic painting of the *quattrocento,* which was concerned with the bulk or empty spaces of things: the painter tried to represent things objectively. Much later came the *impressionists,* who no longer painted things, but sensations; it was subjective painting, not interested in what the artist saw but rather in the very act of seeing. Cubism comes as the last act; these painters are no longer interested in things or sensations, but in ideas. They renounced objective art, like the classic, and subjective art, like the impressionistic; and instead became projective. Turning his back on the world, the painter refused to use his retina as a mirror reflecting everything around him; instead, he closed his eyes and projected his ideas.

This evolution in art runs parallel with the evolution of physics, which passed from investigating things by naturalistic observation to studying the perceptions of things, and ended by analyzing their ideologic scheme. This transition in both the scientific investigator and the artist from external reality to subjectivity and intrasubjectivity—that is, the displacement of the angle from which they viewed the universe—provides the vital interpretive clue to the evolution of scientific method and modern artistic technique.

Futurism, which was born in 1910, is interested in landscape just as cubism is interested in still life. It is an art that glorifies the dynamism of the machine, born in the north of Italy during the years when a gigantic explosion of industrial power took place there. The widespread use of machinery in industry and incipient fascism, together with the worship of power, dynamism, speed, "the dangerous life," all incubated futurism. It is an art of movement and force, of persons and animals in motion, mad streets, whirring machines, factories, and cities, which suck the spectator into their whirlpools. It is not a cloistered art like cubism; it seeks its impetus in the public square and in dynamic interrelations.

After that came *surrealism* with Dali, Ernst, de Chirico, Klee, and Tanguy. A fantastic art, it includes works characterized by deliberate incongruity and inconstancy, having as its principal aim to shock the observer with the unexpected, violating all convention and custom, creating its own laws in a lawless world. The trick of this technique was to paint with great realism each fragment of the unreal taken from a universe of phantasmagoria and nightmare; but the care taken in the painting of the component parts of the dream made the unreality possible. The themes are extraordinary visions fabricated out of ordinary, familiar things, with double images, each one representing something completely different but connected by the nonlogic of dreams. It is an art that exalts spatial, subconscious liberty; it is a visceral art, deep, cavernous, dissecting, interested in the human figure and in landscape. Remotely related to the expressionistic compulsion, it sought dynamic space and organic forms in landscape.[N]

The psychodynamics of abstract art.

Next came purely *abstract* art, which was actually born many centuries ago when the Flemish artists of the fifteenth and sixteenth centuries began to abstract, that is, to eliminate superfluous elements from their pictures, leaving only the basic factors.

That tendency has developed to the maximum in modern abstract art, having four determining factors: (a) the progress of photographic art, which convinced the painter that the camera could in many cases get results objectively superior to those achieved by the paint brush; (b) the influence of music, which inspired the artist to create a universal art, an international language of emotions that would be free in space, as music was free in time, from the provincialism of local themes; (c) scientific discoveries, especially the high-powered microscope and the long-range telescope which widened the visual horizon of man; and (d) the development of stroboscopic cameras that register all speeds.

All these factors, together with the perfecting of machinery and the introduction of cylindrical, conical, and spherical forms to replace forms found in nature, have gradually influenced the artist to abandon the universe at which he has been looking from age-old angles in favor of a universe that reveals itself in fragments and strips but which is growing daily. Not only has the traditional order of space, form, and color undergone a revolution analogous to the scientific revolution, but the factors of time and motion have been added.

In its most intellectual and geometric as well as its most emotional and romantic forms, abstract art has followed various trends that can be summarized as follows: (1) Preference for themes based on mechanical or architectonic forms, still life and inanimate objects, favoring the representation of the mechanical, the mineral, the telluric or lunar, and the machine-like. Except in surrealistic art, rarely does the animal or human figure appear in abstract art, which seems to have turned its back on the external, objective world. (2) Adoption of a limited bidimensional space, which is an end in itself, a finite space such as the Einsteinian universe. (3) The introduction of color as a dynamic element of form itself and the introduction of time and motion in an art that up to our century had been eminently static. Abstract art, like the new physics, enjoys animating the static or inanimate, as if it were attempting a unification of the living and the nonliving. (4) The desire to attain an almost mystical unity.

In abstract art, as in the new physics, there is a contrast between the rigorous austerity of its scientifically objective methods and the mysticism implied in its ultimate aim of understanding—and regulating—the universe.°

Abstract art may be classified according to its main objectives. Some of these are the representation of *abstract geometrical forms, stylized geometrical representations, abstract organic forms,* or *stylized organic forms.*

In the first group we can include pictures without a definite subject, representing only a *geometric form pure and abstract,* intersections of lines and right angles, series of geometric forms the asymmetry of which gives the spectator a pleasant, harmonious impression, like that he receives from certain fugues of Bach, the mathematician of music. It is an art that avoids curves and takes pleasure in lines and right angles, uses great unadorned rectangles of uniform intensity without shading, separated and at the same time united by narrower bands. Pure art is abstract, ascetic, of immaculate whiteness and great mathematical precision. Its supreme exponent was the Dutch painter Mondriaan, creator of an abstract space of primary colors and of pure, almost musical, rhythmic form, with colors that correspond optically to the spatial form desired. His principal apostles were Van Doesburg, Gabo, and Nicholson, their art being symbolic of our era of advanced engineering, obsessed by mathematical order and the mechanization of the universe.

When to the afore-mentioned style is added the representation of an object, an art of *stylized geometric forms* is created. Its objective is to represent objects geometrically, stripping them of everything superfluous, and leaving them reduced to their schematic form, to their skeleton, to the pure symbol of the thing. Vertical and horizontal lines are used to represent objects that are sometimes solid and compact. Not only the inanimate but also the living can be represented geometrically in this group, provided it appears only in mechanical forms meant to accentuate the basic structure of a thing. A jar or a bottle is represented by Morandi as *the* jar or *the* bottle, symbolizing all the jars and bottles of the world. They are not things; they are the telegram of things, the geometric shorthand of things. Instead of lines and straight planes, this art constructs volumes of three dimensions, especially cylinders, cones, and spheres, which according to Cézanne were the basic elements of nature. Light is always theatrical in these pictures, and objects appear in dramatic isolation, or grouped in the form of a cluster of symbols. Fernand Léger was the shining star of this style, and Archipenko and Le Corbusier his satellites.

Sometimes abstract art may utilize *forms* that unmistakably represent or suggest *life* and living things. It is the art of *abstract organic forms* made famous by Calder, Noguchi, Joan Miró, and Jean Arp.

The works of Jean Arp look as if a piece of sculpture, representing a human torso, had fallen on a beach and had been abandoned to the elements: beaten by the waves and whipped by the wind day after day, its edges finally become smooth, its planes soft, its contours vague, its juttings and angles round. There remains, then, what we might call the spirit of primitive art; that which exists in a human torso underneath its angles and its curves, its folds and its edges. Arp has shrunk the work of Nature, proceeding by leaps, all of which coincides with the laws of Planck and the theories of Von Uexküll.

This third group embraces figures painted or sculptured irregularly, figures of fluid contour that avoid the regular geometric curve as well as the straight line; curves are not traced by repeating a basic unity, but rather grow in accordance with the rhythm of changing development. The resulting form cannot be broken up into parts and must be considered as a unique whole. Each unit of these free forms should not be broken up into parts but apprehended as a whole, its parts united by a surface or a contour tension like that of the cells of living beings. Its unifying principle is internal, and each constituent form embodies the possibility of change without losing its identity.

Sometimes organic form is applied to the image, not for the purpose of including objects in a measurable order and rhythm as geometric form would do, but to give things the fluidity of form.

Instead of skeletal structure, this type of *stylized organic form* prefers the bulbous and protuberant outlines of soft and stylized contours, indicating that the most complex forms of life we know derive from simple cellular organisms and resemble each other. They are symbolic forms similar to the natural species from which they evolved, but with their own laws of development. They are, for example, parts of the human being, hands or feet, isolated but alive, tragic or humorous comments on the human being whom they still resemble. Miró, Henry Moore, Picasso, and Paul Klee are the prophets of this style, which sometimes is a mere wandering line, or figures seemingly created from aimless lines, or even an abstract form of a wavering and cabalistic nature, the possibilities of which have been exploited by modern caricaturists.

A commentary on the sense of form in modern art.

The revolutionary change that abstract art represents in comparison with classic art may perhaps be best appreciated in its concept of the human form, which deserves some special observations.

Artistic anatomy has always reflected in its iconography the climate prevailing in each historical epoch, such as the medieval allegorical-religious vision, the architectonic style of the Renaissance, the mechanical movement of the baroque style, and the evolutionism of the past century.[P]

In our times, the change in human morphology reflected in abstract art runs parallel with the change in the concept of scientific anatomy. In the last twenty years, many voices have proclaimed that morphology as a science was suffering from ankylosis and that the anatomy of the corpse should be revived, making of it a fertile synthesis instead of a sterile analysis. Anatomy should be closer to physiology, biologists and anatomists have repeated insistently; it should give up the study of particularities, and be dynamic instead of static. This desire for dynamism in the study of form has manifested itself in dissection halls as well as in artists' studios.

Old anatomists studied the human body from the standpoint of its projection in space, leaving to physiology the study of its projections in time.[Q]

The anatomist of the last century, just like the artist, studied the human being as a self-enclosed whole. The focus was therefore on causality, on studying the living being as a geometric figure, as something already given, in the Platonic sense. It was a mechanistic, static conception which, translated into artistic terms, meant the purely esthetic realization of a stylistic idea. Human beings were thought of in terms of Platonic ontology, matter being modeled after the eternal archetype of ideas.

The new anatomy thinks of the human being as pure process, and it is interested as much in his origin as in his future development and the meaning of his biologic changes. It is an arithmetical, finalistic view that places focus on the living being as a physiologic process; it is a teleologic notion in the Aristotelian tradition, considering every being to be made up of matter which is a potential, and form which is the act or entelechy. This concept has been translated into art through the study of the human form subject to a biologic conformity to plan and with a dynamic tendency to some end. As against the classic notion of form as an idea, modern art posits form as a function or as an end in itself.

Abstract art, like modern anatomy, accepts the fact that form can be an end, a basis of function, or function itself, preceding structure. Form is not conceived as a simple manifestation of the living being in space, but rather as function projected into time. The new artistic morphology is above all physiology. The modern artist can no longer think of pure spatial geometry separated from time, any more than he can conceive of pure temporal physiology liberated from space. For that reason, he has incorporated form and function into his art as supreme manifestations of the living being, just as matter and energy are the manifestations of the inanimate.

Practically speaking, this has meant a revolution in the art of looking at living beings. Bones, muscles, and other anatomic structures are still in the positions they always were, but the point of view from which we regard them is no longer what it was. The object observed has not changed; what has changed is our own vision. Human form is no longer for the abstract artist a mere expression of the living being, or the result of a spatial scheme, but pure dynamic process, motion in time. That is why the abstract artist has given up the staticism of classic art, which prevented him from seizing the functional realities of form, and has become eminently dynamic, constantly striving after form as function in time and space.

THE PSYCHOBIOLOGIC IMPACT OF ATOMIC SCIENCE ON MODERN ART

The psychobiologic process of the formation of the "spatial scheme" of the milieu.

What have been the consequences of the psychologic impact on modern man of this atomistic *nuova scienza*? We can summarize them in a single statement: the result of the conceptions of modern physics discussed previously has been to destroy completely what we may call the mental spatial scheme man had of the universe.

The human being, through the windows of the senses, is constantly receiving from his surroundings impressions that engrave on his nervous system certain structures called engrams, which ultimately become part of his organism. The totality of these impressions made by various engraphic stimuli forms what can be called the *internal correlative of the outside world* and creates in the human mind the spatial scheme of the milieu.

Since the form of the engrams varies in accordance with the internal nervous structure of each organism, we have to accept with Von Uexküll that each animal has its special inner world in which a specific graphic architecture exists and supports its image of the external world. This means that the outside world of the jellyfish differs from that of man, and the outside world of man differs from that of the badger or the butterfly, because each species receives different stimuli—graphic, visual, olfactory, tactile, auditory, thermal, or pressor—which engrave in each species a different internal image and spatial scheme of the world. And so the expression "outer world" is a variable one and depends on the point of view of each species.

The afore-mentioned engrams and the external stimuli that cause them are constantly conditioning the activity of the living being, including his esthetic conduct. The human being therefore forms his universe in the image and likeness of the engrams that he accumulates. Man's idea of the universe varies with the sensory and mental images that man forms of the universe, thanks to his reading and thinking. Although external stimuli may be exactly the same, the organism reacts to them differently at every turn. His reaction is therefore conditioned—in the Pavlovian sense—by external or sensory and internal or biopsychic stimuli.

For thousands of years, the human being has lived with a spatial scheme in his mind from which came his image of a geometrically perfect universe, situated in infinite space, in which matter was all, matter being immutable and obeying laws that were even more immutable. When atomic physics broke up the universe into atoms, it altered its perfect geometry, turning it into a chaos of probabilities; it replaced its perfect continuity with physical discontinuity; it established change by leaps in place of continuous evolution; and it completely undid the spatial scheme of man on which was based his image of the universe. Instead of his former spatial image, which was firm, certain, definite, solid, and continuous, man found himself with the image of a finite sphere in which everything was change, improbability, disorder, and spasm.

Destruction of the bodily image of man.

The consequences of the new biology and psychology were equally cataclysmic for the spatial and bodily schemes of the human being.

Von Uexküll's new biology concept showed that it was necessary to discard Darwinism and in its place establish that the process of life was that of beings whose structure was based on a conformity to plan, and that they progressed by biologic leaps—not very different, in my opinion, from the physical leaps of Planck. Thus, the leap totally replaced uninterrupted evolution in the interpretation of the biologic process.

The new histology, backed by the high-power microscope and finally by the electron microscope, also revolutionized the concept of the *bodily image,* that is, the morphologic scheme that each human being has of himself and of his fellow man.[R]

Until the beginning of our century, anatomy was static, solidified, fixed, rigid, and the human being was conceived of as a small microcosm of solid parts and subject to laws, weights, and measures, just as the macrocosm around him was subject to the laws of physics. The new ultramicroscopic histology, breaking up the human being into elements so far invisible, plus the new physiologic and dynamic concepts of what previously was static human anatomy, destroyed also the bodily image of the human being, and transformed the former orderly conception of the human organism into a confused image of molecular elements in constant change and restlessness.

In the joyous days of pagan art, the skeleton was invisible in painting. In the Middle Ages, gentlemen, ladies, bishops, and pages show their flesh in paintings but neither skulls nor bones appear. Aldous Huxley once asked—and found no answer—why the skeleton appeared so late in art. As a matter of fact, the first work representing a spatial scheme of anatomy and the beginning of modern science did not appear until 1543. This was the *Fabrica* of Vesalius, in which the magic of Calcar's illustrations under the supervision of the brilliant Belgian introduced into art the skeleton as the supreme expression of the human form. In the wake of this work, artists began sculpturing recumbent anatomic figures on tombs. In the seventeenth century these statues stood up and opened their eyes. At their feet there were skulls, perhaps in memory of the syphilis pandemics that destroyed the noses of the infected and reminded artists of the existence of the skeleton. As time passed the skeleton grew and sprouted wings on figures decorating mausoleums.

The psychoanalytic psychology of Freud contributed to this revolution by establishing the supremacy of nonrational life over rational life and by creating an abyssal psychology that gave greater importance to the deep, instinctive, nonrational aspects of the mind than to conscious life. A world of darkness, sex, violence, and aggression took the place of an orderly, moral world created laboriously as psychic superstructures for culture and religion. Thus the third basic image or scheme of the human being, that of order, fixedness, and law in his mental life, was also replaced by the new Freudian scheme in which the instinctive zone of the mind was the decisive factor.

The psychologic impact of atomic science on modern art.

The man of our century reacted to this cataclysmic destruction of the basic values of his life, of the spatial scheme of the universe, of his bodily image, and of his psychologic self image with a vague but often violent restlessness. But the artist, who is always the finest spiritual barometer of an age, reacted even more radically, reflecting in his techniques the disquiet he felt at this breakup of vital schemes.

The aim of the artist is to reproduce the beauty of the external world. But beauty is not, as Kant demonstrated, a predicate of things endowed with objective reality, since the esthetic canon varies from one country to another and from one age to another. A Zulu's conception of beauty is far different from an Eskimo's; El Greco's standards of beauty differ appreciably from those of a contemporary surrealist. Therefore, as the scientific attitude toward external objects —that is, the universe—was altered, and the spatial and bodily schemes of the subject changed, a tremendous change was also wrought in the esthetic canon of our century.

The painter, adopted as the most patent example of this thesis, uses today, as he did two thousand years ago, one of the two great esthetic senses: sight, which perceives external plastic stimuli of a static type, on which are based the spatial or visual arts (painting and sculpture), just as the temporal or auditory arts are based on hearing, which captures rhythmic and melodic stimuli.[8]

The eye gives a simultaneous impression of external things, just as the ear gives the succession of time or rhythm.[7] That is why there is an overlapping of the spatial-simultaneous stimuli on the one hand and the temporal-successive on the other. Visual art requires, under any circumstances, a spatial-temporal correspondence, which already existed for the artist long before Einstein discovered it in his theories of relativity.

The modern painter was exposed to the influences that galvanized our times like a bolt of electricity. When the notion of a stable universe was proved a fallacy, and the image of his own body was altered, the artist's spatial scheme of the world was destroyed.

The key to the meaning of modern art, the art that sometimes strikes us as incoherent and deformed, lies in the fact that the abstract painters, sensing that their spatial scheme of the world is broken, reflect this mental commotion in their pictures, and paint a dislocated universe, with fractured planes, without continuity or solidity, in which space and time blend in plastic relativity. This is a world in which the artist's brush seems to be moved by the same Planckian shock that is disturbing the universe of atomic physics.

Abstract art, then, is the diagrammatic representation of the breakup, wrought by atomic physics and modern science, of the spatial scheme in the mind of modern man, especially in the mind of the artist.

Furthermore, the strange version of man painted by surrealist artists (combining the human being with inanimate objects, as Max Ernst does, or giving it a gelatinous, transparent consistency, as Dali does, or presenting him from within, as Henry Moore does) represents the breakup of the bodily schemes, to which the artist has been drawn by the concepts of modern physiology and biology.[v]

The artistic rebellion against the influence of the new physical science.

The modern artist has reflected in his technique the psychologic impact of atomic physics, but, on the other hand, he has fought against that influence in each facet of his art. First, in order to fight the breakup of the spatial scheme of the universe, the abstract artist has enclosed this universe within the frame of his picture, especially within the finite—Einsteinian—space of the bidimensional universe created by cubism. In this way he has tried to limit the infinite, just as physics has done, so as to be able to impose some order in his artistic cosmos.

Second, he is doing everything he can for the cause of order, harmony, and clarity when he frees himself from superfluous forms, colors, and rhythms and seeks, like Mondriaan, the supreme perfection of order, clarity, and calm in his white, fixed universe of straight lines and harmonious angles. That universe which was converted into a chaos in the artist's mind by the breakup of the spatial schemes of the world about him, he now tries to reconvert into a cosmos of harmony and clarity.

Third, with the breakup of the spatial schemes in his mind, the modern artist ceased regarding the object like Velázquez did; he even ceased to look at light like the impressionists did; he has withdrawn more and more until he has shut himself up within himself, in a voluntary process of progressive psychic blindness. This protest is comparable to hysterical blindness in which form is first lost, then light and color, and finally all vision of things. Scorning the unstable outer world of disintegrated structures and uncertain laws, the abstract artist has created his own world of ideas, as in cubist painting, or has tended to restore a biopsychologic order of his own, as in surrealistic painting.

The solitary figures of de Chirico shivering under a spectral moon in Venetian piazzas, or Dali's lonely figures alone in deserted lunar places, impress one as beings submerged in a cosmic loneliness that the artist himself feels because atomic science has torn apart his universe, leaving him alone with his ideas.

The artist's canvases dramatize his double conflict: his anguish over a universe that has fallen apart, and his profound desire for order, reconstruction, and harmony. This conflict has exploded like a geyser into an art that is incomprehensible till we correlate it with the conceptions of modern physics.

In a hundred years science has proceeded from the study of things to the study of sensations and ideas. At present, physics is attempting, from its fixed world of ideas, to dominate the changing world of things and sensations. Art, working in analogous channels, is trying, from the watchtower of ideas, to create ideologic painting. Modern painting tries to present the chaos that exists in the physical world of today as it appears to men who do not understand its scientific structure; at the same time, it attempts to convert this universe into a pure and harmonious cosmos through the magic of art.

A glance at the future of art.

One can with the mind's eye reconstruct a bridge with half its arch destroyed, the other half describing a semicurve in the air; with the mind's eye one can see the missing half and complete the whole arch. By means of such psychologic extension, it is possible to foresee the trends of art in the future.

The work of the modern artist has reflected the psychologic impact of atomic science, which has destroyed the basic schemes of his existence as man and artist: his spatial scheme of the universe, and his bodily and psychic image of himself.

But a further reaction is already apparent in the art of painters like Dali, one of the most fanatical of surrealists, who in his most recent period is turning his back on surrealistic art and is painting "atomic Madonnas" and a mystic universe where everything floats in phantasmagoric levitation.

The modern artist, in reaction against the disintegration of the universe brought about by the physicists, is reconstructing this universe in his work. If we listen carefully to the voices of abstract artists we can detect in all of them the same note of mysticism, the same transcendental desire for unity and for ineffable communion with eternal, stable, and absolute forces.[v] *Abstract art embraces all techniques, but at its bottom there palpitates as a unifying element and common denominator the desire for integration, for unity, for solidity, for continuity, the desire to find again the lost unity of the cosmos, of man with himself, and of man with the cosmos.*

As his only means of restoring the broken unity of matter and spirit, the artist has chosen the path of integration, oneness, and simplification. *Abstract art is simplification.* It strips the universe of color and form and creates it anew, beginning from the naked, pure idea. Quasi-religious mystical integration of a new universe will be the aim of the new art.

On the basis of that same objective of unity and integration which pulsates in the new atomic science as the philosophic key to its structure, we can anticipate that modern art will tend, in the next half century, toward a new lay mysticism based on the principles of the new physical science and intended to restore the lost unity of the spatial scheme of the universe and man's bodily image. We can indeed foresee it as a tremendous endeavor toward the artistic integration of man and his cosmos.

SUMMARY

The year 1900 marks the beginning of a crisis in the conception of the universe. The new atomic science, Einsteinian physics, the quantum theory of Planck, the new astronomy, and modern mathematics, as well as ultramicroscopic biology, have revolutionized the concepts of classic physics. The new picture of the universe, the acceptance of finite space, the identity of matter and energy, the idea of the relativity of time and its continuity in space—all these have caused a crisis in man's concept of the world around him and of himself.

The work of the artist has reflected this crisis, for there is a historical interrelation between scientific thought and artistic sensibility. Since 1907 the new forms of modern art—surrealism, cubism, and abstract art—have shown the psychologic impact of atomic science, which destroyed the spatial scheme and bodily image of man. The spatial scheme in the human mind is born as a result of the engrams engraved on the nervous system by sensory stimuli and by mental images evoked by meditation; in that spatial scheme lies the key to the concept man has of his milieu. The bodily image in the human mind comes from kinesthetic intraperceptions and the reaction of man's psyche to external sensory stimuli.

Atomic physics and ultramicroscopic biology have destroyed man's spatial and bodily schemes. The modern artist has reacted by representing diagrammatically in his abstract art a dislocated universe. This universe is as disintegrated and discontinuous as that of atomic science. Space and time are fused, matter has been converted into energy in a limited and finite universe—the Einsteinian universe—and mutations are made in leaps of the quanta type. The human figure disappears from the cubist universe to reappear in surrealism, which portrays the disruption of man's bodily image and of his psyche. The technique and the subject of the modern artist have reflected this disintegration of his spatial and bodily schemes. At the same time, the artist has rebelled against such disruption of his world and mind and has reacted with a strong desire for unity, integration, harmony, and order.

We may anticipate that art in the next half century will concentrate on simplification, integration, and quasi-religious endeavor to order, because the artist longs to restore the lost unity between the body and the psyche of man and to reinstate man to his rightful position in the cosmos.

NOTES

A. Leucippus' doctrine was revived with Heisenberg's atom, just as Democritus' was revived with the more deterministic notion of the atom of Rutherford and Bohr. Around his idea of the atom, Democritus created a cosmology based on atomism, which was opposed by Plato and Horace. Lucretius (75 B.C.) and Aristotle contributed to the development of atomic theories; as a matter of fact, Aristotle laid the basis of scientific physics.

B. In 1900, when Newton's theory of space and time was still accepted, "ether, absolutely at rest" was conceived as a substantial vehicle bearing waves of light through interstellar space. In that year, physical research still supported the idea of continuous matter; it was interested in the behavior of gross matter and paid no attention to its atomic structure. Technologic advances were formidable in the fields of thermodynamics, hydrodynamics, electricity, aerodynamics, acoustics, and ultrasonic waves. The most notable difference between the physics of 1900 and 1950 is the complete victory of contemporary atomists, who have revived the old speculations of the medieval alchemists.

In 1900 the history of the atom began. Its milestones have been the discovery of the electron (1894) by J. J. Thomson; of roentgen rays (1895) by W. K. Roentgen; of radioactivity (1896) by Henri Becquerel; of radioactive elements—radium and thorium—by Pierre and Marie Curie (1898); and the identification of atomic nuclei and alpha and beta rays from 1902 on by Rutherford and his school. Today we know that the atom is made up of protons of positive electric charge, neutrons without electric charge, electrons of negative charge, eighteen hundred times lighter than the nucleons, and other subatomic particles.

C. As he developed his equations, Max Planck observed that they could describe the emissions of radiant energy through leaps—which he called *quanta* —that varied with the frequency of light. His equation, now famous in the history of science, was that "a *quantum* of energy equals h times the frequency of light." The h is the so-called constant of Planck.

D. To the theory of the discontinuity of energy, Planck added the idea that just as atoms differ according to the type of matter from which they come, some being heavier than others, energy atoms also differ according to their source. The magnitude or quantum of the energy of radiation was directly in proportion to the frequency of the radiation. Planck's constant was, then, not a quantity of energy, but a *quantum* of kinetic momentum.

E. The quantum theory cleared up the puzzle of atomic stability, and allowed for interpretation of the periodic systems of elements, but both the wave and the corpuscular theories of light remained popular. Planck's formula was as follows: $q = h\nu$, where the constant h equals about 6.6×10^{-27} erg-second and ν is the frequency of radiation of the particle. Louis de Broglie hypothesized that corpuscular particles were associated with wave systems. The unity of both aspects of matter and light was later formulated mathematically by Heisenberg, Born, Jordan, Schroedinger, and Dirac.

F. In 1913, Niels Bohr successfully applied the quantum theory to the phenomena of the atom, describing it as a miniature sun surrounded by electronic planets which leap like waves from one to another orbit emitting (or absorbing) quanta of light without obeying regular laws.

G. The most important Einsteinian law is the one that establishes the equivalence between mass and energy: $E = mc^2$, c representing the speed of light. Later, in 1908, Minkowski established the mathematical theory that space and time fused in a four-dimensional extension in which each point represents an "event" and in which the generalization of regular Euclidian geometry is maintained.

In 1915 Einstein extended the theory of relativity to the accelerated systems, obtaining a theory about fields of gravitation that embraced the Newtonian theory as its first approximation. His principal contribution was the prediction and verification, during the total eclipse of 1918, that the light which came through to us from the stars detoured when it passed near the sun. Astronomers developed the idea of the expansion of the universe, taking as their basis the discovery that distant nebulae or galaxies drew away from our planet at speeds proportionate to their distances. Later, mathematicians developed a modification of the Einsteinian equation, describing a closed, expansional universe of curved spaces.

H. Albert Einstein has said (in his article "Physics, Philosophy and Scientific Progress," J. Internat. Coll. Surgeons, *14*:755–758, Dec. 1950): "As a matter of fact, one easily recognizes certain principal features to which science has firmly adhered ever since those times:

"First, thinking alone can never lead to any knowledge of external objects. Sense perception is the beginning of all research, and the truth of theoretical thought is arrived at exclusively by its relation to the sum total of those experiences.

"Second, all elementary concepts are reducible to space-time concepts. Only such concepts occur in the laws of nature; in this sense all scientific thought is geometric. A law of nature is expected to hold true without exceptions; it is given up as soon as one is convinced that one of its conclusions is incompatible with a single fact which has been proved by experimental investigation.

"Third, the spatio-temporal laws are *complete*. This means that there is not a single law of nature which, in principle, could not be reduced to a law within the domain of space-time concepts. This principle implies, for instance, the conviction that psychic entities and relations can be reduced in the last analysis to processes of a physical and chemical nature within the nervous system. According to this principle there are no nonphysical elements in the causal system of the processes of nature; in this sense, there is no room for free will within the framework of scientific thought, nor for an escape into what has been called vitalism.

"Just one more remark in this connection. Even though the modern quantum theory contains a weakening of the concept of causality, it does not open a back-door to the advocates of free will, as is already evident from the following consideration: the processes determining the organic phenomena are irreversible in the sense of thermodynamics and of such a kind as to eliminate the statistical element ascribed to molecular processes."

I. Astronomy in the last half century has made great strides, such as the analysis of stellar movements, the confirmation of the theory of relativity, the concept of spiral galaxies, the construction of gigantic telescopes, radioastronomy, the birth of modern trigonometric parallaxes, the exploration of stellar structures and of interstellar dust and gases, advances in photocellular astronomy. Immediate objects of study, according to Harlow Shapley, are cosmic physics, stellar spectroscopy, the structure of the Milky Way, drawing of maps of remote galaxies, the origin of the planetary system, and the study, through radio microwaves, of the meteors and cosmic rays.

J. Atomistic physics is the physics of the moment, and tends to treat everything in a fragmentary, atomistic way. According to this theory, the electron passes from one orbit to another through a series of strange leaps because the electron does not pass from one orbit to another through intermediary space, but disappears from one place to appear in another. The electron *does not move* by leaps, but rather *exists* in leaps; it evaporates in one place and appears in another, without having traveled to that other place. Therefore, the electron *is* the series of separate aspects it would present in continuous movement if such a thing existed. As the universe is matter and matter is composed of electrons, it has been suggested that the universe moves by leaps between which it disappears. Perhaps a similar theory might be applied to the human psyche.

K. We admit today that living beings are made up of biogenetic elements of low atomic weight, situated at the start of the periodic scale, and they all —except zinc, arsenic, and iodine—have atomic weights less than that of iron (56). At the other end of the periodic scale, we find the elements of greatest atomic weight, among which we have—beginning with lead (207), radon (222), radium (226), actinium (227), and uranium (238)—elements that, along with their isotopes, are all radioactive, that is, easily disintegrable atoms the fission of which takes place with liberation of energy.

The most unstable atoms are found at both ends of the periodic scale; silver is the only element of perfect stability and is near the middle point of the scale (108). The other elements are metastable in either direction, and liberate energy through the conversion of their atoms either when their nuclear components are added together in the lighter elements or when the nucleus of the heaviest disintegrates.

The biogenetic elements have, on the other hand, a greater nuclear stability. Seaborg compiled in 1944 a list of isotopes known at the time, of which forty-five were radioactive. Tracing the frequency of radioactivity in the isotopes and in normal atoms, in successive groups within the periodic series, and considering the proportion of radioactive bodies in each group, we see that the curve superimposes itself on the curve of stability of the atomic nucleus. Gamow said in 1946: "The best opportunity of producing atomic transformations and liberating their hidden energy lies in both extremes of the periodic system: the heavy isotope of hydrogen (deuterium) or the light isotope of uranium (U 235), both very rare elements on the planet."

L. The changes in physics have led to similar changes in biology and psychology. Medicine today is more interested in intraorganic chemicoenergetic changes than in cruder neurologic alterations. The unity of matter and energy is accepted not only for the universe but also for the human body.

Comparison was made by Langdon-Brown between energy originally developed in the zygote, which proves the impetus that carries the organism like a bullet in its passage through life, to an explosion of atomic energy. At the moment of birth, there remains only two per cent of the initial impetus, which decreases constantly because it is subject to thermodynamic laws, although the functioning of life maintains that evaporating energy at a useful level.

The organic and nervous tissues, like the molecular aggregates that they are, withstand the changes of the individual molecules of their surroundings but are subject to the statistical laws of physics.

Modern physics accepts the human body as a continuum of matter and energy, as electrons charged with energy, the energy content of which varies not continually but by leaps, according to the quantum theory, and moves, according to Schroedinger, in a continuum of space-time of four dimensions. Each organic system has a quantity of energy, the level of which changes by that mysterious event called a quantum leap. Each molecule of said system is made up of atoms and has a certain stability, and its configuration does not vary until it receives from without the necessary energy for said leap. Said difference of level determines quantitatively the degree of stability of a molecule.

These conditions exist in the human being from before birth. Modern physics considers the possibility that a gene or fiber of chromosome may be an aperiodic solid. This conception of a well-ordered association of atoms with sufficient resistance to preserve its order permanently and to make isomeric adjustments may perhaps explain the mystery of how the diminutive particle of the nucleus of the fertilized egg contains, as if written in tiny code, the entire future development of the organism.

After birth, life continues as an incessant biochemical change, although it maintains its unity, integration, and internal organizations against attacks from without.

It is interesting to note that fundamental differences between living and nonliving organisms have been abolished. Small viruses are considered by chemists as molecules and by biologists as cells, to which the quantum theory may also be applied.

M. Human life, it has been said, has developed through the capture of "levels of energy." Up to 5000 b.c. man limited himself to assimilating solar energy through edible animals and plants, resulting in a very rudimentary culture. About seven thousand years ago the agricultural man appeared, planting his fields with edible plants, thus absorbing more energy, a method that in one thousand years created vast civilizations. This stage lasted six thousand years. In 1700, in Western Europe, "fossil fuel"—that is, coal, oil, and gas—was being used.

A new culture came to be when the first atomic bomb was exploded in Alamogordo, New Mexico, July 16, 1945, six years after Otto Hahn and Strassmann discovered the fission of the heavy nucleus of uranium. This scientific event, which had immediate practical applications in the manufacture of radioactive tracers, the treatment of cancer, the prolongation of life, and conversion of hydrogen into helium, will make possible the harnessing of even more energy.

N. The strange game of hide-and-seek present in so many surrealistic paintings, for example, in Dali and Tchelichev, like images of beings infinitely multiplied, is an allegoric representation of the psychologic self-image broken also by the psychoanalytic impact. It is the mind looking for itself.

O. They are sketches that contain implicit movement and are surrounded by an indeterminate space. They have been used on posters, advertisements, furniture, architecture, and ceramics. Because they seem cut from a large drawing, their free organic existence is striking. It is a style used with great success in modern canvas hammocks and chairs and in show-windows.

P. According to Laín Entralgo, it is significant that anatomic nomenclature began in history as numerical and expressed magnitude (*duodenum* = twelve fingers), and in the Renaissance changed to symbols of arrangement and relation (*deltoid* = delta).

Q. An analogous division might be applied historically, as the study of the human being in his spatial projection has been the subject of geography, just as the human being in his dynamic projection has been the subject of history.

R. When this image disappears or is deformed by neurologic lesions, it can be freed from its bodily frame and converted into a hallucination, which has given rise in literature to the legend of the human "double" the sight of which means death, and which is only the perception, without object, of our own bodily image.

S. Of vital importance in the discussion of the impact of atomism on modern art is the fact that psychologic perception is interpreted today as possibly being determined by physical factors. Perception does not receive the movement of matter but the effect of the impact of such movement on our organism.

We construct the world on the basis of messages through the sensorial organs to the brain. The mind weaves an impression using the stimulus that reaches the brain through the sensorial nerves and which lacks color, temperature, sound, and texture, qualities given to it by the brain.

Mental processes are the result of cerebral processes which, in turn, depend on stimuli from the body or the milieu. What the mind contains is determined by the milieu, and vice versa. Organism and milieu are one whole. Our perceptions seize the configuration of situations. The qualities of the objects are those of the entire situation. Physicists and physiologists accept that cerebral stimuli are of atomic nature, but the brain receives separate impressions and the mind does not end but rather *begins* with the global picture of everything.

T. Formerly, artists commissioned by great lords and wealthy men to paint their portraits very often captured in their paintings the chronic illnesses of their models, thanks to which we have today a splendid iconography of great historicomedical value. What the brush of the classic artists reproduced was simply the charming pirouette of the human body in a bronze by Donatello, the explosive anatomy of Michelangelo, or the graceful gesture of the nudes of Boucher and Fragonard. Rembrandt's brush was able to grasp the psycologic depth of a state of mind in his own self-portrait, just as Franz Hals captured on the faces of the burgomasters he painted their rotund, smug middle-class life. But no one could capture the dynamic process of illness, which has a beginning, a development, and a conclusion that is at times the cosmic tragedy of death, nor could anyone depict the unfolding of a psychologic process.

U. William Hogarth (*Analysis of Beauty—Introduction*) said in 1753:

"Notwithstanding I have told you my design of considering minutely the variety of lines which serve to raise the idea of bodies in the mind, and which are undoubtedly to be considered as drawn on the surfaces only of solid or opake bodies: yet the endeavoring to conceive, as accurate an idea as is possible, of the inside of those surfaces, if I may be allowed the expression, will be a great assistance to us in the pursuance of our present inquiry.

"In order to my being well understood, let every object under our consideration, be imagined to have its inward contents scooped out so nicely, as to have nothing left but a thin shell, exactly corresponding, both in its inner and outer surface, to the shape of the object itself: and let us likewise suppose this thick shell to be made up of very fine threads, closely connected together, and equally perceptible, whether the eye is supposed to observe them from without, or within, and we shall find the ideas of the two surfaces of this shell will naturally coincide. The very word, shell, makes us seem to see both surfaces alike.

"The use of this conceit, as it may be called by some, will be seen to be very great . . . and the oftener we think of objects in this shell-like manner, we shall facilitate and strengthen our conception of any particular part of the surface of an object we are viewing, by acquiring thereby a more perfect knowledge of the whole, to which it belongs: because the imagination will naturally enter into the vacant space within this shell, and there at once, as from a centre, view the whole from within, and mark the opposite corresponding parts so strongly, as to retain the idea of the whole, and make us masters of the meaning of every view of the object, as we walk round it, and view it from without."

V. Let us quote the opinions of some American abstract artists: George L. K. Morris: "Can you imagine it in any other time—an artist just putting shapes together—shapes that represent nothing, either alone or in combination? He puts a frame around it, and offers it on the open market, just as a good thing to have around and look at; something that will speak to you as an independent personality, and yet is very quiet." Later on he defends the effort of self-control and pacification of "harnessing of freedom" which is the real strength of the artist. Then he compares an artist who paints nature without selecting his themes to a "pianist who sits down on the keyboard (Whistler) or on the palette." Painting is, basically, an optical experience. Art has an emotional impulse and a structural texture, and produces two forces as different as inhaling and exhaling, and requires the impulse of the painter to activate a picture with life.

Willem de Kooning: "Abstraction first used to designate a still life led the artist to conceive of art not as something in which everything can be eliminated." "It gave some people the idea that they could free art from itself." "The artist turned his back on things in order to take possession of ideas," "social ideas, to make their objects with, their constructions the pure plastic phenomena. . . ." "Man's own form in space—his body—was a private person; and that it was because of this imprisoning misery—because he was hungry and overworked and went to a horrid place called home late at night in the rain, and his bones ached and his head was heavy—because of this very consciousness of his own body, this sense of pathos, they suggest, he was overcome by the drama of a crucifixion in a painting or the lyricism of a group of people sitting quietly around a table drinking wine. . . ." "Kandinsky understood 'Form' as *a* form, like an object in the real world; and an object, he said, was a narrative—and so, of course, he disapproved of it. He wanted his 'music without words.'

". . . Futurists had a simpler sentiment. . . . No space. Everything ought to keep on going!

"The argument often used that science is really abstract, and that painting could be like music and, for this reason, that you cannot paint a man leaning against a lamp-post, is utterly ridiculous. That space of science—the space of the physicists—I am truly bored with by now. Their lenses are so thick that seen through them, the space gets more and more melancholy. There seems to be no end to the misery of the scientists' space. All that it contains is billions and billions of hunks of matter, hot or cold, floating around in darkness according to a great design of aimlessness. The stars I think about, if I could fly, I could reach in a few old fashioned days. But physicists' stars I use as buttons, buttoning up curtains of emptiness. If I stretch my arms next to the rest of myself and wonder where my fingers are that is all the space I need as a painter.

"Today, some people think that the light of the atom bomb will change the concept of painting once and for all. The eyes that actually saw the light melted out of sheer ecstasy. For one instant, everybody was the same color. It made angels out of everybody. A truly Christian light, painful but forgiving."

Alexander Calder: "I think that at that time and practically ever since, the underlying sense of form in my work has been the system of the Universe, or part thereof. For that is a rather large model to work from.

"What I mean is that the idea of detached bodies floating in space, of different sizes and densities, perhaps of different colors and temperatures, and surrounded and interlarded with wisps of gaseous condition, and some at rest, while others move in peculiar manners, seems to me the ideal source of form.

"I would have them deployed, some nearer together and some at immense distances.

"And great disparity among all the qualities of these bodies, and their motions as well.

"A very exciting moment for me was at the planetarium—when the machine was run fast for the purpose of explaining its operation: a planet moved along a straight line, then suddenly made a complete loop of 360° off to one side, and then went off in a straight line in its original direction.

"I have chiefly limited myself to the use of black and white as being the most disparate colors. Red is the color most opposed to both of these—and then, finally, the other primaries. The secondary colors and intermediate shades serve only to confuse and muddle the distinctness and clarity."

[All quotations in note V are from *What Abstract Art Means to Me,* New York, The Museum of Modern Art, Bulletin, Volume 18, No. 3, Spring, 1951.]

THE LIVES OF LEONARDO

A Short Story

Florence, May 1504

To His Excellency, Don Luis de Vergara, Grandee of Spain, at the Court of Her Majesty the Queen of Spain, Doña Isabel la Católica

God keep Your Excellency Don Luis de Vergara, Grandee of Spain, and our Most Exalted Majesty the Queen, Doña Isabel la Católica.

I, Don Lope de Medina, Knight of the Order of Saint James, the humble servant of Her Majesty, and Your Excellency's envoy to Italy, consider the first part of my mission fulfilled, and beg to render an account to Your Excellency so that I may be given further orders and pursue my assignment to a satisfactory conclusion.

In compliance with my instructions, I went first to Milan. This is a lovely city of great culture, although our own cities in Spain far surpass it in beauty and learning.

My first night in Milan I spent at the Osteria della Bella Spagnuola. While ambling through the lonely narrow streets in search of lodging, that name, which under the full moon shone as if incrusted in silver on the board over the door of the inn, called to me like a voice from my distant country. It was late. At the inn, an ill-humored and sleepy-eyed host served me a piece of hard bread and some scraps of mutton. But the red wine was good and the embers in the fireplace gave forth a pleasant warmth, for the nights are chilly. While

---

From *Town & Country* 106:55, 142, 1952.

I gnawed at the bones, the innkeeper had a glass of wine with me. The flickering candlelight danced wildly on his unshaven face and disheveled hair as I proceeded to question him along certain lines of great interest to both Your Excellency and me.

Milan, like Florence, is going through a period of relative calm. The people of Florence still recall with horror the stakes set up in the pubic square by Savonarola's orders, and heretics tremble when the latter's name is mentioned, although it is six years since he left this world. But right now Cesare Borgia provides so much to talk about, that it should wipe out all memory of the past.

The innkeeper was the first person to speak to me of Leonardo da Vinci, the object of my mission. He himself never spoke with Leonardo, but many years ago he lived in Florence and Leonardo had to pass by the innkeeper's house on his way to Andrea del Verrocchio's atelier. The innkeeper evoked his corpulent figure dressed in black velvet, without shoulder belt, sword, dagger, or any other weapon. He walked meditatively, his eyes looking right through people. It is a pensive da Vinci the innkeeper remembered. He recalled Leonardo's stopping to scrutinize a damp spot on a wall or to look up in a trance at the fat white clouds in the Florentine sky, which he later sketched in a notebook. When I was quite convinced that the innkeeper knew little of importance about Leonardo da Vinci, I retired to my room.

The next day I went to Piero della Sagazza's shop. Your Excellency will recall this painter, some of whose canvases were sent to Spain. He is both painter and sculptor and has his own atelier, where he gives classes in painting and deals in pictures with the great lords of the various duchies in Italy.

The letter of introduction that the sculptor Pedro Berruguete gave me in Madrid was of great help. Piero della Sagazza, a great admirer of Berruguete's work, immediately afforded me his hospitality. We spent a pleasant evening in his atelier, surrounded by bronze busts and pink marble torsos, onyx boxes and green jade figurines, lamps and jugs wrought most consummately in silver, and canvases in all stages of completion. Piero della Sagazza is not only the master of the secrets of *al fresco* painting, but also of tempera and oil. The room smelled of clean fresh paint. Through the open window drifted the sound of a lute playing in the distance one of those plaintive compositions so dear to the hearts of all Milanese. A table was laden with silver bowls full of dried fruits, pieces of *caccio* cheese, and flasks of Neapolitan wine of which Piero is very fond. As it grew darker and the square of sky outlined by the window was dotted with stars, Piero told me many things about Leonardo da Vinci.

Leonardo was born in 1452 and is today fifty-two years of age. He has come to that dangerous period in an artist's life when he must surpass himself and reach for fresh laurels, or give everything up and follow the humble path to a monastery. Leonardo is passing through such a period of melancholy that hardly anybody can speak with him. Only a few intimate friends may enter his home, where he rarely sleeps to avoid surprise visits. He has changed radically since the time he was in the service of the Duke of Milan; he would no longer be able to spend fifteen years on the statue of the Duke di Sforza. Piero thinks that Leonardo is now going through that crisis inevitable in the life of all men who, ignoring the limitations of the human being, embrace the entire universe, suffer a tragic disillusionment, and become overconscious of their shortcomings. His natural misanthropy has deepened of late. Only work seems to alleviate his anguish at not being able to extend his creative genius beyond the limits he has reached.

Thirty-five years ago, Piero was a young man of twenty and one of the pupils in Verrocchio's studio in Florence. At that time Leonardo frequented Verrocchio's studio. He was a fine-looking young man with a handsome head of black hair, a lofty forehead, and sky-blue eyes. Piero especially remembers Leonardo's fondness for anatomy. Other disciples still cultivated the manner of Giotto and painted as if their figures were meant for medieval altarpieces, but Leonardo was obsessed by the human body. He loved Masaccio's "Adam and Eve" simply because they struck him as an ordinary Florentine middle-class married couple with all the imperfections of naked flabby flesh; and he went into ecstasy over Fra Filippo Lippi's chubby Virgins and robust little angels. Piero thinks that Leonardo admired the realism of Verrocchio, who painted Virgins with tranquil countenances, long slim fingers, and well-defined anatomy, or chubby children exuding good health. Leonardo also liked the naturalism of Donatello's bronzes and the violent emotions underlying the ferocity on the faces of Signorelli's Virgins.

A LOVELESS YOUTH

In Verrocchio's atelier, Leonardo, with amazing anatomic precision, modeled clay figures which he then painted on canvas, imitating relief with his brushes, thus introducing into painting the sensation of bulk and solidity. When his fellow students saw his maiden work, "The Adoration of the Magi," they had to admire his knowledge of anatomy.

Piero recalls those years with nostalgia. Leonardo was a good friend to all of them, but his kindness and gentleness were dispassionate and strange, as distant as the dates on a palm tree. Nobody dared mistreat an animal in his presence. Behind his back some people made fun of his mania for buying caged birds in the market, kissing their palpitating breasts, and then setting them free to fly on their yellow wings into the morning air.

"No," Piero told me, "no one ever knew whether Leonardo had a mistress or whether he was ever interested in any girl. No one ever saw him in the company of women except when he was working on some painting, and even on such occasions he treated his models with lofty reserve. His was a loveless youth. 'He who does not control sensuality,' he used to say, 'becomes an animal.' Of course—" Piero paused, got up and walked toward the window. With his back turned to me, as if he wished to avoid looking me in the face, he continued, "Of course it was all slander, but because he was seen often in the company of fair adolescent boys there were many nasty rumors and finally the authorities had to intervene. They even suspected his intimacy with the master Verrocchio. The hearing lasted three months, after which he was found innocent of the heinous crime of which he was accused. There could have been no other verdict."

According to Piero, Leonardo has been all his life a man of pure heart and unimpeachable morality. To doubt his virility was an outrageous insult. But Piero does not believe that Leonardo has ever loved any woman. Love in any of its plastic manifestations strikes him as repulsive and degrading, and that is why he depicted it the way he did in one of his sketches, which a friend has put away as one of those creations that can be shown only when its author has passed into the world of shadows. It is said that Leonardo loved only once in his life, and even that was more like a scientific experiment. He prefers to live with a free soul and to cultivate the dreams of a timid man enamored of an ideal.

"THE LAST SUPPER" IN CANDLELIGHT

Piero promised to show me one of Leonardo's paintings called "The Last Supper," which hangs in the refectory of the monastery of Santa Maria delle Grazzie in Milan. As I was too impatient to wait for the next day, Piero della Sagazza and I set out through the labyrinth of deserted streets under a sky already covered with stars. When we reached our destination it was already quite late and even the church bells were sleeping.

The monastery loomed before us, a mass so great and black that it seemed as if the night had frozen into a solid block of darkness. We knocked at the door several times. A little peephole opened. Piero whispered to the monk who kept watch at the door, the door opened, and we entered the courtyard of the monastery. The moon shed splinters of silver over our mantles. We could hear the gurgle of water in an invisible fountain. We passed through another door. More darkness. Corridors. Our boots wakened a thousand sleeping echoes. Finally, guided by the monk, we reached a large room. My nostrils were assailed by the stale smell of cooking and moldy bread. The monk struck a tinder and lit a candle; the bluish flame projected a series of dancing shadows on the walls. The pale face of the monk was like the end of a wax taper. We were in the refectory of the monastery. In a corner there was a pile of hay. On the wall separating the refectory from the kitchen "The Last Supper" was painted.

I could not see very well and I was sorry I had not waited to visit the monastery during the day, although the monk told me that even when the sun is high the light is bad. Vague figures licked by the flame of the candle oscillated before my eyes. I drew closer until my face was almost against the wall. I could see the cracks in the painting caused by the heat from the kitchen. I looked down. To widen a door situated under the mural, the monks had cut the picture, sacrificing the legs of Jesus and of two of the apostles. Piero spoke enthusiastically about this work. Exhaling warm breath into my ear, he whispered how Leonardo had spent many days staring at the painting, incapable of filling in Jesus' face. Finally one day he felt the inspiration. The pale light of the candle revealed that face to me: it had all the gentle fortitude of the Saviour. In the shadows the golden countenance stood out, as if suspended in midair, radiating a diamantine light. When I moved the candle away, the eyes of Jesus kept on staring at me.

Out on the street again, dogs barked at us, and the crow of the cock heralded the first light of dawn.

A GLANCE BACK—THE PASSIONATE MOTHER

On the following day, Piero introduced me to Mona Francesca, a native of Vinci, the town where Leonardo was born. She is a little old woman with silvery hair and a face as wrinkled as a dry leaf and veiled by that golden down that comes from great age. She has a fruit stand and sells to the rich merchants and great lords of the district. When we approached her stand, the fruit wagon had just left and Mona Francesca was surrounded by huge yellow reed baskets overflowing with porcelain-like fruit, among which a few dew-sprinkled leaves had slipped in.

Mona Francesca welcomed us heartily, since Piero has done her a few favors and also buys her merchandise. When she was told that I wanted information about Leonardo because I was considering commissioning him to paint a picture, she became even more enthusiastic and begged us to taste her exquisite plums.

Mona Francesca had been a servant in the very same inn where Catalina, Leonardo's mother, had worked. Mona Francesca nostalgically recalled that inn in the small town of Vinci, on the slope of Mount Albana, not far from the city of Empoli in Tuscany, between Pisa and Florence. It is a hamlet snuggling in the mountain, a group of houses seemingly poised for flight. The surrounding hills are fragrant with thyme and lavender. Mona Francesca said she shared the work of the inn evenly with her good friend Catalina. At dawn both would get up and stuff the fireplace with ginger sticks to make the fire smell sweet. The spacious kitchen was illuminated by oil lamps contained in typical wide-necked clay vessels. ("Everything is Etruscan here in Tuscany," Piero said smiling.)

A Pisan notary by the name of Piero da Vinci used to come to this inn. A love affair blossomed between the gentleman and the serving maid. The fruit of their illicit love was Leonardo, who spent his childhood in the home of his mother's parents until he felt impelled to leave and seek his authentic destiny, which began in Verrocchio's studio. Catalina later married a simple workman who could never, not even by the furthest stretch of the imagination, be called Leonardo's father. Mona Francesca's eyes dimmed with tears as she recalled Leonardo's devotion to his mother.

Leonardo used to pass by the fruit stand occasionally and stare at Mona Francesca with his limpid blue eyes. Sometimes the master took pleasure in drawing flowers and birds on the wall to amuse the children of the neighborhood who came to buy fruit. The things that Leonardo could do! For Mona Francesca he invented a special scale so that she might weigh her fruit; he gave her several sketches he made of her fullface and in profile, and some sort of a knife, which he constructed for her one day in less than an hour, to peel fruit without injuring the pulp. On another occasion he invented a machine that sucked the dust from her stand into a bag that could then be emptied very comfortably. "Yes," said Mona Francesca, "Messer Leonardo is a good man, humble with the humble and proud with the proud."

A MATHEMATICIAN IN FLORENCE—WHEN LEONARDO WANTED TO FLY

On my first evening in Florence I had dinner at the palace of the Duke of Pavoneda; the other guests were a doctor and a mathematician belonging to the court of Cesare Borgia. With me was Piero della Sagazza, whom I had persuaded to accompany me to Florence.

The atmosphere was intimate, the dishes select, the table service of purest gold, the music of the lyres exquisite, and the wine as red and warm as blood. The profusion of Oriental tapestries hanging from the walls muffled our voices and all other sounds to the point that when someone spoke it sounded like a murmur, which gave the conversation a confidential tone. As soon as supper was over, the duke excused himself on the grounds that the duchess was indisposed and he must return to her side. But a lovely half-veiled lady, whom I saw through a mirror as she quickly crossed the hall beyond the dining room, was probably the real explanation for the duke's sudden departure. We were then alone with Messer Paolo Crivelli, the mathematician, and Dr. Bertoldo Rinozzi. Servant girls cleared the table, leaving instead a silver jug with wine, figs, nuts, and a vase of roses so red that they looked almost black. The music of the lyres ceased, and without further ado I began to ask both men questions about Leonardo da Vinci.

"A talented charlatan," answered the mathematician.

Messer Paolo Crivelli had also been in the service of Ludovico il Moro. Evil tongues say that he never forgave Leonardo for winning Ludovico's favor with a multichorded lyre in the form of a horse's head which the artist himself fashioned. At that time, Leonardo offered his services to Ludovico il Moro as "an inventor of war-machines, constructor of moveable bridges and armored cars, engineer, expert in artillery and the art of sieges, sapper-miner, sculptor and painter." It was at that same court that Leonardo triumphed over Paolo Crivelli and other courtiers in a dispute over paleontology and geology. Later, at the court of the Duke of Milan where Crivelli was serving temporarily, both men met again. My feeling is that Leonardo completely ignored the mathematician and manifested a certain scorn for his branch of knowledge, which aroused hatred for Leonardo in Crivelli's heart.

Leonardo, Crivelli told me, never finished the equestrian statue of Francesco Sforza, the founder of the Sforza dynasty, despite the fact that he spent fifteen years at it. He "wasted his time" at a thousand other technical problems "of no importance whatsoever." He constructed a revolving stage for theatrical productions, took part in the competition to construct the dome of the Cathedral of Milan, sketched fortifications for the city of Lombardy, and studied the system of canals and locks which regulated river traffic in the most active province in Italy. At the same time, he was to be seen filling his notebooks feverishly with notes, sketching, working out problems in mathematics, astronomy, physics, architecture, botany, and geology.

"It was impossible for me to make out his notes," Crivelli then told me, "because Leonardo wrote them from right to left, and with his left hand, and I would have needed a mirror to read them. Leonardo is a man who imagines he can master everything because he thinks himself endowed with divine omniscience. There is no science which he does not attempt to master. He does not realize that one single science—mathematics in my case—is enough to occupy an entire lifetime. His pride has no bounds. They say that even now he is submitting plans and maps to Cesare Borgia, and that he has offered to change the course of certain rivers and isolate entire cities from the sea."

What most infuriated Crivelli was Leonardo's audacity in attempting to construct a flying machine. When still a young man, they say, he constructed a machine, a sort of bat heavier than air, with which he claimed to be studying the flight of birds. This strange contraption can still be seen covered with dust in a corner of his studio, together with all sorts of things on which he worked at one time or another, such as models of war tanks and cannons, ships that would sail under water, cranes and diving suits, dark chambers, minerals and crossbows, models of bombs which would reduce the universe to atoms, vehicles propelled by their own motive forces, and a thousand other chimeras. But, above all, flying was Leonardo da Vinci's obsession. "It almost seems," said Crivelli, "as if he wants to escape from men through the heavens, or perhaps to snatch from our Lord the secret of the heights which belongs only to Him." And Crivelli grew pensive as he rubbed the ruby-colored knots on his gouty fingers.

As it was getting late, I arranged a meeting with Dr. Bertoldo Rinozzi for the following day.

AT DR. RINOZZI'S OFFICE—LEONARDO AND THE HUMAN BODY

I found the physician in his study, sitting near a window, wearing a short fur-trimmed coat despite the heat, and holding a tube full of an amber liquid up to the light.

Dr. Rinozzi's study was spacious but dark. The light of the candelabra shone on the ivory bindings and gold backs of the huge volumes enclosing all medical knowledge. On his table, along with flasks containing innards in alcohol, crushed herbs, and diverse amulets, *The Canon* of Avicenna and Galen's *Hygiene* lay open, and several anatomic plates showing the best areas to bleed the human body, undoubtedly for the edification of his barber-surgeon.

The first thing he did was to take from a highly ornamented Spanish chest he has in his study and place on his desk a bundle of papers, hundreds of sheets of various sizes covered with tiny cryptic and unintelligible writing. Among these were all sorts of anatomic illustrations. I am not a physician, not even a learned man, and my modest experience as a diplomat does not embrace medicine, but even I realized the marvelous precision of these sketches.

Dr. Rinozzi said they were all originals by Leonardo da Vinci. They were found in his atelier one day when the crowds, incited by Savonarola who suspected Leonardo of practicing black magic, assaulted the atelier. Compassionate hands rescued these papers, and when they noticed that they dealt with anatomy they gave them to Dr. Rinozzi for safekeeping.

"I do not know Leonardo well enough," said Dr. Rinozzi, "to return them to him personally, although I am waiting for the opportunity to do so; meanwhile I am fully aware that this is a treasure which one day science will fully esteem. Look at this, and this, and this! More than fifty sketches on the heart and the motion of the blood. Of course, there are many errors, for Leonardo is so bold as to contradict the ideas of Galen and to replace the latter's 'hidden powers' by mechanical forces. His study of the mechanics and hydraulics of the heart is incomparable, although I do not claim to understand his theories completely. He says that the function of the heart is to engender body heat. Contrary to Galen's, Avicenna's, and Mondino's principles that the heart has only two ventricles, Leonardo says there are four. He says that the heart is not made of special tissues, that it is a muscle, and he even describes its valves. He must have studied and dissected many dead bodies to have been able to reduce the dimensions of the organs to mathematical formulae. Look at these drawings of bones, muscles, nerves, arteries, cuts of the brain and liver, casts of vessels of the brain, colored blood vessels, sketches of the faces of men condemned to death, of monsters and dwarfs. It is a pity that this man—whom I do not believe to be an atheist or sorcerer, but a mystic in love with all living things—has such scorn for us physicians that he calls us liars and destroyers of life. When Dux Galeas died and his disciple Andrea Salaino fell ill, Leonardo threw the pills prescribed by the doctors out of the window."

THE SAINT AND THE DEVIL—LEONARDO AND SAVONAROLA

Dr. Rinozzi paused and looked at me pensively. "This Leonardo da Vinci," he resumed, "is a very courageous man. Let me tell you a story I have never revealed to anyone. I saw him in church one day, when Fra Girolamo Savonarola was delivering a terrifying harangue to a vast crowd. His fiery words painted the frightful picture of hell with its thousand torments for sinners. The people were petrified on their knees, screaming 'Mercy! Mercy!' Over the sea of trembling people prostrate before that implacable voice announcing the Day of Judgment, I saw Leonardo da Vinci near the door, a solitary figure amidst the masses of kneeling religious fanatics. With pencil and notebook in his hands, he stood erect, staring at the hysterical preacher with eyes sparkling like aquamarines. His face was of almost feminine delicacy, his beard heavy, and his hair soft and wavy. He wore a black tunic which reached down to his knees and covered an ankle-length red mantle. I drew closer to him and when I saw what he was doing, I shook with admiration and fear. Leonardo da Vinci was calmly drawing a grotesque caricature of Savonarola, the priest feared by all!"

THE LADY WHO NEVER SMILED

As I did not wish to speak with Leonardo da Vinci before learning Your Excellency's opinion, I begged Piero della Sagazza, who was still in Florence, to point the master out to me, even from a distance, so that I might add my own impression to those I had garnered from others. Piero smiled enigmatically and told me that as soon as he found out how and when we might see Leonardo da Vinci, he would let me know.

Two days went by. I visited every important church, museum, and palace in Florence. I attended several diplomatic banquets and became acquainted with the ever-growing intrigue in high circles. On the third day, a messenger brought me a note. It read as follows: "This afternoon, at sundown, follow the bearer of this note and you will find me." It was signed by Piero.

Curious and impatient, I waited for sundown. It was one of those afternoons when the Florentine sky appears washed by the angels to allow its blue to shine in all its pristine purity. Wrapped in my cape, I followed the guide. We left behind the main thoroughfare, on which only a few bold passers-by still lingered, for after sunset prudent people dare not venture on the streets which bristle with bandits and drunkards.

We were already outside the city gates when we came up against a wall enclosing the garden of a very old house. A tower bell nearby tolled six strokes, which quivered through the air that hung entranced in the still of twilight. Evening was languidly descending over the noble yellowed stones. A black martin took flight and then remained suspended in midair over our heads, like a bird of ill omen. When we entered the garden through a discreet little door, I was enveloped by the fragrance of roses. On the other side of the little door Piero della Sagazza appeared and raised his forefinger to his lips as if to enjoin me to silence.

"I succeeded," he whispered, "in bribing a maid to let us enter unseen. You shall see the master painting a picture from behind some curtains. Do not speak, make no noise whatsoever, or we may be arrested for housebreaking."

"Where are we?" I asked.

"In the home of Ser Piero di Batto Martelli, deputy of the *signoria*, where Leonardo da Vinci is painting Lisa di Antonio Maria di Noldo Gherardini, a Neapolitan lady. She is the wife of Francesco di Bartolommeo di Zanobi del Giocondo, one of the twelve *buon'uomini* of the city. It is said that he will soon be one of the *priori*."

We advanced on tiptoe through the sand-covered garden among colorful flowerpots. From the house came soft rhythms of music.

"He has been working on this portrait for two years," Piero told me. "He always paints it at the twilight hour, because it is then that the shadows of the face are most definite and the lines stand out in all their purity. Mona Lisa comes to sit daily."

Still on tiptoe we made our way along a corridor ending in a door covered by thick tapestries. There, Piero pressed my wrist in a signal to be especially quiet. Carefully we pushed aside a corner of the tapestries. Through a glass window in the door we could see the studio. Mona Lisa was seated. Near her stood the man I had come to see: Leonardo da Vinci.

Mona Lisa is about thirty, slim but well proportioned, with a soft, delicate face. Her beauty is voluptuous, of antique mold, like those vague scents that brush by us when we open an old chest. Although far from the autumn of life, she is already a ripe woman. I could almost smell the aroma of tuberoses which her body, in the torpor of premature fullness, suggests. Her limpid, dreamy eyes attenuate the sensuality of her countenance. Her hands, like enamored doves, lay crossed on her lap. Mona Lisa! Her sad face fascinated me, because every woman smiles at some time or another, but this was the face of a woman who had never smiled.

LEONARDO AND LA GIOCONDA

Holding my breath for fear of being detected, almost suffocated by the heavy tapestries, I could barely see Leonardo's profile. He is tall, with the corpulence of a wrestler, and has a thick silky beard. His hands are too delicate and his gestures almost effeminate. I could not see the painting too well, for the *leggio* on which it stood was partly turned away from us. When the painter changed its position with one of his quick gestures, I could see him and his work better.

Leonardo da Vinci seems to be, judging from his alert eyes and his firm movements, at the height of his physical and intellectual powers. His body is that of an athlete—they tell me he is a great horseman—but his hands are more those of a zither player—they tell me he is that too—than those of Hercules. His sparkling blue eyes hold a promise of friendship, but his weak chin discernible beneath his beard indicates withdrawal. His is the countenance of a man tormented by deep anguish, a man who craves to do great things and cannot do them, who tired of doing what is possible dreams of doing the impossible. This man is a dilettante who, because he desires so much, can achieve practically nothing. His melancholy, his tremendous yearnings, are expressed in his pale smile full of sadness and renunciation. In the silence while the lute player rested between two songs, I could feel the vibrations in the air, like a tenuous hum, like the beating of wings, between Leonardo da Vinci and Mona Lisa. It was as if the nostalgic lady and the melancholy painter were silently reciting to each other the endless psalm of their sadness. When Leonardo moved away from the easel, I could finally examine the picture of Mona Lisa. And I staggered under the impact of a sudden revelation. Mona Lisa's was really the portrait of Leonardo da Vinci himself!

This was not my senses deceiving me, nor an arbitrary interpretation. Leonardo da Vinci was really painting himself with a woman's face. The face, the body, the garments, all were Mona Lisa's, but the subtle expression of the countenance, the remote melancholy were Leonardo's. And then I noticed something that sent shivers down my spine. The woman seated in that room was a sad woman who looked as if she could never smile. Her expression was one of eternal seriousness. But the woman on the canvas was smiling, the same identical gelatinous smile that never left Leonardo's lips while he painted Mona Lisa.

All this is so strange that I am perplexed and cannot explain it clearly. But this is true, Your Excellency: for years Leonardo has been painting a woman who is only a mirror of his dreams. In her face Leonardo is painting his own portrait, and especially that strange smile that never leaves his lips, but which I dare say never crossed the lips of Mona Lisa.

L'ENVOI

I beg Your Excellency to convey, through the Chief of Protocol, to Her Exalted Majesty the Queen, Doña Isabel la Católica, this testimony about the man who is today one of the outstanding artists in Italy. I await your orders, but my advice is this: Leonardo da Vinci is too close to us for us to judge whether he is a genius or a prodigious charlatan, an admirable artist and scientist or a mad visionary. I can personally vouch for his great artistic ability. Nevertheless, I sincerely and respectfully suggest that no attempt be made to enlist his services to paint the portrait of Her Exalted Majesty the Queen, Doña Isabel la Católica. The man could never paint our sovereign in all her glory, because he is too engrossed in his own tragic personal drama. They tell me that all his works bear the same smile I saw him give to Mona Lisa: Leonardo da Vinci bestows that smile on all his paintings so that they may not cry. It is the smile of one who feels that he could be master of the universe, the equal of the gods, but is held down by his human limitations. Even I, a simple man, was greatly disconcerted when I noticed the contrast between the countenance of Mona Lisa, a solemn, humorless woman, and that of "La Gioconda," that smiling sphinx Leonardo da Vinci has painted. Because the smile worn by the woman in the picture is the smile of the master himself, a smile that hides his deep silent skepticism about a world that he feels is incapable of comprehending the magic of his genius.

PSYCHIATRY LOOKS AT MODIGLIANI

We should no longer regard works of art as isolated objects with a mysterious life of their own in space. A painting is a psychologic projection of the soul of a man who happens to be an artist. Each stroke of the brush, each color, each curve and line acquires its true meaning from the mood of the artist when he applied more pigment here, less pigment there, when he selected black and white in preference to colors, when he decided to do a landscape instead of a human figure. An artist's moods, his selection of tools, subject, technique, lines, colors, are all significant in the study of the intimate texture of his spirit.

Because we know little about these factors, our attitude while standing before the work of a great artist is not one of admiration for the artist himself but for his paintings, as if they were totally independent of the man behind them. Why not look at the paintings as if they were still in the hands of the man who did them? Only then—through the living artist—can we understand his work.

What follows is an experiment in interpreting the life of Amedeo Modigliani through his art, and his art through his tortured life.

Modigliani was born in Leghorn, Italy, on July 12, 1884. His childhood was spent in coughing and ailing, which shortened his school days. At sixteen, when a boy is barely entering life through the biologically explosive door of adolescence, Amedeo, spitting out fragments of lung, had already signed his away. Only his visits to the art school in Rome where his mother sent him succeeded in making him see in art another world stronger than that of death.

From *Gentry* no. 8:92, Fall, 1953.

In 1906 he went to Paris. He was dazzled by Cézanne, who even after death continued to win battles, and by Picasso whose genius was ascending like an impatient comet over the French skies. He exhibited his work first in small galleries and finally at the Salon des Indépendants, bulwark of those immortals not yet recognized by mortals. But the police closed the exhibition, for even in Paris Modigliani's nudes were considered indecent.

This was the heroic period in Modigliani's life. A man who knows that he is going to die, as Modigliani did, knows also that there is only one way to defeat death—to live fast. What is lost in duration must be made up in intensity. Modigliani tried to compress several lives into one. He painted constantly, and between fits of coughing, bouts of drinking, and experiments with drugs, tried to satisfy his insatiable sexual desire with an endless series of women who, naked and immodest, now look down upon us from his paintings with long, narrow eyes.

Every day of Modigliani's fourteen years of struggle, orgy, and tragedy in Paris, under the triple curse of sickness, failure, and poverty, was like every other. He woke late. The sun, when it shone, was the only clean thing to enter his room. His head ached each morning; he was cold, he coughed, and he shivered as though quicksilver were running through his veins. Everything in his room was gray: the covers of the bed and the towels over the cracked washing bowl, the walls into which humidity had eaten its way like leprosy, even the face reflected in the mirror from which the silver had almost disappeared.

Let us reconstruct a single day in Modigliani's life, following him as he leaves his sordid room and steps out onto the pavements. . . .

Slowly he makes his way through the narrow streets. His head is reeling. He vaguely remembers that he drank too much the night before, as he had done the night before that and all other nights, and that he had again taken that drug with music in its name and death in its wake; that his friend Utrillo, an even greater drunkard, had stolen his coat and that he had had to chase after it through half of Paris; that together they had painted, in drunken revelry, a mural on the walls of a lavatory in a café. Utrillo had done the little streets with white walls, and he the figures. And when the proprietress of the café saw it, she had made them wash the walls and had thrown them out on the street. There is a vague scent of flesh about his clothes; he remembers with a tremor the few minutes of passion with some woman during the night.

He arrives at the house of the art dealer in whose cellar he is allowed to work. He takes a long draught from the bottle and the liquid burns. He coughs painfully and the cough seems to tear off strips of lung. He spits and is horrified. He takes another swig and begins to paint. The rain outside is forgotten and so is his disease. Pausing only for another swallow from the bottle, or to wait for a coughing attack to subside, Modigliani paints a woman, her neck like a swan's, her eyes like jade, her mouth set in infinite sadness.

It is late at night when Modigliani finishes his bottle and his painting. He collects the few francs the dealer advances for the day's work. Half-drunk already, trembling with cold, hunger, and fatigue, he goes out through the blue night of Paris and starts all over again the endless search—for fortune? a woman? a friend? God? himself?

In 1918, with the scanty proceeds from fifteen of his paintings sold by a friend, Modigliani went to the south of France. When he returned some months later to Paris, he entered a hospital. In January, 1920, he died. A few hours after his death, his neighbors heard a scream: Modigliani's mistress, in a supreme romantic gesture, had jumped out of the window of his room.

When the man died, the legend began. Fauvism and Cubism stepped aside to make place for the newcomer who, like Utrillo, was his own school—the school of the painter of swan-necked women.

How can psychological projection techniques throw light on Modigliani's complex personality? Can the symbolism of his painting serve as a clue to his fantasies and emotional drives?

One of the most widely used of these techniques is the drawing of a human figure, a method taking as its premise that our personality is revealed through our thoughts, words, gestures, movements, and actions. Ask someone to draw a person, and he will draw a figure which he subconsciously identifies with himself. Such subconscious autoidentification represents what in psychiatry is called the projection of the *body image*—the image of himself that exists in every person's subconscious. The figure drawn is as intimately related to the person who drew it as handwriting is to the writer.

It is possible to understand something of the psychology of an artist through the subject of his work. Exceptions are rare. Picasso in his period of introversion turned his back on the human figure and painted still life. There are those who all their lives kept their backs turned to human intercourse and preferred to face still life; witness Braque's mandolins and Morandi's bottles. But Modigliani was too human to be interested in objects of mineral immobility. He loved life as only a tubercular condemned to premature death can love it.

If Picasso made of the world a watch factory and appointed himself celestial watchmaker, anticipating in his pictures the atomic bomb and the disintegration of the universe, Modigliani turned it into an album of the artistic personalities of his time and the little people around him. He painted sculptors—Brancusi and Laurens; poets—

Cendrars and Cocteau; painters—Soutine and Kisling; the dancer Nijinsky; the fashionable men and women he saw coming out of the opera; he painted *concierges,* maids, musicians, neighborhood children, and particularly his mistresses. He was possessed of a deep desire to immortalize everyone around him.

And there are Modigliani's nudes, the most naked nudes in the history of art. Modigliani's nudes are shamelessly carnal, unreservedly erotic; they are panoramas of that complete abandon and cynical serenity of satisfied flesh.

Almost always he painted single figures; his backgrounds are mere decoration intended to emphasize technically some special quality of the subject. He limited his art through the restricted radius he voluntarily imposed on his technique, yet he attained an unlimited variety by investing each subject with a powerful individual characterization, for he was expressing in each portrait the objective truths of his own compulsions.

Modigliani's figures always give an impression of loneliness, isolation, nostalgia, reflecting the introversive attitude of the artist himself. Their postures suggest recoil, withdrawal within themselves, as if on guard against their environments. Their hands are crossed over their laps in an attitude that might be called maternal, yet seems to be protecting the reproductive organs. Recoil, withdrawal, self-defense: these are impulses of a person who feels himself surrounded by hostile forces. The bare, smoky, rusty backgrounds symbolize the nebulous world of alcohol, drugs, and the undefined nostalgias that possessed the artist.

His women are proud, majestic, with that agelessness of a stone idol which, abandoned on a desert, impassively withstands the attacks of the elements and the passing of the centuries. His men are like Aztec gods—aloof, immutable, eternal.

Psychologically, this is a revealing clue to the complexes in Modigliani's personality: he saw others in the same way children see adults—as powerful giants untouched by the storms in a child's world. Modigliani, who never ceased being a child, symbolized in his women the maternal archetype; he made of every woman in his paintings the woman-mother-goddess type, to be simultaneously loved and respected. For them death does not, cannot exist.

REVEALING CLUES IN MODIGLIANI'S ART

The neck.

The most striking feature in most of Modigliani's pictures is the neck. Long, thin necks have been observed in the drawings of psychosexually undeveloped schizophrenics. When a subject shows an obsessive interest in necks in his projective drawings, it reveals that he is preoccupied with the conflict between his physical impulses and the restraint his mind exercises over them. The neck is the organ that divides his intellectual life (centered in his head) from the instinctive life-impulses of his body.

The fact that Modigliani elongated the necks of his models out of all normal proportion reflects the conflict between his overpowering sexual impulses and his desire to dominate them through asceticism.

The head.

Modigliani's heads are distorted. The head in projective techniques is the center of the ego, of all our social and intellectual power, and of our control of physical impulses. When a subject loses control over himself, he usually compensates for this loss by enlarging the size of the head in his drawings.

The mouth.

Modigliani's mouths are shaped like a Cupid's bow. The recurrence of this type of mouth in his paintings indicates a morbid interest in the oral region, a characteristic of oversexed, alcoholic individuals, and of people suffering from psychosexual infantilism. Subjects of this type usually have a compulsive need to concentrate on the mouth as a pleasure-giving organ.

The eyes.

The half-closed eyes Modigliani painted again indicate emotional immaturity. They are the eyes of one looking at the world without seeing it, except perhaps as a stimulus-producing, nebulous mass. Through the half-closed eyes of his figures, the artist himself, without too much interest, stares out at the world from the distance imposed by his sickness and his alcoholism. On the other hand, those same half-closed eyes express a desire to keep the world out, to concentrate solely on himself and on his obsession with his sick body.

The nose.

The nose is also highly significant in drawings made under projective techniques. In most Western countries, a flat nose has always been a symbol of sexual impotence and of a somewhat tortuous personality. A small nose is considered attractive in a woman; it is not so in a man. Actually, in Spanish countries the word *chata* (literally, *flat nose*) applied to a woman is an endearing term; but to insult a man, one calls him *chato,* implying that he lacks virility.

Modigliani's art reflects the psychological secret of his personality as a man, which in turn determines the characteristics of his art. His longing for intellectual and spiritual self-discipline was constantly struggling with the demands of his overflowing sensual nature; his dreams of physical and sexual vigor were at odds with the failings of his body, his ailments, and his psychosexual infantilism; his desire for glory rebelled against the frustrations and poverty of reality.

Modigliani gave free reign to his instincts until he burned himself out in his own fire, although he never allowed the sordidness of his life to intrude in his art. His choice of the human figure as his only medium reveals his terror of loneliness. His nudes reveal his escape through the flesh. The attempt to immortalize his subjects by imparting to them a semblance of ageless idols reveals his desire to transcend the limitations of ordinary mortals like himself. Modigliani's figures seem beyond death because he has transformed them into sculptured ideals by a process of artistic mineralization. And that unique serenity, that melancholy calm which he imparted to his figures is an attempt to realize the dream of peace which he never attained in his tortured life.

"Nobody dies the day before," says a gaucho proverb. Some people may lament Modigliani's early death at thirty-five. If he were living today, Modigliani would be sixty-eight years old, but he would still be younger than the other living titans of modern art: Picasso, Braque, and Miró.

It is regrettable that Modigliani was not allowed more time and energy and less pain and anguish; but his fourteen creative years were far more productive than half a century of work of some other artists. There is no such thing as premature death for genius. One mystery a departed genius takes with him is whether his creative force would have lasted had it not been cut short by death. Perhaps fate ordains that some geniuses give what they have to give and then disappear, like a comet once it has showered its light across the heavens. Modigliani did not die before his time. Like a candle, he burnt out after having given light. Perhaps if he had not known of his forthcoming premature death, the light of his genius would have been less brilliant.

Some people may even say that to die young in the midst of genial creation, like Modigliani, is a noble fate accorded only to those beloved of the gods.

THE STRANGE UNIVERSE OF GEORGES BRAQUE

*t*he world was created as a magnificent but chaotic conglomerate of forms, colors, sounds, and smells. The Cubist painters have re-created the world by converting the original amorphous chaos into a geometric cosmos subject to law and measure. The qualitative impressions of classic art have been converted into quantitative measurements.

Cubism was created by the Spaniard Pablo Picasso and the Frenchman Georges Braque, who were later joined by Fernand Léger and Juan Gris, making up the original quadrumvirate. That was back in 1907 when Paris *was* Paris, when the satin shoes of the can-can girls were used as much to drink champagne from as to dance in and blue gas flames still lit up the *vie de Bohème* celebrated by Murger and Musset. With the passing of time, however, it was Picasso who with his restless brush became the sun that eclipsed the light of the other stars, while Braque, the authentic artificer of Cubism, was relegated to the background so often reserved for innovators.

In the last few years, however, attention has again been drawn to Braque's work, and the aging French artist has been vindicated as the giant of Cubism who revealed to lesser mortals the beauty hidden in the most insignificant objects.

PICASSO AND HIS NEW TERRA INCOGNITA

When Picasso finished his "Demoiselles d'Avignon" in 1907, he intended in no way to establish a new school of painting; the picture

---

From *Arts & Architecture* 71:16, 32, 1954.

was simply the fruit of his restless Mediterranean temperament avid for new means of expression. Groping his way toward a new style, Picasso developed an interest in the black masks of East Africa, which were the source of inspiration for the two *demoiselles* on the right of his painting, while for the three on the left he was inspired by prehistoric Spanish sculptures. The painting was a great success, for the rebellious Spaniard, brandishing his brush like a sword, had attacked the "pretty" themes of the Impressionists, had abandoned the attempt to capture expression through color so characteristic of Gauguin, and had gone much further than Cézanne in his desire to capture expression through form.

This was the beginning of what Ortega y Gasset has called the "dehumanization" of art, the beginning of two new paths with no room for nature and its themes, the two paths along which the art of our century runs: the "musical" path of the polychromatic harmonies of color, initiated by Gauguin (we need only recall his dictum, "For me painting is like music"), developed by Matisse, who changed the colors of nature into the more varied colors of his palette, and culminating in Kandinsky, who turned his back on models and freely painted the colors that flashed through his mind; and the path of liberation of form, initiated by Cézanne and Seurat, developed by Picasso and Braque, and culminating in Mondriaan. If the former group of painters ran the entire gamut of "musical" emotions, the latter group was primarily interested in geometric sensation. Cubism represented the end stage in the evolution of painting from artistic realism to total abstraction and followed a logical pattern and architectonic order, of which Picasso was the prophet and pioneer and Braque the supreme pontiff.

Cubism was born as an art exercised by architects of the brush whose fantastic desire was to change our tridimensional world into a four-dimensional world by introducing the element of time into painting, thus confirming the fact that Einstein's theory of relativity holds true even in art.

THE YEARS OF INDECISION

Georges Braque was born in Argenteuil-sur-Seine on May 13, 1882. He came from a family of house painters who painted pictures for pleasure on Sundays. As a child he enjoyed wandering along the Seine, which only a few years earlier had been glorified on canvas by Monet. When he was eight years old his family took him to Le Havre, where a new world would for many years unfold before his eyes like a vast water color of changing nuances. There the sails of sloops hovered like butterflies, the salt-laden breezes carried the spice of adventure, and the blue aromatic spirals of smoke rising from sailors' pipes enfolded stories of the seven seas. As night fell, the lights of the city went on and the port resounded with the music of strange tongues. The lighted windows of cafés were a breach in the dark night through which one entered the world of the unpredictable. The painted faces of women smiling at the passer-by from doorways held out promises of unspeakable pleasures. The influence of this port—beaches and sails—is still reflected in Braque's work today, in his apparel (the jerseys he wears still seem to drip the blue of the sea), and in his dark weather-beaten face.

In his early years Braque was a house-painter's apprentice who spent all his spare time making untutored strokes on paper with pencil or brush. Only after he had done his military service did his family consent, contrary to tradition, to his studying painting systematically. The young land-sailor dropped anchor in Montmartre and initiated the engrossing but painful process of self-fulfillment.

He was tormented by doubts. Where did his talent lie? In archaic Greek art? In Poussin's classicism? In Impressionism? The nervous brush of the adolescent attempted many manners before finally succumbing to the magic of the little dots of light painted by Seurat and the flaming colors that characterized the work of Matisse and Derain. Under the influence of the first he painted a little picture called "The Port," and under the spell of the second he painted the landscape of L'Estaque, a small town east of Marseille on a bay encircled by the blue shadows of the Alps. His work was grouped with that of the *Fauves,* exponents of those lively colors and thick profiles that even today mark the work of Matisse and Dufy.

Braque exhibited his first canvases at the *Salon des Indépendants* in Paris: a handful of landscapes and figures in vivid pinks, greens, and purples. Still thrilled by his first sales, he retired to La Ciotat, a small port near Marseille, to continue painting. At this time he was deeply impressed by Cézanne, who had renounced Impressionism and was painting a strange universe made up of cylinders, spheres, and cones. One can guess the impact of Cézanne's work on Georges Braque; one can visualize the young artist attempting to imitate the master-geometrician in oils whose brush was also a ruling-pen and compass and who could re-create nature by painting three humble geometric figures.

When Braque returned to Paris, there was a handful of pale green and brown landscapes under his arm. A young collector, Daniel Henry Kahnweiler, who was buying paintings from Derain and Picasso, purchased everything Braque had done. Then the timid deferential Braque met Picasso, a Picasso still wrapped in boastful Andalusian arrogance like a musketeer in his cloak. Seated at café tables, the two artists would lose themselves in long conversations until the stars were erased from the sky by the pink sponge of dawn.

One autumn day Braque went to Picasso's studio to see his picture "Les Demoiselles d'Avignon." He was strangely moved by the painting: the five nude girls had faces reminiscent of some prehistoric bas-relief and were enveloped in a dynamic aura of disquieting diagonals and obliquities.

As Kahnweiler himself has pointed out, Cubism derives from the black masks of the Ivory Coast so fashionable in Paris during the early part of our century. In African masks and figures the artist found a new art in which he might convey not what he saw but what he knew about an object or person. It was a conceptual art in which the statue was only a sign or emblem of what the artist wished to represent. The spectator had therefore to imagine the face hidden behind the masks. The faces and figures were three-dimensional and the concave replaced the convex. The outside world penetrated the statue rather than gliding over it. The figures were not compact or self-enclosed, hermetically wrapped in the sack of an epidermis as protection against the discovery of the secret of its inwardness; they were open figures with eyes like two wooden cylinders. This was, so to speak, transparent sculpture.

Picasso applied these principles to painting, along with or following his study of African masks, and painted his "Demoiselles." As he viewed this picture, Braque felt he was resisting the pleasure it afforded him. It may have been the resentment any creative spirit experiences when faced by a power that will enslave him, and even admiration is enslaving. But two months later, Braque began to paint a nude woman in gray, beige, and pink, and when he finished it he found himself staring at yet another "Demoiselle," a woman all angles in dynamic combination with planes fascinating in their mobility. Thus, while Fauvism sang its swan song in the latest paintings done by Derain and Matisse, Picasso and Braque were giving to the twentieth century the first creations of a new style in which the world became a whirling geometry of superimposed planes, transparencies, distortions, and writhings, which Braque would later develop to the ultimate and which is now known as Cubism.

Not very long ago Matisse was asked to confirm the anecdote that it was he who unwittingly coined the term "Cubism" when he described Braque's picture of the port as "a series of little cubes." The old magician of the dazzling colors shrugged his shoulders at this anecdote, but whether Matisse is responsible for the name or not, it does not alter the fact that Braque and Picasso created Cubism and that the steel-like edges of whirling planes provided the basis for an extraordinary friendship between these men: the Spaniard with the restless soul of a *saltimbanque* and the orderly Frenchman who constructed his pictures with the meticulous care of a Swiss watchmaker.

CONVEX AND METALLIC IS THE WORLD

The nude that Braque painted in the fall of 1907 is therefore to a certain extent an outgrowth of Picasso's "Demoiselles d'Avignon" and of the angular, cubic planes of Negro sculpture. The painter was drawn to the idea of reconstructing the universe arbitrarily by reducing the capricious curves of a woman's body to a limited number of straight lines and rectangular blocks. When Braque returned to L'Estaque the following spring, he psychologically renounced the violent reds, blues, and violets of Fauvism and confined his colors to pale greens and ochres. When he painted a landscape he rejected everything soft, empty, or round and saw beauty only in the straight, angular, and abrupt. Woods and beaches became cubes and cones, prisms and polyhedrons. The world was no longer a garden catalogue; it had become a treatise on Euclidean geometry.

For Braque, space did not contain red earth, blue skies, and emerald woods; it held only geometric forms and volume. The universe lost its soft concavities and became prickly with gray and brown convexities. But even the vanguardistic *Salon d'Automne* rejected Braque's pictures and, although two of the judges later cast favorable votes in futile vindication, Braque withdrew the pictures. Later they were exhibited at the Kahnweiler Gallery in Paris and came to represent the first great victory in the embattled history of Cubist painting. Astonished spectators stared at these pictures that somehow recalled static Egyptian art. The canvases depicted a self-enclosed universe, convex, metallic, a pyramid of cubes piled up in a space as securely locked as a money-safe but endowed with certain mysterious harmonies. There was a great sincerity and strength in these pictures, two qualities always admired in an artist's work.

Meanwhile, Braque continued working with Picasso. They took walks together and had long talks and drank red wine at twilight while the Seine turned a liquid ruby; and they painted together, an unheard-of phenomenon in the history of art. So similar were their pictures, so close their collaboration, that it was difficult to distinguish between their works.

But nature in its combinations became too monotonous to Braque. The sky was always blue or gray; trees always grew in the same way; there were no vertical rivers. Why not play God a little? Why not imitate the child who arranges his blocks any way he wishes? Why not paint the infinite variety of combinations permitted only in that lawless, limitless, anarchic universe that is the uninhibited human mind? And so Braque embarked on his new phase and marked out the battleground on which Cubism would fight and win its great victory: still life.

"THE GUITAR IS MY MADONNA"

Flemish painters glorified interiors, cozy rooms safe from the inclemencies of weather and the dangers of the world. They exalted opulence in their still lifes by combining fruit, table-settings, fowl, fish, pipes, bread, and rich hangings in splendid demonstrations of good living. To understand the meaning of still lifes, one must remember that we see them every day and interpret them without realizing the tremendous impact they have had on the modern world of advertising, the movies, literature, and ordinary daily life. A high hat, a gold-handled cane, and white gloves in a foyer, all evoke the gentleman who left them behind on his way to the drawing room. Two glasses of champagne, one of them edged with lipstick, and an ash tray bristling with cigarette stubs, one of them in a gold holder, evoke the magic rendezvous that took place at the little table in the discreet café, just as the thick well-gnawed mutton bone, the empty wine bottle, the bread crumbs and cheese rinds, all bespeak the healthy eater who held Rabelaisian communion with the world of gluttony.

The still lives of the classical painters and later of the French Impressionists held a message that consisted of the charming esthetic arrangement of various objects in a friendly artistic group. A Frenchman, Chardin, transmuted the Flemish-Dutch tradition of still lifes into the poetry of the humble objects of daily life. With his brush he related the plastic poem of everyday living. The classical artists preferred painting partridges and seafood; the Impressionists— Manet, Renoir, Cézanne—preferred fruit and flowers. It was Braque who introduced the poetry of musical instruments, for he had played one of them, the accordion, at Latin Quarter dances attended by Picasso, Derain, and Dufy.

In Braque's still lifes we see glasses and bottles, pipes, tobacco, newspapers, playing cards, mandolins, and especially guitars, because the guitar, as Juan Gris pointed out, was Braque's madonna, just as the mandolin would become his mistress. His iconography was later enriched by the addition of players of musical instruments, flutes, musical scores, notes, and piano keys. With these objects Braque was able to paint forms that reminded him of the sphere, cylinder, and cone, all Cézanne's favorites, and also to gratify deep-rooted lyrical appetites, to give vent to that vague musical urge engendered in his soul by the romantic breezes of Paris.

THE SECRET OF BRAQUE'S STILL LIFES

It has been said that Braque painted still lifes only. This is not true. Braque has painted fields and beaches, women and landscapes, but he always came back to still lifes, to groups of objects arranged in his imagination according to an order known only to him. In the pictures belonging to this, his great analytic Cubist period, we see strange figures, superimpositions of blocks, cubes, angles, planes, lines, and polyhedrons in chaotic confusion. But as we study these paintings more carefully the chaos becomes cosmos. There frequently appear single letters or musical notes, representing chance fragments of reality caught by the artist in the course of his daily living. These disparate elements remind us of the snatch of music we chanced to hear one day on the street from a blind man's violin or from an invisible piano, or the advertisement from some show-window that caught our eye briefly, or a piece of newspaper half-buried in a garbage can. The insertion of these bits of the subconscious in Braque's pictures is like the insertion of commercial catchwords in a poem or the shriek of an automobile horn in a symphony. They represent the humble but imperious voice of reality, reminding us that we are still inhabitants and prisoners of the earth no matter how violently we beat our wings in a vain attempt to reach the empyrean or the poetic ideal.

As Jean Cocteau has pointed out, Picasso's Cubism was Spanish, one of the many instruments used by the artist to assert his imperious and inexhaustible genius; Braque's Cubism was French, that is, it was the reason and essence of his life, the method of expression most appropriate to his exquisite nature. Picasso was the "discoverer" of Cubism, Braque its "colonizer." Picasso was the master of a style he later abandoned; Braque fell in love with Cubism and was chained to it for the rest of his life. Picasso was the seducer, Braque the faithful lover.

TWO EVASIONS FROM THE WORLD

Ortega y Gasset once told us students in Madrid that art is escape. I believe that there are two ways of escaping from the world: by exploring exotic uncharted lands and seas or by becoming a monk and retreating to the cell of a monastery. Picasso belongs to the first; Braque to the second. Picasso fled from life in the mad boat of his ever-changing art; Braque in the cloistered solitude of his Cubist cell, in the hermetic niche of each one of his pictures. As one looks upon the tragic merrymaking of his guitars and mandolins, the mechanical perfection of his compositions, one feels shut in, one gasps for air. Suddenly this tridimensional universe flattens into two dimensions and then springs up into four. What we lack in air we make up in time. Braque's pictures have no air because they have no backgrounds; on the other hand, they imprison time in their grays and mauves. Only once in a while does the movie camera technique used by Braque afford us a glimpse of reality through some musical passage or the letters chalked on a bar window or the label on a bottle of rum.

When he wished to carry this idea of mixing the real and fantastic to the extreme, he created his *collages:* here paint was mixed with sand, paper, wood, carton, and wire to produce compositions that are statues flattened by a steam roller, works of sculpture pressed down on canvas by a painter's brush, attempts to capture the changing world in the immutability of the monolith. These *collages* are like the letters of a mysterious alphabet of esthetic emotions, known exclusively to the artist.

BRAQUE'S PRIVATE UNIVERSE

The world captured by Braque is a fascinating one. His Cubist paintings show some object transformed by dint of being broken, deformed, flattened, cut, and made transparent until it becomes a magic bit of the universe thrown around and upset by some schizophrenic god. If the greatness of a work of art is not measured by its theme or development, colors or size, but rather by some unique quality, and if that quality is the function of the truth, liberty, and perfection within the work, then Braque's paintings are great.

Braque proved that he was a master of colors, then gave them all up except for the mono-, bi-, or tri-chromatic tones. He is an artist with a great imagination who cut the wind out of his own fancy, suppressed all impetuousness, and concentrated on showing us the poetry of ordinary things, the charm of the commonplace, the immense possibilities of domestic objects.

As Braque himself has said, he never paints an object until it has lost its functional properties and is ready to be discarded. The Cubist technique initiated by Braque means taking an object—a guitar, a pipe, a bottle, a table, a glass—and breaking it apart with the same loving cruelty shown by an entomologist dissecting a butterfly. Each object is broken up, examined from within (as children, we loved breaking our toys open to see what was in them), and then combined with parts of other objects—dead birds, envelopes, table legs, flowerpots—until a new reality is created out of space.

The title of the painting is misleading because it expresses only the initial idea which was lost as the work developed. Braque starts, for example, with the idea of a table holding several objects. In his mind he regroups these objects and dismembers them. Then he combines them on the canvas, taking a cut of wallpaper, a table leg, guitar strings seen from within, the profile of a mandolin, and placing them all on the table as seen from above. Next, using his palette brush, spatula, and knife, he combs and scratches the colors, mixes them with sand, cement, or graphite, and obtains marvelous pictorial effects of corrugated cardboard, wallpaper, marble, granulated woods, sand, printing ink, marble dust, wire, and cloth.

The objects in the painting are seen from every angle as if the painter were spinning us around with him on some merry-go-round. The unity of an object melts into the unity of other smaller objects inside of it. Transparencies are introduced when two planes are superimposed one on another and small shadows appear within the area of the large shadows, like playing cards that cast no shadows when they are on the table but project ever-growing shadows when they are picked up.

The final result is an intensely decorative painting which also reveals a tremendous curiosity on the part of the artist in everything invisible and mysterious in the inanimate world around us. That is why Braque's Cubism may at first sight strike us as cold, but it slowly becomes—with its soft olive greens, honey-yellows, wax-grays, and silvers used in loving treatment of oyster shells, sliced lemons, flower petals, or violin-bows—the work of a devoutly religious man who executes his work on his knees, so to speak, in an attempt to humanize the enigmatic universe represented by the objects we see all around us.

BELLICOSE INTERMEZZO

After 1913 the vicissitudes of life separated the strong Picasso from the reticent Braque, just as they had come between Van Gogh and Gauguin. When the First World War broke out, Braque exchanged his brush for a rifle. He had dismembered the world in his Cubist canvases; now on the battlefields of France with his own eyes he saw the real world fall apart.

The war left him sick and exhausted. He suffered a serious head wound which almost blinded him and he had to undergo a trepanation. Fortunately he received this wound at the height of his career; otherwise, his enemies might have attributed the origin of Cubism to the bit of shell imbedded in Braque's skull.

It was at this time that Braque attempted a new style of subtler colors and more harmonious compositions. His art became less abstract and more human. Natural objects again appeared in his works. He explored new artistic paths, and several elements of classical Greek art appeared in his pictures like *arpeggios* of some distant symphony. He sculptured, too, and after the horrors of the German occupation in the Second World War his work became more firm, more confident, in the grand tradition of Poussin and Chardin.

In some of his more recent works, e.g., his billiard tables, he tried to introduce a new dimension by adding the element of congealed movement to the illusions and tricks of tactile volume and hallucinatory spaces.

Thus Fauvism comes to its final bifurcations of romanticism and classicism. And we might call Braque a Classicist if by classicism we mean the control of the emotions by reason and logic in a musical, poetic, and architectural arrangement of the universe.

GOD'S GEOMETRICS

If by art we mean the search for the expression of beauty, then one may ask whether Cubism is art. But beauty is something eminently subjective, and in art a theme is a vehicle not only of beauty but of truth and freedom. In this sense there certainly is a similarity between a Madonna by Raphael and a Cubist abstraction by Braque. The Renaissance Madonna was a way of conveying to the spectator ideas of serenity, peace, and goodness; Braque's still life of some cactuses in a flowerpot, for example, seeks to convey to us the idea of greenness and angularity. We may therefore say that the modern work is as beautiful as any classical painting since it, too, fulfills its objective and conveys its message.

From 1919 on, Braque's life has been made up of work and triumph. His record shows one exhibition after another, all crowned by success. All over the world critics have conceded that he is supreme among the moderns in spatial organizations and the magic of color. And we all concur that from his dexterous integration of the figure presented frontally and in profile—he is thus able to show the body and its shadow, the being and the soul—there rises an eloquent musical voice that sings out the beauty of a quiet harmonious art.

Georges Braque is today a man of 80 years, modest, retiring, timid, the very antithesis of his work. He lives in a quiet street, named after the *douanier* Henri Rousseau, who painted enchanting jungles. There the artist works—sometimes on twenty paintings at once—still wearing the blue jerseys, the yellow mufflers, the corduroy trousers of former years, but now snow-white hair crowns the terracotta-colored face, just a bit paler than the reds and ochres of his canvases.

His works are the children of his soul, of a life dedicated to a strange search for the mysterious beauty of ordinary things: a bartender playing cards, a vase of roses, a violin asleep on a sofa. Braque did not seek bulk as did the painters of the *quattrocento;* he did not seek chiaroscuro like Ribera or Caravaggio, or light like Rembrandt, or air like Velázquez, nor did he want to describe sensations like the Impressionists. He strained toward the idea of things. His eyes were not sponges soaked with color, but projectors reflecting a hidden inner sun. Braque penetrated the innards of the universe and there he found pure geometry and harmony and form; there he found the proof of Plato's dictum: "God geometrizes."

Braque, like Saint Theresa among her humble cooking-pots, found in the lowly things of daily life the imprint of a superior order of harmony and beauty.

THE BRUSH AND THE BOTTLE
MAURICE UTRILLO

PRELUDE ON A RAINY DAY

*a*ll my life I have sought poetry where I could, when I could and how I could," said Maurice Utrillo.

One mid-November morning in 1949 I was in Utrillo's tiny studio at 25 Rue des Bouleaux in the village of Le Vesinet not far from Paris. Outside, the rain steadily beat down on the carpet of autumn leaves in the garden. Inside, Utrillo before my very eyes was giving the finishing touch to a small painting of a crooked street in Montmartre splashed with brilliant blossoms and gay red roofs under a blazing summer sun. Laying down his brushes, Utrillo stood staring vacantly at his hands stained with paint, apparently unaware of the marvelous world that had just come to life under his magic brush.

In the history of modern art there is perhaps no life more sordid and no art more enchanting than that of Maurice Utrillo. After more than half a century of painting and a quarter of a century of fame during his lifetime, Utrillo *"l'emmuré"*—immured by both the dominating love of his mother and his wife and his love for absinthe—continues to be a baffling mystery.

MONTMARTRE IN 1900

"I was born in Paris, in a house on the Rue du Poteau, on December 25th, Christmas Day, in the year of our Lord 1883. . . ." Thus Utrillo began his memoirs during one of his enforced retirements in a nursing home.

The Butte Montmartre, one of the most famous hills in the world, was at the beginning of our century a little village shaded by the quiet sails of four old windmills. Plants grew wild and cows wandered unhindered through the streets. But soon town and country were waging a battle on the meadows as artists began to encroach on the domain of farmer and peasant. Dressed in bizarre clothing and speaking strange languages, they sought shelter on the hill where the solitary Rousseau had woven the subtle tracery of his philosophy. Two things they all had in common: an empty purse and a rich store of dreams.

Youngsters most of them, the intruders formed a miniature world of their own, completely isolated from the rest of the universe, like those puddles of water caught in the cavities of rocks after the tide has retreated. In this particular puddle swarmed a fauna yearning for success and power. Theirs was a veritable human jungle, small but fraught with life, quarantined voluntarily, like a colony of lepers, from humdrum middle-class Paris. Theirs was a world of art, its main object not so much to keep on living as to create new life, its most important goal not how to live but how to use what life they had.

These artists of Musset's Montmartre did not regard themselves as waifs and strays but as rebels and crusaders marching, barefooted perhaps but with flying colors, towards the blue horizon. Among them were the Spaniards, Picasso, Bertolozzi, Zuloaga, and Juan Gris; the Italian, Modigliani; the Slav, Soutine; and the Frenchmen, Derain, Pierre MacOrlan, Roland Dorgeles, Segonzac, Vaillant, Dufy, Braque—and Maurice Utrillo.

These brothers-in-penury divided into various camps and each camp frequented a different café. One group met at the Café Fauvet on the Rue des Abbesses; another at Catherine's on the Place du Tertre; still another at Manières on the Rue Caulaincourt. But when night descended upon Montmartre, they all gathered at the corner of the Rue St. Vincent and the Rue des Gaules, in an ancient café squatting under the shade of an old acacia tree, its windows, begrimed by dust and age, casting a circle of light on the ground and around the roof like an old pirate's lantern. The Café des Assassins, as it was then called, later became Le Lapin à Gile.

At this café the *voyous roses,* immortalized by André Salmon, met the *gigolettes* from the Rue Montmartroise, while amateur singers performed under the alert eye of an armed gendarme. The food was excellent; the pink wine of Anjou overflowed the glasses and the hearts; and Apollinaire recited his poem "Alcohol"; while still one more anonymous painter found inspiration in a blue-eyed blonde sitting in front of a green absinthe, just as Nerval found it in Sylvia. Outside, across the street, the sails of the Moulin de la Galette dozed under the stars which, like the amber eyes of hundreds of cats, kept watch over the alleys of Montmartre.

THE DRINKING CHILD

Utrillo started painting at the age of sixteen at the behest of his mother who, under the advice of a physician, wished to interest him in art as an alternative to another more dangerous pastime. For at an age when most boys are barely beginning to glimpse the facts of life, Maurice was already a slave to that "Lady of the Green Eyes," absinthe. At sixteen he was already a drunkard.

This case of the infant drunkard is perhaps unique in the annals of medical psychology. Adults drink to return to the freedom from responsibility of childhood. Maurice Utrillo was already a confirmed drinker in his childhood. While other children were still drinking milk, he was chasing after absinthe. This precocious alcoholism was to keep him all his life in a state of emotional infantilism, like a tragic Peter Pan of the spirit.

Modern psychology looks for the secret of the adult's complexes in his memories of his infancy; but when the complexes already appear in childhood, it then must search further back into the family history to discover the causes. In Utrillo's family tree there were branches strong and verdant and bearing fine fruit next to branches sick and stunted, whose poisoned sap was one of the factors responsible for this drinking child. Only the vigor inherited from his mother's side of the family would enable him to withstand his years of tragedy and ultimately be like a fig tree that renounces the blossoms and bears fine fruit instead.

SUZANNE THE REBEL AND HER LOVE-CHILD

In the year 1884 there came to Montmartre a misshapen youth with stunted legs and a large square head. His red sensuous lips intensified the waxen pallor of his face. He was of gentle birth. In his childhood the bones in his legs had been fractured in a fall, turning him into a pitiful dwarf-like creature. His shattered soul pushed him to seek beauty not in the fine treasures of his family estate but among the human detritus sheltered in the alleys of Montmartre.

But "everything takes its color from the glass containing it." The magic hands of the deformed Toulouse-Lautrec, like the hands of a great conjurer, scraped and scrabbled among the garbage pails and pulled out a wilted cabbage, a rotting orange, which under his impassioned brush turned into magnificent orbs of silver and gold.

In the house on the Rue Tourlaque where he painted street walkers in their tawdry finery, one day Toulouse-Lautrec met a pretty country wench who was scraping together a living as a model. Her real name was Marie Clementine Valadon, but she called herself Suzanne Valadon. She was born at Bessines near Limoges in 1867 and had been a circus performer until she fell off a trapeze, escaping death only by a miracle. The Montmartre artists soon discovered her body, magnificent under the light of the candles. Today she stares down upon us from paintings in museums, her opulent beauty bared and immortalized by the brush of Renoir and Degas.

Suzanne Valadon, breathing art through every pore of her body, took to drawing sketches in charcoal on the walls. Degas, who was completely bewitched by her and called her "ma terrible Marie," urged her to paint. Gradually she developed a style of her own and became one of the leading figures in the art of her period and the second greatest woman painter in the world.

Suzanne at the age of sixteen had a love affair with a man named Boissy, an actuary for an insurance company who dabbled in painting. Boissy was also a drunkard, but with no sign of genius to redeem his weakness. Suzanne soon tired of him and left him. Boissy disappeared forever from her life, leaving no trace other than an unborn child, which he presumably sired * and which was to inherit his father's love for alcohol. This child, born on Christmas Day under the auspicious sign of the Goat, while the bells of the Sacre Coeur were tolling, was called Maurice.

Suzanne Valadon next became the mistress of a tradesman named Paul Mousis, who married her some years later. Mousis showed great affection for Maurice; he nevertheless firmly refused to give the child his own name.

The boy was thus condemned to bear no name at all unless it might be that of Valadon, his mother's maiden name. But Suzanne was a captivating young woman with a host of admirers, among whom there was one elderly but gallant, footloose Spaniard, Don Miguel de Utrillo y Molina, a painter, architect, and journalist, a man of the world, a veritable paragon of good nature who often, when he saw Suzanne worrying about her little Maurice, promised to recognize him as his own. Perhaps he thought it a happy joke; perhaps it just tickled his vanity to confess at his age a sin he had not committed.

In 1891 Don Miguel de Utrillo kept his word. In the company of two witnesses, a waiter and a clerk, he repaired with Maurice to the town hall of the *Dixième Arrondissement,* legally acknowledged Maurice as his own son and gave him his name, which the child of love would in the course of time make famous. Thus Maurice Valadon became Maurice Utrillo.

---

* It has also been said that the father of Utrillo was Renoir or Degas.

Maurice Utrillo, then, was the offspring of a singular family environment: a restless mother, a drunken father who had disappeared even before he was born, a stepfather who in spite of having married his mother would not be a father to him, and a kind stranger who gave him his name although he had never had intimate relations with his mother. To all appearances he had three fathers, yet while still in his childhood his only family was his grandmother and his mother. The possessive love of these two women turned him into a prisoner, and his imprisonment was to last until the moment he died.

Shy little Maurice went to public school at the Place St. Pierre. At playtime he always refused to join the other children in their games, preferring to sit moodily in a corner. When the other children came and made faces at him, he would jump up and beat them off with his bare fists. By the time Maurice moved on to the Collège Rollin, his studies already reflected his bad behavior.

For Maurice had discovered the green magic within the absinthe bottle. Everyday after school he would repair to the Gare du Nord and buy, beg, or borrow a glass of the pearly liquid. Sometimes he was carried home to Pierrefitte, Montmagny, by laborers who amused themselves by hauling little Maurice from café to café to see how many absinthes they could pour down his little throat before he spinned and whirled and finally flopped down in a stupor like a sparrow hit by a bullet.

His grandmother, who herself was not averse to a wee drop, appalled by the boy's condition, would reprimand him, but no sooner did she start to scold than the boy would turn into a raving lunatic, kicking, shouting, tearing his clothes off, ripping up exercise books, until finally he would drop exhausted.

After a family debate, it was decided to send the boy off to learn a trade. Maurice went through several apprenticeships: from errand boy to a flacking tin-maker to clerk at the Crédit Lyonnais, where in spite of his excellent mathematics he was shortly dismissed because of his bouts of drunkenness and unwonted outbursts against his superiors. Other jobs followed, but he kept none more than a few weeks at the most. His gullet craved constantly for wine and his fists for brawls.

Reluctantly his mother admitted that her son was a drunkard and put him away in Saint Anne's Sanatorium for a few months. Upon his discharge, the doctor who attended him told his mother the tragic truth. Maurice must somehow be weaned from his craving for alcohol. Why not try to interest him in painting, since she herself was such a promising artist?

When his mother handed him the brushes for the first time and sat him in front of the easel, Maurice looked at her disconsolately out of his big mournful eyes. Obediently, for his outbursts were unleashed only under the scourge of alcohol, he began without much desire or interest to paint the outside world that had treated him so harshly. Sometimes he would interrupt his painting to read the catechism his grandmother had given him. And mysticism and art combined soon began to spin their tenuous web around the soul of the afflicted lad. One day his mother decided to take him to Paris, and, naturally, Paris to an artist meant Montmartre.

Suddenly Maurice became aware of the world around him: the little alleys sparkling with sunshine, the old houses with ivy-covered walls, the fences draped with flowers, the strange little studios, the tiny shops, the flower stalls, the promenading young women with legions of little imps concealed in their eyes, their flesh redolent of jasmine and sin, and the bistros with their magic bottles, their windows reflecting the sunlight by day, and by night the fancies and dreams in the myriad eyes that peered through them. Maurice would press his adolescent nose against the window pane and breathe in the smell of tobacco and wine and sweat. There was much laughter and shouting and the noise of a piano.

Maurice was delighted with this world and felt the desire to paint it. He set up his easel in the open air and began painting the narrow streets, the squares, the windmills, the churches and bistros. The curtain that formerly concealed the world from him suddenly lifted. One addiction: drinking; one instinct: painting. That was all Maurice had. Through the scarlet tunnel of Beaujolais he plumbed the depths of his own destruction; through the rainbow imprisoned in his brush he ascended the heights of immortality.

But the crowd had no understanding for this human masquerader, this grotesque scarecrow who squatted on street corners making idiotic faces and babbling foolish things while painting the world around him. Children pelted him with stones, women giggled as they passed him, and men threw abuse at him. In vain the harassed artist sought peace and quiet. One after another came the pinpricks of mockery, abuse, and menace. In the end he sought refuge in a bistro, and finally, blind with wine and fury, he would turn on those who had abused and mocked him, battering at everyone within reach, even women and children. To the world's pinpricks, Maurice retorted with blows.

THE WORLD IN PICTURE POSTCARDS

From 1902, when his mother coerced him into painting as a possible cure for his drunkenness, until some twenty years later, Maurice's life was one long struggle between his impulse of self-destruction through alcohol and his yearning, incomprehensible even to him, to fashion on canvas his artistic genius.

He painted Montmagny, Pierrefitte, the Butte Pinson, Montmartre, the Seine. The pictures flowed with astonishing speed from his hands. He was a juggler with his brushes, a conjuror with colors. In seven years he painted more than seven hundred pictures, which he sold for a few coins apiece, swapped for a drink or a mouthful of food in a bistro, gave to a prostitute in return for her favors, or simply forgot in a public lavatory after being sick from his drinking, that is, if he had not already ripped the canvas in the course of one of his brawls.

For all that, Utrillo's real torment had as yet hardly begun. All the enchantment of Paris was captured in his pictures, but his slovenly appearance, his unkempt mustache and hair, his greasy black suit, his general look of degenerate emaciation prevented people from realizing the genius hidden beneath all this. As a revenge, Utrillo made it a practice to station himself outside the Sacre Coeur and pull the hair of the pious old women or abuse the expectant mothers on their way out. Afterwards, tired and lonely, he would start his nightly pilgrimage through the bistros and cafés of Montmartre, craving a glass of wine or absinthe, offering his pictures in exchange, which more often than not were tossed under the counter to become a comfort station for cats.

Though brightened by the tinsel of bohemian life, these were years of frenzied work, torture and solitude. How could anyone explain how this degenerate creature was able to paint at such dizzy speed, one picture every day or so, each one a masterpiece?

Convinced that he could not work in peace outdoors, Maurice shut himself indoors as a flash of inspiration opened the world anew before his eyes. He would paint using picture postcards as models. I saw him doing it in his studio. But the crumpled gray postcard he held in his hand had been transformed on the canvas into a street scene painted by brushes literally dipped in light and sunshine.

At first he copied his favorite artists, Sisley and Pissarro, and later on, Monet and Raphael. On his palette he used five colors from his mother's supplies: two chrome yellows, vermillion, lacquer, and zinc white; to these he eventually added others.

His forced or voluntary retirements from the world date from 1903. As a child Maurice was a prisoner of his mother's and grandmother's love; later he immured himself to evade the mocking crowds in the streets and be able to paint; afterwards because of his drunkenness he was an inmate of hospitals, asylums, and even jails. When I visited him, only some four years before his death, he was still a prisoner in the custody of his wife. I saw the sadness in his eyes as the *emmuré* painted the outside world that was forbidden to him. Perhaps this is why so many of his compositions have an air of loneliness and impending tragedy. And here also may be the secret to the absence of figures in his paintings. In his first period his streets and squares were utterly deserted, walled in by heavy skies, high walls, and closed houses, conveying the loneliness of the man himself, shut in a miserable lodging, tortured by his craving for a drink and without the means to indulge it, trying while undergoing the torments of the damned to re-create a world vibrant with color, sound, warmth, and feeling.

THE WALL

Utrillo's memory was prodigious. Alone in the dimness of his studio, illuminated, like El Greco, only by his inner light, he could reconstruct any street, any house, church, or café in the whole of Montmartre. But the walls he painted, the walls that were his great obsession, which he at once loved and hated because they were both a shelter and a prison, did not seem solid enough, and he set furiously to mixing his whites with sand and plaster. In this way he created on canvas walls so solid that sometimes he defied his friends to destroy them with a hammer. On his canvases he built a hallucinating Paris of grim architecture, he created anew the outside world into a marvelous symphony of whites. At first his skies imitated Corot, but later they became truly the skies of Paris, and his painting developed a bold, vigorous, forthright style, neither "arty" nor artificial. Realism and fancy in his painting became exalted through drink. As the years rolled by, he added pinks and vermillions, light green and vibrant blues to his range of colors. All the output from his magic brushes continued to be sold at from five to twenty francs apiece (the same prices that Renoir's, Monet's, Picasso's and Sisley's paintings commanded between 1870 and 1890). These paltry sums, however, were a fortune to Maurice, who could get a dozen glasses of absinthe for five francs.

The year 1907 marked the beginning of Utrillo's "White Period," in which he painted hundreds of pictures with zinc white mixed with sand. This was also the year when his mother, having been divorced from Paul Mousis for some time, married one of Utrillo's personal friends, a painter called André Utter, who in age might have been her own child.

For a time Utrillo lived with his mother and her new husband in a studio at 12 Rue Corot. He sold his pictures to Libaude, a hard and expert art dealer, and exhibited some of them at the Salon d'Autumne. The next year, Francis Jourdain on a visit to Libaude's galleries brought with him the famous writer and journalist Octavius Mirabeau, who fell victim to the enchantment of Utrillo's pictures. That year human figures appeared for the first time in Utrillo's paintings, a fact deserving of some attention later on in this article.

One item of psychologic interest is that at first Utrillo's paintings were signed "Maurice Valadon." Later on he changed this to "Maurice, Utrillo, V," with three commas, as though he realized the unfolding of his personality into the man, Maurice; the artist, Utrillo; and the *emmuré* walled in by his family, Valadon. So closed in by family walls did he feel that finally he went to live alone in a dilapidated boarding house on the Butte. In the five years from 1911 to 1916 Utrillo lived either at Monsieur Gay's Casse Croûte or at the Belle Gabrielle.

The years passed. Utrillo went on painting. He painted that he might drink, and he drank that he might paint better.

Now, drink creates nothing in a person; it only exaggerates what one already is. Drink can change us into caricatures of ourselves. It can bring repressed inclinations out to the surface. *In vino veritas*. Drink cannot make a dull mind brilliant, nor can it turn a pessimist into an optimist. Drinking turns the flirt into a nymphomaniac, the nostalgic person into a melancholic, the unsatisfied into a resentful person.

Drink helped Utrillo to break the bonds of his natural shyness and unleash his pent up fury against the world he believed was being ruthless with him. All the ridicule and mockery he endured during the day, while painting outdoors, was avenged no sooner he had a few drinks. Year after year (it was a marvel that his frail frame withstood the strain) he followed the same nightly routine: café after café, drink upon drink, quarrels, fights, and brawls. And usually he ended headlong in the gutter, a revolting sprawling creature amidst the garbage cans, his face bloody and raw from fist blows and broken bottles; or else he was dragged, kicked, cudgeled, or buffeted by the gendarmes to the nearest station, there to sleep off his drunken debauch in the safety of a cell.

In the morning his mother would retrieve him, and all aching and with his mind beclouded by alcohol he would return to his paintbrushes to fight another glorious battle on canvas. His hands at night had trembled like aspens when they grasped the glass of cheap Beaujolais; now they hovered in the air, light as a dove's wings, guiding the brushes into creating the cathedrals of Rouen, Paris, Chartres, and Rheims. This was Utrillo, the artist, trying to assuage the unrest that alcohol had failed to assuage with a world gleaming with the colors of the rainbow and the lights of the heavens.

Utrillo wanted to be cured. In 1912 of his own accord he entered the Sannois Infirmary. Libaude, the art dealer, agreed to pay the monthly charge of 300 francs in return for which he collected every week all the paintings Utrillo did while in the hospital.

SAD BOHEMIA

Utrillo left the sanatorium apparently cured. While there he painted a number of pictures of infinite freshness, inspired by the spring scene peeping through the windows and the modest flower beds in the garden of the asylum. Like a frightened stag he now fled from the world and humbly sought refuge in his mother's house. Utter, his mother's husband, bought him a few scraps of yarn to weave into a canvas on which to paint.

But Montmartre still beckoned. Utrillo soon shook off the family trammels and went to lodge at the Casse Croûte. To live within the confines of a café was Utrillo's ideal of freedom. There he spent his happiest years until 1915. He exhibited at the second Salon d'Automne in Paris, paid a visit to Corsica and Brittany, had a private show at Eugene Blot's, and had some of his pictures hung at the first exhibition of the Salon des Indépendants in 1913. In 1914 (a score of his pictures could still be purchased for 575 francs) his "White Period" came to an end. He commenced his period of definite architectural delineation. This phase of his life ended in 1915 when he was called up for the army and discharged immediately after his mother proved the many disabilities from which he suffered.

Utrillo's life meandered happily during those years, moving back and forth from the Casse Croûte on the Rue Paul Feval to the Belle Gabrielle on the Rue St. Vincent. By day he painted, withdrawn from the world around him, a bottle of wine clasped between his legs; by night he ate little and drank a lot, got thoroughly inebriated, came to blows with everyone and was invariably kicked out into the street. Repentant, he returned in the morning to ask forgiveness from Marie Vizier, the landlady of the Belle Gabrielle.

One day, while Madame Vizier was out, simple-hearted Maurice, anxious to please her, painted the lavatory walls with murals. The foul cubicle was transformed by the magic of his brush into a retreat purified by chaste churches, sleepy little streets, and flower-covered pavilions. His job finished, he hid away to watch the result of his well-meant surprise. Like the juggler in the story, he now offered what he could do best with all his heart. Madame Vizier returned home and went into the closet. A few seconds later she came rushing out shouting with anger, her skirts stained with fresh paint. She searched out the guilty party and, barely managing to keep her hands off him, made him wipe off with turpentine the *"cochonneries dégoutantes"* with which he had dirtied her walls. Years later she wept tears of rage to think that Fortune herself had adorned her house and she had had the face of Fortune wiped off.

Unfortunately Maurice did nothing to make peace with the world at large. He continued to shout abuse at expectant mothers. This quirk, not explained in any of his biographies, can be interpreted on psychologic grounds. Utrillo was an illegitimate child. Long gone were the days when to be a bastard was something of a good omen; even in easygoing Paris an illegitimate child was condemned to humiliation and ostracism. Utrillo's subconscious hatred of his mother's misconduct could wreak its revenge by abusing pregnant women who were about to bear still more "children of sin." His hatred for these women was translated during this period into his fondness for painting still life only, as though he wished to eschew all human beings.

One night he returned home half-crazed after a scrimmage with some drunken colliers and besmirched his frightened mother with bits of coal. Other times his hatred turned on Libaude, who had monopolized his whole output for five years hoping to make a fortune after Utrillo's imminent death from drink, particularly since Mirabeau was giving Utrillo so much publicity. Sometimes Utrillo went as far as the door of Dorival, an actor and collector who had cheated him in the payment for some of his paintings, waited until a visitor came along, and then shouted up the stairway, *"Merde pour Dorival!"* running off before the concierge could come out and strike him. Utrillo was still a little boy who did not want to grow up.

During the First World War his physical condition improved, he ate enough for four, and painted some two hundred pictures which now commanded a slightly higher price. But he still refused to believe in his genius and once again he turned to drink and dedicated himself as never before to his favorite passion. His violence when drunk was terrifying. He yelled at soldiers in the cafés and threw himself like a mad bull at one or a score if they contradicted him or made fun of him, thus seeking to erase his inferiority complexes. The gendarmes knew him well and abused him ignominiously. The barkeepers feared his violence. No one would recognize in this drooling degenerate, who in a blind, drunken fury would charge against everyone around, the gentle shy little man who in his lucid hours behaved like a humble friar and with his paintbrushes was the Fra Angelico of Montmartre.

THE SPECTER OF INSANITY

In 1916 Utrillo was again interned, this time in Villejuif, an insane asylum. There he spent four months of damnation, surrounded by mad creatures who snatched away his tubes of colors and ate them as if they were cream.

Utrillo convinced the doctors and nurses that he was not mad. His paintings were more serene than ever, more harmonious and flooded with peace. He always created his gayest works in his most painful moments. The only door to freedom was his pictures of white walls in which black doorways stood out hauntingly like the hook on a gallows tree.

For the first time he heard the definition of his failing: dipsomania, a compulsion to drink in spite of himself. But the word "dipsomania" means little more than, say, "diabetes" or "arthritis." The diagnosis must go deeper than that. Psychiatrists are aware of the fact that dipsomania is a symptom of a profound psychologic process. He who seeks his fancies and his world within the bottle with a frenzy as delirious as Utrillo's is compelled by forces which shall be mentioned later.

Between his stay at Villejuif in 1916 and his readmission to the Picpus Asylum in 1918 stretched a period in which Utrillo, terrified by his experience among the insane, remained housebound like a convalescent child tied to his grandmother's apron strings. Then one day he ran out of the house and perpetrated such a string of outrages that he had to be committed to the Hospital of Aulnoy sous Bois, from which he escaped. Again he voluntarily re-entered the Picpus Asylum, where after a preliminary treatment with bromides and showers he was allowed to paint. When he was discharged, he gave the attendants paintings instead of tips. And upon returning to the Butte he learned to his surprise that he had become famous. He was 35 years old.

The saga of Utrillo spread throughout Montmartre. Now everyone offered him a friendly word, a glass of pernod, a bottle of Beaujolais, in exchange for a little picture by that "mad Utrillo." The crowds greeted him with respect in the streets and the girls offered themselves as models. But Utrillo was not interested in female companionship. He took shelter instead in the Rue Labat, in the house of a secondhand art dealer who offered him board and lodging in exchange for everything he painted. Drink, however, pulled ever more strongly at his coattail and his brawls became bloodier with each passing day. His path pointed only two ways: interment or internment, the grave or the jail. Once more he retired to Picpus and came out all the better for it. And once more his mother welcomed him home and took him to her arms as if he were a wounded fledgling returning to the nest.

Days of great affliction for his family followed. Utrillo when sober was as big a nuisance as when drunk. If he was not rampaging around his room tearing up canvases or smashing crockery in infantile fits of temper, he was outside playing the flute and driving the neighbors to distraction. Sometimes he escaped from the house and as soon as he reached Montmartre the practical jokers made merry by giving him all sorts of horrible concoctions, unspeakable mixtures into which they even emptied the muck from the ashtrays. The end was inevitably a tragic pathologic bout of intoxication, and then after a brawl he was lugged, wallowing in blood, to the police station. The angel of the paintbrushes was also the devil of liquor.

Still once more he went back to Picpus and again was discharged, tranquilized but not cured. *Qui a bu, boira.* His eyes were clear, his heart aflutter. The kindly voice of his brushes called, but the green-eyed goddess once more whispered her sensual promises in his ears.

MODIGLIANI'S COAT

He now sought shelter in Montparnasse, in the home of an old neighbor who was a painter and a drunkard like himself. His name was Amedeo Modigliani.

In Modigliani's studio Utrillo painted at high speed, and with what the two artists earned they got drunk every night. Wine tastes sweeter in the company of friends. The two painters staggered together from café to café. In a café on the Rue Campagne-Première, happy as schoolboys playing hooky and singing away like canaries, they painted a fresco on one of the walls. Utrillo did the scenery and Modigliani the figures. Today it would be a mecca for art lovers from all over the world, except that the landlady, enraged by the "rubbish" on her wall, kicked the two drunks out into the street and furiously wiped off the fresh paint.

At dawn the two artists retired to Modigliani's studio. Utrillo, unable to sleep because of his friend's snoring and assailed by renewed thirst, got up and on tiptoe swiped his friend's overcoat and carried it off to pawn it for more liquor. When the Italian awakened his wrath knew no bounds. In the livid light of early morning he trailed Utrillo through the cafés of Montmartre. It was none too difficult to follow a track bestrewn with broken glass, empty bottles, and all the evidence of violent brawls. When Modigliani finally found Utrillo he had also pawned his own jacket and vest. The meeting ended in more drinks, more singing, and more brawls.

Emerging from a café howling and shouting, Utrillo kicked some gendarmes who called to him to be quiet. Covered with bruises and blood, he was hauled off to the police station and thence to the ward of the mentally afflicted at Picpus.

Utrillo woke up in a veritable hell. Leering faces with foaming mouths bayed and howled like mad dogs. He, too, ended up howling out his prayers for fear that God might not hear him in that inferno.

At last his mother managed to get him discharged on the promise to keep him at home under the constant vigilance of a male nurse. It was the year 1919. Utrillo was 36 years old. From then on until his death he would never again be a free man.

THE CAPTIVE PAINTER FINDS HIS EGERIA

It was a great day for the bastard painter when in 1928 President Herriot himself, at the Château St. Bernard on the Saône, near Trévoux, pinned the Legion of Honor on Utrillo's breast. When the ceremony was over, Utrillo wandered out into the garden humbly showing his beribboned decoration to the flowers and birds. Back in his room he fondled and kissed the blue ribbon and finally fell on his knees and prayed to a little silver statue of Joan of Arc.

The years from 1928 to 1935 were years of captivity and nostalgia. Locked in his studio, deprived even of his favorite toy train when it was discovered that he drank the engine fuel, he whiled away the days, months and years, playing little tunes on a harmonica, indulging in childish pranks (every first of May he shouted out the window, "Vive l'Anarchie," then hid from the view of the gendarmes on the street, bragging afterwards to his family of his daring; and he shot with a toy pistol at the women passing by), and, above all, painting hundreds of pictures, each better than the last, for his hand seemed to grow steadier as his mind grew more unstable.

One day a widow of an art collector, Madame Lucie Pauwels, née Valore, came to visit the painter. She chatted with him and patiently listened to his mystic rantings. A devoted admirer of his art, she ignored all his failings. Turning firmly to Utrillo's mother, she said, "I have been sent by heaven to save Maurice."

The two women sized up one another. Each recognized the other for the stalwart Amazon she was, and, though a sense of antagonism stirred slightly between them (it was to grow considerably in the course of time), each recognized also the other's desire to save the painter from self-destruction. A tacit pact was sealed between them and another wall was erected around the *emmuré*. On May 5th, 1935, at the age of 52, Maurice Utrillo was married to Madame Lucie Valore Pauwels.

THE GILDED CAGE

It was raining when I boarded the train at the Gare St. Lazare that would take me to Le Vesinet to see Utrillo.

I had made the same journey under identical weather conditions the day before. Le Vesinet station stood near a road carpeted with autumn leaves. A taxi bore me along roads bound by hedges and small red-roofed white houses to the Route des Bouleaux. Number 26 was a large villa protected by a high wall. A huge wooden gateway, bolted and locked, bore a sign, La Bonne Lucie. Here Bourdelle once had lived. Now and for the last fifteen years it sheltered the compulsory solitudes of Maurice Utrillo.

I rang the bell. A kindly looking maid peeped through a window and asked me if I wanted to see "Madame."

"Yes, I do want to speak to Madame. No, I haven't got an appointment, but I've come specially from New York on this particular business. . . ."

"Come back tomorrow at eleven in the morning." The window was shut tight and I was left standing on the lane under the chill autumn rain.

I returned the following day. I was resolved to see Utrillo at all costs. There was no taxi at the station and I had to walk a mile and a quarter to the villa. The cold rain followed me all the way.

Again I rang the bell. A man came out, looked me up and down, and inquired about my identity. He added that he doubted very much that Madame could speak to me without a formal appointment. Shutting the door in my face, he left me standing out in the rain. I waited. After a short while he returned. Madame would speak to me but only for a short moment. I stayed three hours. Two and a half hours I talked to Madame; the other half hour with Utrillo himself.

The house was two-storied, with a terrace, huge French windows, and a beautifully landscaped garden. Marble torsos peeped from under the ivy, a small stone fountain gurgled quietly, and in a huge aviary a score or more of brilliantly plumaged parakeets chattered away. Several barking puppies rushed to meet me, followed by a much larger dog not quite so friendly. A manservant silenced them with a wave of the hand and asked me to follow him. There was an air of peace and quiet and rural elegance. Madame Utrillo stood on the threshold of the entrance hall.

She was dressed in a robe which afforded an occasional glimpse of the flimsy stuff of a nightgown. I guessed her to be in her sixties. She had a broad, powerful face with large cheeks and a determined mouth. Her blue eyes had a steely gleam under her saffron-colored hair. As she spoke her whole face was tinged by her various emotions, just as a landscape is tinged by the tones of the sun as the hours pass.

The hall behind her, which one entered directly from the garden, was a fabulous stage decorated with two murals on which the streets of Montmartre wended their crooked narrow way, gilt and satin furniture, crystal chandeliers, and some brilliant paintings of dolls and great vases of flowers slightly reminiscent of Rousseau and Matisse although strangely primitive. These were Madame's own paintings. For indeed the first thing one meets in the home of the painter Maurice Utrillo are the pictures of his wife Lucie Valore.

THE MOTHER AND THE WIFE

On either side of the central hallway, Madame Utrillo showed me two drawing rooms, one devoted to paintings by Utrillo's mother, Suzanne Valadon, the other to Utrillo's own paintings selected from those he had produced since his marriage in 1935. Even this arrangement of the ground floor of the house was symbolic of Utrillo's life.

Madame Valadon's paintings were mostly portraits of herself in all her sensuous nakedness, her body powerful with the litheness of a young lioness. She had also done a portrait of Maurice as a youth, with dreamy eyes and a vague expression on his face.

Madame Utrillo's paintings in the entrance hall struck me as the frolicsome effort of a restless, wayward girl. The two fine murals of Montmartre's byways had been painted by Utrillo for Charpentier's opera *Louise*. "When the curtain rises and the audience sees these backdrops, there will be a roar of applause," Madame Utrillo told me with pride.

Utrillo's own gallery, on the other side of the hall, was as dainty as the boudoir of a fifteenth century marquise. All the paintings were small in size and as delicate as the trill of a nightingale.

"Critics say his 'White Period' was the best," Madame Utrillo remarked to me, "but take a look at these pictures, observe the freshness of their coloring, the vibrancy they have, and then compare them with the others."

Indeed, these paintings from Utrillo's final period were by far superior to those of former periods. They showed a new strength. Gone were the haunting whites and grays; instead, every painting was now a garden of blazing blossoms. With the advent of Lucie Valore, radiant color had erupted into Utrillo's life. The pictures painted during the strange honeymoon of the two artists looked as if the brushes had verily been dipped into sunshine and the blue of the sea. The style perhaps was a little too precious, had more mannerisms, lacked its original spontaneity. Figures dotted some of the canvases, always in pairs, symbolic according to Madame Utrillo of the two of them. These paintings, one felt, had been done by someone with lots of time for little details, something Utrillo never had before his marriage.

We sat on a gold brocade sofa facing the garden. The aviary at the other end of the garden was like a flying rainbow of feathers.

"In this house," said Madame Utrillo, "the master has worked for a good fourteen or fifteen years. Since the second of May, 1935, the day we were married, he has lived at peace with the whole world. People say I keep him shut up like a prisoner. Judge for yourself. Look at this home, the gardens, the art treasures I have surrounded him with. Everything here was designed with his happiness and protection in mind. I live only for him, though at the same time I, too, have followed my own art." She showed me a few more of her own sketches, childish in their primitive style. "People come here to see Utrillo and they go away saying that the real revelation has been to meet me."

She took me into her own studio and showed me her portrait of Utrillo, wild-eyed but with his hair slicked down, his tie properly tied, every button on his dressing gown buttoned up. Undoubtedly Madame Utrillo had been born an orderly person. Or did she just want to forget the sordid, dissipated, abject life her husband had led in his youth?

There were many richly colored paintings in Madame Utrillo's studio, signed photographs of Maurice Chevalier and Marlene Dietrich, a photograph of Rita Hayworth against a turquoise beach and wind-tossed palm trees, a cage with a gorgeous scarlet bird hopping incessantly like a wild flame, books, paintbrushes and paints, and a large window from which hung the trembling silvery fringe of the rain.

I asked Madame Utrillo about the course of Utrillo's life since their marriage. She sighed and her eyes misted with tears. They had been so very happy, she said. Madame Utrillo took very seriously her role of savior of her husband.

Since 1935, when held by the iron hand of his wife he retired from the world, Utrillo's work had all been contracted for by the dealer Petrides. The following year he exhibited his flower pictures at Petrides' galleries and in 1937 at Adams Brothers in London. That same year he went with his wife to live at Le Vesinet. In 1938 he lost his mother, Suzanne Valadon. The year after that his work was exhibited at the Valentine Gallery in New York. In 1944 he gave his fourth exhibition at Petrides'. And the same year in the company of his wife and his dealer he went for a walk on the Butte Montmartre.

It must have been the most nostalgic moment in Utrillo's life. Now he was rich and famous. Now his pictures, which in the past he had swapped for a glass of wine, brought him millions of francs a year. But now all his millions could not buy him a drop of wine.

On his visit to Montmartre, which his wife allowed him to prove to him that he could safely confront his past, he painted a little picture of the Lapin à Gile, which held so many memories of his youth. Perhaps this was the only time in fifteen years that he painted in the open air and directly from the model. The outing over, Utrillo was taken back to his cell. For the first time in his life he had not succumbed to the voices of the green-eyed goddess of Montmartre.

L'EMMURÉ AND HIS CELL

Madame Utrillo consented to my having a word with the Master— such was my insistence! It was indeed a very special favor, extremely difficult to obtain. We went down one flight of stairs and up another, stopping in a small dark corridor before a doorway. Beseeching me to disregard Utrillo's attire ("Sometimes," she warned, "out of sheer mischief he strips down to his underpants."), she unlocked the door and we entered the room.

It was a tiny studio overlooking the garden, with a window that barely allowed a glimpse of the sky. Paintings were piled all over the floor and on two sideboards. I saw a silver statuette of St. Joan, Utrillo's tutelar patroness, images of other saints, reliquaries, scapulars, medals, missals, prayer books, rosaries of silver and copper. Perched on a stool in front of a smallish easel was a little man painting a picture.

He was very small, painfully emaciated, wisps of hair straggling on his forehead, which the plough of time had furrowed deeply. His unshaven cheeks were sunken and the hand holding the brush was fleshless. Near the easel lay a crumpled gray picture postcard of a little street in Montmartre. On the easel stood the same little street transmuted by the magic alchemy of the artist's soul. A street blazing with brilliant flowers and green-leaved trees, the sparkle of spring quivering in the sunfilled air. It was a beautiful little painting. Utrillo, as if unaware of our presence, continued painting. Quietly I watched him immersed in his world of light and color. How baffling, even to a psychiatrist, that this wretched creature, that had wallowed in a world of degradation, could time and again re-create a world all beauty, peace and purity.

At last he rose from his perch and set his brushes down on a dresser. He had no palette. His tubes of colors, five or six at the most, were spread out on a table. He offered me a limp hand, withered and dry as an autumn leaf, and gave me a smile from his clear blue eyes like a timid child. He was dressed in rumpled pyjamas over which his wife had hurriedly tossed a dressing gown. In a hesitant voice he showed me his mystic relics and reminded me of the gallant Spaniard to whom he owed his name. Then he talked of his mother and showed me some faded photographs of her that hung next to the little figure of Joan of Arc. They, his mother and St. Joan of Arc, were his tutelary deities. When Madame Utrillo told him that I was impressed by her portrait of him, he answered that he himself preferred the one painted by his mother—"still, everyone to his own taste."

When he had finished showing me his diminutive cell, with a trembling hand he autographed for me a photograph of himself, "Maurice, Utrillo, V." He was still paying homage to his mother who had opened for him the door to the only world that could afford him a little happiness.

Utrillo sat down again in front of the easel. The postcard had fallen to the floor but he never noticed it. Once more his mysterious creative automatism was at work. The brush in his fleshless hand like a sword of flame seared the canvas with a blazing spot of red. The rain was audible on the roof above. Maurice Utrillo, insensible to the world around him, applied the final brushstroke on still another vision of his own inner world.

THE ARTIST AND HIS ART

Upon what basis does the art of Utrillo rest? It is impossible to pigeonhole him into any particular school. He never varied his themes, but then this is not uncommon among the modern geniuses of painting. Braque clings ever fervently to mandolins and Morandi to his bottles. Utrillo's characteristic symbol is a wall in a little street. His paintings of narrow streets fenced in by deserted houses and these by high walls are actually cells beyond his own cell window, cells like those in which he lived all his life, but electrified with the light and color that he would have liked to have. That is why there are no people in his pictures. For Utrillo hated the people in the street, who had inflicted so much pain on him, almost as much as he loved, with the love of the wandering gypsy, the street itself. His paintings are windows to outside cells filled with blue skies, sunshine, and flowers, all the things lacking in the cells of the boarding houses, asylums, hospitals, and jails, where his young life had frittered away.

The magic of Utrillo's art is that it pleases both the art critics and the street cleaners in Montmartre. This attests to their universal meaning. It is now hard to believe that once Utrillo's paintings hung in the company of hams and sausages in the display windows of the shop of Père Gay at 3 Rue Paul Feval and that now and then some laborer would splurge forty francs on one of the masterpieces for which Utrillo himself had received but a few sous.

An incurable dipsomaniac, Utrillo nevertheless had, like Baudelaire, the faculty, granted only to the elected of the gods, of seeing much more through a barred window than most people can see through a window wide open. He placed imagination, which may after all be the only true reality, before reality itself. His pictures are the children of a childish fantasy, but they overflow with human sentiment. A strange and noble presence inhabits his empty streets. His works are melancholy windows that open onto the heart. They do not strike us with wonder, but they do stir our emotions. They have the mellow nostalgic beauty of a beautiful woman growing old gracefully. They have the solemnity of a Chekhov tragedy or of the poems of Verlaine. They moved Mirabeau to say, "Nobody, not even Raphael, has ever painted the pained endurance and eternal resignation of inanimate things the way he does." Utrillo did for Paris what Whistler did for London and Piranesi for Rome. In his white, red, and green dreams he re-created an unperishable quaint and eerie Paris. As Francis Carco said, he alone "learned to reveal the city as though it were rising from the uttermost depths of the ocean." Yet he was as unconscious of his own genius as the orange tree is of the golden fruit it bears.

What an ironic paradox that this man so ill treated by life should have become the god of his little universe, capable of bending to his will the fog, the snow, the rain, the sun, and all the mysterious gleams of light. "There is poetry in everything," Utrillo once said. "I can see in walls, which others might call leprous, beautiful colors and the marks of time and of humanity. I am neither a madman nor a fool; only a cranky sort of fellow."

UTRILLO'S SECRET

The psychologic roots of Utrillo's tragedy go back to his illegitimacy. It weighed upon him from the very beginning. Against the lack of a proper father, aggravated by the presence of three men who quibbled about becoming his father, against the ribaldry showered upon him by those around him, he sought escape through alcohol. It was the means of attaining that mental regression to childhood which others attain through the mechanism of a neurosis. Alcohol returned him to the child's world of fantasy and irresponsibility, which perhaps cloaked the more intimate tragedy of sexual incapability.

The first period of his life was dominated by his mother and was characterized by retirements into hospitals, asylums, or within his own family circle. The second phase was dominated by his wife and lacked all contact with the external world and alcohol. He now created paintings ever more brilliant in coloring. Each year the critics licked their lips in anticipation of the definite failure of his creative talent which would bring higher prices for his work, and each year he dumbfounded them with still another batch of paintings more beautiful than ever. In Coquiat's words, "That devil of a Maurice is forever coming up with a fresh batch of masterpieces."

Utrillo's whole life was a harrowing mea culpa in which can be glimpsed the guilt feelings and complexes that poisoned his life: his sexual mother fixation, his sexual impotence, and his horror of the world in which he had suffered so much.

There is perhaps no better way of analyzing the sexual aspect of Utrillo's character than by considering his paintings in which women appeared for the first time. Either they stand with their backs towards one, or their faces are blurred and indistinct. These are signs of an abnormal sense of modesty and of sexual shyness. These women, moreover, are always large, broad-hipped and buxom, suggesting a vigorous sexuality. With something of the devil in him, Utrillo would tell his drinking companions in the old days when he was finishing one of these pictures: "I certainly handed that one a bottom."

Like Rubens, Maillol, and Renoir, Utrillo painted wide-hipped women symbolizing the fact that for him, who had been dominated first by his mother and later by his wife, there never existed such a thing as the weaker sex. In them he also symbolized his erotic ideal inspired by the maternal figure, just as the sign *"Vin Liqueurs Café Tabac"* in many of his pictures symbolized his other great passion, wine.

The exaggerated pelvis and the abstract profile of his women represented for Utrillo undisguised shameless sex. These thick-haired women are wrapped in a cloak of sexual aura. It is as though Utrillo's moral infirmity were aggravated into a violent libido and a primitive type of sexuality. To Utrillo painting one of these women was the same as possessing her, as was the case with the Spanish painter Romero de Torres.

Utrillo's sexual obsession rebelled against the monkish continency imposed on him by his erotic mother-fixation and his alcoholism by painting coarsely sexual women, who were the subconscious portrayal of his own mother, whom he loved and hated at the same time and whose shameless sensuality he had simultaneously envied and condemned in his boyhood. These feelings were translated into his abhorrence of expectant mothers, for in them Utrillo subconsciously saw his own mother carrying her illegitimate son. His mind revolted against women bringing into the world other children who might be subjected to the same tortures he had suffered. His wife told me that he had forbidden women to enter his home, whereas he always welcomed priests, an exaggeration of his mystical delirium.

Alcohol and painting were in Utrillo's case inseparable and complementary means for the child-man and the man-child to evade a cruel and hostile world. No doubt without alcohol Utrillo would never have painted and without painting he would have soon gone completely mad. The picture postcard I saw him copying in his studio was his only contact with external reality. Painting was at once his escape and his salvation. His streets are deserted because that was how he would have preferred the world to be—without the people who had abused him while he had painted outdoors.

Utrillo's ideal world had room only for streets filled with light and color and protective walls and nothing else. Hence the feeling of infinite loneliness that permeates his paintings. Barring those instances when his erotic obsession with broad-hipped women prevailed, with one sweep of his brush he banished all people from the face of the earth. This was his revenge on a wicked world.

L'ENVOI

The secret of an artist's greatness is not to be explained by psychiatry or endocrinology, by complexes or by glands. The divine spark we call genius is a manifestation of the celestial spheres of the mind revealed to us only through their reflection in the artist's work. Utrillo's tragic story, reconstructed here from information I gathered from relatives, friends, critics, and admirers, casts a tainted light which only increases the greatness of his art. An art as peaceful, as graceful, as spontaneous as the doves I saw, upon leaving the house, fluttering in the rainwashed air above the painter's cell.

THE THEATRE IN OUR AGE OF ANXIETY

OUR "AGE OF ANXIETY"

To write about our "age of anxiety" is to study a romantic theme. And I will start off by making that most romantic of gestures—protest. For I don't believe that ours is *the* age of anxiety. To believe this is to admit that we are facing inevitable disaster. Fortunately, this is not true. Longevity is increasing all the time; the Crusade of Medicine is conquering the stronghold of many illnesses; and we have made astounding progress in technology.

If we often say that we are living in an "age of anxiety," it is because we like to think that we have been chosen by the gods to witness great historical events. To be part of the human chorus attending a great historical event is the same, we feel, as to participate in it, just as to belong to the chorus is also to be an actor.

Our age *is* a critical one, but History tells us that there have been other critical periods. Mankind lived through the invasions of pre-historic monsters, the sinking of entire continents into the sea, world-wide epidemics, and hundred-year wars. At those times, men enjoyed the feeling of acting in a historic tragedy, just as there are people today who would like to have two livers so that they might complain about both of them.

We cannot, therefore, call ours *the* age of anxiety, for the word "anxiety" can be found even in the Bible. Anxiety has always been

---

Two lectures delivered at forums sponsored by the American National Theatre and Academy, New York, 1952 and 1953.

an integral part of History, and today it is no more recurrent than in previous times. Today, however, we are more preoccupied with anxiety than formerly. We have discovered that this word provides a high-sounding name for a frequent garden variety of emotional disturbance. And to discover the name of a thing is tantamount to discovering the thing itself. But the difference between past times and ours is the difference between the prompter and the actor, the difference between the echo of the word and the word itself. Formerly people paid the minimum price for suffering from anxiety; now we pay the exorbitant price of having found a name for it. The difference between their price and ours is like the difference between friends who go out to dine: the fellow who takes the hat check is the one who doesn't intend to pay the bill for dinner.

But if this is not *the* age of anxiety, we are, however, living in *an* age of anxiety. States of anxiety today outnumber all other types of neuroses put together. This anxiety manifests itself in the four fundamental spheres of human life: The sphere of the *I,* whose immediate problem is work; the sphere of the *I* and *you,* whose basic problem is love; the sphere of the *I* and *we,* whose essential problem is our place in society; and the sphere of the *I* and the *It,* which takes in our relation to God.

To attempt a succinct definition of anxiety is as difficult as trying to impale a butterfly with a telegraph pole; and to think that we know everything about anxiety because we have experienced it in our personal lives is like thinking that we know all about the fires in hell just because we have read all the advertisements on match covers.

THE CONCEPT OF ANXIETY

However, we must provide a cage for the wild bird of this concept. What we call "fear" is a reaction to a more or less objective danger. But *anxiety* is a subjective fear of oncoming danger; a painful sensation of apprehension. It represents the reaction of the *ego* to the inner pressure of impulses which, if satisfied, would make us suffer from a conflict with ethical standards. It is a subconscious fear of a conscious fear. An attack of anxiety is a sort of radar warning that an enemy air force is approaching. If, instead of meeting the warning with fortitude and preparedness, we react in panic and confusion, the result is anxiety.

Each psychoanalyst has his own interpretation of the cause for anxiety. Freud attributed it to the repression of the sex impulses and fear of their being discovered; Adler attributed it to the frustration of the instinct for domination; Karen Horney to ill-repressed hostility. But I never like overloaded explanations. Frequently psychoanalytic interpretations are like overdecorated rooms, or like the faces of elderly noblemen in my native country, Spain, crowded with sideburns, mustache, spectacles, gold teeth, and a wart like a volcano. Let us accept the simplest definition of anxiety: fearful expectation due to a conflict with repressed impulses.

Anxiety seems to forewarn some cataclysm, but it may also portend a happy event. Crises of collective anguish have often preceded wonderful happenings, as for instance in the years before the birth of Christ or the discovery of the New World. Then, as now, that collective anguish manifested itself in a devaluation of life and in a longing for material pleasures, in orgies and in wars. We struggle against the fear that the world will fall apart by seeking intense but transitory sense-gratifications. Or we fight anxiety with melancholy sedatives, instead of using the strength that comes from understanding.

Man reacts to anxiety by undertaking a vast program of collective devices with which to combat his fear. And since there is no better way of eliminating the fear of death than by killing death, man is making the most astounding advances ever achieved in two thousand years of medicine. Among the defenses being set up against death, we must emphasize the great role played by amusement: we attempt to forget death through lavish spectacles. That is why we have today more physicians and hospitals, more artists and more expensive shows than ever before.

Of course, the expensive spectacle is in keeping with the swift pace of our times, which in turn explains why the most prosperous arts are the dynamic arts, like the movies and its stepdaughter television, and the least prosperous are the more static arts, like sculpture, the theatre, and literature. The triumphant arts today are bidimensional, like the movies and painting; but the tridimensional, like sculpture, architecture, and the theatre, suffer. The speed of the airplane and the automobile has forged a bidimensional world in which there is no time to inspect things closely to get to understand them better intellectually. We have no time to walk around a statue slowly in order to grasp its meaning better, nor to plumb the tridimensional depths of a theatrical work. The advent of tridimensional movies may mark a Renaissance of sculpture, theatre, and the other tridimensional arts which proceed more slowly and require the spectator to pause and reflect.

THE PSYCHOLOGIC ORIGIN OF THE THEATRE

When the curtain goes up in a theatre, those seated in the first rows experience a gust of cold wind. It is the wind of Immortality.

The theatre was born when man located himself in time and space and needed representation to be able to evaluate his own spiritual dimensions. The first theatre was created in the brain of primitive man who, by the golden light of his fire, dreamed of his past actions and planned future ones. He was his own play and his own spectator. From these fantasies, born in the neuron jungle of his brain and projected upon the walls of his cave as if on a screen, the first plays were born. Since the dimension of space was lacking, man compensated for it by extending his thoughts in time.

The first actual theatre crystallized as a collective act, and from the very beginning had the majesty of all great epics. If history was the search for the epic, the theatre was the record of that search. That collective sense that informed the theatre was its salvation during such times when everything tended to disperse men; only acts based on a solid collective unity survived. That is why the theatre is today a magic hope contained within three walls that reflect the outburst of man's spiritual strength, and a fourth transparent wall through which the audience contemplates the image of its own defeats and reconstructions, as if staring in a mirror. To borrow from Hamlet, the theatre holds the mirror up to mankind.

THE CHORUS THROUGH THE AGES

From the very beginning the public has actively participated in the theatre. Every spectator is a frustrated actor, just as the cork of a champagne bottle is a "frustrated" bullet. We can best appreciate the participation of the public in the theatre if we consider the Oedipus trilogy of Sophocles. The three dramas are fine examples of group psychology. The chorus reflects the attitude of the public and converts Oedipus into a scapegoat by bringing down upon the hero the wrath of the gods. In this way the guilt-feeling of the audience created by its own subconscious incestuous desires is alleviated. The hero of Oedipus, like the hero of any drama, represents the collective ego and is created to do things that the community would like to do but dare not do. The chorus was created in the theatre in order to explain the reactions of public moral indignation. What is true for the hero as individual, for the chorus as community, and for the relationship between them is true for the public.

In modern times the chorus as such has disappeared except in certain experimental works, in García Lorca, and in Tennessee Williams. But it has been replaced by the narrator, the "funny-man," the "double," or a musical motif. In 1950 at the International Psychiatric Convention in Paris, I witnessed some experiments on the possibility of combining the theatre with movies that would reveal to the public the mysterious inner world of the actors, which they convey with their gestures but seldom in their words. There are some who demand that the new theatre reveal everything at once, the conscious and the subconscious; but we should not demand the impossible, for to do so would be to become like those people who have the knack of always ordering the only dish on the menu that is no longer available.

Because the playwright is not an isolated phenomenon in the community, but a collective crystallization, he requires a public. A book is a book even without readers, but a play does not fulfill itself until it has an audience. This fact distinguishes the theatre from the economy, the culture, and the science of a country: whereas the latter represent the conscious mind of a nation, the theatre is its subconscious.

THE THEATRE AS PSYCHODRAMA

The question arises whether the theatre should become today a collective psychotherapy, a psychodrama of nations. In my opinion, not at all. What we call therapeutic medicine is always an art, but art is not always therapeutic. Science uses general knowledge to cure an individual case; art uses the creative power of an individual— the artist, to please a collective entity—the public. Science is the general answer to a concrete and measurable problem. Art is a concrete answer to general imponderable questions. The scientist uses reason; the artist uses passion. The scientist does not care whether his truth is ugly so long as it is true; the artist does not care if his truth is imaginary so long as it is beautiful. The scientist seeks substance; the artist seeks form. From the Middle Ages on, art became divided into pure or fine arts, cultivated by the artist, and applied or industrial art, cultivated by the artisan. But the theatre cannot be merely artisanship, for were it so, it would betray itself. Artisanship in that case would mean that art bears a message. I don't object to that, provided that the "message in a bottle," which is as important as the message the shipwrecked man casts in the sea, can be read by many at the same time, and provided the bottle is full of artistic champagne.

The theatre today is both visual *answer* to the image of our era and a rebellious *recoil* from it. The theatre is an answer in so far as it reflects, like a mirror, the problems of an epoch. The dramatist is a man whose hand is guided by a brain bathed by the cultural currents of his time. In this sense—in this sense only; for the playwright who is not true to himself prostitutes his art—he is influenced by the preferences of his public. All works of art at a given period seem to be related, just as all the vases fashioned by the same potter look alike until we examine them closely and see that their contours betray the tender touch of his fingers when he was happy or the heavy pressure of his thumb when he was angry.

THE ACTOR AS HERO

The modern public has influenced the theatre in two ways. First, it has reduced the social prestige of the author and actor. In the past, actresses, like Talma, Rachel, Bernhardt, or Duse, occupied an important position in society. They belonged to that category of happy mortals favored by the gods. In those times the salvation of men and nations was measured in terms of the poetry, painting, and theatre they created. Today these activities are considered of minor importance. Such an attitude lowers the stature of art to a very low level.

Today the electronic engineer, the radar and the television expert are the most valued of men, and the artist per se means little. Such a monstrous subversion of spiritual values imperils Art and makes it imperative to call a halt to the progress of technology for the good of civilization. Nations have often been saved by poets. I respect technology, but I recognize its inferiority to Art in the scale of spiritual values. A hundred years from now no one will remember the names of the manufacturers who produce thousands of refrigerators or television sets a day, but as long as the world remains civilized, people will remember with great emotion the artists who are weaving with the wicker of their art the ideal basket of future glories.

Second, the public's attitude has changed not only toward the actor, but also toward the theatre. In the past, people would go to the theatre to be moved by what was happening on the stage, and they measured the esthetic quality of a work by the laughter or tears it provoked. The diamonds on ladies' throats did not sparkle so brilliantly as the tears in their eyes. A hundred years ago esthetic sense was based mostly on emotion. A work was evaluated in terms of the sentimental reaction of the public. An author's main ambition was to arouse the spectator even if he had to sacrifice the esthetic quality of his art. The public liked to forget their little daily worries and wanted to acquire spiritual stature by associating themselves with the majestic sufferings of dramatic heroes. They probably thought that by forging their souls from the same metal as the heroes they saw on the stage, they would end up by becoming just as heroic. This was, of course, a false assumption. They might as well have believed that since smoking pipes do not burn, by building houses and furniture of the same wood as pipes, they could put an end to fires.

That public attributed to the theatre a philosophic importance that it does not enjoy today. The theatre was not merely a diversion but a salvation, a plank people held on to when they felt that the vessel of their period was sinking. Today things have changed. Art no longer enjoys that importance, and the public, with noble and notable exceptions, goes to the theatre simply to enjoy itself. Life today is so rich in emotion that we do not have to go to the theatre in search of more emotion. At best, we seek to spend three hours in a pleasant stupor. The theatre reflects this tendency and produces works that, for the most part, aim only at amusing. Poetry is sacrificed to prestidigitation. Fortunately, because the theatre is also *reaction,* a minority is reacting against this influence and is creating a pure art, uncompromising and austere. That is why the authentic artist is a rebel who seeks not only to reflect the reality of his time but also to escape it through the magic window of his dreams, or to reform the world by struggling against it. His conflicts with his times and country are the key to his creative energy. They move him to create beings who suffer, live, and struggle through the battles that the author himself experienced in the dark night of his soul. The playwright's work, which is revolt and escape, is his answer to his tremendous inner questions. The restoration of the dignity of the theatre and of the artist, which is being undertaken by a small minority, is the measure of the spiritual salvation of our time.

Debased art is the expression of a public which, for lack of national myths and legends—that supreme food for the soul—tries to an-esthetize itself with the sorry drugs of musical comedies and whole-sale murder over television. As a reaction to this, an avant-garde group of artists is creating a good theatre; they are helping the public to air its conflicts in a gigantic collective psychoanalysis, with the stage taking the place of the psychiatrist's couch.

The theatre today must not limit itself to being simply an *answer,* if it wants to continue being theatre. It must be *reaction,* above all! It should not limit itself to satirizing or making fun of our problem. Problems are serious and must be taken seriously.

The anxiety theme reached the theatre through the existentialist movement of Sartre and even through isolated works like those of Miller, O'Neill, and Tennessee Williams; now we must let the theatre go down into the lower depths of the popular soul where anxiety festers. Signs of the movement to break down even the physical barriers that limit the theatre are theatres in the round, arenas where the actors mix with the public, thus encouraging greater identification with the conflicts treated by the play. The great tragedy of the theatre has been its limitation in space by four walls. The walls of the theatre mark off a parcel of the real and imaginary world and allow it to grow out only through the open door represented by the footlights. When the tension is too great, it rises upward. During periods of anxiety, the theatre, to prevent its high-voltage emotional charge from breaking through its walls, stands on its toes and, since it cannot stretch out horizontally, stretches up vertically—towards God.

THE TRIPLE MISSION

The theatre can and must have a triple mission in our time: *amusement, education,* and *inspiration.* We have already spoken about theatre as amusement. If the actor is good, the theatre is a magic force that stirs us. Madame Modjeska in London made her public cry just by reciting multiplication tables in Polish. Ernesto Rossi created an atmosphere of terror with his gestures while declaiming the prices of a menu. But that is not enough: magic is only one component of theatre. We must stress the theatre's function as educator, not of our minds, but of our emotions. To see other men act is one of our deepest passions. That is because in our daily lives we are taught to train our muscles but not our souls. We learn to pretend, to use an identical tone of voice and the same facial expression when we greet a friend or an enemy, when we are happy or sad, when we are bored or excited. Our life is an endless poker game with the rest of the world. But we all dream of doing quite the opposite. We dream of having personality, the basic key of which is sincerity and courage. To have personality is to escape deadly uniformity, an ankylosis more paralyzing than arthritis. That is why the human heart beats for the theatre, which is a hinterland of energy, a vast land of dreams, a domain of natural action where the actor does what we are all dying to do: he laughs when he is happy, whereas we all smile wanly; he weeps when he is suffering, while we have to be satisfied with nonchalantly lighting a cigarette; and he makes passionate love to his neighbor's wife when the best of us have to be content with leering at her out of the corner of our eye.

The theatre is a school of emotional sincerity, in contrast to our stereotyped feelings and repressed emotions in daily life. The objective of the theatre is truth and not pretense: the exploration of the soul and free flow of the emotions.

Emotional sincerity is the best explanation of why the theatre cannot prosper in an atmosphere of oppression. Modern psychology looks upon the human mind as an iceberg whose lower part or subconscious is submerged, and, although invisible, is greater and more important than the visible zone of consciousness. The individual mind is a pyramid with a wide base and a very narrow apex.

The light on this apex reaches only part of the rest of the pyramid. To some psychoanalysts, the lower part, the subconscious and unconscious, is a sewer full of the mud of undesirable impulses, and if we descend to those lower depths we must wear high rubber boots; to other psychoanalysts, it is an attic full of fabulous mythologic treasures where we have to proceed with the delicate hands of the antique dealer.

MAGIC AND MYTH

In prehistoric times, the human being lived in a universe full of cosmic myths and collective legends which were projections of his own soul. In modern times, that soul has withdrawn and has become bottled up within the mind. Myths and legends have become individual fantasies and rituals of the daydreamer, the neurotic, or the artist. Under a dictatorship, the world returns to primitive magic and collective myth. People do not have to create anything new, because their external national life is saturated with myths and legends created by the dictators solely to exploit those fantasies of the collective soul. National life under a dictatorship is a mythologic theatre, and the members of the military hierarchy are the actors who force the public to identify itself emotionally with those myths. That is why a good theatre can never emerge in such an atmosphere; such an organized collective mythology can only produce bad theatre and make of the people a compulsory audience.

The theatre in our democracies is free creation and individual mythology. It educates our emotions, but it also undertakes to inspire us. This is what we call "carrying a message," even though the message is not presented through solemn gestures, black costumes, and sorrowful faces, but laughingly, with waltz music and camellias. It is in the form of such a message that God now reappears in the theatre and presents Himself to the eyes of mere mortals.

GOD IN HISTORY

What happens to God in the course of History is an interesting thing. When I speak of God, I also include what some call Fate and Nature. Humanity draws near God and away from Him periodically, just as the earth, turning on its orbit, draws near and away from the sun. Man has always before him his entire spiritual universe, but he looks at only a portion of it, just as the reflector of a boat illuminates parts of the coast line but leaves the rest of it in darkness as it sails along. During periods of crisis God is again in sight. When man is threatened on the horizon of his material existence, he automatically shoots up vertically through prayer and ideals. Thus, in Periclean Greece man rose vertically through philosophy. In the

Middle Ages he proceeded horizontally in the Crusades. In the Renaissance he enclosed himself in the worship of the beauty of his own body. In the nineteenth century he rose on the whirlwind of his philosophic theories. In our day he is rising in a vertical line to God. Our interest in interplanetary navigation is another psychologic sign of our desire to escape to other planets where we may find greater mental sanity.

We are today in great need of aid from the theatre. Modern man feels he is caught between two tremendous forces, which represent two diametrically opposed conceptions of life, and around whose battering-rams are grouped all the other powers in the world. And man feels terrified. Do you know what we might compare the situation of modern man to? Just imagine that one night you step out onto the terrace of your house, but instead of looking up into a peaceful star-studded heaven, you see with horror that the stars have banded into two separate tremendous groups. Like soldiers of two apocalyptic armies, separated only by a dark zone like a heavenly no man's land. They are motionless. Silent. Menacing. As if awaiting the sign to start a final cataclysmic attack which will destroy the universe. Terrified, you rush back to the warmth of your apartment, where the light and pictures and music make you forget the nightmare in the heavens. That is what is happening to people all over. Terrified by the spectacle of the world divided into two camps, they take refuge in the warm, glittering magic of the theatre.

On that brilliantly lit stage, men can re-create a world where they live and love, work and play, like human beings. A world where they can convert every spotlight into a morning star that heralds the dawn of a new day, not only inside, but above all outside the theatre.

FOREIGN THEATRE VERSUS AMERICAN THEATRE

Let us consider now another aspect of theatre in our age: foreign theatre versus American theatre. I have been asked, "Is foreign theatre superior to American theatre?" This question gives rise to another: Is there such a thing as a foreign theatre and an American theatre? Wouldn't this be the same as asking if there are two types of measles just because its victims may be, say, Eskimos and Gauchos?

Thus that question brings up another problem. How many theatres are there? The answer is: There are as many theatres—with a small "t"—as there are stages in the world, but there is only one Theatre—with a capital "T"—through which man, wherever he may be, expresses his artistic impulses. *Externally* the theatre may be different in different countries; *basically* it is the same all over since it reflects this universal creative impulse.

Some time ago I was in Paris and I went to the theatre. Later I visited Andorra, a tiny country on the French-Spanish border, and I went to the theatre there. In Paris the theatre was fragrant with the perfumes of women and ablaze with cut–crystal chandeliers. In Andorra a crude stage had been improvised in the middle of the unpaved village square, and I sat on a bench and watched the play while dogs and even goats sniffed at my shoes. But both theatres were alike in that they pointed out similar moral implications.

THE PSYCHOLOGY OF AMUSEMENT

Before we discuss the differences between American and foreign theatres, let me point out that the best way to know people is to study the way they amuse themselves. Serious activities are similar everywhere because life forces them upon us. It is only when people dream that any difference between them is revealed. Our dreams are the personal trousseau we bring into the world.

There are two types of periods in history. One of them, like the Gay Nineties, is when people are more concerned over finding pleasure than avoiding pain and pay greater prices to entertainers than to doctors. The other, to which our own aspirin age belongs, is when emphasis is laid upon removing pain through melancholy drugs instead of seeking out happiness. We have excellent hospitals but few good theatres. We keep inventing new analgesics but we monotonously repeat our theatrical fare. To treat our ailments we are satisfied with nothing less than the latest antibiotic, but we resign ourselves to plays in which the unfaithful wife flirts with her husband's best friend just as she did hundreds of years ago.

AMERICAN THEATRE AND FOREIGN THEATRE

In the American theatre the psychology of the characters is vague because the audience is more interested in *what* happens to the characters than in the characters themselves, whereas in the foreign theatre the audience is not so much interested in what happens to the characters as in what they feel, in their emotions and passions. This is why foreign actors are not ashamed to give free vent to their emotions. They laugh madly when they are happy, they roar with fury, and they weep when in grief. American actors usually express these emotions by turning their backs to us and staring stolidly through a window, brushing imaginary specks of dust from their lapels, or lighting the inevitable cigarette, in a trite show of unnecessary stoicism.

The foreign theatre reduces action to a minimum. Events serve only to state moral problems. It is a theatre not of adventures, but of reactions to the great problems of life. Passion is restrained only by grammar. The heroes are seldom burdened with everyday pre-occupations, the alarm clock or the monthly rent, and so they are free to devote themselves body and soul to moral suffering. It is a theatre choked by moralistic dispositions.

The American theatre, on the other hand, piles up incident on incident in an effort to entertain a public fond of motion and difficult situations. The psychologic anatomy of feelings is not so important. Characters are used as a diving board from which the action of the play takes its great leap.

The American theatre is a theatre of motion. The foreign theatre is a theatre of words. Abroad, the theatre competes with books; in America, it competes with movies. That is why the American theatre has to move faster than the movies, while abroad it has to be more interesting than books.

Psychologically the theatre is escape from reality. We therefore don't want it to remind us too much of the home we leave for an evening to escape from everyday life. The theatre should be an image of life rather than life itself. Part of the magic of the theatre is the decor and costumes, which should be nature improved by art and not a *copy* of nature. In this respect, the American theatre succeeds magnificently.

THEATRE SYMBOLS AND THEMES

So much for the external differences between American and foreign theatres. As I said before, the law of universality applies to the Theatre with a capital "T." Because symbols and themes are always the same, they repeat themselves through the centuries as regularly as the song of the cuckoo in a well-behaved clock. Only their interpretation by authors, actors, and audiences varies.

The hand of a playwright when writing a play is guided by a brain influenced not only by his personal background but also by that of his country and by his time. But the playwright has always managed to escape the prison of his time. He usually expresses what he doesn't find in the bare cold room of his life and his time. He wouldn't be a playwright otherwise. He does not live in the external truth among salts and acids but, as Stevenson said of the writer, "in the warm phantasmagoric chamber of his brain with painted windows and storied walls." And at the bottom of his work we can hear the nostalgic refrain of a blind nightingale who longs for the lost blue skies.

The most popular theme is that of a man and a woman alone in a garden with the serpent hidden behind a tree. It is the story of Adam and Eve in the Garden of Eden. Today this story is called *The Voice of the Turtle* or *The Moon Is Blue*. Another perennial theme is that of the aging husband who goes off on a trip and entrusts his lovely young wife to a young friend of his. These two are thrown together, drink too many cocktails, and she is unfaithful to her husband. Now, if you substitute love potions for the dry martinis, you have the story of *Tristan and Isolde* and *Pelléas and Mélisande*. The theme of Electra and Orestes has been revived by Giraudoux and O'Neill. Brünnhilde, the Wagnerian Amazon who was looking for a man stronger than herself, reappeared in *Lady in the Dark* by Moss Hart, and Antigone in the play by Anouilh.

And if you were to ask what sort of plays will be staged in the year 2000, I would answer: Plays with the same themes from the Bible, Homer, Sophocles, Molière, and so on, themes that incarnate man's conflicts—conflicts universal in time and space.

Of course there are plays without themes, like some of the musicals, which succeed thanks only to the power of propaganda. No one takes the trouble any more to propagandize the classics. Which reminds me of the hen that lays one egg a day and makes so much noise that everyone knows about it. On the other hand, a codfish lays millions of eggs a day and no one on earth hears about it. The result is that everybody eats chicken eggs but nobody eats codfish eggs.

THE PLAY AS PSYCHOANALYSIS

We are back at the question, "Is foreign theatre superior to American theatre?" What does one mean by "superior" theatre? To me "superior" theatre is that theatre which tries to meet the challenge of our age. In every age the theatre has had two functions: the obvious one of entertaining the public, and the hidden one of crystallizing the anxieties, fears, and dreams of its time. Sometimes the theatre has saved the spirit of a nation. The theatre of Lope de Vega maintained a sense of national pride in the Spanish people after the defeat of the invincible Armada.

The theatre is the key to the secrets of the soul of a people. Why? Because such activities as politics, industry, science make up the conscious life of a people, but the theatre is its subconscious mind. Into that magic box the playwright, the actors, and the directors project their dreams, desires, complexes, and fears. Against these the audience projects its own fears and dreams. A play is a gigantic psychoanalysis. The stage is the couch and the actors the psychoanalysts who bring our conflicts out in the open, allowing us to get rid of them. From this point of view the theatre takes on its maximum value in times of anxiety like ours. *That* theatre which helps its audience to experience the freedom that comes with emotional catharsis *is* the superior theatre.

VIII. editorial messages

THE FABRIC OF A DREAM

*t*he first anniversary of *MD,* which the medical profession has so generously turned in such a brief period into a beloved companion, is a good time to answer the numerous inquiries about when, where, how, and by whom this magazine was conceived, and above all to say something about its guiding philosophy.

MD has been called "an editorial miracle," "an unbelievable phenomenon," "a fairy tale of medical publishing." The editorial praise in thousands of letters received has an impressive emotional dimension. All agree that *MD* is a favorite source of enlightenment and entertainment. To them and to the pharmaceutical and allied industries, whose support has contributed to the success of *MD,* are dedicated the first editorials of this year, presenting the birth, fabric, and perspectives of a dream. For *MD* crystallizes a dream that was born when the writer was studying medicine beneath the azure skies of Spain and that was to be fulfilled beneath the smoke-and-silver skies of Manhattan.

Every physician, wherever he may be, has in his student days gone through the stage of dreaming of an ideal image of himself and an ideal program of future achievements. We all nurse a "project" for our future life that takes precedence over all other ideas and decisions and *is* truly our authentic being and destiny. We are free to realize it or not, but we cannot change it. As Ortega y Gasset once said: "We are indelibly a unique programmatic person who needs to realize himself."

From *MD Medical Newsmagazine* 2:7, January, 1958.

Human life is the drama of our passionate struggle to become in reality what we are only in prospect. To live is to realize our own self, and a fulfilled life is that of the man who eventually becomes himself and whose ideal profile of existence, because he was faithful to his authentic destiny, is fully filled in with realizations. On the other hand, there are those in whose programmatic profile life makes deep dents, leaving among the remains but the stump of what once was their ideal profile of life. Life is endeavor, and authentic life means to do what we were born to do and not just anything, to discover our true destiny and follow it, always being faithful to one's self.

Often this ideal program of life is envisioned in our youth's dreams. That these dreams are frequently an anticipation of inner potentialities was once expressed by Goethe: "Our dreams are presentiments of the faculties latent within us and signs of what we may be capable of doing. What we can do and what we wish to do loom in our mind as something belonging to the future and outside us; we crave for what we already possess."

In the program of life envisioned in my student days, I saw the physician as the living paradox of an intellectual who, by vocation or because of an interest in science, chose a profession that made of him a man of action, concerned more with occupation than with pre-occupation, with quick vibrant professional reflexes instead of the spiritual apraxia of the preoccupied or "pure" intellectual. Such a physician is forced by his profession to bury his "unlived lives," to anesthetize his inner vocations, to let his other artistic gifts grow rusty, thereby shutting out many of the marvelous vistas of the world around him. The physician often lives in an enclosure with mirrored walls that reflect only the uniform images of his professional interest. Instead of so many mirrors, he needs open windows, allowing him to see the sunny lands of the world beyond.

Thus began the dream of integrating the unlived lives of the physician—as a universal man, a professional, and a member of society—into a single concept, for concepts are the compasses that orient our life amid the things and events in the world. This concept consisted basically in adopting a *total perspective* of people, things, and events in the world and of that living history we call "our times." History, I felt—especially the history of medicine, which is a *social* science that uses the methods of the natural sciences—could become, if properly used, a dynamic force that would lend reason and meaning to this concept.

Later I would realize that the best vehicle for this concept was a magazine that, like a castle atop a hill, had windows open to all winds; a magazine that would bring the physician information about medicine and about all aspects of life. He could then look at life and at art with the analytic eyes of the scientist and at medicine with the esthetic eyes of the artist. For history shows that the physician and the artist were originally one and the same person, and that art and medicine are but two of the many sides carved from the monumental quarry of civilization.

It took many years to fulfill this dream. These waiting years nurtured the desire to *communicate* with physicians as widely and as pleasantly as possible. Communication, furthermore, had to be done with "a judicious amount of levity," a decision prompted by the psychology of my native people, with whom persuasion must always be preceded by a little seduction. To put across the exactness of an idea, it is indispensable to express it with charm and that magic quality that bullfighters call *garbo*. For a magazine expressing without charm and humor such a concept as this one would be—to borrow Brillat-Savarin's description of a wonderful meal without cheese—like a one-eyed beautiful woman.

Such was the stuff from which was woven the fabric of *MD*. The goal was a magazine with a historical vision, at once realistic and romantic, of the modern physician's world and times; a magazine that would convey truth and beauty and would look with medical eyes at the Humanities and with humanistic eyes at Medicine. It is a tribute to the humanistic sense of American physicians that this dream of a medical student in Spain was accomplished in this land, with their kind encouragement.

A romantic is a man whose heart has gone to his head. That great romantic, G. K. Chesterton, once said: "Nearly all the best and most precious things of the universe may be bought for a half penny." He was referring to such things as a little bag of jewel-toned drugstore candy, a ride in the flying castle that was an old omnibus, or a small painted cardboard theatre. "I make an exception," he added, "of the sun, the moon, the earth, stars, thunderstorms, people and other trifles. You can get them for nothing." To these great things that one cannot pay for, I wish to add the generous encouragement *MD* received from our colleagues, which has given meaning and substance to the fabric of a dream.

THE *MD* CONCEPT

*t*he purpose of the medical newsmagazine *MD* is to satisfy the physician's curiosity about the vast, rich tapestry of medicine *and of life.*

MD regards the physician as a man of many personalities. He is not only a professional but also an individual and a member of society. As a professional he is interested in the art and science of healing; as an individual he feels the need to increase his general cultural knowledge; as a member of society he wants to understand the political, economic, and sociologic, as well as the public health problems of his community, his country, and the world in general. A physician is not only a social person; he is also a *historical* person. The interests of the world therefore are his interests.

MD embodies a new concept of medical journalism. Medical journals are usually dedicated to satisfying the professional needs of the physician, leaving his many other interests to lay journals. *MD* is dedicated to satisfying *all* the needs of the physician—medical, cultural, and social.

Through word and image—the word simple, the image vivid—*MD* presents all the important news in medicine, travel, sports, personalities, the arts, science, politics, and economics as seen through the eyes of the physician. It also portrays the role of the physician as *man of action*—artist, writer, sportsman, traveler, statesman—in today's world.

The section *World of Medicine* reports all the important news in

From *MD Medical Newsmagazine* 1:7, January, 1957.

medicine. *Medicine in the World* presents world events affecting the physician and medicine. *Medicine in the Arts* describes the contribution made by the arts—man's proudest heritage—to medicine and medicine's contribution to the arts.

MD guarantees exhaustive research on every story. The most modern methods of communication and the graphic arts will be harnessed. Dynamic correspondents in leading medical centers throughout the world, skilled photographers and medical artists, and science researchers—all these are collaborating under the direction of an editorial board of leading world authorities in each medical branch.

True to Osler's words, *MD* will "create, transmute and transmit" news and events for the physician. It will inform him, guide him, and entertain him.

Beyond the office and the microscope throbs a wide, exciting world. From its brightly lighted chambers *MD* provides the physician with a picture window on this world.

CHILDREN OF APOLLO

*t*the initial success of this magazine amply confirms the need for the concept that inspired it—to assist the physician in his triple personality of human being, professional, and member of society. The praiseful letters received from all over the country reveal how deeply our colleagues feel that *MD* has interpreted their professional needs, their social duties, and their cultural ideals.

We all accept today the idea that Medicine is Art and Science. The key of Science is analysis; the essence of Art is synthesis. *MD* endeavors to conciliate analysis with synthesis. The physician's mind is like a series of rooms that are filled with knowledge but sometimes lack communication among themselves. *MD* attempts to link the vast knowledge in the modern medical mind as a corridor in a hospital links all rooms without interfering with their privacy. Because *MD* believes that unless a physician is a kind and cultured man he cannot be a good physician, it presents the world of today as seen by the physician possessing a clear mind and a simple heart.

Years ago the physician in this country was primarily a family doctor who exercised his deep understanding and practical wisdom within the patient's home. Medical education was rather elementary; hospitals were scarce; research was pioneering and heroic. But in our days the physician is no longer the practitioner, isolated with his patient, as Robinson Crusoe with Friday, on the island of disease. Today the whole world is his world. Besides being a healer and a "knower," he is also a preventer and an organizer. A preventer be-

From *MD Medical Newsmagazine* 1:9, February, 1957.

cause medicine is concentrating on prevention as the ultimate way of combatting disease. An organizer because he counsels and guides his community in matters of public health, instruction, law formulation, urbanization, social service, and politics. Thus the physician has come to fulfill the four basic objectives of medicine—to promote health; to prevent disease; to restore health; to rehabilitate the sick.

Disease is nowadays more than ever a social phenomenon, since it is influenced by environment. It is also a *historical* event, since it is a dynamic process that develops in time and is inserted through its chronologic dimension into the patient's personal biography.

Hence the emphasis that *MD* places on the historical background of every current problem. Proof of the value of this historical approach is that the most important medical document has always been the clinical case *history,* not only of unusual but also of ordinary cases, that "small change" of medicine that constitutes the rich capital of the physician's experience.

We are faced daily with peptic ulcers and schizophrenia, acute hypertension and rheumatoid arthritis. To diagnose we use auscultation, radioactive isotopes, roentgenograms, and psychologic and laboratory tests. We cure through antibiotics and steroids, psychotherapy and surgery. But if we are to prevent future sickness, we must also know those social and historical dimensions of disease—the economic, social, and cultural state of a man or of a people. The physician must be able to feel the cultural pulse of his time. *MD* seeks to aid him in this endeavor.

In our world, shrunken by the jet plane and enlarged by the electron microscope, men and nations are so closely related that the physician's interests must be universal. With great joy and simple pride, *MD* is at the service of physicians, the children of Apollo, god of healing and poetry, who today are already contemporaries of the physicians of tomorrow.

THE STRINGS OF THE LYRE

$t$he continuing avalanche of letters of applause received by MD lavishly assures us that it is fulfilling its purpose: to interpret the physician both as a professional and as a human being.

The mind of the modern physician is like a lyre, the instrument of Apollo, of which often only the professional string is struck. To strike all the strings and produce harmonious sounds—this is the endeavor of MD.

What we mean was once expressed simply by that great architect of brain histology, Santiago Ramón y Cajal. When he was a child his father, a country doctor, asked him what he wanted to be when he grew up. "I want to be a man," he answered. By the time he grew up into a noble figure, pensive of brow and silver-bearded, familiar to all of us, Cajal was truly a man. He lived a full life as physician, histologist, investigator, teacher, writer—and Nobel Laureate; yet besides the world of neurons and neuroglia he was also interested in his fellow man and in everyday events.

Because we believe that the ideal of wholly "being a man" is shared by many physicians today, because we believe that these physicians want not only to be outstanding in their profession but also to participate actively in the life of their world and times, MD is dedicated to their service.

Many voices are raised daily in favor of or against our Age of Specialization. We are *for* specialization—provided it does not entail

---

From *MD Medical Newsmagazine* 1:13, March, 1957.

renouncing other intellectual endeavors because they are not directly related to our specialty. *MD* would like to provide one of the answers to the problem of excessive specialization by helping the physician to integrate his technical knowledge with general culture and his professional work with world personalities and events. We do not enjoin a Utopian encyclopedism; but we do believe in a humanistic way of life.

We have been asked by correspondents whether "we can keep it up," whether we can maintain the cultural level of the previous issues. The answer is *yes! MD* is but a mirror of the complex and dynamic image of the physician of today, who, in turn, closer than ever to the Platonic ideal of the *Asklepios politikos,* the medical statesman, is an important figure in every area of modern life.

MD will join the physician in his daily search for wisdom. This search has been expressed, from Spinoza to Will Durant, as a search for a total perspective, an integrated universal vision of persons, things, and events with all their relevant relationships in time and space. This means accepting the fact that the picture of the world and of things in general that every one of us has in his mind is only an *image* and not the outer objective reality. It also means accepting the idea that this world of ours is reflected in millions of mirrors—the minds of people—each one reflecting a different image because of its different curvature. To achieve wisdom, then, is to be able to consider the total perspective of each thing or person and to accept one's own individual image as only a part of that perspective. Only when we accept this is it possible to add to knowledge those two supreme attributes of science that are also a part of the *MD* concept—order and clarity.

And lastly, through its various sections, *MD* attempts to stimulate all those "reserve" occupations—whether writing or gardening, chess playing or travel—without which the physician slaving at his professional occupation would become a technical automaton. These reserve occupations are like the organic reserves of fat and sugar that protect the body against the dangers of fasting; they help the physician to develop those muscles of the mind that otherwise might become atrophied.

MD joins the physician in striking—in search of a richer melody—all the strings of the Apollonian lyre.

AESCULAPIUS IN THE KITCHEN

*T*he millenary empiricism of the cook and the modern knowledge of the dietitian have faced each other through the centuries. Today the physician is concerned with cooking both as a professional whose advice is sought by his patients and as a human being who relishes the pleasures of the table, for gastronomy is not totally irreconcilable with dietetics.

Cooking, like enjoyment of art, is tradition. That is why old countries, those along the Mediterranean, for instance, combine artistic feeling and superb cooking; while young countries, predominantly industrial and technologic, are characterized by simplicity in their cooking. To be excited to emotional heights by artistic beauty or by exquisite food requires many centuries of apprenticeship. Few will deny that French cooking has always reigned supreme, followed by Italian and Spanish cooking. This type of cooking is more typical of countries characterized by a certain technologic backwardness, which in turn enables them to concentrate on the culinary and other arts.

Brillat-Savarin emphasized the difference between the pleasures of eating and the pleasures of the *table*. The first entails only hunger and its appeasement; the second includes not only the food itself but its quality, how and where it is served, and with whom it is enjoyed. Eating merely satisfies the pangs of hunger; the *table* excites the appetite and combines—to borrow George Bernard Shaw's definition of matrimony—maximum temptation with maximum opportunity.

From *MD Medical Newsmagazine 1*:7, April, 1957.

Italian and Spanish cooking cater to hunger, which like sex is a call of the instinct. French cooking caters to the appetite, which is a fine, intellectual "emotion" demanding more than merely eating. According to Brillat-Savarin, hunger is an instinct of animals; appetite, an attribute of humankind. Italian and Spanish cooking possess an empiric meaning and a natural flavor; French cooking is independent of hunger and is pure, marvelous artifice and *mise en scène*. Italian and Spanish cooking, which trust somewhat to chance, cannot compete with the artistico-scientific characteristics of the French cuisine; they are, however, far superior to the dinner without tablecloth, on counters, of industrial towns, or to the semisynthetic food of very young countries.

Physicians should take an interest in cooking and the pleasures of the table. Good cooking does more for home unity, to keep the man of the house and the entire family united, than the best television. Good cooking should bring out, not drown, the natural flavor of food, just as a dress should outline, not conceal, the graceful lines of a woman's figure. Good cooking need not be insipid when it is "scientific." In every meal there is a factor as important as calories, vitamins, and amino acids—the psychologic element. A good meal should leave us *psychologically* satisfied. This was easy when cooking, a long time ago, was a slow, leisurely art. It became impossible when man began to be transported at vertiginous speeds by new locomotive methods, forcing him to eat quickly food prepared even more quickly. To complicate matters, canning and refrigeration were invented, with the result that modern man, unlike his prehistoric ancestors, no longer chases after food. Food now chases man. For he can today have tropical papaya in the icy Arctic wastes and Scottish salmon in the sandy African plains. The kitchen has been defeated by the laboratory.

It is important to revive the old love for fine, gracious dining, today limited perhaps to transatlantic liners, which often offer the traveler all the marvels of international cooking, and to an occasional automobile trip that may unexpectedly lead to one of those old inns buried in the byways, effaced from the gastronomic map by the railroad, that other invention that years ago destroyed human contact with the landscape.

Cooking is a revealing key to the culture of a country. "National" dishes reflect a country's soul. The Spaniards' tendency to violence and their flair for bright colors are evident in their sharp-flavored, polychrome *paellas*—the water color of the Spanish kitchen—and their encyclopedic *cocidos*. The Japanese love for order and cleanliness is translated into those dainty miniature gardens that make up their favorite soups and dishes. The aseptic robustness and reserve of the

British are transmuted into wholesome roast beef and Yorkshire pudding. The Scandinavian seafaring nature is reflected in their smorgasbords teeming with marine creatures. Gallic subtlety finds expression in their delicate sauces; Italian earthiness in their *pastas,* seasoned with endearing onions, tinted with the scarlet of tomatoes, and crowned with the gracious touch of cheese. The American cuisine is assimilating in its melting pot the best of international cooking, just as it has assimilated all beverages in that often overpotent democratic fraternity of spirits, the cocktail.

Spanish cooking I know best. Consequently, I know its defects. But its excess of oil and garlic, its lethal rich sauces, its overuse of bread —all these are compensated by its rich variety, ranging from the cheese and chestnuts consumed by Don Quixote with the goat shepherds beneath the oaks of the Sierra Morena to the lavish extravagances prepared for Camacho's wedding. Spanish cooking has been for centuries basted by Mediterranean sunlight, breeding such exotic dishes as *arroz a banda,* rice cooked in concentrated fish and seafood broth, which imparts to every little grain all the essence of the Mediterranean sea; Andalusian *gazpacho;* trout and partridge *en escabeche;* and *turrón* of Arabian tradition, made with almonds, eggs, and honey. Spanish food demands the company of wines: sherry, dignified as an hidalgo; amontillado, solemn as a philosopher; manzanilla, gay as a dancing girl; and the *vinos de mesa,* which more than warm the stomach, and also tickle the heart.

The physician must be something of a gastronomer for his patients' and his own sake. Did not Hippocrates stress equally pleasure and wholesomeness in eating? An Italian glutton once said, *"Dello buono poco, ma questo poco abondante"* ("Of the good just a little, but of this little in abundance"). The physician must perforce choose moderation in food, but why sacrifice quality and style?

No one can orient cooking as the physician can. He knows that taste and smell are functionally a unit. He knows therefore that it is better to replace the floral centerpiece—which finally makes the flowers smell of food and the food taste of flowers—by fruits, whose aroma does not interfere with that of food. The physician knows that the gourmet's instinct anticipated scientific knowledge by including in every meal butter, salad greens, cheese, and fruits, thus guaranteeing an ample ration of vitamins, proteins, and other basic nutritive factors. He knows that the fatigue of the hunt improves the quality of game flesh; that broiling meat carbonizes the fat and caramelizes its sugar content; that the preparation of mayonnaise involves electric forces that act upon the egg and oil suspension molecules; that the same difference exists between fried and boiled food as between an oil painting and a water color, the oil and water drying up in each case, leaving but the polychrome image of the cooked food.

The physician knows as well that a good meal should consist of *one* basic dish, preceded by two dishes to tone up the stomach and tantalize the palate, and followed by two dishes as a transition to the dessert. And he appreciates the value of wines, which do not anesthetize the palate as cocktails do, and which, just like very old people, should be kept for better preservation in a horizontal position. Wine should be poured in a wide-rimmed glass that it may be improved by the greater oxygenation, and the glass should be colorless that it may transmute the wine into a glowing gem to be lovingly looked at, smelled, "dreamt on," and talked about before it is drunk.

Above everything else, the physician realizes the importance to health of initiating a crusade—beginning in his own home and continuing with his patients—to cultivate not the habit of eating but the pleasures of the table. This crusade would revive the spiritual pleasures inherent in fine dining, such as leisure, courtesy, and graciousness in presentation and service, a pleasant atmosphere, and the music of feminine voices instead of the radio. A crusade to turn us into cosmopolites in our gastronomic tastes is the best way to develop brotherhood between men and nations. The physician, who has presided over many a banquet, from the days of Eryximachus at Plato's Symposium to our times, knows that an occasion of gracious commensality is also an occasion of true confraternity.

TO WALK AND TO SEE

*N*otes on Walking and Seeing," was the title the classical Arabian authors gave their travel books. And the Greek philosopher Solon also recommended travel in order "to see."

Man is the most restless of all living beings. From the beginning he has roamed the earth, on foot and horseback for millennia, only recently in steamboats and motor vehicles. Perhaps travel holds such fascination because living is traveling through time just as traveling is living through space.

Today we travel far more than ever. But we no longer travel forced by hunger and cold as prehistoric man was, or by epidemics and wars as medieval man was, or by the passion for exploration as Renaissance man was. Today we travel because we want to know every corner of this world of ours, which, as Chesterton said, has expanded with the microscope and contracted with the airplane.

We also travel to flee our habitual milieu and daily worries, to cease temporarily from being participants and to become instead spectators of life on different geographic stages. A journey is motion through space; but it is also a jump toward that precious anonymity of the traveler that affords the opportunity to become, to quote Hazlitt, "the gentleman in the parlour."

The physician through the ages has been a traveler in his own right as well as a counselor to travelers. Hippocrates traveled far and wide and compiled a splendid treatise on public health for the wandering

---

From *MD Medical Newsmagazine* 1:9, May, 1957.

physicians of his time. The first great physician-traveler and explorei of the ancient world was Democedes of Croton who traveled through Asia carrying in his knapsack the legacy of Greek medicine.

The list of physician-travelers is extensive and distinguished. There was the Portuguese Garcia de Orta, who explored India in the sixteenth century; the surgeon Monkhouse, who overcame scurvy on Cook's expedition to the South Seas in 1769; Walter Russell, who accompanied Captain John Smith on his explorations of the Chesapeake region; the two Scottish surgeons, James Bruce who discovered the source of the Blue Nile, and Mungo Park who explored Senegal and Kaarta; and Dr. Livingstone, who discovered the Zambesi River and Victoria Falls.

Surgeons are also listed among the conquerors of the sea, men like James Lind, who subdued the scurvy that had caused ten thousand deaths, according to Admiral Hawkins' reports; Thomas Dover, who on the island of Juan Fernández, facing the Chilean coast, rescued Alexander Selkirk, later immortalized as Robinson Crusoe by Daniel Defoe; Eugene Sue, equally famous as a novelist; and of course the great Tobias Smollett. These mighty men of the past wore their combined medical, nautical, and literary laurels with the greatest of ease.

In the air the first pioneers were also physicians. After the Montgolfier brothers conceived the poetic idea of "imprisoning a cloud in a cloth bag," which culminated in the balloon, the first human being to ascend in it was the Frenchman, Jean Pilâtre de Rozier, a physician-apothecary. He subsequently became the first martyr to aeronautics when he perished in an attempt to emulate a Boston physician named Jeffries who, with Pierre Blanchard, for the first time crossed the English Channel in a balloon. And it was Paul Bert, a pupil of Claude Bernard, who founded aeronautic medicine.

In some respects travel is more dangerous today than in the past. The old slow way of traveling—on foot or on horseback, or in a lazy slow boat—allowed the traveler time to adapt himself mentally and physically to new environments. The airplane has revolutionized all this. The mind no longer arrives, as in the stagecoach era, many days before the battered body. Now the body arrives almost anywhere in the world in a few hours, while the mind may "arrive" days later, thereby suffering great stress through lack of time to adapt itself to the sudden change. There is also the danger of disease carriers—birds, rodents, flies, mosquitoes—stowed away in fast vehicles, traveling as unwanted guests.

The demand for counsel on travel from physicians increases daily. *MD* therefore features travel medicine in this issue, calling attention to problems of stress, malnutrition, infection, intoxication, and traumas. The traveler ever more is able to take with him everything that will help him—food, clothes, artificial climate, even adequate psychologic preparation—to enjoy travel without pain and without fear, and to return home the richer for his experiences. In this lies the joy of traveling.

As the Greek Argonauts, who symbolized life as incessant sailing, said: "The essential thing is not to live; the essential thing is to travel."

THE ENDEAVOR OF WILLIAM HARVEY

Greatness in medicine may be attained by discovering a drug or by formulating a principle. William Harvey attained greatness by formulating a principle that changed the face of medicine. His scientific method replaced qualitative impression by quantitative mensuration. For introducing accurate calculation into medical research, Harvey deserves to be called the father of modern physiology.

Harvey's chief claim to fame rests not so much in his discovery of the circulation of the blood, which had already been described by Colombo and Cesalpino, as in his having *demonstrated* it scientifically. Harvey's historical hour was not in 1628 when he published a little book that revolutionized medicine, but in 1616 when he enunciated, before an audience that failed to understand him, the principles of the circulation of the blood. With admirable scientific honesty, Harvey did not publish his findings until twelve years later, after he had verified them conclusively.

The secret of Harvey's achievement can be traced back to his youthful years in the sun-drenched Italian town that Shakespeare called "Fair Padua, nursery of all arts." There Harvey, already enriched by the anatomic heritage left by Vesalius, watched the great Fabricius dissect the venous valves in his famous anatomic theatre, a dark cavernous wooden box lit only by flickering candles held aloft by the students. There also, many a night, he watched through Galileo's telescope the glittering stars in the Paduan sky, learning from the

From *MD Medical Newsmagazine* 1:7, June, 1957.

master the laws that regulate the motion of the celestial bodies, laws that he would later apply to the motion of the blood.

Harvey was a man of the Baroque, the seventeenth century art style characterized by excessive ornamentation, emotion, and movement that wrenched the stone of cathedrals from its Gothic placidity and twisted it into dizzying whirlpools. *Movement* in the Baroque was expressed with the curved line and the *circle*. Is it surprising, then, that Harvey, who lived in and breathed this dynamic atmosphere, transplanted to science the concept of the circle and the dynamics of motion? That is how Harvey became interested in the two movements in man that last from birth until death: respiration and the heart beat.

All of man, body and mind, abhors a vacuum. Just as the body must fill with fat and connective tissue the void created by the extirpation of an organ, so must the mind replace one belief by another if it is to avoid a crisis. The Renaissance uprooted man's medieval convictions, thrusting him into a crisis when new convictions were not promptly forthcoming. Harvey lived through this crisis, and he did what every human in a crisis does: he "undressed." A man in a crisis sheds everything, hat and coat, that may hinder action. Harvey shed the old Galenic ideas and tried to solve the ideologic crisis of his time by developing new scientific convictions.

Harvey lived in two countries that were ideal ground for his endeavors. In every historical period there are "visceral" countries, that is, countries that become the vital organs around which the rest of the world is organized. In Harvey's time the visceral countries were Italy, where he spent his youthful years, and England, where he lived his years of assertion and maturity.

In the beginning perhaps Harvey, as does every young man, sought glory merely by emulating someone great—Vesalius or Fabricius; but later the way to glory lay in creating an "open"—Baroque—vision of the human body instead of the "closed" architectonic—Renaissance—vision of Vesalius. Harvey's physiologic work was pure Baroque action, *anatomia animata,* that is, moving anatomy *in space,* just as his embryologic work was moving anatomy *in time.* Without an understanding of this Baroque influence upon Harvey, one cannot fully understand the historical meaning of his endeavor.

There is still much to be studied about Harvey. His little-known years of research in London, prior to his discovery, were the same years in which Shakespeare presented his plays at the Globe Theatre. No other plays mention the words "heart" and "blood" as often as do Shakespeare's. In *Hamlet, Macbeth, Coriolanus,* the poet's intuition seemingly anticipated the scientist's concept of the motion of the blood. Shakespeare's work is as Aristotelian in its concept of the heart as the source of life and of the emotions as was Harvey's in the scientific world. One can well imagine the impact of the bard's verses upon the mind of Harvey.

William Harvey will always be one of the greatest examples of the scientist who lives to seek the truth in science. In this issue *MD* pays homage to this simple man who crossed the threshold to greatness on that memorable day in April, 1616, when he wrote in his notes for his second Lumleian Lecture that the blood circulates and that it does so in a *circle*.

A PLACE IN THE SUN

$\mathcal{W}$ hen summer comes, man loves a place in the sun and the physician can help him to enjoy it.

The human being is a biologic system capable of reacting adequately to new situations or to internal needs. The functional activities of the organism are subject to a periodic rhythm related to external factors and endogenous influences.

Recognition of seasonal rhythms in the reactive capacity of the human organism demands that the physician systematize them into new concepts. Individual responses to summer atmospheric and biosocial factors justify the creation of a new body of knowledge that might be called "Summer Medicine."

The thirteenth century compilers of the *Regimen Sanitatis Salernitanum* recommended the adoption of special measures in the summer months: "In Summers heat (when choller hath dominion)— Coole meates and moist are best in some opinion . . ."

We know today that a "person" is composed of two factors: biopsychic organism and "circumstance." Under the last term the philosopher Ortega y Gasset included the double dimension of space and time. In this sense each person is at once a spatial and a historical being.

The surrounding landscape exerts a powerful influence on "persons." The influence of the landscape *color* is a fact. Green and blue —sea and sky, the summer colors—are pleasant and sedative; white (snow), tranquilizing; red and yellow, exciting. Landscape *form* also

From *MD Medical Newsmagazine* 1:7, July, 1957.

influences us. The plainsman feels confined when transplanted to the valley, while the city dweller sometimes feels an indefinable anguish when confronted with a wide horizon.

Hegel classified landscapes into *highlands, valleys,* and *coast.* These landscapes are characterized by the relation between earth and water. The highlands are dry. The valley is born of the river. On the coast "trembles the sea," as Dante once said.

In the valley the identification between man and earth is complete, allowing individuality and agricultural races to attain maximum expression. Monotonous nature divorces the highlander from the landscape, rendering him more companionable and creating races of town dwellers and sometimes of immigrants. The coast with its beckoning sea, symbol of mutability, makes men adventurous but lacking in permanent roots.

To the landscape must be added the *climate. Meridional* climate has a languishing effect physically while it sharpens man's intuition and instincts; *continental* climate, with its extremes of heat and cold and dryness and wetness, and *coastal* climate, with its strong winds and humidity, have a stimulating effect; artificially created *city* climate tends to reduce reproductive capacity and to increase intellectual life.

To the permanent climatic conditions are added *climatic rhythms* (daily, lunar, and seasonal). Summer, with its high temperatures and intense light, decreases vitality to its lowest point.

In homeothermic animals, high *temperatures* dilate the skin blood vessels, cause physical lassitude (hyperthermia, thermal polypnea, tachycardia), and reduce appetite and fur thickness.

Light generally provokes positive phototropic reactions in some birds and mammals. The *weather* acts through its elements: atmospheric temperature and pressure, humidity, light, air ionization. Summer heat induces depression, restlessness, anxiety, and insomnia, and it reduces work capacity.

Man has been described as a "cosmic sounding board," and weather as a cosmic effector mechanism governing organic reactions. Studies (Wheeler) have suggested that each climatic phase (heat-humidity, heat-dryness, etc.) may stimulate a certain type of historical period. Bonanza years, it is claimed, are "humid," depression years are "dry," dictatorships bloom in "hot-dry" years, and periods of democratic stability are "cool" and "humid."

"Summer Medicine" as a *corpus doctrinalis* can be of positive value to our profession. It can be of greater value to man, who in the summer forsakes artificially weathered modern life and renews contact with outdoor life and nature. Instead of being harmful, this should, under adequate medical guidance, restore to man the joy of living in a place in the sun.

THE ANGELIC CONJUNCTION

*t*he "country doctor," that solid tradition in American medicine, is not really disappearing; he is only changing into counselor and statesman. He is becoming the rural incarnation of the classical *Asklepios politikos*.

This combination of professions in a rural physician is not new. As far back as the time of the "Mayflower" there was among the valiant survivors one Samuel Fuller, "deacon and physician." Indeed, the combination of preacher and physician, called by Cotton Mather "the angelic conjunction," was the rule in the heroic days of American medicine, when the exercise of one profession alone failed to provide an adequate livelihood. In those days a physician was sometimes "pastor, schoolmaster and physician"—as John Wilson, a graduate in 1642 at the first commencement of Harvard College, signed himself—sometimes a lawyer, and nearly always a farmer. Perhaps this is why the country doctor has had so great an influence on the evolution of American medicine.

The country doctor is a glorious figure in the history of medical progress in America. A rural physician was the first to treat surgically the dreaded vesicovaginal fistula; another was the first to ligate by flickering candlelight the common carotid artery; still another in the woods of Kentucky performed the first extirpation of an ovarian tumor. Few medical branches indeed can boast of such an honorable tradition of merit and service.

But the country doctor today is in a period of transition. With the

_____

From *MD Medical Newsmagazine 1*:9, August, 1957.

rise of large urban centers, which ruled American life the second half of the past century, just as progressive expansion of the Western frontier ruled the first half, physicians, following the flux, concentrated in the big cities.

Another decisive factor in the emigration of physicians from country to city was specialization, which has always paralleled the growth of large cities. The enormous medical progress achieved in our century has led to specialization, first in research and then in medical education. In the times of the country doctor, the specialist was only a consultant, but as the patient became more educated he began to consult the city specialist directly, thus weakening the social function of the country doctor.

Young physicians today, impelled by these historico-social factors and by the fear of not being able to survive in small towns, gravitate ever more to the large cities. Aware though they are that competition in the city is greater, they nevertheless feel that the opportunities to advance their career are also greater. Further, while still students they learn to depend on the assistance of city specialists and laboratories. In the country they would be forced to depend a great deal more on themselves. Some of them also fear the routine and the lack of scientific stimulus that they believe rule in rural areas.

Medical practice is far simpler in the city, in spite of its apparent complexity, than in small towns, for the city physician may enjoy the benefit of close contact with clinical research centers, and also need not know all of medicine, but may specialize in one field.

Lacking the technical facilities afforded by the city, the country doctor is forced to render his action more elemental and dynamic, and to rediscover the curative powers of nature. He knows his patients from birth to death, and he knows their families and their environment. This helps him to make a better diagnosis. More than a physician, he is a counselor who guides his patients in matters of health and life. Ilis presence, his word, may save entire communities from the threat of epidemics or other afflictions. Thus, rural medicine can certainly provide the observant physician with a unique field for research and study.

That the country doctor is usually addressed by his first name— "Doctor Jim" or "Doctor Peter"—indicates that he is regarded as a symbolic being and beloved representative of an archetype, like the angel in folk tales, and not just as a citizen with a bureaucratic identification, as he is in the city.

Because the atmosphere of the city is uniform and the circumstances surrounding pain and disease are nearly always alike, the ailments of city patients lack nuances. The heart of the mighty labyrinth that is a big city is of stereotyped simplicity. In contrast, rural life, simple and uncomplicated though it appears, entails fundamental differences that lend identity to the diseases of its people.

The truly local is truly universal, for the authentic dimension of universality is not of time or of space, but of *depth*. That element in a country that is truly universal, because it is eternal, is found not in its big cities, but in its small towns, wherefrom spring the roots of its traditions.

The real America is not constituted by its great cities, but by its little towns, where the nation was forged. The inhabitants of rural areas are the tradition of this nation, just as country doctors once constituted the most dynamic force in its medical progress.

The country doctor is a sympathetic participant in the great emotional storms—economic and social—of his patients. This privileged role affords him an intimate view of his patients, which on occasions he has transmuted into the pure gold of literary creation.

More and more every day medicine becomes the art of promoting health, preventing disease, restoring health, and rehabilitating the invalid. In this great medical scheme the country doctor is established as the basic factor both in rural health centers and in health stations in factories and in industrial and residential districts. To achieve these goals, in the future, rural health stations may lead to district health stations, and then to teaching hospitals. At the core of this system there looms that heroic infantryman of medicine, the country doctor, with whose help our profession will continue to reach new heights of dignity and grandeur.

THE NEURON JUNGLE

an's quest for mental health is now opening new paths through the neuron jungle.

Medical attitudes are always preceded by social attitudes. For several millennia the attitude of terror of primitive societies toward insanity made them bury the insane alive to protect themselves from the demons that possessed his soul. Eventually, this drastic fatal "therapy" was changed to isolation in chains and in dark cells. But man then began the search for a path through the neuron jungle. Isolation was followed by the use of drugs and physical methods; then by seismotherapy (fevers, chemicals, malaria, convulsants, coma, and shock); and finally by the present physiodynamic and psychopharmaceutical therapies. Thus physical isolation, so much in vogue before Pinel with his own hands delivered the insane from their chains, has become chemical isolation. And man continues the search for new paths across the neuron jungle.

In the field of diagnosis, Kraepelinian interest in the psychiatric *nosos* was replaced by post-Kraepelinian curiosity about the *semeios,* or symptoms, exemplified in the Freudian concept of psychodynamics or symptom formation. The current tendency is to seek the *aitia,* or the hidden cause of mental sickness, so as to adopt the best treatment. This tendency will be accelerated by a physiodynamic perspective. There can be no mental illness if there is no functional disruption of one of the underlying organic structures due to metabolic, psychogenic, and pathophysiologic changes. Since the mind itself

---

From *MD Medical Newsmagazine 1*:7, September, 1957.

can exist only as an expression of cerebral activity, physiodynamic psychiatry claims that there can be no psychosis unless there are metabolic disturbances affecting the organic structures.

The physiodynamic therapies are replacing the philosophic hypotheses of the past century by a healthy naturalistic tendency. But in psychiatry it is essential to *know,* if we are to cure. In the past, empiric therapy prevailed over diagnostic classification. Today we admit that every medical or psychiatric action is cognitive as well as conative. Like the general practitioner, the psychiatrist must be above all a naturalist capable of observing with a researcher's eye the deep organic processes that cause the "surface" symptoms of the patient.

Modern psychiatry has reintegrated clinically the psyche and the soma, which Descartes separated after Plato had united them; it has included in the clinical history the *time* element and the *biographic* component, so essential to anamnesis and vitally important in prognosis; and it has introduced biochemical and chemotherapeutic elements in the solution of etiologic, diagnostic, and therapeutic problems. The new psychobiology, or physiodynamic psychiatry, employs the latest hallucinogenic agents and studies hormonal equilibrium, cerebral lipoproteins, cerebral circulation and oxygen consumption, adrenal changes, and nervous tissues and their possible hormones. The "nervous juice" or brain hormones, which back in the Spain of Don Quixote already intrigued the great physician and humanist, Sabuco, and the activity of the pituitary-hypothalamic-adrenal axis are perhaps the *terra incognita* wherein lies hidden the secret of psychoses.

Sixteenth century man craved an ideal art form, and seventeenth century man a philosophy of science. Twentieth century man craves mental peace. Ataraxis, or mental peace, the dream of the classical Chinese philosophers, today haunts man more than ever. But while "accidental" diseases—trauma, infections, intoxications—have decreased, "personal" diseases of internal origin—mental, sclerotic, degenerative, and tumoral—have increased. To cope with this situation, we, more intent on curing than on knowing, have devised blind therapies, thus creating a fast and shallow science.

The history of psychiatry can be summarized thus: 5000 years of demonology and 1000 years of search for a scientific principle based on the Hippocratic concept that mental disease has only one physical cause and one effect (mania-melancholia), and that the cure is elimination of the *materia peccans,* or "foreign body." Today the physiodynamic therapies pursue three historical objectives: *to eliminate the symptoms* (hallucinations, agitation, and negativism) that make the patient "different" and therefore difficult to treat; *to establish communication* with the patient—isolated as though on an island by the walls of his disease—and to treat him as if he were suffering from any other illness, maintaining his contact with the outside world and hospitalizing him only during the acute phase; *to understand what is happening to the patient,* not in a philosophic but in a scientific sense.

As a result of Virchow's theories, the microbe was the dictator of medicine until the day when the patient was again regarded as a human being instead of as a "thing." The old constitutional pathology, *idiosynkrasia* and *temperies,* was then rediscovered, and the symptom was regarded as the response to the biologic situation created in the organism by disease. Totality, responsiveness, and constitution became the new viewpoint, together with the principle that the patient was situated in a certain environment in space and at a certain moment in time, that is, that he was a *social* and a *historical* person, and that the psychiatrist should explore the *total* person.

The psychobiologic revolution was caused by Cajal, Pavlov, Sherrington, Kraepelin, Bleuler, Freud, Adler, Jung, and Meyer, all born in the most creative period (1849–1866) in the history of psychiatry. As a result of their work, mental illness now has a physiochemical substratum; neurosis can be "heard," and not only "seen" as in Charcot's day; the patient is regarded as a human being living a painful way of life; psychiatric medicine is becoming medical anthropology; disease constitutes a chapter in biographic evolution; the person and his environment have been integrated; the total personality of the patient, his psychobiology, and the psychosomatic roots of his disease are carefully studied, and so are the normal person and diseases in general as biologic and biographic processes. Psychobiology has triumphed over Cartesian dichotomy.

The new ataractic drugs have fostered the attitude that "the mental case" *is* a patient, have reduced the patient's agitation, and have improved his communication with the psychiatrist. These drugs leave the patient *ataraktos,* calm and mentally peaceful, the longed-for objective of the Epicurean philosophers. We do not yet know how the ataraxics work. Perhaps they work on the hypothalamus, that islet of nerve tissue, refuge of the primitive instincts inherited from our hirsute ancestors who ranged the primeval jungles; or perhaps they affect the neurovegetative system, especially the reticular formation of the cerebral cortex, that archaic paleo-cortical-hypothalamic-mesencephalic system that adapts man to the spatial circumstances of the exterior world and that contains a condensed representation of the peripheral structure. Perhaps the ataraxics imitate and complete the autopharmacologic efforts of the human body to combat the stress of disease.

Psychochemical therapy and psychosis-inducing hallucinogenic drugs may one day explain the similarity between the imagery of literary geniuses and mystics and that of persons under the influence of mescaline and other "phantastica" drugs. They may also explain the similarity that has been demonstrated experimentally to exist between the artistic work of writers like Baudelaire, De Quincey, Poe, and Coleridge, of painters like Braque and Picasso, and of persons under the effect of hallucinogenic drugs. Perhaps schizophrenia is the result of a gigantic biochemical error in the organism, in which case genius might be the end result of *small* metabolic errors!

Meanwhile, it is pressing that psychiatry and scientific medicine be integrated, so that we may benefit from the new methods and techniques, and that the physician understand psychiatry better, so that he may apply it in his practice with as much precision technically as he already does empirically.

The next few years may witness this integration of Medicine and Psychiatry under one single scientific standard. Freudian theories will then find their legitimate but not overestimated historico-medical place, not as the basic answer to psychiatric problems or to knowledge of the human mind, but as a tool of incalculable psychologic value.

It is important to remember that since psychiatry is dedicated to the study of alterations in human communication, it, more than any other medical discipline, should render its own communication system less pedantic and confusing. Psychiatry should be approached with the simple healthy criteria of a naturalist, and its phenomena should be described with the simplicity with which Darwin in his later years counted and described the leaves of a plant. Replacement of the current esoteric psychiatric jargon by a simple, clear language will contribute much toward improving communication between psychiatrists themselves, psychiatrist and physician, and psychiatrist and patient. Transparency of language indicates clarity of thought, which is indispensable in this branch of science.

Finally, let us never forget that in psychiatry, as in medicine, pathology is also physiology. There is nothing as physiologic as the pathologic, pathology being the reverse of the physiologic coin and pathologic changes the accelerated phases in that most physiologic process of life—the inexorable course toward death.

An organicistic approach, integration with other branches of medicine and science, clarity of communication—these should be the continued objectives of the science of the mind, if it wishes to add fresh laurels to the wreath of glory woven, since Pinel's days, by the giants of Psychiatry.

PER ARDUA AD ASTRA

m edicine's intervention in business is fairly recent, though since the last century Medicine has helped in organizing industrial workers' health programs.

Businessmen paid little attention to Medicine in their professional life until they realized that medical advances could help them to increase their output by protecting their health, checking incipient illnesses, and improving working conditions. Collaboration between Medicine and business signaled the latter's acceptance not of offices or buildings, but of the *human* element as the basic factor in their enterprises.

Medicine entered the business world late, probably because until the high Middle Ages medical practice was not a salaried profession in a business sense. From the fall of Rome until the thirteenth century physicians were almost always priests. Since the Church supported its clerics, the physicians among them could exercise their healing ministry without pay. Medical services were first rewarded an honorarium in the high Middle Ages. Thus what some still considered the gratuitous efforts of amateurs was raised to the dignity of a true profession.

Business emerged on the historical scene when direct barter between craftsmen or laborers and lords, burghers, or consumers was widened to include the business manager as intermediary between the workers who provided skill and the capitalist who provided money. The modern capitalistic system in business began with the

From *MD Medical Newsmagazine* 1:9, October, 1957.

advent of this intermediary, who pushed business to the foreground, creating a special world, partly industrial, partly commercial, but above all a business world dealing in physical and mental manpower and the fruits of its efforts.

Leading industries, such as steel, clothing, oil, automobiles, recognized early the need for Medicine to safeguard the workers' health, but business executives were late in acknowledging that *they* too are human and need medical assistance in their work. This awareness began with the first disturbing statistics on the high rate of illness and mortality among businessmen. Only then did they, who believed themselves stronger mentally and physically than their subordinates, begin to seek medical assistance not only in the home but also in the office.

Medicine has eliminated many of the "external" diseases—infections, intoxications—that formerly plagued mankind. Two other types of illness now prevail: *internal* (hypertension, ulcers, allergies, arteriosclerosis, degenerative diseases, nephroses, psychoses), and *occupational,* caused by physical and mental tension, a confined sedentary life alternating with periods of intense activity and sudden travel, overeating alternating with hasty snacks, tobacco and alcohol excesses, and general stress. To these may be added disorders due to poor lighting, acoustics and sitting conditions, and bad circulation caused by inactivity.

Medicine has integrated the factors that affect the life of the businessman, which flows from one tightly shut box, his office, to other similar boxes, other offices and his home, alternating prolonged physical inactivity with inordinate mental and physical activity and emotional expenditure and sudden air and motor trips. Commuting— a twice-daily Olympic marathon—symbol of social success, like Cadillacs and mink coats, contributes another source of worry, speed, and stress to the businessman's existence.

Much has already been done to render business offices more hygienic from the viewpoint of space, lighting, ventilation, acoustics, temperature, comfort, and elimination of noise. But much has yet to be done to improve the executive's physical and mental health. Periodic medical checkups, frequent vacations, wise eating and drinking habits, avoidance of overexertion in anything, including golf, moderate physical exercise and rest, preventive medication, and timely treatment of incipient affections are of vital importance physically. It is also important to take more time to enjoy life and make equilateral, instead of isosceles, the life triangle of work, play, and rest, and to eliminate fear and tension, transforming the competitive urge for material gain into a sporting spirit to prove one's skill. All this will make of the businessman a more efficient and above all a healthier man.

Sickness and death are not more prevalent in business circles than in other branches of human endeavor, including Medicine. They are in direct relation to the businessman's negligence of his health and to his ambience and way of life. The physician must teach the executive to live better, for he is an artisan of the world and time in which we live. The executive can attain heights of fame and glory as a builder of a new world. Let him learn to accept medical counsel and he will reach the stars with his toil. *Per ardua ad astra.*

HALF WOMAN AND HALF DREAM

It is no longer a secret, as the ethnographers have shown, that work as unremitting daily toil is an invention of woman.

In primitive society, man was drawn to hunting in times of peace and to battle in times of war, that is, to enterprise and action, to *discontinuous* sport and adventure. But *continuous* and specialized tasks were the creation of woman, who was the first agriculturist, harvester, ceramist, weaver, and metallurgist.

The highly *public* nature of male psychology drives man, whatever his profession may be, to act all the time on the social stage, with his fellow human beings as audience. In contrast, the *private* nature of female psychology impels woman to view her intimate inner life alone or, at the most, with only the one she loves. Man in history was always a restless and wandering adventurer; woman, the creator of routine and customs.

Until the late Middle Ages woman was conspicuously absent from History. The early Middle Ages was an epoch of great adventures—crusades, tournaments, and pilgrimages—from which woman was excluded; but in the late Middle Ages a feminine star ascended the historical horizon and woman began to exert a profound influence on the ethnic destiny of mankind. From mere servant and slave, she gradually became helpmate and companion to man. In the love courts of Provence, woman chose as her favorite he who was *prou et courtois,* courageous and courteous, thus creating a male ideal that subsists, though a bit ragged at the edges, to this day. On this

From *MD Medical Newsmagazine, 1:9,* November, 1957.

male ideal the stone Madonnas on the portals of medieval cathedrals bestowed their Gothic smiles, as today, in the physician's office, the dedicated and loyal assistant bestows upon him, her professional ideal, her bright smile.

The salient difference between male and female psychology is that man wants to *know;* woman, to *feel.* Man's mission is to *do;* woman's, to *be.* Man is measured by what he *does;* woman, by what she *is.* Man's goal is to attain perfection in science, art, and technology; woman's, to attain the concentric perfection of her being. Consequently, woman's role in the building of society has been peripheral, but in spiritual self-development she has vastly outdone man. Whereas the difference between the quasi-anthropoid who roamed the prehistoric jungles, with barely a spark of intelligence in his brain, and modern man is based mainly on what the latter knows and can do today, between prehistoric and modern woman the difference consists primarily in the latter's great spiritual development as a human being, to which end she throughout history has dedicated her efforts. On the other hand, woman has made history with her personal preferences, choosing neither the strongest nor the wisest male but he who attracted her. Thus she has maintained the male species on a healthy mediocre level, preventing him from sinking back to the level of the anthropoid or rising dangerously to the heights of the archangel.

All this makes it even more remarkable that woman should figure so actively in medicine. There is a woman at the physician's side around the clock, be it his nurse, secretary, assistant, collaborator, or wife. The gentle sex has established a bridgehead in the medical citadel, and every day she strengthens this new historical position. Let the physician welcome this fair invasion, for woman always brings with her qualities that the male lacks, qualities that contribute sensitivity, humaneness, and gentleness, so necessary in medicine.

The second "oldest profession" in the world is nursing, for this is really what the Mesopotamian priestesses did when they comforted and ministered to temple visitors. Medical history abounds with distinguished women who were nurses: the noble Fabiola who renounced wealth and pomp to attend the poor at the first hospital in Rome, which she founded; the Abbess St. Radegunda de Poitiers, daughter and wife of kings, who founded a convent and dedicated her life to nursing lepers; St. Hildegard, Abbess of Bingen on the Rhine, who consecrated her life to medicine; Trotula, Rebecca, Abella, and the other "ladies of Salerno"; St. Clare, founder of the Franciscan order of "Poor Clares"; Elizabeth of Hungary, who was immortalized in paintings showing her carrying a basket of food for the poor that turned miraculously into roses when she was surprised by her irate husband, and who was founder of the "Gray Sisters," thus called because St.

Francis of Assisi gave her his threadbare gray cloak; the Dominican St. Catherine of Sienna, heroine of the Black Death and patron saint of nurses; and many others down to the lay saints of our times, among whom Florence Nightingale stands out so nobly.

Woman's participation in medicine has changed with the evolution of the profession. In ancient and medieval times, woman's contribution to medicine was taking care of the sick; today she also helps the physician. With diligence, dignity, and authority she labors in offices, hospitals, laboratories, statistical departments, technical auxiliary services, administrative offices, complex communication systems, and many other areas of vital importance to the physician and medical progress. Perhaps in no other profession has woman established herself with as much dignity and authority as in the medical profession.

There is one other woman who makes a vital contribution in the life of the physician—his wife. To marry a physician is to marry a profession, not a man. It is to marry his obligations without his rewards. It is to renounce a wife's rights to a normal regulated life. She may offer him help and inspiration, hope and consolation, but she knows that she will never shine in the hall of honor of medicine. We may applaud the scientific music composed by the physician, but we neglect the muse that inspired it. Her noninterference in his work and duties, her renunciation of everything except sharing his endeavors and their fulfillment and his search for greatness make the physician's wife his most valuable collaborator.

To this modest and invisible helpmate and to the other women in the physician's life whose sensitivity, devotion, and inspiration have contributed the greenest leaves on Medicine's laurel crown of greatness, we render a tribute. To them we say, with the poet Rabindranath Tagore, "Woman, you are half woman and half dream."

THE HOLIDAY AND THE HOLY DAY

J oy to the world. Christmas bells are tolling, announcing the arrival of the King of Kings. Once again the miracle unfolds. Rosy flesh trembles on the golden straw in the humble manger, bemisted by the breath of ox and mule. Christmas cards depict snowclad hamlets beneath star-spangled skies, flying sleighs with tinkling bells, tables groaning under the weight of brown roasts, golden bread loaves, steaming puddings, casks of cider and spiced punch, recalling memories of the season as immortalized by Charles Dickens, that gay, benevolent dictator of Christmas. In every corner, like a formidable challenge to the Atomic Age, Santa Claus shakes with laughter, the jolly snow of his beard spilling down his scarlet-clothed paunch. Shops brim with festive wares; man's soul, with renewed childhood.

Town and village glitter in their gorgeous Christmas wrapping; yet, is this very glitter impairing the warmth innate to the season? Is there too much scenery and not enough performance? Christmas conserves its original prestige as a religious and pagan homage to God and to the gods, since it combines the four most popular human activities: eating, drinking, merry-making, and praying; but for many people it has become merely a *holiday* instead of a *holy* day.

Christmas is a children's holiday, and children are the kings of tomorrow. It is a homage to the mystery of man's origin, so important to the physician, in which every child becomes a King and every adult a Wise Man. In these times of drastic surgery and cautery,

From *MD Medical Newsmagazine* 1:7, December, 1957.

children are constantly receiving a lesson in facts. Christmas affords them the opportunity to step through the lighted window of legend into the world of myth. And myths are the purest rain with which to water the garden of a child's soul. Were parents aware of this, they would never put away the Christmas tree with the tinsel and the cotton and the crystal bells, and the house would never be free from the fragrance of pine needles.

But children will always have a Christmas tree. Should there be no room for a Christmas tree in the rigid geometry of the atomic cities of tomorrow, it will suffice to take children out on the terrace carpeted with the silvery petals of snow and let them gaze upon the night sky. And there they shall behold the most wondrous of all Christmas trees, glittering with millions of celestial stars.

For adults, Christmas revives the old conflict between the two most powerful human instincts: to walk the open road in quest of adventure; and to retire to one's cave to enjoy its warm comfort. These two instincts for the cave and the road have always clashed in man's mind. At Christmas the instinct of the cave wins. Man gathers around him those he loves, turns night into day with festive lights and roaring fires, and challenges winter's scarcity of food with lavish abundance. Crushing for a few days the roaming instinct that has taken him, yesterday by stagecoach, today by stratocruiser, to the confines of the earth, he is content to remain behind his frosted windowpanes, while the logs crackle on the hearth, the table sparkles with fine damask and cut glass, and fair ladies as resplendent as a morning in May smile upon him. Thus the unconscious primeval archetype of the cave wins at Christmastime over the unconscious archetype of the road.

These psychologic motives inherent in Christmas and its influence upon the mind can cause the depressive episodes known as Christmas neuroses. Modern Christmas inherited the holly from the Roman Saturnalia, the mistletoe from the Druids, the ivy from the Saxons, the Santa Claus myth from the Germans, and the manger from the Latins; but its basic substratum is a universal myth of death and resurrection, depression and joy, the year's and Nature's death agony and the new year and Nature's rebirth in spring.

The proximity of the new year renders us conscious at Christmas of the passage of Time, and we then realize that it is not Time that changes but we ourselves. Man created the calendar and the clock— cages of Time—to establish his own biologic rhythms and deliver himself from those of Nature. But all he achieved when he imprisoned Time—Time that is Tyranny—was to imprison himself behind the crossbars of the calendar and the clock's hands. Christmas' greatest gift to man is the opportunity it affords him to escape his clock- and calendar-regimented world through the magic fourth dimension of legend.

The true poetry of a physician's soul is his devotion to the mystery of Life and of the human being, whose best guardian he is. Christmas affords him the chance to get close to that mystery and to offer man not myrrh—a symbol of Medicine—as one of the Wise Men, a physician, offered the Child Jesus, but words of peace and happiness. Words—the "country doctor's" gospel—to perform his work without covetousness or fear, secure in the knowledge that in work lies the secret of man's strength and fortitude; to oppose the relativity of Time and Space with the eternity of Being; to balance the insecurity of environment with the greatest security there is, that of a confident mind and a stout heart; to accept that to love, to work, to dream, and to wait is man's destiny; to live *deeply* instead of fast and take roots so that he may bear fruit; to learn, as Pindar counseled, to be what he is, otherwise he shall be nothing.

How can these principles be applied? By reviving the symbolic message of the original Christmas in all its simplicity—greatness is simplicity—that legendary Christmas that Mother, Father, and Child spent in a stable warmed only by love and the breath of a mule and an ox. That Christmas that was not a holiday, but a *holy* day.

THE PHYSIOLOGY OF AN ENDEAVOR

*t*here are only three pleasures in life pure and lasting, and all derived from inanimate things: books, pictures, and the face of Nature," said William Hazlitt. These three things are contained in a medical magazine: words, images, and that face of Nature revealed in health and disease. To turn these things into a source of pleasure besides enlightenment—this was the dream that gave birth to *MD*.

In old Canton there were magicians called "bewitchers of the night" who, with the help of lanterns, Bengal lights, cymbals, exotic perfumes, and balls of jade, which they circulated among the spectators, succeeded in casting them into a dream world that turned a placid evening into a night of delicate fantasy and revelry. *MD* wanted "to bewitch the night" of the readers. But, barring the fleeting sensations of the touch of paper, the smell of ink, and the rustling of the pages, it had only two tools—words and images, which in scientific journals had always been technical and factual—adequate indeed for informing and evoking medical concepts, but certainly not for bewitching anyone.

"By the power of the written word to make you hear, to make you feel . . . before all, to make you see." *MD* wanted to do what Joseph Conrad said. A luminous style, unafraid of metaphor and paradox, rich in humor and color, in salt and sun. The language of science, like the distant stars, sheds light but not warmth. *MD* wanted to shed both the light and the heat of the flame.

From *MD Medical Newsmagazine* 2:11, February, 1958.

Images, the second tool, would have to be relevant, but there would also be others to create an atmosphere, a mental mood, relating medical subjects to people from exotic lands or to their historical roots, helping the physician to become an ocular athlete, to look at his world with the eyes of wonder of a child, keeping one foot in the twilight world of fairy tales and another in the bright world of reality, in that harmonious balance that only great poets, scientists, and the wholesome, simple man of the street can attain. Thus the physician might have eternal youth, even when his head is as gray as the walls of a hospital and his arteries almost as hard.

But "the mellow voice of words and a picture crisp and bold" demanded by Leonardo da Vinci was not enough to build a bewitching vision of Medicine. A new approach to medical subjects was imperative. This, only *living* history could provide. For a man has no Nature; he has History. Man is what he has done. He is his past. He is his experiences, which he carries on his back as the vagabond carries his knapsack. What Nature is to things, History is to man. Let History then be hidden in the subjects, subtly impregnating them with its flavor, as the truffles do in a pie.

Words, images, and the fabric of History: these guide the pen and camera of *MD*. With them it endeavors to bewitch the night of the physician, opening for him the treasure chest of life, conjuring around him a polychrome screen of Coromandel.

Despite the success of the new auditive methods of medical communication, the medical journal remains the best method, for it alone offers the gift of communing with words in solitude and silence—two things more precious today than ever.

G. K. Chesterton paid a tribute to journals when he said: "The roar of the printing wheels weaving the destiny of another day. . . . Here is the school of labor, and of some rough humility, the largest work published anonymously since the great Christian cathedrals."

Only by listening to its beats—the medical journals—is it possible to know the condition of the heart of Medicine.

TO NAVIGATE—THE ESSENTIAL THING

Our last two editorials depicted two panels of a triptych: the past and the present of *MD*. This third panel looks at the future. We have no desire to prophesy, a task as discredited as it is dangerous, commanding at first applause and later abuse. But we do harbor the hopes of the navigator who, guided by the silvery caravan of stars, sets out to new promising lands. We believe that the byword of the legendary Greek Argonauts is a good one for any journal: "The essential thing is not to live; the essential thing is to navigate."

Our future work is simple and clear. Above all, we wish to continue to enrich the leisure of the physician. We also wish the doors of the physician's often-isolated mental compartments—professional, social, and human—to open, as hotel rooms do, to one unifying corridor: a historical purpose in life. Thus the physician may come to replace the twentieth century cult of anguish by a happy and serene equanimity. A life culturally enriched is the best way to attain ataraxia. Not the ataraxia that meant to the stoics and Epicureans tranquility through absence of perturbation; but that which twenty-four centuries ago a physician named Democritus defined as calm alertness and happiness of soul. In modern terms this can be translated into self-control and presence of mind in any emergency, akin to that supreme quality of the physician that Osler called *aequanimitas*.

In our world of atoms and sputniks, equanimity and ataraxia signify wisdom and total perspective. These things *MD* has endeavored

---

From *MD Medical Newsmagazine* 2:11, March, 1958.

to stimulate in the past by feeding the cultural stream of the physician's personality, which runs parallel, though with a different rhythm, to his professional and social personalities, just as river, road, and railroad run parallel, though at different speeds.

For the future, *MD* has two new aims: to present monthly a vivid panorama of events in clinical medicine, and to cover the economic problems of the medical profession, for medicine did not cease to be mostly gratuitous experiments of *aficionados* and become a regulated profession until the late Middle Ages, when it was granted the right to dignifying remuneration.

MD aspires to be an educational tool at the service of medicine. It is already used to stir in students the romantic ambition to be better physicians by being better men. To further our progress in this direction and develop a closer contact with our readers, we are planning to invite our colleagues to join the craftsmen in our happy literary workshop.

MD has also made an unprecedented decision. A journal cannot be only lean flesh and quick bones, like a hound. It should also contain advertisements. Years ago advertisements were mere propaganda in the worst taste; today they constitute a reliable source of medical information. The evolution of pharmaceutical literature has followed the same course as painting in history. Classic art represented the bulk of things; impressionism, the quality; and abstract art, the idea. Pharmaceutical advertising began by presenting the physical iconography of drugs; later it dramatized their properties; and now it presents the concept encompassed by each product. Ethical in principles, educational in aims, the pharmaceutical advertisement has become more informative and less self-praising. It is renouncing the showy, full-blossomed rosebush in favor of the flowerless but fruit-bearing fig tree.

To be fully informative, *MD* like other medical journals must carry advertisements. But wishing to spare our readers the unlimited encroachment of advertisements on editorial matter, advertising pages in future issues will be limited to an average of one hundred a month. Thus *MD* hopes to continue being, ever-increasingly, the open window through which the physician may contemplate the wondrous world around him in a state of alert ataraxia.

DE L'AMOUR

N owadays we talk too much about loves and not enough about Love. Love has been outmoded by the insecurity of modern life and the distorted heritage of Freud. Stendhal's *De l'Amour*, once as much a part of a lady's boudoir as a treatise on kidney diseases was of the physician's office, is now a museum piece. We are therefore happy to dedicate this issue to reinstating the meaning of Love.

Everyone, especially lovers, thinks himself qualified to pontificate on love; but the best authority on this subject is perhaps the physician, for he comes most into contact with the problems—and consequences—of the tender passion. Besides, to know a thing is not to be it, any more than to be it is to know it. It is unnecessary for a zoologist to be a kangaroo to be able to speak authoritatively on kangaroos.

Stendhal evolved the "crystallization" theory of love: the sedimentation on one person of imaginary perfections projected by another. Just as a twig cast into the Salzburg salt mines, he said, is slowly coated by a myriad tiny iridescent salt crystals until transfigured into a glimmering wand of silver, so is the loved one transfigured into a vision of graces by the lover's imagination.

Stendhal was wrong, as proved by Ortega y Gasset, whose concepts of love we fully endorse. True love is born suddenly and lasts forever. It is a motion of the soul toward something incomparable. To be in love is to feel bewitched by someone who is or seems perfect.

From *MD Medical Newsmagazine* 2:11, April, 1958.

Love first starts with a centripetal stimulus aroused by another person, which when it finally strikes the core makes love blossom centrifugally until it becomes a psychic current flowing endlessly toward that person.

We all carry deep within us a preformed imaginary profile of the beloved that we try on most persons we meet. Therefrom springs the arrow, the French *coup de foudre,* the Spanish *flechazo,* love at first sight, when we suddenly meet someone who fits this ideal model.

Although love is a dynamic feeling, it narrows our world; it is a psychic angina that begins with a change in our attention, which becomes obsessively fixed on one person. The image of the beloved fills our world completely. Hence, we do not "crystallize" on the object of our love, but set it apart and stand hypnotized before it as a lion before a lion tamer. A lover's soul, filled with one single image, is like a sick man's room filled with the smell of flowers. In this sense, love impoverishes our world "horizontally," while enriching it "vertically" with knowledge of another human being.

Love, however, is not the same as sexual instinct. Whereas love is born from another being whose qualities trigger the erotic process, sexual instinct pre-exists the object of desire, cares not for perfection, and insures only the continuation of the species, not its improvement. Sexual instinct is sometimes selective; love is always so and excludes all desired objects but *the* one. There is no love without sexual instinct, but in true love such instinct merely serves the same purpose as the wind in sailing.

Love, Ortega y Gasset said, is "surrender by bewitchment," not a will to surrender, but surrender despite oneself; one is engulfed as if by magic by the beloved. This is not so of desire, which entails no surrender, only the capture of the quarry. In desire the object of desire is absorbed; in love the lovesick one is absorbed. We can desire without loving, but we cannot love without desiring. Desire dies with fulfillment; love is never fully satisfied. Thus, love is the most delicate reflection of a person's soul, a wondrous talent granted to only a few.

Being man's supreme aesthetic experience, love in its essence may never be fully understood. But we can always hope to experience the same passionate feeling that inspired Don Quixote to roam the sun-baked plains of La Mancha in quest of great feats to perform as a tribute to his beloved Dulcinea.

THE SUN QUEEN

Sun and water are the oldest curative agents. Since time immemorial, they have put new life into frozen limbs and have abated the fires of fever in man and beast.

In no other country perhaps were sun and water so important as historical factors as in ancient Egypt, that "gift of the Nile," in Herodotus' words, "Egyptians being all those who drank of its waters."

The periodic inundations of the sacred river compelled the Egyptians to become versed in mathematics, geometry, and jurisprudence, in order to be able to delimit anew the boundaries of their lands when washed away by the Nile. Likewise a gigantic bureaucracy had to be organized to record the changes caused by the floods. Water to the Egyptians was as vital economically as therapeutically.

The sun, however, was even more important. To the Egyptians, dwellers in a sun-parched land, the sun was a venerated deity known as Ra. The cult of the sun-god developed in Egypt, where six thousand gods crowded the religious pantheon, indicating that to the Egyptians the Beyond was the most important thing, their home on earth being but a transient rest and the tomb the chief dwelling place of man. The story of how a bold King, Amenhotep IV, established the monotheistic cult of the sun-god in opposition to the ruling polytheism and how his consort Nefertiti came to be Queen of the Sun lies like a delicate, still-fragrant rose pressed between the yellowed pages of the book of History.

From *MD Medical Newsmagazine* 2:13, May, 1958.

Some relics of the glory of her ancient civilization still endure in modern Egypt. The pyramids, huge paperweights clamping down the desert so that it shall not be swept away by the sirocco, and the Sphinx, surrounded by crowds of sightseers, still stand "like two indestructible film stars signing autographs." But the most beauteous symbol of all is the bust of Nefertiti, who after more than three thousand years still bewitches us with her veiled gelatinous smile.

Nefertiti was wife of Amenhotep IV, whom Breasted called "the first individual in the history of mankind" and Sigmund Freud, "a remarkable and unique man, worthy of the greatest interest." Amenhotep IV (c. 1375–1359 B.C.) belonged to the XVIIIth Dynasty, when Egypt became a world power, and during his seventeen year reign he achieved an extraordinary politico-religious feat—the establishment of a "heliotherapic" cult, with the sun as "official" source of health, life, religion, and beauty. In this rare enterprise he was supported by Nefertiti, whom he wedded when he was twelve and she ten, a shy girl with a profile like a gazelle in flight, whose bust at Berlin's Dahlem Museum is, together with La Gioconda, the subtlest interpretation of the feminine enigma.

From childhood Amenhotep was an ardent devotee of Ra, the sun-god of Heliopolis, but still more so of Amon, another sun-god of later origin regarded as an incarnation of Ra, particularly in his manifestation of Aton, which was the solar disk visible to the human eye, considered by Amenhotep as the visible source of life, growth, and action.

Under the young Pharaoh's dynamic initiative, temples to the sun flourished everywhere. So much did the sun obsess him, that he changed his name Amenhotep IV (which dedicated him to the god Amon) to Akhenaton or Ikhnaton (glory of the sun Aton). The priests of Amon, who already viewed with cold eyes the Pharaoh's heretical tendencies, were horrified when with unprecedented audacity he broke with millenary tradition and transferred his residence from priest-ridden Thebes to Akhet-Aton (Aton's horizon), halfway between Memphis and Thebes (now Cairo and Luxor). So carried away by the reformation impetus was Akhenaton that he decided there could be only one god in heaven just as there was only one Pharaoh on earth, he had the name of Amon removed from all monuments and papyruses, he dismissed the priests of Amon, and he refused to be considered as a god, proclaiming instead the monotheism of Aton, the disk of the sun.

Akhenaton was barely thirty years old when he died, and his politico-religious revolution died with him, though according to Freud it was revived by an Egyptian called Moses, who transmitted to the

Jewish people a monotheistic religion founded on Akhenaton's solar cult.

In addition to this monumental political exploit, Akhenaton stimulated the Amarna period of Egyptian art, during which, in contrast with the preceding agoraphobic, hieratic art, artists were authorized to paint what they *saw*. A product of that period was the bust of Nefertiti, the Sun Queen, whose sweet, shy grace softened the years of surgery and cautery during which Akhenaton wrought his bold reform.

Nefertiti apparently was the daughter of Amenhotep III, Akhenaton's father, and an Indo-European princess of his harem, which would make her a half-sister to her own husband. That explains why on Akhenaton's death, Nefertiti sought an alliance with an Indo-European prince of her own race. This was looked upon as treason, and she was assassinated. The mummy of her body, slender as a wheat stalk, has never been found.

Proud of his gentle companion's beauty, the Pharaoh often allowed artists to depict them together. In art Akhenaton appears as a brachycephalic adolescent with sensitive features, dreamy eyes, and a flaccid pot-bellied body. At his side, both of them bathed in the rays of Aton the sun, is always Nefertiti, her features delicate, her contours fleeting like the reflection of the moon on the Nile.

Perhaps Akhenaton—this is my own personal hypothesis—suffered from rachitism, as his iconography suggests, and that may be why the sun meant so much to him biologically. In any case, he established the sun as a symbol of health and purity, creator and preserver of human life, this being "a portentous anticipation of present-day scientific concepts regarding the effect of sunlight," as Freud said.

Of the singular medico-religious experiment by this Pharaoh, the bust of Nefertiti remains as its symbol. Lofty and dreamy her brow, a grain of sun glowing in her eyes, her lips parted in a half smile–half kiss, her neck swanlike, the Sun Queen from among the mists of antiquity still casts a ray of sunshine upon us, justifying the meaning of her name Nefertiti—"The Beautiful One Has Come."

GIVE ME OF YOUR DREAMS

*a*rt and Medicine down the centuries have virtually been parallel excavations in the gigantic quarry of Civilization. Like artists, physicians too are children of Apollo, god of Art and Medicine. Art and medicine have often combined in the person of the physician, perhaps because medicine, which is professionally a service, must be creative if it is to yield its maximum harvest. This may be why physicians, artists, and philosophers have always enjoyed one another's company, as illustrated by Plato's immortal *Symposium,* so brilliantly illuminated by the thoughts of the physician Eryximachus.

For several years now we have been giving much thought to the intimate correlation, still inadequately explored, between artistic trends and medical progress. That as a rule medical novelties in any epoch appear subsequently to artistic innovation is as much a fact, though unnoticed by many, as the parallelism between the arts and the structure of medical learning in any one period. Let us review briefly some of the correlations at different moments of history that we have observed.

Seeking to defeat amorphous nature, where there are no straight lines, ancient Egypt created an art of pyramids and colonnades (optical crutches for the Egyptian eye) that was agoraphobic, funerary, geometric; likewise, her medical systems were rigid and monolithic. These systems obviously based their concept of a "canal" carrying the blood through the body on the water-bearing canals that were so vital a factor in Egypt's daily life. By contrast, Greek art was

From *MD Medical Newsmagazine* 2:11, June, 1958.

a noble craftsmanship of blue skies and open seas. No longer mere dwellings for gods, temples like the Parthenon, for instance, were wide open places accessible to both the sun and all people. And so also was the philosophy of Greek physicians—wide and open, bathed by the sunshine of Hippocratic thought.

Byzantine art was precious and full of mannerisms. Unable to venture into space in a city bristling with gilded domes, as Constantinople was, escape was sought in time, through workmanship that demanded the greatest patience and application, such as illuminated miniatures, stained glass, and enameled jewelry. Similarly, Byzantine medicine fled into time, replacing "spatial" exploration of the patient by the compilation of ancient learning. Arabian art shunned the representation of the human form, favoring instead arabesques and floral designs on their majolica ware, tapestries, and rugs; in surgery, they refused to cut into the body with the scalpel, preferring cautery instead. In medieval monasteries they practiced "library medicine," dogmatic and heavy with the dust of Galenism, a medicine that was "bidimensional," like the altarpieces, paintings, and allegories of the pre-Raphaelites.

In the Renaissance, with Leonardo da Vinci's *saper vedere,* with the cult for the naked form and the craving to explore the human body, which paralleled the craving to explore the unknown lands beyond the seas, art and medicine were united once more in the incomparable work of Vesalius. For Benvenuto Cellini the object of painting was "to paint properly a naked man or woman." From bodies stripped for dissection da Vinci derived inspiration for his fine drawings, as did Michelangelo for the colossi he painted in such felicitous poses on the ceiling of the Sistine Chapel. Similarly, Vasari's artistic biographies are comparable in their psychobiographical approach to the *observatio,* or Renaissance clinical records (which replaced the medieval *consilia*), made for instance by Fernel (whose *magnum opus* has been likened to a Florentine *palazzo* erected on medieval foundations), Montanus, and Benivieni. Baroque art, the two leading characteristics of which were motion and emotion, expressed in an ornate architecture that was a veritable whirlpool of stone, had its parallelism in the work of the Baroque physiologists, whose studies concentrated on organic "local movement." In fact, while the Globe Theatre in London rang with the echoes of the words "blood" and "heart," which, like an incessant *ritornello,* constantly recurred in the works of the immortal bard, Harvey in his laboratory not too far away was working on the theory of the motion of the blood. Later, the poetic and philosophical movement in art, impelled by a hunger to visualize the infinite, was reflected in the passion for exploring the infinitely small with the microscope, a craving that had been increasing in the seventeenth century ever since Galileo. In fact, in the quiet town of Delft, Holland, while Leeuwenhoek, a master polisher of magnifying glasses, was investigating the minute structures of the invisible world, his neighbor Vermeer was at the same time depicting the world of the minute in his exquisite paintings. The Enlightenment, founded on the Encyclopedia, had its parallel in the medical encyclopedism of the great medical figures of that age. Again, the positivistic naturalism of the last century was translated into experimental realism in the lectures of Claude Bernard, and Émile Zola, who attended the lectures, transmuted it into *L'Assommoir* and his other realistic novels.

In our own times, Seurat's pointillism, which split light into colored dots on canvas, ran parallel to the discoveries on the refraction of spectrum light passing through a prism and the advances in ophthalmology. The new concepts of physics on form and light were born at the same time as the impressionism of Manet, Monet, and Pissarro, who depicted their subjective impressions of the outer world; the psychologic expressionism in Van Gogh's tortured paintings ran parallel with Freud's exploration of the subconscious; the fragmentation of the human form and penetration of its deeper planes by radiology after Roentgen coincided with Braque's and Picasso's cubism; atomic physics disintegrated the universe, and so did the work of Dali and other abstract painters; Kandinsky's non-objective art and the surrealism of Miró, Tanguy, Klee, and de Chirico are mirrored in the advances since Freud in psychiatry and psychology, just as the modern concept of a single space-time continuum had its counterpart in Picasso's later work depicting figures simultaneously full-front and profile, thus introducing a new time dimension into the until then spatial world of painting.

This series of intriguing correlations between universal, historical attitudes in medicine and in art does not mean that one has been responsible for the character of the other in any particular epoch. Sometimes this has been so, but generally both have been merely facets of the civilization of their time. Artists and physicians as men have been influenced by the cultural and social breezes of their times, which they reflect in their artistic work or medical concepts. The modern physician should remember this correlation, for it will help him to understand philosophically his scientific concepts and even to anticipate new trends in medicine simply by observing the path chosen by the rest of the culture of his time.

W. J. Mayo has beautifully expressed this unity of the real with the imaginary, of science with art, in his words inscribed on a stained-glass window at the Mayo Brothers House: "Take of my experience but give me of your dreams."

THE JOY OF LEISURE

Loafing is the last shred of Paradise left us. For the trivial pleasure of nibbling the apple, Adam condemned us to a life of toil in which the art of loafing has been virtually lost.

In Andalusia, Spain (very near where I was born, which makes me an authority on the subject), loafing has been raised from a sin to a virtue. In contrast to our way of life, with its prolonged intense efforts and short feverish recreations, they have adopted a life of little toil and little but continuous recreation, perhaps because they feel that a little fiesta all the time is better than a big holiday once a year. But here we must seek other solutions to the problem of how to reconcile *otium,* the respite from the pressures of life, with *nec-otium,* the negation of rest that our work represents.

Man is the only living creature that needs to *di*-vert himself, to escape his everyday personality and at least for a while become traveler, fisherman or golfer. This temporary occupation is often more tiring than his normal one, but excels it in that it is a happy occupation.

There is no better way of knowing people than by studying how they amuse themselves. Of the three points in life's triangle—toil, rest, and recreation—two are oppressively monotonous: work and sleeping. "Serious" activities are similar everywhere. Only when a person tries to fill his leisure is the difference between him and others revealed. Our dreams are the personal dowry we bring into this world.

Mankind's recreations reveal two types of periods in history: when people are more concerned with seeking pleasure than with avoiding

From *MD Medical Newsmagazine* 2:11, July, 1958.

pain and gladly pay higher prices to entertainers than to physicians as in the "Gay Nineties"; and when there is greater concern in eliminating anxiety and pain by means of drugs than in actively seeking happiness. Today we have excellent hospitals but little good theatre. We keep on discovering new ataraxics but monotonously repeat our theatrical fare. For therapy only the latest antibiotic will satisfy us, but we still sit through plays where the wife is unfaithful to her husband with his best friend just as she was a hundred years ago.

Reducing to a simple equation what man does to occupy his leisure, I would say he escapes either into nature or into himself. Some people escape into nature because they unconsciously feel that man is a fugitive from nature. Eons ago man fled from nature, where he did things only within a fragment of space, and into history, where he could do things in a time-dimension. But ever since he ceased to be a child of nature to become a maker of history, man has often felt the need to return to nature and do the things—hunt, fish, swim—that will bring back his primitive happiness. Other people escape inward, into that intimate self lost in the daily anxieties. Man began by being nature, but essentially he was and is spirit. Lost are those two precious kingdoms—nature and spirit—in the daily struggle for life. And when we do not seek nature we seek the spirit, through music or reading or the lost art of conversation. When in such moments of leisure man finds himself again, he feels the same joyous shock he would feel should he probe with a lamp the depths of a mine—his own soul—and stumble upon a heap of rare gems sparkling in the darkness.

These two gateways to Paradise still remain open to modern man, but it is not enough to use them only during idle hours. We must also learn to live guided by two simple rules: to preserve an inner calm even amid storms; and to have always a little *fiesta* or sense of humor in that sunlit little corner of Paradise that we all carry in our hearts.

BRIGHT TWILIGHT

In contrast to the years that were devoted to the worship of youth after the First World War, the Western World now reveres maturity. Historically, gerontocracy has certain advantages. History has recorded times for the young and times for the aged. The former have nearly always been periods of crisis; the latter, of stability. For centuries Greece glorified her youth only to succumb politically at the hands of Alcibiades, a young man of dictatorial ambitions. Rome, on the other hand, sought the support of the mature, and that Rome of *patres* and senators became mistress of the world.

This country is now bound toward an age governed by silver-haired men. Medicine's contribution to these men must not be solely "adding years to life and life to years"; it must also teach them that gray hairs are a reward, not a penalty. But gray hairs must be deserved.

When young, no one stops to think that one day he too will be old; old age then is only a reflection in the mirror of somebody else's old age. As André Maurois said, we rebel at the biological injustice that allows a carp to live three hundred years while Byron and Mozart died at thirty. To those two attributes of old age, acceptance and serenity, must be added gymnastics not only of the mind and body, but also of the heart, for the secret of prolonging youth lies in knowing how to preserve Hope so that its bright light may shine upon the twilight of life.

Age has not always been looked upon as the last station but one on life's journey to the land of shadows. In the Renaissance, "old men,"

From *MD Medical Newsmagazine* 2:11, August, 1958.

because of their experience, were sought after in the arts and in war, as occurred in the *Tercios* in Flanders. This concept of the experienced old man was replaced in the eighteenth century by that of the "autumnal," a literary concept of some biological value, which yielded in our own time to that of "involution," or the process of man's physical and mental adaptation to those new circumstances that arise during that turbulent crisis known as the climacteric, when man is no longer capable of strenuous physical effort and, sometimes, of procreation. But these losses are compensated by a stronger and more efficient dynamism derived from the consolidation of his ideas, and from a superior mental activity in politics, science, and art. Even in love the older man has learned that it is possible to replace successfully youth's greater frequency of passion by skill and imagination, as proved in his old age by the immortal rascal Casanova.

There is an enchanting book called *The Art of Long Life* by Luigi Cornaro, a sixteenth-century Venetian nobleman. Cornaro loved life with ever-increasing intensity to the end of his days. Until the age of 40 he was an overindulgent hedonist; but thereafter he made sobriety his rule for a long, happy life and reached the ripe old age of 95, having written in his last few years four books on the art of long living, wherein he describes his famous diet of *panado* (a clear broth with a coddled egg), veal, and wine, which he called "the old man's milk." This dynamic old man said that there was no reason why *after* 90 one should abandon the idea of a paradise on earth, a noble ambition revived in modern geriatrics.

Medical advice, however, is not all that is needed in old age. It must be supplemented by a simple philosophy founded on a conscious and willing renunciation of the superfluous and an increased sense of responsibility and curiosity regarding the marvel of Life. Therein lies the secret of how to continue creative work and preserve Hope in senescence, two things that can render life's autumn into a bright springtime.

FASHION AS DIMENSION AND SYMPTOM

O ur thesis on fashion is simple. Fashion is in every epoch not something arbitrary and capricious but an important historical dimension. Though externally fashions, whether in hats, automobiles, songs, or dances, may be superficial and frivolous, intrinsically they reveal the biologic and historical reasons governing the social habits and feelings of human beings in every epoch. Fashion is an external reflection of the biologic mechanism that regulates the historical development of human life. The woman who today hides her graceful figure in the amorphous monstrosity called the "sack," or the young man who prefers the temporary *petit mal* of "rock and roll" to the celestial spheres of the waltz is not yielding to the social impact of a fashion but anticipating imminent social phenomena.

Two different instincts underlie fashion: imitation and class distinction. The woman who blindly adopts every fashion does so because, although fashion actually destroys individuality by making all people alike, it also bolsters those with a weak or no individuality by upholding them in the mass. In this sense fashions have the same effect as replacing the national costume that distinguishes one people from another by a common universal costume that makes all people look alike. In Turkey, Kemal Atatürk, desirous of "westernizing" his people, made them substitute western headgear for the picturesque *chechias* of Anatolia. In the Roman Empire, from the Caucasus to Britain, the Latin attire was politically *de rigueur*. In the Madrid of Charles III, the people revolted when the government decreed that

From *MD Medical Newsmagazine* 2:11, September, 1958.

they cut down their huge cathedral-like sombreros and sweeping capes introduced a century earlier by the Flemish guards. In all these instances, fashion was used to usher in "on the twirl of a cape," in bull-ring parlance, a political concept in a nation.

Fashion "socializes" and differentiates at the same time, often originating as a reflection of the more powerful psychologic impulses of an age. During the romantic period, bereaved women swathed themselves completely in solid black. With the austerity of mourning they artfully clothed their bodies, just as with their extreme pallor (caused by hypochromic anemia or chlorosis, the great "romantic malady") they veiled their smoldering romantic passions. Mourning attire was a sign of grief for the deceased, but it was also exploited for its mysticoerotic potentialities. The mysterious black wall of silk, which cloistered her as though in private communion with the departed husband, invested the attractive widow with a provocative charm. Often these bereaved ladies ended up, like Lehar's "Merry Widow," in places like Maxim's, dancing in the arms of some gallant swain to the dreamy strains of a waltz.

Clothing was born of three different imperative requirements: as a defense against the weather; as a sign of social rank; and as a sex stimulant. Today this last factor determines the changes in fashion. No sooner has one fashion exhausted its powers of suggestion upon the male than another one is contrived.

Fashions have been at times compensatory. Medieval pointed shoes and the farthingale fulfilled the respective functions of hiding unshapely feet and unwanted pregnancies. Women's clothes became more concealing in times of full-fleshed women, and tight-fitting in times when women's figures were, like the Equator, an imaginary line. Medieval woman's social unimportance, typical of an epoch when man excluded woman from his life of hunting, feasting, and orgy, fostered a solemn hypertrophy in dress. By contrast, whenever woman has been dominant in an historical period, she has abbreviated her apparel to the minimum, which is what everybody does in a moment of crisis demanding direct attention—strip off and discard everything that might hinder action. In this light, nudism would be the maximum expression of a woman's personality, a woman who is not afraid to be what she is and wants to be nothing more.

Clothes therefore were not really born of the need to combat the weather. Some tribes discard their clothes when it rains. Clothes are a way of attracting attention, in imitation of those tropical birds whose brilliant plumage makes them more sought after by the opposite sex. Modern fashions indulge in the element of surprise. Hence the violent contrasts and the fact that fashion "comes from abroad," a distant country, nearly always Paris. This is what the natives of the

Solomon Islands did when they imported "from the outside" the fashion of paying in oyster shells.

The woman bent on following all the fashions does so to break the established order, to attract attention, or as a rebellion against the male, who, poor thing, is always more conservative. But the female fashion plate is hardly ever an interesting woman. Fashion becomes the core of her personality, a hard and constant slavery. All day long she must pay service to elegance and must trot from place to place so that men and, even more important, other women may notice her. This usually turns her into a bored and boring creature.

On the other hand, there is the woman who can select from the vast common stock of possibilities. In that divine faculty of knowing which costume will enhance, not drown, her personality lies the secret of the interesting woman, the woman who can work her will on fashion, adopting only what will complete her personality and transform her into a true thing of beauty.

The important point to remember is that fashion is a revealing dimension and symptom of an epoch, which allows a precise prognosis of its historical course. The postwar bangs, switches, and hair pieces with which women concealed not only part of their faces but their thoughts were indicative of the state of mind that led to the social crises previous to the Second World War. Today's "sacks," "rock and roll," and "angry young men" are signs of an attitude that borders between contrition (sackcloth and ashes) and discontent (revolt against the pirouette), an attitude far more dangerous than the hydrogen bomb.

DISEASE AS BIOGRAPHY

*t*he most revealing historical document on the medical progress of an epoch is not a list of its foremost figures or discoveries, but any clinical *case history* made by a conscientious
physician at his patient's bedside. Hippocratic *catastases,* medieval
consilia, Renaissance *observationes,* seventeenth-century *historia
morbi,* anatomicoclinical protocols by Bichat, Laennec's clinical case
histories with new "auditive" data, in brief, the history of the clinical
case history—this is the most authentic form of making medical
history.

The clinical case history fully reveals the concept of disease that
prevailed in a given epoch and portrays the physician's search for
the nature of disease. In that search nothing has been so important
as the advent of the *biographic* concept of disease, which considers it
a dynamic process that develops across time in the patient's life, as
against the ontological concept, which considers disease an autonomous entity endowed with a natural history.

Why is this biographic concept of disease, which was strengthened
by Adolf Meyer's and Freud's work, of value to the practicing
physician? If the present holistic approach of treating the patient as a
whole person is not enough to indicate its value, we should then recall
the intriguing assertion made by the Hamburg clinician, Arthur Jores,
that, of the two thousand affections known in human pathology, we
know the etiology of less than half, these being precisely those that
man has in common with higher mammals. The rest, of which we

From *MD Medical Newsmagazine* 2:11, October, 1958.

know the pathogenesis but little or nothing of the etiology, are *specifically human* diseases. This means that in order to solve their etiological secret we must have a greater knowledge of man. Hence the ever-increasing tendency to make of Medicine *medical anthropology,* that is, knowledge of the human being living that anomalous and painful way of life represented by disease.

Consequently, therapeutics will never again be a chess match in which by playing our pieces with mathematical precision we inexorably checkmate disease, but an effort to understand the "whole person" of the patient, his environment and his biography, of which his disease is but one chapter. We therefore must not focus our magnifying glass on a single facet of the patient, but we must look at the whole man as if through a reducing glass.

The late Victor von Weizsäcker considered disease as a "biographical crisis," and proposed dividing diseases into three groups: (a) *neuroses,* or atemporal functional disorders in the rhythm of vital phenomena; (b) *bioses,* or reversible temporal alterations in the organic structures, manifested in the individual's corporeal totality; and (c) *scleroses,* or irreversible structural modifications, representing the "historicity" of the disease. Recently I verified that in the seventeenth century Thomas Sydenham had already classified diseases into "acute," biologic or *animal* (epidemiological, we would say now); and "chronic," biographic or *human* (which we now call psychosomatic). In his turn, Karl Jaspers established the contrast between eminently *biological* and predominantly *biographical* diseases, showing again the growing tendency to create a *graphia* of the human *bios,* or a "biographical" medicine.

Today the city physician has little opportunity to learn thoroughly the person and environment of his patients, that is, their biography. On the other hand, the "country doctor," who sees his patients even more often when they are well, gradually accumulates a vast store of knowledge about them of inestimable value when he has to face the biographic accident of disease. All this is not "psychosomatic" medicine, a term so abused that, like a much-handled coin, it is all but worn out. It is simply a way to look at patients in this age of technology, statistics, and the laboratory with the same curious, penetrating, understanding, and, above all, human eyes with which over two thousand years ago a great, kindly physician looked at them in the shade of a plane tree on the sun-drenched island of Cos.

LADY WITH THE LAMP

I remember her as one of the most impressive memories of my childhood. From the rose-clad balcony in our home in Cartagena, a sun-drenched ancient seaport in the south of Spain, I would watch her emerge from the house across the street, a small black bag in her hand, and slowly disappear in the night, her blonde hair burnished silver by the moon. I never saw her by day; she always called on her patients at night. The neighbors affectionately called her *la Samaritana*, and they said that she came from distant lands and that healing the sick was her mission in life. My memory of her is as vague as that of the sky in those serene summer evenings, but I can still see her swinging lantern lighting her path through the dark velvet of the night.

In those days I was under the magic spell of Robert Louis Stevenson's tale, "The Lamp Bearers," about children playing at hiding belt lamps inside their coats. Perhaps that is why I was all the more impressed by the pale, silent figure setting forth in the dead of night to help the ailing, accompanied only by the bright tiny moon of her lantern.

Years later I learned that woman's oldest profession was that of nurse-priestess in the Mesopotamian ziggurats. Later came such great female medical figures as Fabiola, who, renouncing her considerable worldly possessions, founded the first civil hospital in Rome; the Abbess St. Radegunda of Poitiers, daughter and wife of kings, who dedicated her life to nursing lepers; St. Hildegard, medical abbess at Bingen-on-the-Rhine, whose tormenting migraines inspired her fa-

From *MD Medical Newsmagazine* 2:11, November, 1958.

mous polychrome paintings of her mystic visions, and whose life was consecrated to philosophy and medicine; the medical ladies of the School of Salerno, Trotula and Rebecca; St. Clare, foundress of the Franciscan sisterhood of "The Poor Clares" and follower of the teachings of St. Francis of Assisi; Elizabeth of Hungary, who founded "The Gray Sisters" after St. Francis of Assisi presented her with his threadbare gray cloak, and who was immortalized in paintings depicting her with a basket of food for the poor that miraculously turned into a basket of roses when her irate husband bade her open it; the Dominican St. Catherine of Sienna, heroine of the Black Death; Heloise, medical paladin of the twelfth century, just as Maria Colinet was of the Renaissance; Anne Hacket of the Baroque Age; and Ana Morandi Manzolini of the Age of Enlightenment. There are many more before we come to the pioneer women of modern medicine, outstanding among whom was Florence Nightingale, whose white Samaritan shade I conjured not too long ago as I sat on a terrace in Istanbul facing the scene of her ministerings, across the mystery-fraught waters of the Bosphorus. And endless also is the list of modern women physicians who, since Elizabeth Blackwell, Lydia Folger Fowler, and Mary Putnam Jacobi in nineteenth century America, gave their minds and their hearts to our profession.

To our profession woman has contributed, besides her talent, a quality inherent to her sex and indispensible in medicine—sensitivity, which is perhaps the reason she has asserted herself in this profession more than in others. At first she tried—and succeeded in—the female specialties par excellence, pediatrics and obstetrics, and, later, laboratory work. Finally her inquisitive mind plunged into the world of the minute, antibiotic research and microbiology, and into the world of mists of psychiatry, where she is already shedding her bright light.

Such light makes her worthy of Longfellow's verse, once quoted by Harvey Cushing in praise of a great noble nurse: "A lady with a lamp shall stand/In the great history of the land/A noble type of good/ heroic womanhood."

A LIGHT IN THE WINDOW

man, like the primates, is a creature of daylight. While apes sought shelter in trees and other Mammifera went marauding in the dark as soon as night descended upon the earth, paleolithic man took refuge in the golden rooms of a fire, which at once provided warmth, protection, and, above all, light.

In the beginning, dawn was man's reveille and sunset his "lights out" bugle. This diurnal phase of man's existence has endured to this day. In prehistoric times, and even today among primitive peoples, man moved around only from dawn to dusk. Later, fires and torches lengthened his hours of activity. Then the Phoenicians invented the wax candle, which reached its zenith in the eighteenth century, when forests of candles turned temples and palaces into glowing suns, emphasizing the fearsome darkness of field and road. The advent of gas and electricity finally turned night into eternal day, freeing man at last from the centuries-old tyranny of darkness.

Pliny the Elder said that we live only while awake. Electricity has lengthened our conscious life. The rhythm of human life no longer follows Nature's. Except for country folk, we no longer go to bed at the fall of night or rise by the sun. But long and peril-fraught was the road to light, for only churches and the rich could afford candles. Even longer for lack of light were the long winter nights. People slept longer, which was good for the illiterate but bad for those who, craving knowledge, for hours pored over the yellowed pages of ancient tomes by the light of a tiny flame, pale and flickering like the tongue of a tired

From *MD Medical Newsmagazine 2:11,* December, 1958.

hound. Lighting by day was hardly better, for, though discovered before Christ, glass was rarely used for windows or if used was colored or opaque. In cold weather, windows were tightly shuttered, plunging dwellings into solid darkness. Until one day light became the heritage —one of the most precious—of civilized man.

The fairy tales of Perrault, Grimm, and Andersen dramatize the importance of light to man. One of their favorite themes is the single lighted window, a rectangle of gold glowing in the distance, dispelling the night bristling around it like an angry cat, beckoning the weary traveler with promises of rest and warmth.

This theme of the lighted window is perhaps the richest in feeling for modern man. In man's soul there constantly struggle two primitive urges—the cave and the open road, the impulse to sit by his hearth, where the leaping flames invite him to dream, and the impulse to ride the frosted roads flashing in the moonlight. Sometimes the open road wins, and sometimes the cave. At Christmas the cave impulse triumphantly prevails. From the outside, the lighted windows beckon irresistibly, offering human kindness and faith; inside, suppressing with a sigh the ever-lurking urge to the open road, we relish, after eons of darkness, the magic of light.

Light there is, perhaps too much, in our cities, converted by those deadly enemies of the moon and the stars—neon and electricity—into landscapes of flashing diamonds, but there is no more beautiful light than that of the humble candle in the window on Christmas night. For in the tiny flame there once again shines the lonely star that lighted a humble stable glowing with golden straw and pink flesh long ago on the first Christmas night.

BIBLIOGRAPHY

BOOKS IN THE PHYSICIAN'S LIFE

1. LAIN ENTRALGO, P.: Vestigios, Madrid, Espasa, 1941.
2. DOYLE, A. C.: Through the Magic Door, Leipzig, Tauchnitz, 1907.
3. BUCHAN, J.: Mountain Meadow, Cambridge, Houghton Mifflin, 1941.
4. STEVENSON, R. L.: Books which have influenced me. *In:* The Essays of Robert Louis Stevenson, London, McDonald, 1950.
5. EDELSTEIN, L.: Sydenham and Cervantes. *In:* Essays in the History of Medicine, Baltimore, Johns Hopkins Press, 1944, p. 55.
6. CERVANTES, M. DE: Don Quijote, Mexico, Seneca, 1948.
7. SIGERIST, H. E.: Civilización y Enfermedad, Mexico, Fondo de Cultura Económica, 1943.
8. PACK, G. T., AND GRANT, F. R.: The influence of disease on history, Bull. New York Acad. Med. *24:*523, Aug., 1948.
9. CASANOVA DE SEINGALT, G. J.: Mémoires de Casanova écrits par lui-même, Paris, Garnier, 8 vol., 1949.
10. CARTER, H. S.: Medicine and literature, Glasgow M.J. *30:*147, April, 1949.
11. KIMBROUGH, R. A., JR., AND KIMBROUGH, A. M.: The physician in current fiction, Am. J. Obst. & Gynec. *65:*472, March, 1953.
12. CARTER, H. S.: Robert Burton and "The anatomy of melancholy," Glasgow M.J. *35:*202, Aug., 1954.
13. MAUGHAM, W. S.: The Summing Up, New York, Doubleday & Co., 1938.
14. VILAR, E.: El médico en la literatura, Valencia, Archivos, 1953, p. 18.
15. WECHSLER, I. S.: S. Weir Mitchell, Neurology *5:*242, 1955.
16. ANON.: Doctors as writers, J.A.M.A. Spectrum *157:*24, March 5, 1955.
17. MUNTHE, J., AND MEXKULL, G.: The Story of Axel Munthe, London, John Murray, 1953.
18. BROWNE, T.: Religio Medici, London, Smith, Elder & Co., 1898.
19. MAJOR, R. H.: Some important books in medicine, Mississippi Valley M.J. *74:*9, Jan., 1952.
20. MARAÑON, G.: Crítica de la medicina dogmática, Madrid, Espasa, 1950.
21. MARAÑON, G.: Prólogo a la anatomía microscópica, por Dr. Rodríguez Pérez y Dr. Correa Henao, Antioquía Médica *1:* May, 1951.
22. PITTIS, W. M.: Some Memoirs of the Life of John Radcliffe, 1715 (Anon).
23. FLAXMAN, N.: How to keep up with medical literature, J.A.M.A. *154:* 1409, April 24, 1954.
24. MAUROIS, A.: Un Art de vivre, Paris, Plon, 1939.
25. ANON.: Humanism in modern medicine (editorial), Quart. Bull., Northwestern Univ. M. School *25:*176, 1951.
26. Selected Writings of Sir W. Osler, London, Oxford Univ. Press, 1951.
27. OSGOOD, C. G.: Poetry as a Means of Grace, Princeton, Princeton University Press, 1941.

MINERVA AND AESCULAPIUS: THE PHYSICIAN AS WRITER

1. ANON.: Anton Chekhov, physician and literary artist, Clin. Excerpts *19:*99, 1945.
2. ANON.: Dr. Oliver Goldsmith (editorial), Clin. Excerpts *19:*35, 1945.

3. ANON.: Doctors as writers (editorial), J.A.M.A. Spectrum *157*:24, March 5, 1955.
4. ANON.: Editorial, St. Thomas's Hosp. Gaz. *53*:61, April, 1955.
5. ANON.: François Rabelais, M.D. (editorial), Brit. M.J. *1*:831, April 11, 1953.
6. ANON.: Humanism in modern medicine (editorial), Quart. Bull. Northwestern Univ. M. School *25*:176, 1951.
7. ANON.: John Keats (1795–1821) (editorial), Clin. Excerpts, p. 3.
8. ANON.: Medical journalism (editorial), J. Internat. Coll. Surgeons *26*:118, July, 1956.
9. ANON.: Oliver Wendell Holmes (editorial), Clin. Excerpts *19*:131, 1945.
10. ANON.: William Somerset Maugham: his career and medical background (editorial), Clin. Excerpts *19*:259, 1945.
11. BAYON, H. P.: René Descartes, 1596–1650. A short note on his part in the history of medicine, Proc. Roy. Soc. Med. *43*:783, April 5, 1950.
12. CARBALLO ROF, J.: El Hombre desde su Enfermedad, Valencia, Archivos, p. 185.
13. CARTER, H. S.: Medicine and literature, Glasgow M.J. *30*:147, April, 1949.
14. CARTER, H. S.: Eccentrics in medicine, Glasgow M.J. *34*:259, June, 1953.
15. CARTER, H. S.: Robert Burton and "The anatomy of melancholy," Glasgow M. J. *35*:202, Aug., 1954.
16. CARTER, H. S.: Dr. François Rabelais, Glasgow M.J. *36*:267, Aug., 1955.
17. DINGLE, H.: René Descartes, Nature *165*:213, Feb. 11, 1950.
18. HARNSBERGER, C., EDITOR: The Lincoln Treasury, Wilcox and Follet.
19. HILLMAN, C. C.: Observations on tropical medicine in the United States Army, Clin. Excerpts *19*:139, 1945.
20. JORDAN, S. M.: Medicine and the doctor in word and epigram, New England J. Med. *248*:875, May 21, 1953.
21. KIMBROUGH, R. A., JR.: The physician in current fiction, Am. J. Obst. & Gynec. *65*:472, March, 1953.
22. MARAÑON, G.: Estudios de endocrinologia, Madrid and Buenos Aires, Espasa-Calpa, 1940.
23. MARAÑON, G.: Les ideas biológicas del Padre Feijoó, Madrid and Buenos Aires, Espasa-Calpe, 1941.
24. MARAÑON, G.: Cajal, Madrid and Buenos Aires, Espasa-Calpe, 1951.
25. MARAÑON, G.: La medicina y nuestro tiempo, Madrid and Buenos Aires, Espasa-Calpe, 1954.
26. MARAÑON, G.: Efemérides y comentarios, Madrid and Buenos Aires, Espasa-Calpe, 1955.
27. MARTI-IBAÑEZ, F.; SACKLER, A. M.; SACKLER, M. D., AND SACKLER, R. R.: The quest for Freud, J. Clin. & Exper. Psychopath. & Quart. Rev. Psychiat. & Neurol. *17*:117, April-June, 1956.
28. MOUCHOT, G.: Co-operation in the profession, Letter from France, p 447.
29. PLITCHET, A., AND PLITCHET, P.: Shakespeare et ses connaissances en médecine, Presse méd. *53*, no. 86, 1945.
30. QUENNELL, P.: Writer and physician: a literary alliance? Med. World *84*:443, May, 1956.
31. ROBERTS, F.: Lingua medica, a study in medical semantics, Brit. M.J. *1*:1444, June 27, 1953.
32. SIGERIST, H.: La enfermedad en la literatura. *In:* Civilización y Enfermedad, Mexico, Fondo de Cultura Económica, 1943.

33. SIGERIST, H.: The historical aspect of art and medicine, Bull. Inst. Hist. Med. *4*:271, April, 1936.
34. VALLERY-RADOT, P.: Un évadé de la médecine—Eugène Sue, Presse méd. *62*:1677, Dec. 1, 1954.
35. VAULTIER, R.: La médecine dans Madame Bovary, Presse méd. *62*:825, May 26, 1954.
36. VILAR, E.: El médico en la literatura, Valencia, Archivos, 1953, p. 18.
37. WARREN, R.: François Rabelais, New England J. Med. *253*:376, Sept. 1, 1955.
38. WECHSLER, I. S.: S. Weir Mitchell, Neurology *5*:242, 1955.

THE PHYSICIAN AS TRAVELER

1. ROBINSON, V.: The physician as explorer in Asia, Ciba Symposia *2*:626–632, Nov., 1940.
2. ROBINSON, V.: Medical explorations in Africa, Ciba Symposia *2*:633–642, Nov., 1940.
3. SCHAEFER, G., AND NAUMANN, W.: Physicians as pioneers of air travel, Ciba Symposia *3*:1026–1032, Nov., 1941.
4. SCHAEFER, G., AND NAUMANN, W.: Physicians as inventors of steam engines, Ciba Symposia *3*:1033–1036, Nov., 1941.
5. SCHAEFER, G., AND NAUMANN, W.: Medical men as investigators of magnetism and electricity, Ciba Symposia *3*:1037–1042, Nov., 1941.
6. SCHAEFER, G., AND NAUMANN, W.: Physicians as builders of optical instruments, Ciba Symposia *3*:1043–1046, Nov., 1941.
7. ACKERNECHT, E. H.: Naval surgery from 1500–1800, Ciba Symposia *4*:1394–1404, Dec., 1942.
8. ACKERNECHT, E. H.: Naval surgery since 1800, Ciba Symposia *4*:1405–1409, Dec., 1942.
9. ACKERNECHT, E. H.: The care of sick and wounded sailors in the United States, Ciba Symposia *4*:1410–1418, Dec., 1942.
10. ACKERNECHT, E. H.: The naval surgeon, Ciba Symposia *4*:1419–1424, Dec., 1942.
11. ROBINSON, V.: Discovery of the balloon, Ciba Symposia *5*:1618–1623, Dec., 1943.
12. ROBINSON, V.: Origin of aviation medicine, Ciba Symposia *5*:1624–1638, Dec., 1943.
13. ROBINSON, V.: Aviation medicine in AEF, Ciba Symposia *5*:1639–1646, Dec., 1943.
14. ROBINSON, V.: Aviation medicine in America air-marks: 1903–1943, Ciba Symposia *5*:1647–1651, Dec., 1943.
15. MARAÑON, G.: El Príncipe explorador. *In*: Meditaciones, Santiago de Chile, Cultura, 1937.

PADUA AND LONDON: A HARVEIAN TALE OF TWO CITIES

1. BLALOCK, ALFRED: The nature of discovery, Ann. Surg. *144*:289–303, Sept., 1956.
2. BAYON, H. P.: William Harvey (1578–1657). His application of biological experiment, clinical observation, and comparative anatomy to the problems of generation, J. Hist. Med. & Allied Sc. *11*:51–96, Winter, 1947.
3. BLUM, LESTER, AND NELSON, WILLIAM M.: The antecedents of blood transfer, Bull. New York Acad. Med. *31*:671–681, Sept., 1955.

4. CASTIGLIONI, ARTURO: Bologna, Ciba Symposia 7:70–100, Aug.-Sept., 1945.
5. CASTIGLIONI, ARTURO: Medical school of Padua, Ciba Symposia 10:958–992, Nov.-Dec., 1948.
6. CASTIGLIONI, ARTURO: The origin and development of the Anatomical Theater to the end of the Renaissance, Ciba Symposia 3:826–844, May, 1941.
7. CABOT, BLAKE: The Motion of the Heart, New York, Harper & Brothers, 1954.
8. COHEN, HENRY: Harvey and the scientific method, Brit. M. J. 2:4690, Nov. 25, 1950.
9. CHAUVOIS, L.: Un "colloque": Harvey, Riolan, Descartes, Chroniques 63: 129–130, Jan., 1955.
10. CHAUVOIS, L.: Molière, Boileau, La Fontaine et la circulation du sang, Chroniques 62:1219–1220, Sept., 1954.
11. DALE, HENRY: Scientific method in medical research, Brit. M. J. 2:4690, Nov. 25, 1950.
12. WHITE, PAUL DUDLEY: The ways of life and heart disease, J. Maine M. A. 47:329–334, Nov., 1956.
13. DURAN ARROM, D.: Ensayo Médico-Histórico de la Circulación de la Sangre desde la Protohistoria hasta 1550, Arch. Enf. Cor. y Vas. 56:123–171, 1954.
14. FLEMING, DONALD: William Harvey and the pulmonary circulation, Isis 146:319–327, Dec., 1955.
15. FLEMING, DONALD: Galen on the motions of the blood in the heart and lungs, Isis 46:14–21, March, 1955.
16. FRANKLIN, K. J.: Fifty years of physiology, Proc. Roy. Soc. Med. 27:789–796, May 3, 1950.
17. GERLITT, JOHN: The development and effects of Harvey's theory, Ciba Symposia 1:87–93, June, 1939.
18. GOTFREDSEN, EDV.: The reception of Harvey's doctrine in Denmark, Acta med. Scandinav. 142:75–86, Feb. 3, 1952.
19. GRAHAM, JAMES M.: William Harvey and the early days of blood transfusion, Edinburgh M. J. 60:65–76, Feb., 1953.
20. GUTHRIE, DOUGLAS: Harvey in space and time, Brit. M. J. 1:575–579, March 9, 1957.
21. HARVEY, WILLIAM: Anatomical Studies on the Motion of the Heart and Blood. Translation by Chauncey D. Leake, Springfield, Ill., Charles C Thomas, 1941.
22. HOLMAN, DELAVAN V.: Venesection, before Harvey and after, Bull. New York Acad. Med. 31:661–670, Sept., 1955.
23. IZQUIERDO, J. J.: On Spanish neglect of Harvey's "De motu cordis" for three centuries, and how it was finally made known to Spain and Spanish-speaking countries, J. Hist. Med. & Applied Sc. 3:105–124, Winter, 1948.
24. KEYNES, GEOFFREY: The Personality of William Harvey, Cambridge, Cambridge University Press, 1949.
25. LAIN ENTRALGO, PEDRO: Harvey, Madrid, Talleres de Artes Gráficas "Diana," Feb. 28, 1948.
26. LAIN ENTRALGO, PEDRO: La vida de Guillermo Harvey, Medicamenta 7:81–84, 1947.
27. MALUF, N. S. R.: History of blood transfusion, J. Hist. Med. & Applied Sc. 9:59–107, Jan. 1954.
28. MARTI-IBAÑEZ, FELIX: Un médico inglés y su gran descubrimiento, Horizontes méd., pp. 538–540, June, 1943.

29. MARTI-IBAÑEZ, FELIX: Towards a history of medical thought, Internat. Rec. Med. & G. P. C. *165*:484–503, 523–538, Sept., Oct., 1952.
30. MARTI-IBAÑEZ, FELIX: Antibiotics and the problem of medical communication. *In*: Antibiotics Annual 1956–1957, New York, Medical Encyclopedia, Inc., 1957, pp. 4–14.
31. OSLER, WILLIAM: The Growth of Truth, London, Henry Frowde, Oxford University Press Warehouse, 1906.
32. OSLER, WILLIAM: The Evolution of Modern Medicine, London, New Haven, Yale University Press, 1921.
33. PAGEL, WALTER: Giordano Bruno: the philosophy of circles and the circular movement of the blood, J. Hist. Med. & Applied Sc. *6*:116–124, Winter, 1951.
34. PI-SUÑER, J.: Joan D'Alos and the doctrine of the circulation of the blood, Yale J. Biol. & Med. *28*:415–418, nos. 3–4, Dec.-Feb., 1955–1956.
35. ROBINSON, VICTOR: Anatomical dissection in the 18th century, Ciba Symposia *3*:845–853, May, 1941.
36. ROBINSON, VICTOR: Hygiene in the dissecting room of the 19th century, Ciba Symposia *3*:854–860, May, 1941.
37. SANCHEZ DE LA CUESTA: Evolución del Pensamiento Cardiológico en la Península Ibérica, Ciencias Médicas Hispano-Americanas, p. 483.
38. SELYE, HANS: Stress and psychobiology, J. Clin. & Exper. Psychopathol. *17*:370, Dec., 1956.
39. SIGERIST, H.: The Great Doctors, New York, Norton, 1933.
40. SIGERIST, H.: The historical aspect of art and medicine, Bull. Inst. Hist. Med. *4*:271–296, April, 1936.
41. SINGER, CHARLES: How medicine became anatomical, Brit. M. J. *2*:Dec. 25, 1954.
42. STENN, FREDERICK: William Harvey and the Spirit of Inquiry, Postgrad. Med., April, 1951.
43. ZURBACH, KARL: Early ideas and theories on the motion of the blood, Ciba Symposia *1*:71–77, June, 1939.
44. ZURBACH, KARL: William Harvey's discovery of the circulation of the blood, Ciba Symposia *1*:78–86, June, 1939.

MEDICINE IN THE SPAIN OF DON QUIXOTE

1. ALTAMIRA, R.: Historia de España y de la Civilización Española, Barcelona, Espasa, 1914.
2. BAAS, J. H.: Outlines from the History of Medicine and the Medical Profession, New York, Vail & Co., 1889, pp. 484, 515, and 523.
3. BLANCO JUSTE, F. J.: Un lienzo al óleo, desconocido retrato del famoso médico Andrés Laguna, Libro de Actas *1*:236, 1935.
4. CHACON Y CALVO, J. M.: Cervantes y El Quijote, La Habana, Cultura, 1945.
5. CIGNOLI, F.: El bálsamo de fierabrás, Escuela de Farmacia, *11*:15, May-June, 1948.
6. EDELSTEIN, L.: Sydenham and Cervantes. *In:* Essays in the History of Medicine, Baltimore, Johns Hopkins Press, 1944, p. 55.
7. FERNANDEZ DE ALCALDE, A.: Enseñanzas que toma la Medicina de la lectura de "El Quijote," Libro de Actas *1*:275, 1935.
8. FORGUE: Historical Sketch of Spain (Medicine), Gaz. d. Hôp. Civils et Militaires, March 19, 1932, pp. 415–422.

9. GARRISON, F. H.: Epitome of History, Bull. New York Acad. Med. 7:589–634, Aug., 1931.
10. GONZALEZ DE AMEZUA, A.: Tres humanistas españoles del siglo XVI frente a la Medicina, Medicamenta 8, no. 136.
11. GRANJEL, L. S.: Boticarios en el escenario de la literatura picaresca, Medicamenta 15:137.
12. GRANJEL, L. S.: La figura del médico en el escenario de la literatura francesa, Arch. iberoam. de hist. de méd. 2:493, 1940.
13. GUTIERREZ-NORIEGA, C.: Cervantes y la psicología médica, Rev. neuro-psiquiat. 9:107, June, 1946.
14. GUTIERREZ-NORIEGA, C.: Contribución de Cervantes a la psicología y a la psiquiatría, Rev. neuro-psiquiat. 7:149, 1944.
15. GUTIERREZ-NORIEGA, C.: La personalidad y el carácter en la obra de Cervantes, Rev. neuro-psiquiat. 10:516–541, Dec., 1947.
16. GUTIERREZ-NORIEGA, C.: Significado y transcendencia del humorismo en Cervantes, San Marcos 8:43, 1948.
17. KRENGER, W.: La medicina en España durante el siglo de oro, Actas Ciba 12:415, 1939.
18. LAIN ENTRALGO, P.: La anatomía de Vesalio, Arch. iberoam. de hist. de méd. 3:85, 1941.
19. LEJEUNE, F.: La cirugía española en su época de esplendor (1550–1650), Actas Ciba 3:71, March, 1936.
20. LEJEUNE, F.: Spanish anatomy before and about the time of Vesalius, Janus, Sept., 1927, pp. 413–422.
21. MARAÑON, G.: La Literatura Científica en los Siglos XVI y XVII, Madrid, 1954.
22. MARTI-IBAÑEZ, F.: La extraordinaria historia de Thomas Dover y Alejandro Selkirk, Horizontes méd. 1:16, 1943.
23. MORENO, A. R.: Introduction to the study of medicine in the Renaissance, Semana méd. July 9, 1942, pp. 89–92.
24. NASIO, J.: La Ciencia Médica Hispánica de los Siglos XVI, XVII y XVIII y su Contraste con la Ciencia Extranjera (Hispanic Medical Science of the 16th, 17th and 18th Centuries Compared with Foreign Science), Hispalis Medica, Feb., 1955, pp. 65–72.
25. NASIO, J.: La ciencia médica hispánica en los siglos XVI, XVII y XVIII y su contraste con la ciencia extranjera, Medicamenta 23:221, 1954.
26. OLIVER, W. W.: Stalkers of Pestilence, New York, Paul B. Hoeber, 1930.
27. PAZ SOLDAN, C. E.: El cuatricentenario de la "Fábrica" de Andrés Vesalius, y las bases anatómicas de la escuela médica de Lima, Reforma med., Feb., 1944.
28. PRIETO, L. A.: España y su historia ante los doctores Finlay y Delgado (Spain and its history before Finlay and Delgado), Med. colon., Madrid 21:20–37, 1953.
29. QUIJANO, OLIVERA, J.: Historia de los hospitales españoles en América durante los siglos XVI, XVII y XVIII, Arch. iberoam. de hist. de méd. 2:529, 1940.
30. RAMOS, F.: La obra pictórica de Pedro Rojas, médico, histólogo y profesor universitario, Actas Ciba no. 3:86, March, 1936.
31. DEL REAL, E. G.: Historia de la Medicina en España, Madrid, 1921.
32. RICO-AVELLO Y RICO, C.: Las enfermedades y los médicos en la vida de Felipe II, Madrid, Gráficas González, 1950.

33. RICO-AVELLO Y RICO, C.: Madrid en el Siglo XVII. Algunos Datos sobre Higiene Urbana, Madrid, Gráficas González, 1948.

34. SAUNDERS, J. B. DE C. M., AND O'MALLEY, C. D.: Bernardino Montaña de Monserrate, J. Hist. Med. & Allied Sc. *1*:87, Jan., 1946.

35. SERIAFINO, R.: La medicina en los libros de caballería andante, Public. de la Cát. de Hist. de Med. *6*:225, 1943.

36. SUBIZA, E.: Los médicos de Felipe II, Arch. iberoam. de hist. de méd. *6*:1954.

37. VALBUENA PRAT, A.: La vida Española en la Edad de Oro, Barcelona, Editorial Alberto Martín, 1942.

38. DEL VALLE INCLAN, C.: El léxico anatómico de Bernardino Montaña de Monserrate y de Juan Valverde, Arch. iberoam. de hist. de med. *1*:121, 1949.

39. El mito de la decadencia científica española desde el siglo XVI al XIX. (The myth of scientific decline in Spain from the sixteenth to the nineteenth century), An. r. Acad. nac. de med. 1955, pp. 231–257.

40. Sanguijuelas y ventosas, Actas Ciba no. 3:96, March, 1936.

THE HISTORY OF ENDOCRINOLOGY AS SEEN THROUGH THE EVOLUTION OF OUR KNOWLEDGE OF THE ADRENAL GLAND

1. ANON.: The action of cortisone, Brit. M.J. *2*:1325, Dec. 1, 1951.

2. ANON.: The adrenal gland (editorial), Brit. M.J. *2*:373, Aug. 13, 1949.

3. ANON.: The history of endocrinology, Brit. M.J. *1*:1033, May 15, 1937.

4. ANON.: Réunion des endocrinologistes de langue française, Presse méd. *59*:1640, Dec. 8, 1951.

5. ANON.: Surgery of the adrenal cortex, J.A.M.A. *149*:934, July 5, 1952.

6. BEACH, F. A.: Hormones and Behavior, New York, Paul B. Hoeber, 1948.

7. CARBALLO, J. R. El Hombre a Prueba, Madrid, Editorial Paz Montalvo, 1951.

8. CASTEX, M. R., AND SCHTEINGART, E.: El valor diagnóstico de los andrógenos y 17-cetosteroides en los trastornos endocrinogénicos, Prensa méd. argent. *38*:2979, Nov. 26, 1951.

9. CAWADIAS, A. P.: The history of endocrinology, Proc. Roy. Soc. Med. *34*:303, April, 1941.

10. CAWADIAS, A. P.: Tendencias modernas en la endocrinología clínica, Medicamenta *21*:399, June 10, 1952.

11. Co TUI: Somatologic perspectives in psychiatric research. Part VI. Endocrinologic orientation to psychiatric disorders, J. Clin. & Exper. Psychopath. *12*:35, March, 1951.

12. COVIAN, F. G.: Hacia una bioquímica de la individualidad, Medicamenta *21*:353, May 20, 1952.

13. DALE, H.: Thomas Addison, pioneer of endocrinology, Brit. M.J. *2*:347, Aug. 13, 1949.

14. DECOURT, P.: Le rôle de la cortico-surrénale dans les phénomènes de Reilly, Presse méd. *60*:663, May 7, 1952.

15. DODDS, E. C.: Stories of endocrine research, Lancet *1*:699, May 24, 1947.

16. EVANS, G.: Inaugural Langdon-Brown lecture, Brit. M.J. *1*:175, Jan. 26, 1952.

17. FERREIRA, A. C.: Les stéroides du cortex surrénal en psychiatrie, J. Brasileiro de Psychiat. *1*:2, Jan., 1952.

18. FOX, J. DE W.: ACTH and cortisone: Miracle therapy or medical tool?, M. Arts & Sc. *6*:31, 1952.

19. GEILING, E. M. K.: Théophile de Bordeu, London, Oxford University Press, 1930.
20. GOLDSTONE, B.: The general practitioner and the general adaptation syndrome, South African M.J. 26:88, Feb. 2, 1952.
21. GUILLEMIN, R.: Alarm reaction and the general adaptation syndrome, Ann. West. Med. & Surg. 6:347, June, 1952.
22. GUTHRIE, D.: A History of Medicine, Philadelphia, J. B. Lippincott Co., 1946.
23. GUTHRIE, D.: The search for a philosophy of medicine, Lancet 1:405, March 23, 1946.
24. HAWKER, R. W.: Synopsis of Endocrinology, Bribance, 1950.
25. HENCH, P. S.: The potential reversibility of rheumatoid arthritis, Proc. Staff Meet., Mayo Clin. 24:167, March 30, 1949.
26. HENCH, P. S.; KENDALL, E. C.; SLOCUMB, C. H., AND POLLEY, H. F.: The effect of a hormone of the adrenal cortex (17-hydroxy-11-dehydrocorticosterone: compound E) and of pituitary adrenocorticotropic hormone on rheumatoid arthritis, Proc. Staff Meet., Mayo Clin. 24:181, April 13, 1949.
27. JENNINGS, P. B.: Adrenal cortical function at death as measured by level of circulating eosinophils, Brit. M. J. 1:1055, May 17, 1952.
28. KENDALL, E. C.: The adrenal cortex and rheumatoid arthritis, Brit. M.J. 2:1295, Dec. 1, 1951.
29. KENDALL, E. C.: The development of cortisone as a therapeutic agent, Antib. & Chemo. 1:7, April, 1951.
30. KENDALL, E. C.: Hormones of the adrenal cortex in clinical medicine, Edinburgh M.J. 59:1, Jan., 1952.
31. KENDALL, E. C.: Some observations on the hormone of the adrenal cortex designated compound E, Proc. Staff Meet., Mayo Clin. 24:298, May 25, 1949.
32. KENNEAR, T. W. G.: The diagnosis of Addison's disease, Chir. 64.
33. LANGDON-BROWN, W.: The birth of modern endocrinology, Proc. Roy. Soc. Med. 39:507, May 22, 1946.
34. LANGDON-BROWN, W.: The evolution of modern therapeutics, Brit. M.J. 1:35, Jan. 13, 1945.
35. LANGDON-BROWN, W.: The Integration of the Endocrine System, Cambridge, Cambridge University Press, 1935.
36. LANGDON-BROWN, W.: Thus we are men, Brit. M. J. 1:206, an. 26, 1952.
37. MAJOR, R. H.: Classic Descriptions of Disease, Springfield, Ill., Charles C Thomas, 1948.
38. MARAÑON, G.: El caso más antiguo conocido de enfermedad de Addison, Siglo méd. 20:605, 1922.
39. MARAÑON, G.: El sentido defensivo de algunas enfermedades tiroideas, Bol. d. Col. municipal de méd., June 21, 1951.
40. MARAÑON, G., and NOGUERA, J. FERNANDEZ: La enfermedad de Addison, Espasa-Calpe, Barcelona, 1949.
41. MARTI-IBAÑEZ, F.: Evolución histórica de la teoría de los chackras, Rev. de Información Terapéutica, Oct.-Nov., 1936.
42. MARTI-IBAÑEZ, F.: Historia de la Psicología y Fisiología místicas de la India, Madrid, Universidad de Madrid, 1934.
43. MARTI-IBAÑEZ, F.: El Pensamiento Médico en la Historia, Guatemala, Universidad de Guatemala, 1947.

44. MARTI-IBAÑEZ, F.: Towards a history of medical thought, Internat. Rec. Med. & G.P.C. *165*:484, Sept., 1952.
45. MARTI-IBAÑEZ, F.: Towards a history of medical thought, Internat. Rec. Med. & G.P.C. *165*:523, Oct., 1952.
46. McGAVACK, T. H.: The Thyroid, St. Louis, C. V. Mosby Co., 1951.
47. McNEE, J. W.: Cortisone and ACTH: The present position in America, Brit. M.J. *1*:113, Jan. 4, 1950.
48. MEANS, J. H.: The integrative action of the endocrine system, Ann. Int. Med. *34*:1311, June, 1951.
49. MOTT, J. R.: La hormona adrenocórticotrófica (ACTH) y las glándulas suprarrenales en estado normal y patológico, Semana méd. *57*:67, Jan. 19, 1950.
50. NEUBURGER, M.: Essays in the History of Medicine, New York, Medical Life Press, 1930.
51. ONE HUNDRED EIGHT AUTHORS: The Biology of Mental Health and Disease, New York, Paul B. Hoeber, 1952.
52. PENDE, N.: Origini ed Evoluzione dell' Endocrinología, Rome, 1950.
53. PINCUS, G.; HECHTER, O., AND ZAFFARONI, A.: Second Clinical ACTH Conference, Philadelphia, The Blakiston Co., 1951.
54. PICHET, A.: Histoire de la maladie d'Addison, Presse méd. *58*:568, May 17, 1950.
55. RIDDLE, O.: The Promise of Endocrinology, The March of Medicine, New York, Columbia Univ. Press, 1941.
56. ROLLESTON, H.: History of endocrinology, Brit. M.J. *1*:1033, May 17, 1937.
57. ROSSI, R.: Schizophrenia and the pituitary-adrenal mechanism, Tufts M.J. 9.
58. SACKLER, A. M.; SACKLER, M.D.; SACKLER, R. R., AND VAN OPHUIJSEN, J. H. W.: The research background of a system of neuroendocrinologic formulation. Part I of physiodynamics and some major metabolic disorders, J. Clin. Psychopath. *2*:1–14, Jan., 1950.
59. SACKLER, A. M.; SACKLER, M. D.; SACKLER, R. R., AND VAN OPHUIJSEN, J. H. W.: A system of physiodynamics and its application to the neuro-endocrinology of psychiatry. Part II of physiodynamics and some major metabolic disorders, J. Clin. Psychopath. *2*:15–33, Jan., 1950.
60. SACKLER, A. M.; SACKLER, M. D.; SACKLER, R. R.; VAN OPHUIJSEN, J. H. W., AND CO TUI: Sex steroid therapy in psychiatric disorders. The therapeutic effect of testosterone and estradiol on hospitalized psychotics, Acta psychiat. et neurol. *26*:415, 1950.
61. SACKLER, A. M.; SACKLER, M. D.; SACKLER, R. R.; VAN OPHUIJSEN, J. H. W.; CO TUI, AND LA BURT, H. A.: Some physiologic common denominators of histamine, sex steroids, insulin, and electric convulsive therapies, Psychiatric Quart. *25*:1–24, April, 1951.
62. SELYE, H.: Endocrinología, Barcelona, Salvat, 1952.
63. SELYE, H.: The general adaptation syndrome and the diseases of adaptation, J. Southern Med. & Surg. *103*:515, Oct., 1951.
64. SELYE, H.: Story of the General Adaptation Syndrome, Montreal, ACTA, 1952.
65. SIMPSON, S. L.: Some recent advances in endocrinology, Brit. M.J. *1*:725, April 5, 1952.
66. SOFFER, L. J.: Diagnosis of endocrine disease: clinical and laboratory considerations, Bull. New York, Acad. Med. *29*:101, Feb., 1953.

Bibliography 681

67. THORN, G. W.; BAYLES, T. B.; MASSELL, B. F.; FORSHAM, P. H.; HILL, S. R., JR.; SMITH, S., III, AND WARREN, J. E.: Studies on the relation of pituitary-adrenal function to rheumatic disease, New England J. Med. *241*:529, Oct. 6, 1949.
68. TUCHMANN-DUPLESSIS, H.: Etat actuel de quelques chapitres de physiologie, physiologie de l'antéhypophyse, Presse méd. *59*:1065, July 28, 1951.
69. WILSON, J. R.: An historical sidelight on Addison's diseases, Middlesex Hosp. J. *52*:104, Sept., 1952.
70. YOUNG, J. Z.: The evolution of the endocrine system, Proc. Roy. Soc. Med. *4*:463, June, 1951.
71. YOUNG, J. Z.: Thomas Addison and the background to cortisone, Brit. M.J. *2*:1535, Dec. 29, 1951.

PHILOSOPHIC PERSPECTIVES OF MOTION SICKNESS

1. HOROWITZ, E.: Motion sickness, East African M. J. *31*:13, Jan., 1954.
2. DE WITT, G.: Seasickness (Motion sickness). A labyrinthological study, Acta oto-laryng. *108*:11, 1953.
3. MARRIOTT, H. J. L.: Medical Milestones, Baltimore, Williams & Wilkins Co., 1952, p. 270.

WORDS AND RESEARCH

1. LAIN ENTRALGO, P.: España como problema, Madrid, Seminario de Problemas Hispano-americanos, 1949.
2. SINGER, C.: History and Technology, London, Oxford University Press, 1954.
3. ROF CARBALLO, J.: Segismundo Freud y los problemas de la medicina actual, Bol. d. Inst. Pat. Med. *12*:129, May, 1956.
4. HILDEBRAND, J. H.: Science in the Making, New York, Columbia University Press, 1956.
5. MELICOW, M. M.: Interrelationships of Medicine and Art, Bull. New York Acad. Med. *33*:347, 1957.

THE HISTORICAL AND PHILOSOPHIC BACKGROUND OF PSYCHOBIOLOGY

1. ANON.: Chemistry of mind (editorial), South African M. J. *29*:461, May 14, 1955.
2. ANON.: Colloquio internacional sobre narcobióticos, Barcelona, April, 1955. *In:* Rev. psiquiat. y psicol. méd. *2*, no. 3, July, 1955.
3. ANON.: Meyer (editorial); Psychiatric Bulletin for the Physician in General Practice, sponsored by the Texas Department of Health *2*:33, May, 1952.
4. DELGADO, H.: Impresiones acerca de la psiquiatría en los Estados Unidos, Rev. neurol. y psiquiat. *18*, no. 2, June, 1955.
5. DELGADO, H.: El Médico, la Medicina y el Alma, Madrid, Paz Montalvo, 1952.
6. FABING, H. D.: Adventures in clinical neuropharmacology, Internat. Rec. Med. & G.P.C. *169*:115, March, 1956.
7. FABING, H. D.: The new pharmacologic attack in psychiatry, Internat. Rec. Med. & G.P.C. *169*:177, April, 1956.
8. JARVIK, M. E.: Mechanism of action of lysergic acid diethylamide, sero-

tonin, and related drugs. *In:* Psychopharmacology, Publ. 42, American Association for the Advancement of Science, Washington, D. C., 1956, p. 145.

9. KEYES, B. L.: Psychiatric Perspectives. Read before the American Pharmaceutical Manufacturers Association, New York, Dec. 14, 1955.
10. KLINE, N. S.: Clinical applications of reserpine. *In:* Psychopharmacology, Publ. 42, American Association for the Advancement of Science, Washington, D. C., 1956, p. 81.
11. KRAPF, E. E.: El medio siglo de la medicina psicosomática, Cursos y Conferencias *21*:367, 1952.
12. LAIN ENTRALGO, P.: Introducción Histórica al Estudio de la Patología Psicosomática, Madrid, Paz Montalvo, 1950.
13. LIEBOW, A.: Medicine taught as human biology, Brit. M.J. *1*:305, Feb. 11, 1956.
14. MARTI-IBAÑEZ, F.: The biophilosophical significance of artificial hibernation, Internat. Rec. Med. & G.P.C. *167*:309, June, 1954.
15. MAS DE AYALA, I.: Bases neurofisiológicas de la patología psicosomática, Medicamenta, *23*, no. 270, 1954.
16. MERENCIANO, F. M.: La enfermedad como experiencia de la vida, Medicamenta, *21*, no. 251, 1952.
17. OVERHOLSER, W.: Has chlorpromazine inaugurated a new era in mental hospitals?, J. Clin. & Exper. Psychopath. & Quart. Rev. Psychiat. & Neurol. *17*:197, April-June, 1956.
18. PERAZA DE AYALA, T.: La Psiquiatría Española en el Siglo XIX, Madrid, Consejo Superior de Investigaciones Científicas, 1947.
19. RIESE, W.: Philosophical presuppositions of present-day medicine. Read before the Twenty-eighth Annual Meeting of the American Association of the History of Medicine, Detroit, May 13, 1955. *Abst. in:* Bull. Hist. Med. *30*:44, Jan.-Feb., 1956.
20. SARRO, R.: Actitud del especialista español ante la psiquiatría dinámica norteamericana. *In:* La Medicina Norteamericana Actual a través del Médico Español, Barcelona, Instituto de Estudios Norteamericanos, 1955.
21. SOLE SAGARRA, J.: La directriz biológica de la psiquiatría, Medicamenta *22*, no. 263, 1953.
22. SOLE SAGARRA, J.: Estudio crítico de la psiquiatría a través de los principales autores germanos, Rev. neurol. y psiquiat. *18*:91, 1955.
23. TORRES NORRY, J.: Notículas para la historia de la psicología psicosomática, Arch. iberoam. de hist. de med., *2*, no. 1, June, 1950.
24. VALLEJO NAGERA, A.: Los prejuicios y falsos dogmas psiquiátricos, Medicamenta *25*, no. 285, 1956.
25. VIDAL TEIXIDOR, R.: El enfoque experimental en la patología psicosomática norteamericana. *In:* La Medicina Norteamericana Actual a través del Médico Español, Barcelona, Instituto de Estudios Norteamericanos, 1955.

THE PHILOSOPHY OF ORGANICISM IN PSYCHIATRY

1. ANON.: Progress in psychiatry, Brit. M.J. *1*:66, Jan. 7, 1950.
2. ANON.: Shock therapy, Psychiatric Bull. *1*:38, Spring, 1951.
3. BAILEY, P.: Cortex and Mind ("Midcentury Psychiatry"), Springfield, Ill., Charles C Thomas, 1953.
4. BOMFORD, R. R.: Changing concepts of health and disease with particular reference to "psychosomatic medicine," Brit. M.J. *1*:633, March, 1953.

5. CASTIGLIONI, A.: A History of Medicine, New York, Alfred A. Knopf, 1947.
6. CAWADIAS: Clinical science in the light of history, Proc. Roy. Soc. Med. *40*:453, June, 1947.
7. CERLETTI, U.: "L'électrochoc," Rapports du Congrès International de Psychiatrie, IV. Thérapeutique biologique, 1950, p. 1.
8. COBB, S.: One hundred years of progress in neurology, psychiatry and neurosurgery, Arch. Neurol. & Psychiat., p. 63, 1947.
9. DELGADO, H., AND MONTALVO, P.: El Médico, la Medicina y el Alma, Madrid, 1952.
10. GALDSTON, I.: Psychiatry in Medical History, in Modern Attitudes in Psychiatry, New York, Columbia Univ. Press, 1947.
11. GUTHRIE, D.: A History of Medicine, Philadelphia, J. B. Lippincott Co., 1946.
12. LAIN ENTRALGO, P.: La obra de Freud y el cristianismo primitivo, Rev. Univ. Madrid *1*: No. 4, 1953.
13. LAIN ENTRALGO, P.: La psiquiatría española en el siglo XIX. *In:* Vestigios, Madrid, Espasa, 1945.
14. MARTI-IBAÑEZ, F.; SACKLER, A.M.; SACKLER, M. D.; SACKLER, R. R.; Co Tui, AND VAN OPHUIJSEN, J. H. W.: Neuroendocrinologic basis for a metabolic concept of several psychiatric disorders, Part I. Historic background to current psychiatric trends, Internat. Rec. Med. & G.P.C. *166*:81, March, 1953.
15. MIRA, E.: Psiquiatría Clínica, Buenos Aires, El Ateneo, 1952.
16. SACKLER, A. M.; SACKLER, M. D.; SACKLER, R. R.; AND MARTI-IBAÑEZ, F.: The Great Physiodynamic Therapies in Psychiatry: An Historical Reappraisal, New York, Paul B. Hoeber, Inc., 1956.
17. SCEOPUL, T. N.: Progresos terapéuticos en la psiquiatría moderna, Prensa méd. argent. *38*:694, 1951.
18. SIGERIST, H. E.: A History of Medicine, Oxford University Press, Oxford, 1951.
19. ULLERSPERGER, van, J. B.: Die Geschichte der Psychologie und der Psychiatrik in Spanien, A. Stuber's Buchhandlung, 1871. Translated into Spanish by V. Peset as "Historia de la Psicología y de la Psiquiatría en España," Madrid, Alhambra, 1954.
20. VALLEJO NAGERA, A.: Tratado de Psiquiatría, Barcelona, Salvat., 1949.
21. WHITEY, L.: Progress and present aspects of medical science, Lancet. *1*:895, June 28, 1947.
22. ZILBOORG, G., AND HENRY, G. W.: History of Medical Psychology, New York, W. W. Norton & Co., 1941.

THE QUEST FOR FREUD

1. ARLOW, J. A.: The Legacy of Sigmund Freud, New York, International Universities Press, 1956.
2. BRAIN, R.: The future of clinical neurology, Lancet *2*:1109, Nov. 28, 1953.
3. COBB, S.: One hundred years of progress in neurology, psychiatry and neurosurgery, Arch. Neurol. & Psychiat. *59*:63, Jan., 1948.
4. DELGADO, H.: La idea del hombre según Freud y según Jaspers, Rev. psiquiat. y psicol. méd. *1*:471, 1954.
5. FREUD, S.: Obras Completas, Madrid, Editorial Biblioteca Nueva, 2 vol., 1948.

6. FREUD, S.: An introduction to narcissism. *In:* Collected Papers, vol. 4, London, Hogarth Press, 1925.
7. GONZALEZ GARCIA, A.: Nietzsche y Freud, Medicamenta *21*:254, 1952.
8. JELLIFFE, S. E.: Emil Kraepelin, the man and his work, Arch. Neurol. & Psychiat. *27*:761, April, 1932.
9. LAIN ENTRALGO, P.: Estudios de Historia de la Medicina y de Antropología Médica, Madrid, Ediciones Escorial, 1943.
10. LOEWENSTEIN, R. M.: Freud: man and scientist (Freud anniversary lecture), Bull. New York Acad. Med. *27*:623, Oct., 1951.
11. MARTI-IBAÑEZ, F.; SACKLER, A. M.; SACKLER, M. D., AND SACKLER, R. R.: The challenge of bio- and chemotherapy in psychiatry, J. Clin. & Exper. Psychopath. & Quart. Rev. Psychiat. & Neuro. *17*:15, March, 1956.
12. MARTI-IBAÑEZ, F.; SACKLER, R. R.; SACKLER, A. M., AND SACKLER, M. D.: The philosophy of organicism in psychiatry, J. Clin. & Exper. Psychopath. & Quart. Rev. Psychiat. & Neuro. *15*:179, Sept., 1954.
13. MERENCIANO, M.: Neurosis, Actas luso españ. neurol. y psiquiat. *Abst. in:* Rev. psiquiat. y psicol. méd. *2*:403, 1955.
14. MIRA Y LOPEZ, E.: Psicoanálisis y medicina, Cultura méd. *7*:254, April, 1946.
15. DE MONCHAUX, C.: The theories of Freud: A reevaluation, The Listener, Sept. 30, 1954.
16. MUNROE, R. L.: Schools of Psychoanalytic Thought; an Exposition, Critique, and Attempt at Integration, New York, The Dryden Press, 1955.
17. NATENBERG, M.: The Case History of Sigmund Freud, Chicago, Regent House, 1956.
18. OBIOLS VIE, J.: La historia clínica antropológico-existencial, Medicamenta *23*:269, 1954.
19. RICKMAN, J.: Development of psychological medicine, Brit. M.J. *1*:30, Jan. 7, 1950.
20. SCHOENWALD, R. L.: Freud, the Man and his Mind, New York, Alfred A. Knopf, 1956.
21. SINGER, C.: Medical progress from 1850 to 1900, Brit. M.J. *1*:57, Jan. 7, 1950.
22. STERN, K.: Psychiatry and Religion, Hosp. Progr. *36*, 62, Nov., 1955.
23. WHITE, W. A.: Professor Freud's seventy-fifth birthday, Ment. Hyg. *15*:527, July, 1931.
24. ZILBOORG, G.: Sigmund Freud: His Exploration of the Mind of Man, New York, Charles Scribner's Sons, 1951.

THE CHALLENGE OF BIO- AND CHEMOTHERAPY IN PSYCHIATRY

1. ANON.: Chlorpromazine, Brit. M.J. *1*:338, Feb. 5, 1955.
2. ANON.: Chlorpromazine, Psychol. Bull. *5*:9, Winter, 1954.
3. ANON.: Largactil, Bibliographie Paris, Specia, 1955.
4. ANON.: Pharmacology of chlorpromazine, Lancet *1*:337, Feb. 12, 1955.
5. DECOURT, P.: Acciones farmacodinámicas y fisiológicas asociadas de los narcobióticos, Rev. psiquiat. y psicol. méd. *2*:233, July, 1955.
6. DECOURT, P.: Ensayos de estudios teóricos sobre ciertos problemas planteados por la aplicación de la terapéutica narcobiótica en psiquiatría, Rev. psiquiat. y psicol. méd. *2*:3:290, July, 1955.
7. HOPKIN, D. A. B.: The action of chlorpromazine, Lancet *1*:605, March 19, 1955.

8. Sackler, A. M.; Sackler, R. R.; Marti-Ibañez, F., and Sackler, M. D.: Contemporary physiodynamic therapeutic trends in psychiatry, J. Clin. & Exper. Psychopath. & Quart. Rev. Psychiat. & Neuro. *15*:382, Oct.–Dec., 1954.
9. Seguin, C. A., and Castro de la Mata, R.: La clorpromazina y su empleo psiquiátrico, Rev. Hosp. Obrero, Lima, p. 126, June, 1954.
10. Trummert, W., and Boehm, G.: Problemas terminológicos concernientes a los narcobióticos, Rev. psiquiat. y psicol. méd. *2*:223, July, 1955.

ON CHRISTMAS AND NEUROSES

1. Boyer, L. B.: Christmas neurosis, J. Am. Psychiat. A. *3*:467, July, 1955.
2. Chesterton, G. K.: Charles Dickens, The Last of the Great Men, New York, Readers Club, 1942.
3. Martin, P. W.: Experiment in Depth, New York, Pantheon Books, 1955.

THE PSYCHOLOGIC IMPACT OF ATOMIC SCIENCE ON MODERN ART

1. Barr, A. H.: What is Modern Painting?, New York, Museum of Modern Art, 1946.
2. Cajori, F.: A History of Mathematics, Cambridge, Cambridge University Press, 1919.
3. Dampier-Whetham, W. C.: Cambridge Readings in the Literature of Science, Cambridge, Cambridge University Press, 1928.
4. Dampier-Whetham, W. C.: The Recent Development of Physical Science, Cambridge, Cambridge University Press, 1924.
5. Driesch, H.: The Science and Philosophy of the Organism, London, 1908.
6. Eddington, A. S.: The Nature of the Physical World, Cambridge, Cambridge University Press, 1943.
7. Jeans, J.: The New Background of Science, Cambridge, Cambridge University Press, 1945.
8. Joad, C. E. M.: Guide to Modern Thought, London, Faber & Faber, 1943.
9. Kahnweiler, D. H.: The Rise of Cubism, New York, Wittenborn, Schultz, 1947.
10. Kaufmann, E.: What is Modern Design?, New York, Museum of Modern Art, 1950.
11. Lhermitte, J.: Visual Hallucination of the Self, Brit. M.J. *1*:431–434, March 3, 1951.
12. Moholy-Nagy, L.: The New Vision, New York, Wittenborn, Schultz, 1947.
13. Ortega y Gasset, J.: Obras Completas, Madrid, Revista de Occidente, 1948.
14. Ortega y Gasset, J.: Papeles Sobre Velázquez y Apuntes en Torno a Goya, Madrid, Revista de Occidente, 1950.
15. Planck, M. K. E. L.: The Origin and Development of the Quantum Theory, Oxford, Oxford University Press, 1922.
16. Rafols, J.: Historia del Arte, Barcelona, Editorial Spena, 1936.
17. Raynal, M.: History of Modern Painting, Geneva, Skira, 3 vols., 1949.
18. Reinach, S.: Apolo. Historia General de las Artes Plasticas, Madrid, Editorial Gutenberg, 1911.
19. Richtie, A. C.: Abstract Painting and Sculpture in America, New York, Museum of Modern Art, 1951.

20. SARTON, G.: Introduction to the History of Science, Baltimore, Williams & Wilkins Co., 1927.
21. SCHROEDINGER, E.: What is Life?, London, Cambridge University Press, 1945.
22. SHERRINGTON, C.; et al.: The Physical Basis of Mind, Cambridge, Blackwell, 1950.
23. SINGER, C.: A Short History of Science to the Nineteenth Century, Oxford, Oxford University Press, 1941.
24. WHITE, L. L.: Aspects of Form, London, Lund Humphries, 1951.
25. WOLF, A.: A History of Science, London, 1935.
26. Les Impressionistes: Leurs précurseurs et leurs contemporains, Paris, Musées nationaux, 1948.

SUBJECT INDEX

Abstracts, medical, 18–21
Acetylcholine, in mental disease treatment, 444
sympathetic nerves and, 323
Acromegaly, described, 226
ACTH, 241–242, 245
adrenal glands and, 240, 247, 253
cortisone and, 240, 253
Adaptation, diseases of, 324
syndrome of, 245–246, 253
Addison-Biermer disease, 224, 225–226
Addison's disease, 232, 236
Addison's description of, 224, 226–227
adrenal cortex and, 237
adrenalectomy and, 229, 230
earliest empirical report on, 250
therapy for, 233–234, 239, 251–252
Adrenal glands, ancient references to, 217–220
"antitoxic function" of, 229
artificial hibernation and, 378
correlation of clinical syndrome with, 224, 226–227, 250
cortex of, 231, 232–233, 236, 237, 251
cortisone and, 238–242, 251–252
"defensive" phase in history of, 243–246, 252–253
first active extract from, 232–233
hormones of, 232–233, 237–238, 251, 252, 253, 322
"morphologic period" in study of, 219–221
nervous system and steroids of, 240
neuroendocrine philosophy, 247–248, 254–255
physiology of, 229–230, 231–232
pituitary extracts and, 240
psychiatry and, 246–247, 253
function of, in schizophrenics, 247, 253, 254, 422
as sex glands, 253
steroids isolated from, 238–240, 251–252
stress and, 254
sympathetic nerves and, 235–236, 237, 251, 323
syndrome associated with, 224, 250
therapy with extracts of, 233–235, 444
Adrenalectomy, effects of, 228–229, 230

Adrenalin, change in chemical structure of, in blood, 236–237
isolation of, 232–233, 234, 237–238, 251
secretion of, 253, 323
in treatment of Addison's disease, 234
Advertising, medical, 20–21, 651
Aeronautics, Leonardo da Vinci and, 548
motion sickness and, 382
physicians and, 116–117, 341, 625
Agranulocytic angina, 196
Alcalá de Henares, University of, 174, 176, 195, 205, 209
Alchemy, Arabic medicine and, 97, 108
in Middle Ages, 304
physicians and, 81–109
Alexandria, medical school of, 88, 214, 218, 301
Allergies, 244, 245
endocrinology and, 324
treatment of, 468
American Academy of Arts and Sciences, 325
American Philosophical Society, 325
Amputations, Albucasis on, 98
Daza Chacón on, 193
in Spain, in Golden Age, 189
Anamnesis, Freudian concept of, 425–426, 461
Anatomy, Avicenna and, 108
at Bologna, 123
form in, 526–527, 535
Harvey and, 134–135
history of development of, 77–78
Hunter and, 315
in Koran, 82
Laguna and, 200
Leonardo da Vinci and, 73, 74, 75–79, 543, 548–549
Lobera de Avila and, 201
in Middle Ages, 305
modern art and, 526–530, 538
in nineteenth century, 316
at Padua, 124–127, 128–130
printing and, 124–125
in Renaissance medicine, 65, 66, 68–70, 78
at Salamanca, 174
at Salerno, 307
in Spain, 150, 182–188
Vesalius and, 134–135, 142 148

Anemia, pernicious, 224, 225–226
Anesthesia, discovery of, 258
  potentiated, 469
Aneurysms, Fragoso on, 190
  López de León on, 192
Angina, salvarsan and, 267
Aniline dyes in tissue staining, 260–261
Animals, fantastic, 491–493
  motion sickness in, 386
Animism, 436
Anthrax, Avicenna on, 108
Antibiotics, discovery of, 320–321
Antihistamines, 430, 469
Antipyrin, synthesized, 259
Antiseptics, discovery of, 258
Antitoxins, 263, 316, 318–319
Anxiety, causes of, 596–597
  chlorpromazine and, 430
  reactions to, 597
Aptitude, Huarte y Navarro on, 203–204
Aqueducts of ancient Rome, 303
Arabia, before Mohammed, 83–84
  bubonic plague in, 84
  civilization of, 85–86
  culture of, 85–86
  Greek culture in, 86, 309, 310
  language of, 86
  translation schools in, 88
Arabic medicine, alchemy and, 97, 108
  Avicenna and, 89, 90–92, 108
  contributions of, 103–106, 311–312
  Copts in, 87, 88, 107
  fourteenth century, 82–83
  Indian medicine and, 89
  influences on, 309–310
  Jews and, 107
  ophthalmology in, 105–106, 369
  organicism in, 435, 445
  origins of, 86–87
  Persians in, 87, 88, 107
  pharmacology in, 89
  Rhazes and, 89–90, 107–108
  Spaniards in, 87, 88, 107
  Spanish medicine and, 93–102, 108–109, 151, 308–312
  Syrian translators and, 86, 87–89, 107
  translations from, 308
  in Western Caliphate, 93–102, 108–109
Arabs, conquests of, 309
  explorations of, 115–116
  expulsion of, from Spain, 309, 311
  in history, 102–106
Arsphenamine, discovery of, 266–267

Art, anatomy and, 66, 68–70, 78, 526–530, 538
  in ancient Greece, 68
  in Baroque Period, 134–135, 137–138, 658
  in Byzantine Empire, 658
  medicine and, 65–66, 415–416, 657–659
  in Middle Ages, 66, 68, 291
  physicians and, 30–31, 59–79
  primitive, symbolism in, 490–491
  Renaissance, 64, 66–70, 134–135, 369, 658
  science and, 55–56
  in Spain, in Golden Age, 168, 175
  symbols and, 498
  see also Modern art
Artificial feeding, Avenzoar on, 108
Artificial hibernation, 373–379, 448, 469–470
Association, technique of, 461–462
Astrology, anatomy and, 78
  in Middle Ages, 304
Astronomy, advances in, 536
  heliocentric, 63, 313–314
  in Middle Ages, 304
Ataraxics, importance of, 637
  physiology of, 431
  use of, for mental diseases, 430–432
Atomic nuclei, discovery of, 534
Atomic science, historicophilosophic roots of, 511–518
  modern art and, 511–540
Atomic theories, 515, 534
  in ancient Greece, 513–514
Atoxyl, sleeping sickness and, 266, 320
  trypanosomiasis and, 266
Auscultation, 231
Autonomic nervous system, chlorpromazine and, 469–470

Babylonia, medicine in, 296–297
Bacteria, chemotherapy and enzymes of, 321
  dyes and reproduction of, 265–266
  infections and, 259
  sulfonamides and, 321
  toxins of, 263
Bacteriology, 316
Baghdad, Caliphate of, 85, 87
  sack of, 309
Barbitals, discovery of, 429
Baroque Period, art of, 134–135, 137–138, 658
  England in, 136–137, 138, 139–142
  Harvey and, 142–143, 628

London theatre in, 144–145
medicine in, 137, 364, 658–659
movement in, 142–143, 145–146, 628
Baths, of ancient Rome, 303
Maimonides on, 102
in Moslem Spain, 96
Behavior, Freudian theories on, 462
Berbers in Moslem Spain, 93
Bertillon system, 76
Biochemical therapy in psychiatry, 444
Biology, psychiatry and, 449–450, 467–471
Birds, as symbols, 491, 492
Blood, chemical structure of hormones in, 236–237
Blood pressure, adrenal extracts and, 232, 233
Body temperature, adaptation of, by poikilotherms, 375
neurovegetative system in regulation of, 373–374
Bologna, University of, 87, 179, 307, 312
foreign students at, 125
medical teaching at, 123
Book publishing in Spain, 150
Botany, Laguna and, 200
Brain, history of theories of, 364
"hormones" of, 422
importance of, 400
Bromides, discovery of, 429
Bufotenin, use of, for mental disease, 430
Bull, as symbol, 491–492
Burgueses of Spain, 174
Business, medicine and, 639–641
Byzantine Empire, art in, 658
medicine in, 306, 658

Cambridge University, 312
Camels, seasickness from riding, 381–382
Cancer, hormones and, 324
Cante jondo, 97, 108
Carbolic acid, introduction of, 396
Carbon dioxide for mental patients, 443
Cardiazol, convulsive shock therapy with, 443
Castration complex, in chess, 504, 506
psychological meaning of, 503–504
Cautery, Arabic medicine on, 98, 108, 311
Celestina, La, or La tragicomedia de Calixto y Melibea (Rojas), 151–166, 211

Cell theory, Cajal's contributions to, 273
Central nervous system, inhibition of, 469
Cerebral arteriosclerosis, treatment of vomiting caused by, 386
Cerebral palsy, 435
Chemistry, Arabic contributions to, 103, 104
in Middle Ages, 304
Chemotherapy, Ehrlich's contributions to, 263–265, 320
in psychiatry, 444, 467–471, 638
in twentieth century, 319–322
Chess, history of, 502
psychology of, 501–508
Chloroform, introduction of, 396
in treatment of psychotics, 443
Chlorosis, myth of, 33–34
Chlorpromazine, discovery of, 468
effects of, 468–470
in mental disease, 430, 444, 467
nervous system and, 378
Cholera, epidemics of, 337
Cholinergy, 323
Christians, in Arabic medicine, 88–89
in Spain: in Golden Age, 169, 170;
medicine and, 150; Moslem, 93;
religious tolerance of, 85–86
Christmas, historical origin of, 478–480
mortality rate at, 476–477
neuroses and, 475–481, 646
paganism and, 478–480
physicians and, 647
psychology of, 645–647
"Chronophages," 22, 54
Church, The, on mental disease, 435–436
in Middle Ages, medicine and, 305, 306–308
Circulation, discovery of, 132–134, 146–148, 314
movement and, 145–146, 148
study of, at Padua, 130
Climate, effects of, 631
respiratory diseases and, 338
temperament and, 346
Clinical case history, 411–413
importance of, 52, 667–668
as literature, 51–53
steps preparatory to, 413–414
Cold, in hibernation, effects of, 378
survival and, 374
Colloidoclastic shock, 443
Colonial America, medicine in, 352–354
Communication, in medicine, 405–407

Constantinople, fall of, 306, 313
Convulsive shock therapy, 443–444
Cooking, importance of, 620–623
Copts in Arabic medicine, 87, 88,
  107
Cordova, Caliphate of, 85, 150
  described, 94–97, 108
  medicine in, 94–102, 108–109
  school at, 88
Corticosterone, 238, 239, 240, 241
Corticotropin, 241–242
Cortisone, 239
  ACTH and, 240, 253
  biosynthesis of, 241
  effect of, 245
  isolation of, 238–240, 324
  reactions to toxic stimuli and, 247
  for rheumatic fever, 241–242, 248
  in therapy, 240–242
Cos, school of, 299
Council of Ephesus (431 A.D.), 87
Council of Vienna, 107
Craniotomies by primitive man, 362–
  363
Cretinism, thyroid extract for, 394
Crimean War, 259
Crusades, 60, 96, 131
Cultural factors in disease, 343–344
Curare, history of, 277–289
  origin of term, 279–280
  primitive man and, 281–284
  Spanish contributions to knowledge
    of, 282–289
  in therapy, 278

Damascus, hospital at, 105
Darwinian evolution, 258–259
"Defense planes" in stress theory, 395
Dehydrocorticosterone, 238
11-Dehydrocorticosterone, 239, 252
11-Dehydro-17-hydroxycorticost-
  erone, 252
Dementia, syphilis and, 439
Demerol, effects of, 378
Desoxycorticosterone, 239, 251–252
Desoxycorticosterone acetate
  (DOCA), 253
Diabetes mellitus, ancient knowledge
  of, 218
  Avicenna on, 108
Diagnosis, advances in, 231, 258
  Freudian theories on, 461
  principles of, in Arabia, 82
  in psychiatry, 439, 449–450
  psychobiology and, 422
Dialectic materialism in Renaissance,
  313
Dialectic method in medicine, 227

Diazol, convulsive attacks and, 444
Diencephalon, 322–323
Dietetics, Avicenna on, 108
Dimenhydrinate in treatment of motion sickness, 386
Diphtheria, antitoxin for, 263, 318–319
  in Spain, in Golden Age, 180, 196,
    198, 207
Disease, biography of, 667–668
  clinical reports of, 411–413
  cultural factors and, 343–344
  described, 617
  ecology of, 342–344, 390
  environment and, 343
  in galleys of Philip II of Spain, 193
  genotype and, 343
  germ theory of, 316, 390, 512
  and history, 393–394
  history and geography of, 341
  neurologic concepts of, 363–364
  phenotypes and, 343
  postoperation, 246
  stress theory and categories of, 396
  theories of, 263–264, 318, 358, 389–
    392, 667–668; early, 389–390,
    393; history of, 424; neurologic,
    363–364; nineteenth century,
    315–320, 390, 459–461; present-
    day, 390–392, 393–394; primitive,
    295; in twentieth century, 317
  transportation advances and spread
    of, 114–115, 339–340
  travel and, 402
Disinfectants, infections and, 401
Dissection, history of, 78, 108, 124,
  126–127
Djondisapur, school at, 87, 107
Dogmatism in medicine, 19
Dolosal, 469
Don Quixote (Cervantes), 25, 26, 48,
  333–334, 497
  balm of Fierabras in, 205
  on galley service, 193
  lessons taught by, 10
  on number of clericals, 172
  on peccancy of Spain, 172, 205
  poverty described in, 171
Dreams, Avicenna on, 108
  Freud's interpretation of, 458
  myths and, 494
Drugs, antitoxic activity of, 263
  hallucinogenic, 429–430
  in mental disease treatment, 429–
    432, 467–471
  mental imagery and, 431
  semantics of, 468–469
Dyes, bacteria and, 264–266
Dysentery, 259

Ear, labyrinths of, motion sickness and, 385–386
Earth, circumnavigation of, 63
man and, 335–336, 384–385
Egypt, ancient: art in, 657; eye, theories on, 369; medicine in, 297; neurology in, 362; sun cult in, 654–656
Electrolytic balance, steroids and, 252
Electron, discovery of, 534
Electroshock, history of, 442–445
Embryology, Renaissance advances in, 314
Emotion, study of, 428–429
Endocrine glands, adaptation syndrome of, 245–246, 253
ancient references to diseases of, 217
as defense against tensions and trauma, 244–246, 252–253
function of, 394
nervous system and, 243, 248, 323, 422
neuroendocrine philosophy, 247–248, 254–255
regulation of body by, 374
shock and, 374
syndromes correlated with lesions of, 215, 216, 224, 226–227, 250
Endocrinology, Addison's contribution to, 221–227
adrenal gland and psychiatry, 246–247
adrenal hormonotherapy, 233–235
advances in, 15
allergy and, 324
Brown-Sequard's experiments and, 227–231
Claude Bernard on, 250–251
cortisone and, 239–242
critical analysis of Addison's monograph, 225–227
experimental method in, 229–230
history of, 213–255
holistic principle in, 227
modern concepts of, 322–324
neurology and, 324
organic chemistry and, 255
psychiatry and, 323, 324
stress theory and, 394
Energy, conservation of, 258
discontinuity of, 534
quantum theory and, 515–516, 534–535
England, in Baroque Period, 136–137, 138, 139–142
cooking in, 622
expansion of, 140

Renaissance, surgery in, 189
Environment, disease and, 343, 390
effect of, 346, 630–631
races and, 345–346
tissues and, 400–401
Enzymes, bacterial, chemotherapy and, 321
Ephesus, Council of, 87
Epidemics, advances in transportation and, 114–115
of fever, Arabs' knowledge of, 311
travel and, 337
Epilepsy, schizophrenia and, 443–444
Epileptic coma, experimental production of, 443
Epiphyses, ancient knowledge of, 218
Eruptive fevers, Rhazes on, 108
Ether, treatment of psychotics, 443
Etiology, Sabuco de Nantes on, 203
Evolution, Darwinian, 258–259, 316
Exploration, 336–337
of Arabs, 115–116
by physicians, 115–117
Eye, history of theories of, 105–106, 109, 367, 368–369
motion sickness and, 385–386
in religion, 367–368
symbolism of, 367–368

Fashion, clothing and, 665–666
instincts in, 664–665
Fears, anxiety and, 596
of primitive man, 502–503
Fenestration, treatment of vomiting caused by, 386
Fertility, religions of, 491
Filariasis, 259
Firearms, invention of, surgery and, 189
First World War, medical geography and, 339–340
Flame photometry, 254
Forensic medicine, Fragoso on, 190
Fractures, Albucasis on, 98, 108
France, cooking in, 621, 622
theatre in, 605
Free association, 440, 461–462

Galleys of Philip II, medical practice on, 192–194
General adaptation syndrome, 324
stress theory and, 395
theory of, 391, 392, 393, 394
Genius, definition, 456
Genotype, disease and, 343
Geography, of Arabia, 83–84
of health, 345–346
history and, 344–346

of Spain in Golden Age, 167, 168–169
Germ theory of disease, 316, 390, 512
Gerontocracy, in Renaissance, 662–663
  in twentieth century, 662
Gibraltar, 85, 309
Glucocorticoids, 253
Goiter, Albucasis on, 108
  ancient knowledge of, 218
Gonorrhea, in literature, 32
  Rhazes on, 107
Gout, Mercado on, 196
  in Spain, in Golden Age, 180
  Valles on, 195
Granada, conquest of, 64, 169
  school at, 88
Grandees of Spain, 173
Greece, ancient: animal symbolism in, 492; Arabs as translators of manuscripts from, 86, 87–89; art in, 68, 657–658; atomic theories in, 513–514; culture of, 297; medicine in, 297–300, 336, 338, 352–353, 354, 359, 389, 429, 625; myths in, 494; neurology in, 362; organicism in, 433–435, 445; philosophy in, 298–299, 603; references to endocrine glands, 217–218
Growth, hormones and, 324
Guadelete, battle of, 150
Gunpowder, invention of, 63, 313
Gunville and Caius College (Cambridge), 128
Guy's Hospital (London), 221, 222, 225
Gynecology, Albucasis on, 98

Hallucinogenic drugs, history of, 429–430
Hashish, 33, 430
Health, geography of, 346
  travel and, 399–402
Hegira, the, 84
Hellenism, in Alexandria, 62
  Arabs and, 86, 309, 310
  Crusades and, 131
  in Renaissance, 62, 65
  theology and, 60
  in West, 306
Hematosonography, 328
Hemoclastic crisis, 246
Hemorrhages, Albucasis on, 108
Herbalists, in Spain, in Golden Age, 197, 199
Heredity, disease and, 390, 438
Hernia, Avenzoar on, 108

Hibernation, artificial, 373–379, 448 469–470
Hiccough, Rhazes on, 107
Hidalgos of Spain, 173
Hippocratic medicine, 206, 214
Histamines in mental disease treatment, 444
Holism, in endocrinology, 227
  in psychiatry, 428
  stress theory and, 395
  in therapy, 667–668
Homeostasis, 246, 374
  neuroendocrine defense of, 376
  in travel, 399
Homeothermic animals, defined, 373
  high temperature of, 631
Homosexualism displayed in chess, 504
"Homunculus" of Paracelsus, 206
Hormone(s), of adrenal glands, 232–233, 233–235, 237–238, 251, 253
  cancer and, 324
  first isolation of, 233
  growth and, 324
  in mental disease treatment, 444, 450
  nerve fibers and, 235–236
  peripheric, 236–237, 322
  in psychiatry, 444
  secretion of, 251
  study of, 231–232
  term introduced, 249
  theories of, 322, 323–324
  in therapy, 233–235
  vitamins and, 324
Hospitals, Arabic founding of, 105–106
  growth of, in nineteenth century, 315
  for mental diseases, 445
  in Spain, 96, 150, 198, 199, 445
Humanism, in medical journalism, 49
  origin of, 61, 306
  in Renaissance, 313
  in Spain, 199–204
Hydrocortisone, 252
  identification of, 241
  in therapy, 242
17-Hydroxydesoxycorticosterone, 252
Hygiene, infections and, 401
  Maimonides on, 100–102
Hyperexis, 376–379
Hypnosis in psychiatry, 439, 440
Hypo-orchidism, 218
Hypo-ovarism, 218
Hypothalamus, artificial hibernation and, 378
  disorders of, 323

importance of, 322, 400
regulation of body by, 374
shock and, 374
tissues of, 248
Hysteria, hypnosis in, 440

Immunology, advances in, 231, 259
development of, 319
philosophy of, 262–264
"side-chain" theory in, 263–264
India, ancient references to endocrine
glands in, 217
Arabic medicine and, 89
Indians, use of curare by, 281–284
use of poisoned arrows by, 277–284
Industrial research, 326, 414–415
Infection, bacterial origin of, 259
dangers to body from, 244, 245
Laguna on, 200
mechanisms of combatting, 318–319
present-day treatment of, 401
travel and, 401, 625
Inquisition, factors in, 174–175, 205
Instincts, concept of, 440
exploration of, 426
in fashion, 664–665
Insulin, original preparation of, 234
shock therapy with, 443, 444
International Association of Psychoanalysis, 461
Invisible College (London), 413

Jews, Arabs and, 107, 310, 311
in Moslem Spain, 93, 94, 98–102
as physicians, 94, 98–102, 107, 149–
150, 202, 204, 310, 311
in Spain: expulsion of, from Spain,
170, 311; in fifteenth century,
149–150; in Golden Age, 168,
169, 170, 202, 204
as translators, 107
Jundi, medical school at, 309
Justice, in Spain, in Golden Age, 173

Keloid sclerodermia, 224
Kitasato Institute (Tokyo), 326
Koran (The), anatomy in, 82

Laboratories for industrial research,
326
Language, of symbols, 483–486
Largactil—see Chlorpromazine
Lateral-chain theory of Ehrlich, 320
League of Physicians and Apothe-
caries, 78
Leisure, man and, 660–661
Lenses, in Spain, in Golden Age, 197

Lepanto, battle of, 169, 170, 182, 191,
192, 193, 209
Letrados of Spain, 174
Leyden, University of, 307
Liberation cocktail, 377–379, 469
Libraries, of Arabs, 310, 311
medical, at Padua, 125
in Moslem Spain, 310
effect of, 631
theories of, 515–516, 534–535
Literature, approach to, 24–25
basic importance of textbooks in,
14–17
Claude Bernard and, 34
early, on travel, 338
Elizabethan, medicine in, 33
Freud and, 35
influence of physicians as writers
on, 35–42
medicine and, 29–30, 31–33
in Middle Ages, 36–37
physicians in, 10–11
of Renaissance, 314
science and, 519–520
Lithotomy, Albucasis on, 98, 108
London, in Baroque Period, 139–142
theatre in, 144–145
Louvain, University of, 92
Love, described, 652–653
LSD, 33, 422, 429
Lytic cocktail, 377–379, 469

McCormick Institute of Infectious
Diseases, 325
Machífaro tragedy, 284
Magic, in Middle Ages, 305
myth and, 603
origin of rites, 490–491
in primitive medicine, 293–296
"Magic bullet" of Ehrlich, 265–267,
319–320
Magnetism, Renaissance interest in,
314
Makushi Indians, 282
Mal de caderas, salvarsan and, 266
Malaria, 259
Roman empire and, 393
therapy with, in psychiatry, 439,
448
treatment of, 468
Malnutrition, travel and, 625
Man, bodily image of, 528–531, 538–
539
earth and, 335–336, 384–385
Freudian contributions to knowledge of, 464–465
as history, 349–350
intellectual, 43

leisure and, 660–661
light's importance to, 671–672
occupied, 43
preoccupied, 43
problems of, 409–410
psychology of, 642, 643
spatial relationships of, 527–528
symbols and history of, 498–499
travels of, 336–337
see also Primitive man
Marañone expedition, 284
Matter, quantum theory and, 515–516,
534–535
Measles, Rhazes on, 107
Meclizine hydrochloride in treatment
of motion sickness, 386
Medical abstracts, value of, 18–21
Medical advertising, 20–21, 651
Medical ecology, Avicenna on, 108
disease and, 342–344, 390
Rhazes on, 90
Medical geography, ancient Greece
and, 338
First World War and, 339–340
history and, 335–347
transportation advances and, 339–
340
see also Geography
Medical journalism, concepts of, 405–
407, 614
lucidity in, 416–417
Medical journals, 5
of abstracts, 18–20
importance of, 648–649
mission of, 17–18
Medical literature, of Albucasis, 97–
98
of Avicenna, 92, 98–99, 108
books as, 3–6, 13–14
basic textbooks, 14–17
clarity in, 49, 50–51
early history of, 3–6
Fabricius and, 129–130
first American medical book, 352
first textbook on psychiatry, 438
of Maimonides, 100, 108–109
of Rhazes, 90
translations of, in Moslem Empire,
4, 86, 87–89
types of, 5
Medical teaching, at Alcalá de Henares University, 174
in America, 326
at Bologna, 123
at Padua, 124–127, 128–130
at Salamanca, 174
at Salerno, 306–307
in Spain, 97, 150

Medicine, advertising and, 651
American: 325–326, 328; birth of,
352; in Colonial times, 352–354;
pioneering spirit in, 354–355;
present-day, 350
in ancient Egypt, 297
in ancient Greece, 297–300, 352–
353, 354, 359
in ancient Rome, 300–304, 354, 359
art and, 65–66, 415–416, 657–659
in Babylonia, 296–297
in Baroque Period, 137, 658–659
business and, 639–641
in Byzantine Empire, 306, 658
communication as problem in, 405–
407
culture and, 292–293
dialectic method in, 227
dogmatism in, 19
experimental method in, 227–228
Freud and, 461–462
history and geography of, 342
in India, 89, 217
literature and, 3–6, 29–30, 31–33
magic thought and witchcraft in,
293–296
in Middle Ages, 65, 304–313, 353–
354, 358, 359
problems in, 409–410
psychoanalysis and, 462
psychosomatic, 428–429
religion and, 66
specialization in, 326–327, 618–619,
633
stress theory and, 395–396
in summer, 630–631
surgery and, 189–190
"time-axes" in, 214
in twentieth century, 316–328, 536,
659
in universities, 306–307, 312–313,
328
women in, 643–644, 670
Meniere's syndrome, treatment of
vomiting caused by, 386
Mental diseases, changing attitudes
toward, 635–638
the Church on, 435–436
heredity in, 438
history of treatment of, 447–453
hospitals for, 445
theories on: ancient Greek, 433–
435, 445; ancient Roman, 435,
445; in Arabic medicine, 108,
435, 445; eighteenth century, 437;
Freud's concepts of, 425–426,
427; medieval, 435–436, 445;
Meyer's concepts of, 426–428;

nineteenth century, 437–440, 459–461; Renaissance, 436–437, 445; seventeenth century, 436–437; in Spain, in Golden Age, 198, 207; twentieth century, 422–423, 441–445
therapy for: 439, 637–638; biochemical, 444; chlorpromazine in, 467, 468–470; drugs in, 429–432; Freud and, 440; history of, 423–432, 447–453, 459–461; insulin shock, 443, 444, 450; pharmacologic, 444; physiodynamic, 447–453; somatotherapy, 441–445
Mental hygiene, 427, 635–638
Mescaline, 33
  effects of, 422
  use of, for mental disease, 430
Metabolism of bacteria, 321
Methylene blue, Ehrlich's work with, 261
  nervous system and, 265
Middle Ages, alchemy in, 304
  animal symbolism in, 492–493
  art in, 66, 68, 291
  astrology in, 304
  astronomy in, 304
  bubonic plague and, 393
  Byzantine medicine in, 306
  chemistry in, 304
  disease in, 393
  epidemics in, 114–115
  exploration in, 336
  fashion in, 665
  Golden Age in, 131
  hallucinogenic drugs used in, 430
  Hebrew physicians in, 107
  Hellenism in, 60–61
  literature in, 31–32, 36–37
  medical thought in universities in, 312–313
  medicine in, 31–32, 65, 304–313, 353–354, 358, 359, 364
  organicism in, 435–436, 445
  philosophy in, 604
  physicians in, 639
  scholasticism in, 123
  science in, 62
  surgery in, 304
  symbolism in, 485, 492–493
  travel in, 112
  women in, 642–643
Minoan culture in Periclean Athens, 62
Minotaur, myth of, 494
Modern art, abstract, 523–526, 530–533, 537–540

atomic science and, 511–540, 659
beauty in, 530–531, 538–539
of Braque, 561–571
cubist, 521–522, 557, 561–571
Fauvism, 563, 564, 565, 570
form in, 526–527
future of, 532–533, 539–540
futurist, 522–523
history of, 521–523
of Modigliani, 556, 558–560
of Picasso, 557, 561–562
psychohistorical profile of, 521–523
psychology and, 527–531
surrealist, 523, 524, 537
symbolism in, 485
of Utrillo, 578, 579–581, 588–590, 591–594
Mohammed, 84–85
Mohammedans, Jews and, 107
  in Moslem Spain, 93
  religious tolerance of, 85–86
Monasteries, medieval, medicine in, 306–308
Monograph, defined, 16
Monte Cassino, medicine in, 307–308
Montpellier, University of, 92, 107, 307, 312
Moors, in Spain, 93, 169
  expulsion of, from Spain, 64, 170, 172
  influence of, on Spanish medicine, 150, 179
Motion sickness, aeronautics and, 382
  clinical studies of, 383–384
  equilibrium and, 384, 385
  as health problem, 399–400
  philosophy of, 381–387
Motivation of behavior, 440
Movement, in Baroque Period, 142–143, 145–146, 628
  circulation and, 145–146, 148
  motion sickness and, 383
  in neurology, 364–365
Mystery, religions of, 491
Myxedema, first described by Gull, 224
  thyroid extract in treatment of, 215, 323

Naples, University of, 307
Narcobiotic action, 469
Nature, study of, in Renaissance, 61–62
Nausea, derivation of word, 383
Naval physicians, 116, 341
Neo-Platonism in Renaissance, 62
Neosalvarsan, 267
Nerve fibers, hormones and, 235–236

Nervous system, adrenal steroids and, 240
anatomy of, 362
Cajal's contributions to knowledge of, 272, 273-274
chlorpromazine and, 378
endocrine function of, 422
endocrine glands and, 243, 248, 323
history of theories of, 364
methylene blue and, 265
Nestorians, 86-87
Neuroanatomy, Cajal's contributions to, 272-273, 273-274
Neuroendocrine system, artificial hibernation and, 378
Neurology, dichotomy in thought about, 361
endocrinology and, 324
history of, 361-365
psychiatry and, 363
Neurons, anatomic individuality of, 272-273
Neuroplegia, 469
production of, 376-379
Neuroses, anamnesis and, 425-426
autumn,477
chess and, 506-507
Christmas and, 475-481, 646
Freudian theories of, 458, 459-461
spring, 477
Sunday, 477
sunset, 477
in twentieth century, 394
Neurovegetative system, artificial hibernation and, 378
blocking of, 376-379
inhibition of, 469
in motion sickness, 383
regulation of body by, 374
North America, discovery of, 64-65, 313, 324
medicine in, 325-326
Nursing, history of, 643-644
importance of, 669-670
Nutrition, travel and, 401-402

Obstetrics, Albucasis on, 98
in Spain in Golden Age, 187, 197
Oedipus complex in chess, 503, 504, 506
Old age, theories of, 662-663
Ophthalmology, Agüero on, 190
Arabic contributions to, 105-106, 109, 311
history of, 367-370
in Spain, in Golden Age, 189
Opium, 443

Organicism, in ancient Greece, 433-435, 445
in ancient Rome, 435, 445
in Arabic medicine, 435, 445
history of, 433-445
in psychiatry, 433-445
in Renaissance, 436, 445
somatotherapy and, 441-445
Organotherapy in endocrinology, 216-218
Oriental rugs, psychology of symbolism in, 483-495

Padua (Italy), described, 120-123
epidemiological center at, 124
medical library of, 125
medical teaching at, 124-127, 128-130
Padua, University of, 65, 87, 179, 307, 312
students at, 122-123, 125, 627-628
Paper chromatography, 254
Pathology, in nineteenth century, 316
origin of clinical, 390
Valles on, 195
Patricide, psychological meaning of, 504
Peccancy, in Spain, in Golden Age, 172, 205
Percussion, 231
Persians, Arabic medicine and, 86-87, 88, 107, 309, 310
Pethidine, effects of, 378
Phallic symbolism in chess, 504
Pharmacology, advances in, 15-16, 319
Arabic contributions to, 89, 103-105, 311
clinical studies of, 406
in La Celestina, 161-162, 163-165
in Middle Ages, 305
in Spain, 151, 199
Pharyngeal paralysis, Avenzoar on, 108
Phenergan, 378, 469
Phenothiazine, 468, 469
Phenotype, disease and, 343
Philosophy, in ancient Greece, 297-299, 603
in ancient Rome, 302-303
of artificial hibernation, 373-379
of atomic science, 511-513, 513-518
of Avicenna, 91-92
of (the) circle, 143-144
of Ehrlich, 268
in Middle Ages, 604
in neurology, 361

of organicism in psychiatry, 433–445
of Paracelsus, 268–269
in Renaissance, 313, 314, 604
of rugs, 486–488
of Sánchez, 204
of Sigerist, 329–334
Physician(s), aeronautics and, 116–117, 341, 625
as alchemists, 81–109
in ancient Greece, 336, 338
in ancient Rome, 300–303
artists and, 30–31
as artists, 59–79
in Babylonia, 296
Christmas and, 647
city, 668
in colonial America, 353–354
cooking and, 620–623
country, 632–634, 668
culture and, 650
described, 616–617
as explorers, 115–117
Jews as, 94, 98–102, 107, 149–150, 202, 204, 310, 311
medical abstracts and, 18–20
medical journals and, 17–18
in Middle Ages, 639
mind of modern, 618
naval, 116, 341
personality of, 614
present-day American, 350
as readers: books in life of, 3–28; finding time to read, 22–25; history of medicine for, 25–26; reading for improvement and, 21–22, 24–25; types of reading, 6–28
satirists of, 32
as travelers, 111–117, 336, 338–339, 340–343, 624–625
women as, 670
as writers: 11–12, 29–56; activity of life of, 42–44; classical writings of, 36; in clinical case history, 51–53; duty of writing, 47–48; finding time for writing, 53–54; history of literature and, 35–42; psychologic motives of, 44–47
Physics, advances in modern, 513–518, 534–537
Physiology, of adrenal glands, 229–230, 231–232
of ataraxics, 431
hibernation and, 378–379
of motion sickness, 383–384, 385–386
of nervous system, knowledge of, 361

in nineteenth century, 315
Pituitary gland, ancient knowledge of, 218
artificial hibernation and, 378
extracts from, adrenal glands and, 246
importance of, 322
Pituitary somatotropic hormone (STH), effects of, 378
Plague, in Arabia, 84
epidemics of, 337
Laguna on, 200
in literature, 32
Lobera de Avila on, 201
Middle Ages and, 393
in Spain, in Golden Age, 180, 194, 196
Planck's constant, 534
Platonic Academy, 300
Poikilothermic animals, adaptation of, to environment, 375
defined, 373
Poisoned arrows, 277–281
Poisons, immunity reactions to, 263
Polypeptidetoxic syndrome, 246
Polyps, Daza Chacón on, 191
Prefrontal lobotomy, discovery of, 444
Primitive man, animal symbols and, 491–492
craniotomies of, 362–363, 442
curare and, 281–284
fears of, 502–503
habits of, 294
hallucinogenic drugs used by, 429–430
medicine and gods of, 66
religion of, 295
research of, 324
symbolism of, 483–485, 490, 491–492
theories of: on disease, 295, 389; on eye, 369
therapy by, 295–296
use of poisoned arrows by, 278–284
Primitive society, women in, 642
Printing, anatomy and, 124–125
invention of printing press, 4, 63, 124, 313
in Spain, in Golden Age, 205
Promethazine, effects of, 378, 468, 469
Proprioceptive system, motion sickness and, 385–386
Psyche, "structural" stratification of, 440
Psychiatry, adrenal gland and, 246–247, 253

advances in, 16, 416, 635–638
biology and, 449–450
chemotherapy in, 444, 467–471, 638
diagnosis in, 439, 449–450
endocrinology and, 246–247, 253,
323, 324
first textbook on, 438
Freud and, 425–426, 440, 455–465
hallucinogenic drugs and, 429–430
hematosonography in, 328
history of, 423–432, 636–637
holism in, 428
hypnosis in, 439
Meyer's concepts of, 426–428
neurology and, 363
neuroplegia in, 377
physiodynamic therapies in, 447–453
psychobiology and, 421–422
psychosomatic roots of, 428–429
somatotherapy in, 449–450
symbols in, 498–499
symptoms in, 470
terminology of, 14
tranquilizing drugs and, 430–432
Psychoanalysis, 259, 317
contributions of, 462
discovery of, 461–462
theatre as, 607
Psychobiology, Freudian concept of
anamnesis in, 425–426
hallucinogenic drugs and, 429–430
historical and philosophic background of, 421–432
Meyer's concepts of, 426–428
origin of, 439–440
psychiatry and, 421–422
psychosomatic roots of, 428–429
Psychodrama, theatre as, 599–600
tranquilizing drugs and, 430–432
Psychology, advances in modern,
518–519, 536–537
of amusement, 605
of atomic science and modern art,
511–540
of chess, 501–508
of Christmas, 645–647
consciousness in, 440
of man, 642, 643
of modern art, 511–540, 555–560,
592–594
of Modigliani, 555–560
of motion sickness, 386
of physician-writer, 44–47
religion and, 480–481
of Renaissance anatomic art, 68–
70, 78
symbolism in, 488, 491–493

of symbolism in oriental rugs, 483–
495
of the theatre, 599–600
of the unconscious, 461
of Utrillo, 592–594
Psychoses, tranquilizing drugs and,
431
Psychosexual development, 440
Psychosurgery, 243–244, 444
Public health, history of, 357–359
Pupilary reflex, Rhazes on, 107
Purification of water, Avicenna on,
108
Pyretotherapy, 448

Quantum theory, 515–516, 521, 534–
535

Races, environment and, 345–346
Radioactivity, 259
discovery of, 534
treatment of vomiting caused by,
386
Rationalism, 63
Rauwolfia serpentina, 430, 444
Reading, defined, 6
in history of medicine, 25–26
for improvement, 21–22, 24–25
professional and scientific, 13
Recurrent fever, 259, 267
Reformation, 64, 313, 324
Refrigeration, of body, effects of,
376–377, 469
Reilly's phenomena, 469
Rejuvenation, experiments in, 251
Relativity, theory of, 516–517, 535,
562
Religion(s), anatomy and, 78
in Baroque Period, 136
eye in, 367–368
in fifteenth century Low Countries,
62
history of, 603–604
of Leonardo, 79
medicine and, 66
of mystery, 491
of Nestorius, 86–87, 308–309
of primitive man, 295
psychology and, 480–481
in Renaissance, 313
Religious tolerance, of Christians, 85–
86
of Mohammedans, 85–86, 310
in Spain, 93, 169–170, 205, 311
Renaissance, art in, 66–70, 70–77, 78,
134–135, 658
as crisis, 63–64, 131, 134, 628
exploration in, 336, 337, 338

gerontocracy in, 662–663
Hellenism in, 62, 65
literature of, 32, 314
philosophy in, 313, 314, 604
psychologic meaning of anatomic
art in, 68–70, 78
religion in, 313
science in, 61–62
in Spain, 62
syphilis and, 393
theology in, 60–61, 313
travel in, 112
Renaissance medicine, 59–64, 313–
314, 354, 359, 658
anatomy in, 65, 66, 77
art and, 64, 66, 67–70, 70–77
geography in, 338
in literature, 32
organicism in, 436–437, 445
purposes and orientation of, 64
surgery in, 189–190
textbooks for, 64–65
theories in: on brain, 364; on disease, 389–390; on eye, 369
Research, of Addison, 222–225
in eighteenth century, 325
in neurology, 365
psychobiology and, 422
in Renaissance, 324–325
in Spain, in Golden Age, 176
in twentieth century, 317, 324–328
words and, 409–417
Reserpine, use of, for mental diseases,
430, 444
Rheumatic fever, 241–242, 248
Rheumatoid arthritis, 241
Rhinoplasty, Arceo on, 190
Roentgen rays, 316, 534
Romantic Period, medicine in literature of, 33–34
Rome, ancient: architecture in, 303;
culture of, 300; disease in, 393;
medicine in, 300–304, 354, 359;
organicism in, 435, 445; philosophy in, 302–303; sanitation engineering in, 303
Royal College of Physicians (London), 138, 313
Royal Society of London, 324
Rugs, history of, 486–488
oriental, psychology of symbolism
in, 483–495
philosophy of, 486–488

Salamanca, University of, 150, 174,
176
Salerno, University of, 87, 107, 306–
307, 312

Salicylates, synthesis of, 467
Salvarsan, discovery of, 262, 266–267
for spirochetes, 319–320
trypanosomes and, 320
Sanitary engineering, 303, 359
Schizophrenia, adrenal function in,
247, 253–254
epilepsy and, 443–444
organic changes in, 422
stress response in, 247, 254
Scholasticism, in Middle Ages, 123
in Renaissance, 313
Science, art and, 55–56, 511–540, 659
atomic: modern art and, 511–540;
philosophy of, 511–513; roots of,
513–518
experimentation in, 389
Freud on, 462–463
in nineteenth century, 258, 316
religion and, 62, 316
requirements for, 175, 206
symbols and, 497
Scientific method, introduction of, 324
Scientific organizations, foundation of,
325–326
Scurvy, conquest of, 341
Seasickness, causes of, 381–382
Sedation in treatment of mental diseases, 448
Seismotherapy, discovery of, 429
Serums, 317
infections and, 401
search for, 231
therapy with, 264, 319
Sex glands, ancient knowledge of, 218
endocrine glands as, 253
Shock, artificial hibernation and, 378–
379
effects of, 374–375
psychiatric, 317
treatment of, 377
Shock therapy, 429, 443–444, 448
history of, 442–445
with insulin, 443, 444, 450
"Side-chain" theory in immunology,
263, 320
Sleep, therapy by prolonged, 443, 450
Sleeping sickness, atoxyl and, 266, 320
Smallpox, epidemics of, 337
vaccine for, 396
Somatotherapy for mental diseases,
441–445, 449–450
Somnifene for therapy by sleep, 443
Sorcery, in La Celestina, 157–161
in Middle Ages, 305
South America, discovery of, 64–65,
313, 324
medical schools in, 326

medicine in, 328
use of curare-poisoned arrows by
Indians of, 277–279, 281–289
theory of relativity and, 516–517,
535
Space, in universe, 527–528
Spain, Academy of Medicine in, 150
Arabic medicine and, 87, 88, 107,
308–312
book publishing in, 150
cooking in, 621, 622
culture of, 93–94, 310, 331
expulsion of Arabs from, 85
fifteenth century, 62: atmosphere
of, 165; medicine in, 149–66—
see also Spanish medicine
hospitals in, 96, 150, 198, 199, 445
medical teaching in, 150
pharmacology in, 151
religious tolerance in, 311
Renaissance in, 62
universities in, 150
Spain in Golden Age (1500–1648),
167–209
arts in, 168, 175
care of insane in, 198
described, 167–173, 209, 210–211
diseases in, 180–181, 206
ethnic groups in, 168–169
geography of, 167, 168–169
hospitals in, 198, 199
individualism in, 175–176, 206
justice in, 173
peccancy in, 172, 205
population of, 170–171, 172–173
poverty in, 171, 175, 198
printing in, 205
religious tolerance in, 169–170, 205
research in, 176
science in, 175–176, 180
structure of society in, 173–174
typhus in, 180, 196, 207
universities in, 174–205
Spain, Moslem: baths in, 96; compared with Renaissance Italy, 94–
95; culture in, 93–94, 310; ethnic
groups in, 93; hospitals in, 96;
Jewish physicians in, 94; medical
teaching in, 97
Spanish medicine, Arabic medicine
and, 151, 308–312
Cajal and, 271
fifteenth century: 149–166; Celestina, La (Rojas) and, 151–166;
influences on, 149–150; wine in,
156
Golden Age: anatomists in, 182–
188; contributions to knowledge

of curare by, 282–289; epidemiologists in, 194–196; humanists
in, 199–204; influences on, 179–
180; laws regulating, 179; magic
and, 179–180; pediatrics in, 197;
practiced on royal galleys, 192–
194; quackery in, 179, 206; royal
protection for, 176–179, 206;
specialists in, 196–199; superstition in, 178; surgeons in, 189–
192; urology in, 189, 197–198;
wounds in, 189
influences on, 149–150, 151, 179–
180
in Moslem Spain, 93–102, 108–109
superstition in, in Golden Age, 178
Specialization, in medicine, 326–327,
618–619, 633
in Spain, 196–199
Sphinx, symbolism of, 492
Spirochetes, discovery of, 266
salvarsan and, 266, 319–320
Staining, aniline dyes in, 260–261
Cajal's contributions to, 273
Ehrlich's contributions to, 260–261
stains as bacteriocides, 320–321
Static electricity, use of, by Addison,
223
Statistics, Agüero on, 191
Steroids, electrolytic balance and, 252
isolated from adrenal cortex, 238–
240, 251–252
reactions to toxic stimuli and, 247
Stress, artificial hibernation and, 378–
379
effect of, 374
reactions to, 254
schizophrenics' response to, 247,
254
therapy for, 401
as travel problem, 400–401, 625
Stress theory, basic principles of, 394–
395
"defense planes" in, 395
formulation of, 391, 392, 393, 394
general adaptation syndrome and,
395
holism and, 395
medicine and, 395–396
therapy and, 397
Suicide at Christmas, 476
Sulfonamides, 319, 320–321
Sun, cult of, in ancient Egypt, 654–
656
"Suprarenin," isolation of, 232–233
Surgery, in Arabic medicine, 98, 108,
311
in Babylonia, 296

history of, 362–363
in *La Celestina,* 162–163
in Middle Ages, 304, 312–313
origin of psychosurgery, 444
in Renaissance, 189–190
in Spain, in Golden Age, 189–192
in twentieth century, 317
Symbolism, animals in, 491, 492, 493
in art, 485, 490–491, 498, 523, 537
culture and, 494–495
of eye, 367–368
language of symbols, 483–486
life and, 497–499
in Middle Ages, 485
in oriental rugs, psychology of, 483–495
of primitive man, 483–485, 490, 491–492
in psychiatry, 498–499
science and, 497
symbol defined, 484
in theatre, 606–607
in watermarks, 485
in words, 411
in writing, 498
Sympathetic nerves, acetylcholine and, 323
adrenal glands and, 235–236
adrenalin and, 237, 323
irritation of, 469
Sympathine, discovery of, 235
Symptoms, of motion sickness, 386
in psychiatry, 470
Syndrome(s), of adaptation, 245–246, 253
associated with adrenal glands, 224, 226–227, 250
correlated with lesions of endocrine glands, 215, 216
Synthetic compounds in treatment of adrenal insufficiency, 239–252
Syphilis, Calvo on, 190
control of, 359
dementia and, 439
Fragoso on, 190
in literature, 32
Lobera de Avila on, 201
naming, 383
Renaissance and, 393
salvarsan and, 267, 319–320
in Spain, in Golden Age, 180, 181, 206
spread of, 337
Syrians, in Arabic medicine, 86, 87–89, 107

Tachyphylaxis, 246
Talmudic literature, dissection in, 78

Teacher(s), Freud as, 463
of Padua, 124–125
Technology, words and, 410–411
Temperament, climate and, 346
Temperature, chlorpromazine and, 470
effect of, 631
low, survival and, 375
Tensions, endocrines in defense against, 244–246, 252–253
Terminology of psychiatry, 14
Testosterone in mental disease treatment, 444
Tetanus, Avicenna on, 108
Textbooks, 14–15
Thalamus, regulation of body by, 374
Theatre, actor as hero, 600
foreign versus American, 604–605, 605–606
history of, 597–599
in London in Harvey's day, 144–145
as psychoanalysis, 607
as psychodrama, 599–600
as salvation, 601–602
symbols in, 606–607
Theology, Hellenism and, 60
in Renaissance, 60–61
science and, in Middle Ages, 62
Theory of relativity, 516–517, 535, 562
Therapy, for Addison's disease, 233–234, 239, 251–252
with adrenal extracts, 233–235
advances in, 231–232, 258, 259, 317–322
artificial hibernation in, 377, 469
biotherapy in psychiatry, 444, 467–471
chemotherapy in psychiatry, 467–471
of cretinism with thyroid extract, 394
cortisone in, 240–242
curare in, 278
holism in, 667–668
insulin coma, 443, 444, 450
medical journalism and, 406–407
for mental diseases: 439, 637–638; drugs in, 429–432, 467–471; Freud and, 440; history of, 423–432, 447–453; somatotherapy, 441–445
present-day: concept of, 262–264; criteria in, 364; for infections, 401; twentieth century advances in, 317–322
by primitive man, 295–296

psychobiology and, 422
for shock, 377
sleep, 443, 450
for stress, 397, 401
Thorium, discovery of, 534
Thymus gland, 218
Thyroid extracts, 259, 316
for cretinism, 394
in mental disease treatment, 444
in treatment of myxedema, 215, 323
Thyroid glands, 218
cancer of, Albucasis on, 108
hormones of, 322
Tic douloureux, Avicenna on, 108
Time, knowing how to "find," 53–54
sources of, 22–23
theory of relativity and, 516, 535
"Time-axis," theory of, in history, 213–214
Tissues, environment and, 400–401
Tobacco, motion sickness and, 383
Toledo (Spain), La Celestina's vogue in, 155–156
as translating center, 108
Tracheotomies in Arabic medicine, 108
Tranquilizing drugs, by Arabs, 86, 87–89, 108, 309, 311
by Constantine the African, 308
by Jews, 107
of medical literature, 4
Transmission, advances in transportation and, 114–115
Transportation advances, medical geography and, 339–340
medicine and, 114–115
Trauma, Agüero on, 191, 207
endocrines in defense against, 244–246, 252–253
travel and, 625
Travel(s), 336–337
in ancient Greece, 336, 338
dangers in, 114–115, 625–626
disease and, 401, 402, 625
early books on, 337–338
health and, 399–402
motion sickness and, 399–400
of physicians, 111–117, 336, 338–339, 340–343, 624–625
in prehistoric times, 112
sea, nausea and, 381–387
stress and, 400–401
Trepanation, Daza Chacón on, 191
primitive man and, 442
in Spain, in Golden Age, 189
Trional for therapy by sleep, 443
Trypanosomiasis, 259

atoxyl and, 266
salvarsan and, 266, 320
treatment of, 468
trypan red and, 265, 320
Tuberculosis, Avicenna on, 108
therapy of, 319
Turkey, chemotherapy in, 317, 319–322
gerontocracy in, 662
medicine in, 316–328, 536, 659
public health in, 317
science in, 511–513
theatre in, 595–607
Typhoid fever, control of, 359

Ulcers, Albucasis on, 98
Unconscious, definition of, 440
motivation, Freud on, 458
psychology of, 461
United States, medicine in: in Colonial times, 352–354; country doctor in, 632–634; medical schools, 326; present-day, 350; spirit of, 349–355
theatre in, 604–605, 605–606
Urethral medication, Avicenna on, 108

Vaccines, infections and, 401
search for, 231
Venesection, Maimonides on, 102
Venous valves, discovery of, 129–130, 134, 145
Vitamins, hormones and, 324
in therapy, 317

Water, purification of, Avicenna on, 108
supply system of ancient Rome, 303
Women, chess-playing by, 501, 506, 507–508
in medicine, 643–644, 670
Words, ideas and, 49–51
medicine and, 410
research and, 409–417
Writing, clarity in, 48–49, 50–51
in clinical case history, 51–53
communication by, 49–51
as escape from professional life, 45
by physicians, 11–12, 29–56
symbols and, 498

Xanthine derivatives, clinical use of, 406

Yaws, salvarsan and, 267

NAME INDEX

Abano, Pietro d', 124, 338
Abel, John J., 232
Abu-Bakr Muhammad ibn-Zakariya al Razi, 89–90, 107–108
Acosta, Cristóbal de, 197
Acosta, José de, 199
Adams, 233
Addison, Thomas, 214, 215, 216, 221–227, 249, 411–412
Adler, Alfred, 424, 461, 596, 637
Agüero, Bartolomé Hidalgo de, 190–191, 192
Aguirre, Lope de, 284
Akhenaton, 655, 656
Albertus Magnus, 60, 65, 131, 312
Albucasis, 94, 97–98, 311
Alcazar, Andrés, 190
Alcmaeon of Crotona, 248, 298, 433–434, 435
Alderotti, Taddeo, 123
Aldrich, 232–233
Alexander of Tralles, 306, 310
Al-Hakim II, 95, 96, 311
Ali al-Tabari, 89, 107
Allbutt, Sir Thomas Clifford, 315
Alphonso VIII, 150
Alphonso IX, 150
Alphonso X, 150, 176, 501
Alvárez de Chanca, Diego, 199, 285
Amenhotep III, 656
Amenhotep IV, 654–655, 656
Anouilh, Jean, 607
Archagathus, 300
Aretaeus of Cappadocia, 90, 218, 300, 435
Arfe y Villafañe, Juan de, 187–188
Aristotle, 36, 47, 90, 91, 123, 124, 195, 201, 202, 217, 298, 299, 302, 311, 312, 314, 338, 434, 435
Arlt, 460
Arnold of Villanova, 150, 307, 312
Arnott, 376
Arp, Jean, 525
Arrington, George E., Jr., 367–370
Asclepiades, 299, 389, 434, 435
Atatürk, Kemal, 664
Auenbrugger, Leopold, 390, 443
Augustus, 303
Aurelianus, 478
Avenzoar, 94, 95, 96, 98-99, 311
Averroës, 93, 94, 99, 202, 312
Avicenna, 13, 44, 65, 89, 90-92, 95, 98, 156, 195, 201, 257, 304, 311, 313, 549
Avogadro, Amadeo, 514

Bacon, Roger, 100, 269, 312, 389
Bacon, Sir Francis, 26, 64, 140, 195, 202, 292, 313, 314, 324, 325, 389
Bacq, 236
Balzac, Honoré de, 34, 210, 458
Banting, Sir Frederick, 234, 382–383
Barba of Valladolid, Pedro, 197
Baroja, Pio, 12
Bartholomew, 337–338
Bastidas, Rodrigo de, 284
Baudelaire, Charles, 32, 430, 431, 503, 638
Bayley, Harold, 485
Becerra, Gaspar, 186
Beers, Clifford, 427
Bell, Joseph, 41, 226, 376
Beltraffio, Giovanni, 75
Benavente, Jacinto, 334
Benedetti, Alessandro, 124
Berengario da Capri, 183
Bernard, Claude, 14, 25, 27, 34–35, 39, 116, 145, 243, 246, 247, 257, 258, 269, 278, 292, 314, 315, 325, 341, 346, 373, 374, 375, 379, 390, 395, 399, 412, 428, 453, 464, 465, 519, 625, 659
Bert, Paul, 341, 625
Berthold de Göttingen, 218
Best, Charles H., 234
Bettany, 222
Bichat, M. F. X., 325, 390
Bigelow, Henry J., 377
Bini, L., 444
Blackwell, Elizabeth, 670
Blake, John B., 351
Blanchard, Pierre, 116, 341, 625
Blasco Ibáñez, Vicente, 51
Bleuler, Eugen, 424, 440, 449, 456, 470, 637
Boccaccio, Giovanni, 32, 151, 199, 210
Boerhaave, Hermann, 56, 108, 195, 257, 315, 325, 390, 441
Böhm, 278
Boisson, Jacques, 34
Boissy, 576
Boswell, James, 32, 38
Botticelli, Sandro, 70
Bouillard, Jean-Baptiste, 230
Bourget, Paul, 35
Boyer, L. Bryce, 477–478
Braque, Georges, 415, 431, 521, 557, 560, 561–571, 574, 638, 659
Bravo, Francis, 182
Breasted, J. H., 655

Brengger, 143
Bright, Richard, 221, 222, 224, 225
Brillat-Savarin, Anthelme, 401, 620, 621
Briot, 468
Britsch, 443
Brontë, Charlotte, 386
Browne, Sir Thomas, 13, 25, 27, 436
Brown-Séquard, Charles Edouard, 215, 227, 228, 230, 249, 390
Bruce, James, 115, 341, 625
Brücke, 463
Bruno, Giordano, 137, 143, 436
Burrows, G., 443
Burton, Robert, 11, 12

Cabeza de Vaca, Alvaro Núñez, 285–286, 289
Caesar, Julius, 300
Caius, John, 11, 125, 128
Cajal, Santiago Ramón y, 14, 15, 24, 25, 27, 46, 49, 145, 260, 262, 268, 271, 276, 333, 424, 426, 437, 441, 452, 456, 457, 618, 637
Calcar, Jan Stephen von, 64, 74, 128, 313, 529
Calderón de la Barca, Pedro, 137, 168, 169, 171, 173
Calvin, John, 64, 133, 201, 308, 314
Calvo, Juan, 190
Canano, Giambattista, 129
Cannon, Walter B., 235, 236, 244, 246, 374, 395, 428, 460
Carballo, Rof, 412
Carbón, Damián, 197
Carco, Francis, 592
Cardano, Gerolamo, 119, 312
Carliner, 386
Carlos, Don, 96, 191, 198, 202
Carrel, Alexis, 325
Carroll, Lewis, 501, 503, 504
Casanova, Giovanni, 10, 16, 37, 46, 51, 121, 138, 663
Casserio Giulio, 128, 129
Castagno, Andrea da, 75
Castiglione, Baldassare, 63, 67, 330
Castillo, Alonso del, 96
Catalina, 545–546
Cattel, James, 477
Cejador, Julio, 159
Cellini, Benvenuto, 63, 68, 69, 95, 312, 658
Celsus, 36, 218, 300, 301, 315, 435
Cerletti, Ugo, 442, 443, 444
Cervantes Saavedra, Miguel de, 10, 24, 37, 42, 48–49, 64, 137, 167, 168, 171, 173, 174, 182, 193, 197, 209, 210–211, 333–334, 497

Cesalpino, Andrea, 64, 130, 133–134, 143–144, 627
Cezanne, Paul, 415, 521, 525, 556, 562, 563, 566
Charcot, Jean Martin, 14, 39, 425, 438–439, 440, 459–460, 519, 637
Chardin, Francois, 566, 570
Charlemagne, 105, 310, 501, 502
Charles V, 64, 169, 177, 180, 181, 187, 191, 194, 199, 201
Charpentier, Gustave, 468
Chaucer, Geoffrey, 10, 64, 128, 210, 312
Chauliac, Guy de, 98, 312
Chekhov, Anton, 12, 36, 39–40, 41, 592
Chesterton, G. K., 8, 112, 331, 337, 476, 493, 613, 624, 649
Chiarugi, Vincenzo, 437
Chirico, Giorgio de, 415, 523, 531, 659
Chirino, Alphonso, 163, 197
Cicero, 199, 300, 312, 382, 413
Cirlot, J. Eduardo, 368
Claus, Émile, 460, 462
Cleopatra, 297, 487
Cocteau, Jean, 558, 567
Coleridge, Samuel Taylor, 33, 37, 431, 638
Collado, Luis, 185
Colombo, Realdo, 128, 130, 133, 145, 185, 199, 201, 627
Columbus, Christopher, 63, 169, 183, 284, 285, 337, 338
Conrad, Joseph, 42, 648
Constantine the African, 98–99, 108, 308, 435
Copernicus, Nicholaus, 63, 64, 65, 130, 313, 514–515, 518
Coriat, 503
Cornaro, Luigi, 663
Cornutus, Manilius, 303
Corral, Leon, 363, 391
Cortés, Hernando, 64, 169
Corvisart, 390
Co Tui, 247, 328
Courbet, Gustave, 521
Courvoisier, Madame, 430, 468
Cox, James Mason, 442–443
Crile, George W., 377
Cushing, Harvey, 14, 39, 146, 248, 268, 323, 670

Dacque, Edmund, 491
Dakin, Henry Dripdale, 233
Dale, Sir Henry, 226, 236
Dali, Salvador, 368, 415, 523, 531, 532, 659
Dalton, John, 514

Dante Alighieri, 37, 42, 63, 65, 72, 73, 124, 199, 329, 338, 448, 513, 515, 631
Danzing, Liek, 161
Daquin, Joseph, 437
Darwin, Charles, 244, 246, 258, 316, 391, 425, 460, 529
Da Vinci, Leonardo, 16, 37, 64, 65, 66, 69, 71, 73, 74, 75–77, 78–79, 90, 94–95, 124, 136, 183, 313, 369, 392, 414, 459, 541–553, 649, 658
Da Vinci, Piero, 546
Daza Chacón, Dionisio, 191–192, 193
Daza Valdés, Benito, 197
De Bordeu, Théophile, 218, 230, 312
Defoe, Daniel, 11, 32, 116, 341, 625
Delay, Jean, 377, 430, 470
Democedes of Crotona, 114, 340, 625
Democritus, 298, 301, 514, 650
De Mondeville, Henri, 184, 312
Deniker, Pierre, 430, 470
De Quincy, Thomas, 33, 431, 638
Derain, André, 563, 564, 566, 574
Descartes, René, 7, 47, 63, 202, 204, 218, 219, 314, 390, 436, 457, 636
Deschamps, 470
De Wit, 385, 386
Díaz, Bernal, 285
Díaz, Francisco, 197–198
Díaz, Pedro, 152
Dickens, Charles, 10, 11, 38, 475, 479, 481
Diderot, Denis, 503
Dilthey, Wilhelm, 344, 349
Dioscorides, 88, 152, 200, 280, 301
Domagk, Gerhard, 269, 319, 320–321
Donatello, 69, 70–71, 543
Dorival, 583
Dostoevski, Feodor, 10, 12, 40, 210
Doughty, Charles M., 116
Dover, Thomas, 11, 116, 341, 625
Doyle, Sir Arthur Conan, 7, 12, 28, 40–41
Drake, Daniel, 326, 339
Dubos, René J., 321
Ducrot, 468
Duffy, John, 351
Dufy, Raoul, 563, 566, 574
Duns Scotus, John, 268, 304
Dürer, Albrecht, 63, 76
Dustin, 246

Edison, Thomas, 326
Ehrlich, Paul, 257–269, 319, 320, 321, 325, 394, 412, 439, 467
Einstein, Albert, 47, 516–517, 530, 531, 532, 562
El Greco, 47, 64, 137, 168, 169, 182, 210, 333, 426, 530, 580

Eliot, Thomas Stearns, 480
Elliot, 236
Emerson, Ralph Waldo, 26–27, 457
Empedocles of Afrigentum, 298, 389
Entralgo, Laín, 189
Epicurus of Samos, 514
Eppinger, Hans, 246
Erasistratus, 132, 301, 434
Erasmus, Desiderius, 10, 61, 63, 125, 313
Ernst, Max, 368, 523, 531
Eryximachus, 409, 623, 657
Esquirol, Jean, 348, 459
Eustachius, Bartolomeus, 55, 219, 250
Evans, Herbert, 240

Fabing, Howard, 431
Fabiola, 643, 669
Fabricius of Aquapendente, 126, 128, 129–130, 132, 133, 134, 145, 146, 147, 189, 627, 628
Fallopius, Gabriel, 133, 189
Falret, 439
Feijóo, Menito, 50–51
Ferdinand of Spain, 63, 96, 169, 177, 183, 194
Ferenczi, 477
Fernández de Oviedo, Gonzalo, 199
Fernel, Jean, 201, 341
Finke, Leonhardt Ludwig, 339
Finlay, Carlos, 316, 328
Fintan, 280
Firor, 238
Flacher, 233
Flaubert, Gustave, 34, 519–520
Fleming, Sir Alexander, 321, 327, 412
Flexner, Simon, 324, 325
Fliess, Wilhelm, 461, 463
Florey, Sir Howard Walter, 321, 327
Foerster, O., 273
Forel, François A., 273, 274
Forster, E. M., 517
Fournel, 468
Fowler, Lydia Folger, 670
Fracastoro, Girolamo, 32, 64, 130, 146, 267, 383
Fragoso, Juan, 190
Francesca, Mona, 545–546
Francis of Assisi, St., 67, 644, 670
Frank, Johann Peter, 339
Franklin, Benjamin, 32, 325, 326
Frederick II, 307
Freud, Sigmund, 14, 27, 35, 39, 53, 268, 393, 394, 415, 416, 424–428, 440, 449, 452, 455–465, 470, 529, 530, 596, 637, 652, 655, 659, 667
Friedman, 233
Fuller, Samuel, 632
Furth, 232, 233

Name Index   707

Galen, 4, 13, 19, 44, 64, 65, 75, 103, 124, 132, 133, 145, 146, 148, 195, 201, 202, 203, 204, 214, 218, 219, 268, 300, 301, 304, 311, 313, 315, 353, 389, 411, 412, 424, 435, 441, 549
Galileo Galilei, 63, 64, 65, 124, 128, 130, 132, 136, 137, 142, 147, 180, 314, 324, 389, 390, 413, 425, 627, 659
Gall, F. J., 437
Garcia de Orta, 115, 199, 340, 625
García Lorca, Federico, 598
Garcilaso de la Vega, 171, 284
Gaskell, 248
Gauguin, Paul, 415, 562, 569
Gautier, Théophile, 166
Gay, 386
Geber, 95, 103
Genghis Khan, 487
Georget, 348, 459
Gerard of Cremona, 150
Gerhardt, Carl, 261, 262
Gherardini, Lisa di Antonio Maria di Noldo, 550–551, 552
Ghose, Aurobindo, 24
Gibbon, Edward, 24
Gilbert, William, 314
Gill, Richard C., 278, 281, 282
Gimbernat, Antonio de, 271
Gimeno, Pedro, 182, 184, 185
Giocondo, Francesco del, 76, 79, 550–551
Giordano, Luca, 330
Giotto di Bondone, 64, 68, 78, 543
Giraudoux, Jean, 607
Girón, Pedro, 188
Glaidus, 443
Gley, Eugène, 236
Goethe, Johann Wolfgang von, 14, 22, 74, 90, 211, 458, 462, 484, 498
Goldsmith, Oliver, 12, 38
Gomara, Francisco López de, 283
Gómez Pereira, Antonio, 199, 202
Goncourt brothers, 32, 35, 520
Góngora y Argote, Luis de, 171
Gossouin, 337
Goya y Lucientes, Francisco de, 168, 196, 210
Gracian, Baltasar, 407
Granada, Fray Luis de, 188
Greene, Robert, 144
Griesinger, Wilhelm, 427, 438, 443
Grimm, 672
Gris, Juan, 561, 574
Grocyn, William, 125
Groddeck, 429
Grollman, Arnold, 238
Gross, 348

Guinart, Robert, 173
Gull, William, 224, 225
Gunville, Edmund, 128
Gutenberg, Johann, 63
Guthrie, Douglas, 119
Gutiérrez Angulo, Nicolás, 207

Hacket, Anne, 670
Hahn, Otto, 537
Hakluyt, Richard, 281
Hall, Courtney R., 351
Haller, Albrecht von, 37–38, 316, 390, 413
Halpern, 468
Haly Abbas, G., 89, 308
Hammurabi, 296
Hamon, 470
Hanrahan, 470
Harl, 470
Haroun of Alexandria, 88
Harris, G. W., 240
Harris, Raymond, 430
Hart, Moss, 607
Hartmann, 237, 239
Harun-al-Rashid, 88, 105, 310, 502
Harvey, Thomas, 127
Harvey, William, 11, 14, 33, 65, 74, 119–148, 180, 214, 226, 273, 292, 314, 316, 324, 325, 390, 413, 627–629, 658
Haslam, J., 437
Hawke, Joan, 127
Hawkins, Sir John, 116, 341, 625
Hazlitt, William, 13, 41, 113, 624, 648
Hegel, Georg Wilhelm Friedrich, 35, 211, 344, 345–346, 465, 631
Heinroth, 437–438
Helmholtz, Hermann von, 514
Heloise, 670
Hemingway, Ernest, 51
Hemphill, 246
Hench, Phillip S., 240, 241
Henle, Jacob, 231
Henley, William Ernest, 458
Hernández, Francisco, 198–199, 289
Herodotus, 114, 654
Herophilus, 78, 301, 302, 434
Herrera, Antonio de, 283, 284
Herriot, Édouard, 586
Hertz, Gustav, 512
Heynes, 302
Highmore, N., 74
Hildebrand, Adolf von, 414
Hilton, John, 224
Hippocrates, 3–4, 13, 27, 53, 90, 113, 195, 201, 204, 218, 227, 298, 302, 310, 316, 338, 353, 362, 382, 389, 411, 434–435, 441, 459, 514, 622, 624

Hirsch, August, 339
His, Wilhelm, 273, 274
Hitzig, 443
Hoagland, 246, 247
Hoffman, 429
Hoffmann, 266
Holbein, Hans, 63
Holmes, Oliver Wendell, 12, 14, 24, 38–39, 41, 246, 326, 328, 460, 486, 506
Homer, 31, 210, 280, 607
Honein (or Johannitius), 88
Horace, 281, 534
Horney, Karen, 596–597
Hoskins, Roy G., 246, 247, 444, 447, 451
Huarte de San Juan, Juan, 182, 197, 199, 203–204
Hudson, Henry, 139
Huerta, 162
Hufeland, Christopher, 164
Hugo, Victor, 519
Huguenard, 376, 377, 378, 469
Humboldt, Alexander von, 278, 279
Hunain ibn Ishaq, 88, 107, 109, 311
Hunter, John, 55, 164, 226, 292, 315, 325
Huss, John, 501
Huxley, Aldous, 48, 50, 529

Ibsen, Henrik, 35
Ikhnaton, 655, 656
Imhotep, 297
Irving, Washington, 475
Irwin, J. A., 382
Isabella of Spain, 63, 150, 169, 177, 194, 283

Jablonski, 443
Jackson, J. Hughlings, 425, 461
Jacobi, C. W. M., 437
Jacobi, Karl, 513
Jacobi, Mary Putnam, 670
Jakob, 273
James, William, 244, 428
Janet, 439, 519
Jaspers, Karl, 62, 213, 429, 486, 668
Jáuregue, Juan de, 210
Jeffries, 116, 341, 625
Jekels, 478
Jenner, Edward, 11, 13–14, 315
Jentzer, 375, 379
Jibrail, 88
Johnson, Samuel, 32, 38, 224
Jones, Ernest, 478, 506
Jores, Arthur, 412, 667
Joshua Ben Nun, 88
Jourdain, Francis, 580–581
Joyce, James, 10, 35

Julius Caesar, 487
Jung, Carl G., 424, 461, 481, 637
Justinian, 300
Juvenal, 218

Kadereit, 265
Kahlbaum, 439
Kahnweiler, Daniel Henry, 563, 564
Kandinsky, Wassily, 415, 562
Kant, Immanuel, 42, 530
Keats, John, 11, 37, 38
Kendall, E. C., 238, 239, 240, 241, 249, 324
Kepler, Johann, 64, 137, 143
Kierkegaard, Søren, 464
Kipling, Rudyard, 24
Kisling, 558
Klaesi, 443, 444, 469
Klee, Paul, 415, 523, 526, 659
Klemperer, G., 443
Kline, Nathan S., 430
Koch, Robert, 260, 264, 292, 325, 390
Koetschet, 468
Kolsky, 468
Kooning, Willem de, 539
Korsakow, 440
Kraepelin, Emil, 14, 424, 425, 428, 439–440, 449, 450, 452, 456, 460, 470, 637
Krafft-Ebbing, Richard von, 438, 439
Kraus, Fredrick, 390
Krehl, Ludwig, 429
Kretschmer, 390
Krogh, August, 377
Kublai Khan, 112, 336

Laborit, Henri, 373, 375, 379, 430, 448, 469–470
La Burt, H. A., 247, 328
La Condamine, Charles Marie de, 282
Laënnec, R. T. H., 14, 223, 390, 411, 425
Laguna, Andrés, 183, 194, 199–201, 207
Lamartine, Alphonse, 33
Lancisi, Gioranni Maria, 219
Landouzy, 71
Lang, Andrew, 30
Langdon-Brown, Sir Walter, 243, 248
Langley, John N., 235, 237, 323
Langlois, Jean-Paul, 230
Laplace, Pierre-Simon, 325
Larbaud, Valéry, 7
Lardon, 239
Lasker, Emanuel, 502
Latimer, Hugh, 125
Latini, Brunetto, 338
Laurens, Henri, 558

Name Index   709

Lavoisier, Antoine, 325, 514
Lawrence, T. E., 112, 116, 381
Lecomte de Nouy, 379
Le Corbusier, 525
Leduc, 443
Leeuwenhoek, Anton van, 369, 370, 659
Léger, Fernand, 525, 561
Lehmann, 430, 470
Leikind, Morris C., 351
Leiva y Aguilar, Francisco, 198
Leriche, R., 246
Le Sage, Alain-René, 11
Leucippus, 514
Lewandowsky, Max, 235
Libaude, 582, 583
Liebeault, 438–439
Linacre, Thomas, 11, 16, 25, 37, 125, 128, 313
Lind, James, 116, 341, 625
Lippi, Fra Filippo, 70, 543
Lister, Joseph, 321
Livingstone, David, 115, 341, 625
Lobera de Avila, Luis, 183, 188, 193, 194, 199, 201
Loeb, Jacques, 251, 325
Loevenhart, A. S., 443
Loewi, 235, 236
Long, Crawford W., 326
Longfellow, Henry Wadsworth, 506, 670
Lope de Vega, Félix, 42, 53, 64, 137, 169, 182, 197, 210
López de León, Pedro, 192
López Madera, 193
Lorn, Hieronymus, 53
Lorry, Anne-Charles, 459
Lowenthal, 505
Lucretius, 117, 300, 534
Ludovico il Moro, 547
Lully, Raymond, 99, 150, 202
Lumley, Lord, 147
Lusitano, Amato, 152
Luther, Martin, 64
Lyautey, General Pierre, 24

McDaniel, W. B., II, 351
McDowell, Ephraim, 326
McIntyre, T. S., 279, 280, 283
Machiavelli, Niccolo, 63, 67, 69
MacOrlan, Pierre, 574
Maeterlinck, Maurice, 44
Magellan, Ferdinand, 64, 284
Magendie, François, 220
Magnan, 348
Magritte, René, 368
Maillol, Aristide, 593
Maimonides (Moses ben Maimon), 94, 95, 99–102, 150, 202, 311

Major, Ralph, 13, 330, 351
Malik-al-Afdal, 100, 109
Malpighi, Marcello, 219, 314
Manet, Edouard, 415, 521, 566, 659
Mann, Thomas, 10
Mantegna, Andrea, 137
Mantovani, 137
Manzolini, Ana Morandi, 670
Marañón, Gregorio, 14, 19, 33, 46, 49, 174, 176, 245, 275, 330, 334, 390
Marco Polo, 336, 337, 338, 489
Marcus Aurelius, 306
Marie, Pierre, 226
Marlowe, Christopher, 144
Martelli, Piero di Batto, 550
Martin, P. W., 480
Martire d'Anghera, Pietro, 282–283
Mary of Portugal, 181
Masaccio, 70, 78, 543
Maser Djawah Ebu Djeldjal of Basra, 88
Mason, 238
Massa, Laurentius, 125
Mata, Pedro, 12
Mather, Cotton, 353, 632
Matisse, Henri, 560, 562, 563, 564
Maugham, W. Somerset, 12, 41–42, 113, 330
Maurois, André, 22, 662
Maximilian, 124
May, Jacques, 342–344, 346–347
Mayer, 514
Mayo, W. J., 28, 292, 659
Medina, Cosme de, 188
Meduna, Laszlo Joseph, 443, 444
Meletio, Juan de, 178
Melicow, 415
Mendoza, 171
Menendez y Pelayo, 26, 152, 159
Mercado, Luis, 195, 196
Merck, 252
Merezhkovski, 414
Meyer, Adolf, 273, 424, 426–428, 637, 667
Meynert, Theodor, 438, 460, 463
Michelangelo, 63, 66, 67, 69, 71, 72–73, 137–138, 186, 658
Miller, Henry, 601
Mira, Emilio, 55
Mirabeau, Octavius, 581, 583, 592
Miranda, Luis de, 172
Mirandola, Pico della, 63
Miró, Joan, 415, 525, 526, 560, 659
Mitchell, S. Weir, 12, 39
Modigliani, Amedeo, 555–560, 574, 585
Modjeska, Madame, 602
Mohammed, 83, 84–85, 102, 309, 310

Moindrot, 468
Molière, 11, 32, 36, 54, 607
Monardes, Nicolás, 182, 197, 286–289
Mondino de Luzzi, 123, 549
Mondriaan, Piet, 524
Monet, Claude, 415, 562, 579, 580, 659
Moniz, Egas, 444
Monkhouse, 115, 625
Montaigne, Michel de, 101, 204, 210, 328
Montaña de Monserrate, Bernardino, 183–185, 188
Montano, Arias, 190, 195
Montanus, 658
Montgolfier brothers, 116, 625
Montiño, Martínez, 180
Moore, Henry, 439, 526, 531
Morales, Ambrosio, 195
Morandi, 525, 557
Morel, 348
Morgagni, Giovanni Battista, 13, 316, 325, 390, 411
Morgan, John, 223
Morphy, Paul, 505–507
Morton, W. T. G., 326
Moses, 655–656
Mousis, Paul, 576, 580
Mozart, Wolfgang Amadeus, 662
Mueller, G., 443
Muirhead, 234
Müller, Johannes, 325, 428, 464
Muñón, Sancho, 152
Munthe, Axel, 12, 46
Murger, 561
Murillo, Bartolomé Esteban, 137
Murray, G. R., 215, 316, 323, 394
Musa, Anthonius, 303
Musset, Alfred de, 29, 561, 574
Mutawakkil, 89

Napoleon, 307, 501
Nash, 144
Naumann, W., 278
Nazari Mohammed V, 96
Nefertiti, 654–656
Neinroth, 348
Nerval, Gerard de, 574
Nestorius, 86–87, 308–309
Neuburger, Max, 330
Newton, Sir Isaac, 137, 140, 324, 413, 457
Nicholson, 524
Nietzsche, Friedrich Wilhelm, 460, 465
Nightingale, Florence, 644, 670
Nissl, Franz, 273, 437
Noguchi, Hideyo, 325, 439
Noguchi, Isamu, 525

Norwood, William F., 351
Nothnagel, 460
Nyro, 443

Olivares, Duke of, 173
Oliver, George, 232, 233
Olschki, Leonard, 337
Omar I, 85
Omar Khayyám, 91
O'Neill, Eugene, 35, 601, 607
Orellana, Francisco de, 284
Oribasius, 304, 306, 310
Ortega y Gasset, José, 51, 93, 134, 210, 216, 292, 299, 334, 337, 352, 396, 423, 520, 562, 567, 611, 630, 652, 653
Osgood, C. G., 26
Osler, Sir William, 14, 17, 24, 25–26, 27, 39, 49, 62, 65, 119, 120, 237, 316, 327, 464, 615, 650
Ovid, 34, 281, 312
Oviedo y Valdés, Augustin Maria, 283, 284

Pagel, Walter, 143
Palacio Valdés, Armando, 12
Palgrave, W. G., 116
Papini, Giovanni, 53
Paracelsus, 19, 37, 59, 94, 214, 218, 268–269, 313, 314, 319, 324, 338, 390, 438
Paraire, 470
Paré, Ambroise, 64, 98, 190, 191, 257, 354
Park, Mungo, 115, 341, 625
Pascal, 443
Pasteur, Louis, 225, 258, 268, 292, 316, 325, 390, 394, 412
Patanjali, 217
Patin, Guy, 17
Paul of Aegina, 98, 306, 310
Paul of Tarsus, 24, 86, 308
Pauwels, Madame Lucie, 586–591
Pavlov, Ivan, 27, 55, 275–276, 424–425, 441, 452, 456, 637
Peele, George, 144
Pegolotti, Francesco Balducci, 338
Pellico, Silvio, 210
Pepys, Samuel, 11, 120
Père Gay, 591
Pereira, 180
Pérez, Antonio, 196
Pérez de Herrera, Cristobal, 193, 198
Perrault, 672
Petrarch, 63, 151, 199, 313
Petrides, 589
Pfiffner, 234, 238, 239
Philidor, 505
Philip II, 96, 115, 128, 167, 169, 176,

Name Index

177, 180–182, 190–192, 194–196, 198–200, 202, 284, 289, 339, 426
Philippeaux, 230
Philocalus, 479
Picard, Auguste, 112
Picasso, Pablo, 20, 415, 431, 521, 526, 556, 557, 560–567, 569, 574, 580, 638, 659
Pigafetta, Antonio, 284
Pilâtre de Rozier, Jean, 116, 341, 625
Pincus, 246, 247
Pindar, 274, 647
Pinel, Philippe, 437, 438, 459, 635, 638
Pinturicchio, 64, 71
Pissarro, Camille, 415, 521, 579, 659
Pizarro brothers, 43, 64, 169, 284
Planck, Max, 457, 515–516, 525, 529, 532
Plato, 10, 31, 91, 123, 227, 298, 299, 376, 409, 426, 435, 498, 534, 636, 657
Pliny, 162, 217–218, 300, 493, 671
Plutarch, 303, 312
Poe, Edgar Allan, 25, 431, 638
Poincaré, Raymond, 24
Pollaiuolo, 69–70
Polo, Marco, 16, 43, 112, 284
Polycrates, 114
Ponce de León, Pedro, 197
Porcell, Juan Tomas, 194, 196
Porphyrius, 91
Postell, William Dosite, 351
Poussin, Claude, 563, 570
Prester John, 338
Prochaska, Georg, 218
Proust, Marcel, 35, 210
Ptolemy, 64, 91, 313
Pushkin, Alexander, 40
Pyrrhus, 381
Pythagoras, 248, 298, 434

Quarles, Francis, 32
Quelch, 278
Quevedo, Francisco Gómez de, 6, 210
Quincey, 506

Rabelais, François, 10, 12, 37, 42, 64, 312
Radcliffe, John, 17
Radegunda de Poitiers, St., 643, 669
Raleigh, Sir Walter, 128, 277, 281, 289
Ramakrishna, 24
Rangone, Tomasso Gianotti, 129
Rank, 461
Raphael Sanzio, 64, 69, 71, 570, 579, 592

Raphaelian, Harry, 488–489
Rasputin, 503
Raven, 233
Rebecca, 643, 669
Reichstein, Thaddeus, 238, 239, 324
Reil, J. C., 437
Reilly, 374, 375, 469
Reiss, 246
Rembrandt van Rijn, H., 12, 458, 570
Renan, Joseph Ernest, 34, 42, 519
Renoir, Pierre Auguste, 566, 576, 580, 593
Rhazes, 89–90, 98, 104, 311
Ribera, 570
Richards, Dickinson W., 376
Richardson, Samuel, 38
Richet, Charles, 297
Richmond, Phyllis Allen, 351
Ridio, 129
Riese, Walther, 361–365
Rimbaud, Authur, 430
Rinozzi, Bertoldo, 547, 548–550
Riolan, Jean, 129, 180, 219
Robinson, Victor, 116
Rodríguez, Barbosa, 279
Rodríguez de Guevara, Alonso, 183
Roentgen, William Conrad, 659
Roger of Palermo, 218
Rogoff, 234, 237
Rojas, Fernando de, 151
Rolland, Romain, 24
Romains, Jules, 35
Romero de Torres, 593
Roselli, 78
Rosen, George, 351, 358–359
Ross, Ronald, 12
Rossi, Ernesto, 602
Rouault, Georges, 560
Rousseau, Henri, 505, 570
Rousseau, Jean Jacques, 312
Rubens, Peter Paul, 71, 137, 593
Rudio, Eustaquio, 130
Ruiz, Hipólito, 289
Ruiz, Juan, 151, 166
Rush, Benjamin, 326
Russell, Walter, 115, 340, 625

Sabuco de Nantes, Miguel, 199, 202, 203
Sabur ibn Sahl, 89
Sackler, Arthur M., 247, 328
Sackler, Mortimer D., 247, 328
Sackler, Raymond R., 247, 328
Sagazza, Piero della, 542–546, 550
Sainte-Beuve, Charles Augustin, 34, 211
Sakel, Manfred, 444, 445
Salaino, Andrea, 549
Salicetus, 98

almon, Andre, 574
Sánchez, Francisco, 180, 199, 204
Sánchez Valdés de la Plata, Juan, 185
Santorio, Santorio, 128, 145
Sarett, L. H., 239, 240
Sargent, 486
Sarpi, Paolo, 130
Sartre, Jean-Paul, 383, 601
Savonarola, Girolamo, 63, 66, 72, 77, 548, 549–550
Sayers, 240
Schafer, E. A., 232, 233, 249
Schaudinn, Fritz, 266
Schiller, J. C. F. von, 12, 37
Schleiden, M. J., 273, 316
Schliemann, Heinrich, 24
Schnitzer, Eduard, 115, 341
Schnitzler, Arthur, 12, 36, 37
Scholastica, St., 307
Schomburgk, Sir Robert Hermann, 278, 282
Schwann, Theodor, 273, 316
Schwarz, 429
Schweitzer, Albert, 12, 36, 46
Scotus, Michael, 150
Scribonius Largus, 442
Segonzac, André Dunoyer de, 574
Selkirk, Alexander, 11, 116, 341, 625
Selye, Hans, 216, 243–246, 249, 254, 324, 374, 391–397, 431
Semmelweis, Ignaz Philipp, 39
Seneca, 93, 150, 202, 300
Servetus, Michael, 64, 133, 180, 182, 200, 201, 308, 314, 333
Seurat, Georges, 370, 415, 521, 562, 563, 659
Sforza, 63, 547
Shaftel, Norman, 351
Shakespeare, William, 10–11, 12, 24, 33, 37, 42, 64, 136, 137, 140, 144–145, 148, 210, 628–629
Shaw, Christopher, 385
Shaw, George Bernard, 35, 620
Sherrington, Charles S., 14, 27, 248, 275, 424, 425, 441, 456, 461, 637
Siebeck, 390, 429
Sigerist, Henry E., 10, 31, 329–334, 339, 342, 343
Signorelli, Luca, 69, 70, 543
Sigüenza, Father José de, 178
Simenon, Georges, 53
Simpson, 376
Singer, 411
Sisley, Alfred, 579, 580, 596
Smith, Captain John, 115, 340, 625
Smith, Edwin, 297
Smollett, Tobias, 11, 12, 116, 341, 625

Socrates, 298, 299, 435
Solander, 115, 340
Solomon, 101–102
Solon, 624
Sophocles, 598, 607
Soriano, Jerónimo, 197
Sotomayor, 202
Soutine, Chaim, 558, 574
Spector, Benjamin, 351
Spengler, Oswald, 206, 293
Spenser, Edmund, 140
Speransky, 390
Spielmeyer, 273
Spigelius, 219
Spinoza, Baruch, 417, 619
Stahl, Georg, 390, 436
Steiger, 239
Steinitz, 505
Stendhal, 5, 10, 210, 503
Steno (Stensen), Niels, 436
Sterne, Laurence, 11
Stevenson, Robert Louis, 11, 479, 606, 669
Stewart, 234, 237
Stockman, 233
Stoll, 429
Stolz, F., 233
Strassmann, 537
Sue, Eugène, 116, 341, 625
Swift, Jonathan, 41, 113
Swingle, 234, 238, 239
Sydenham, Sir Thomas, 10, 17, 53, 90, 202, 315, 316, 317, 389, 390, 424, 459, 464, 668
Sylvius, 129, 185, 199
Syrski, 462

Tabari, 89, 107
Tagliacozzi, Gasparo, 190
Tagore, Rabindranath, 644
Taine, Hippolyte Adolphe, 24, 34, 67
Takamine, Jokichi, 232, 233
Talma, 600
Tanguy, Yves, 415, 523, 659
Tarik, 85, 92–93, 309
Tartakower, 505
Terence, 199
Testut, Leon, 15
Thackeray, W. M., 11
Theophilus of Antioch, 479
Theophrastus, 281
Theresa, St., 431, 570, 641
Thessalus, 354
Thévenot, Melchisédech, 436
Tintoretto, 69, 71
Titian, 63, 69, 71, 124, 128, 313
Tizzoni, Guido, 230
Toller, Ernst, 332
Tolstoi, Leo, 42, 210

Name Index 713